W9-CDG-560

BIO 309 Pathophysiology

Scott Dube, DO

BIO 309 Pathophysiology

University of New England

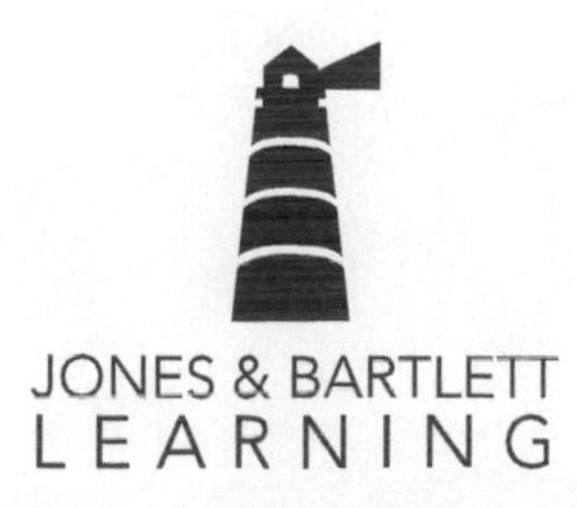
JONES & BARTLETT
LEARNING

World Headquarters
Jones & Bartlett Learning
5 Wall Street
Burlington, MA 01803
978-443-5000
info@jblearning.com
www.jblearning.com

Jones & Bartlett Learning books and products are available through most bookstores and online booksellers. To contact Jones & Bartlett Learning directly, call 800-832-0034, fax 978-443-8000, or visit our website, www.jblearning.com.

This book is produced through PUBLISH – a custom publishing service offered by Jones & Bartlett Learning. For more information on PUBLISH, contact us at 800-832-0034 or visit our website at www.jblearning.com.

Copyright © 2013 by Jones & Bartlett Learning, LLC, an Ascend Learning Company

All rights reserved. No part of the material protected by this copyright may be reproduced or utilized in any form, electronic or mechanical, including photocopying, recording, or by any information storage and retrieval system, without written permission from the copyright owner.

Disclaimer

This publication is sold with the understanding that the publisher is not engaged in rendering medical, legal, accounting, or other professional services. If medical, legal, accounting, or other professional service advice is required, the service of a competent professional should be sought. The authors, editor, and publisher have designed this publication to provide accurate information with regard to the subject matter covered. However, they are not responsible for errors, omissions, or for any outcomes related to the use of the contents of this publication and make no guarantee and assume no responsibility or liability for the use of the products and procedures described, or the correctness, sufficiency, or completeness of stated information, opinions, or recommendations. Treatments and side effects described in this publication are not applicable to all people; required dosages and experienced side effects will vary among individuals. Drugs and medical devices discussed herein are controlled by the Food and Drug Administration (FDA) and may have limited availability for use only in research studies or clinical trials. Research, clinical practice, and government regulations often change accepted standards. When consideration is being given to the use of any drug in the clinical setting, the health care provider or reader is responsible for determining FDA status of the drug, reading the package insert, and reviewing prescribing information for the most current recommendations on dose, precautions, and contraindications and for determining the appropriate usage for the product. This is especially important in the case of drugs that are new or seldom used. Any references in this publication to procedures to be employed when rendering emergency care to the sick and injured are provided solely as a general guide; other or additional safety measures might be required under particular circumstances. This publication is not intended as a statement of the standards of care required in any particular situation; circumstances and the physical conditions of patients can vary widely from one emergency to another. This publication is not intended in any way to advise emergency personnel concerning their legal authority to perform the activities or procedures discussed. Such local determination should be made only with the aid of legal counsel. Some images in this publication feature models; these models do not necessarily endorse, represent, or participate in the activities represented in the images.

Cover Image: © Photos.com

6048
Printed in the United States of America
19 18 17 16 15 13 12 11 10 9

Contents

1 General Concepts of Disease: Principles of Diagnosis
From: *An Introduction to Human Disease: Pathology and Pathophysiology, Ninth Edition by Leonard Crowley* 1

2 Cells and Tissues: Their Structure and Function in Health and Disease
From: *An Introduction to Human Disease: Pathology and Pathophysiology, Ninth Edition by Leonard Crowley* 21

3 Inflammation and Repair
From: *An Introduction to Human Disease: Pathology and Pathophysiology, Ninth Edition by Leonard Crowley* 43

4 Neoplastic Disease
From: *An Introduction to Human Disease: Pathology and Pathophysiology, Ninth Edition by Leonard Crowley* 53

5 Immunity, Hypersensitivity, Allergy, and Autoimmune Diseases
From: *An Introduction to Human Disease: Pathology and Pathophysiology, Ninth Edition by Leonard Crowley* 93

6 Abnormalities of Blood Coagulation
From: *An Introduction to Human Disease: Pathology and Pathophysiology, Ninth Edition by Leonard Crowley* 117

7 Circulatory Disturbances
From: *An Introduction to Human Disease: Pathology and Pathophysiology, Ninth Edition by Leonard Crowley* 132

8 The Cardiovascular System
From: *An Introduction to Human Disease: Pathology and Pathophysiology, Ninth Edition by Leonard Crowley* 149

9 The Hematopoietic and Lymphatic Systems
From: *Essentials of Human Disease, Second Edition by Leonard Crowley* 227

10 The Respiratory System
From: *An Introduction to Human Disease: Pathology and Pathophysiology, Ninth Edition by Leonard Crowley* 246

11 The Liver and the Biliary System
From: *An Introduction to Human Disease: Pathology and Pathophysiology, Ninth Edition by Leonard Crowley* 281

12 The Pancreas and Diabetes Mellitus
From: *An Introduction to Human Disease: Pathology and Pathophysiology, Ninth Edition by Leonard Crowley* 318

13 The Gastrointestinal Tract
From: *An Introduction to Human Disease: Pathology and Pathophysiology, Ninth Edition by Leonard Crowley* 337

14 The Nervous System
From: *Essentials of Human Disease, Second Edition by Leonard Crowley* . . . 379

15 The Musculoskeletal System
From: *Essentials of Human Disease, Second Edition by Leonard Crowley* . . . 405

16 The Urinary System
From: *An Introduction to Human Disease: Pathology and Pathophysiology, Ninth Edition by Leonard Crowley* . . . 427

17 Index . . . 465

General Concepts of Disease: Principles of Diagnosis

LEARNING OBJECTIVES

1. Define the common terms used to describe disease, such as lesions, organic and functional disease, symptomatic and asymptomatic disease, etiology, and pathogenesis.
2. List the major categories of human disease.
3. Explain the approach that a practitioner uses to make a diagnosis and decide on a patient's treatment.
4. Describe the various types of diagnostic tests and procedures that can help the practitioner make a diagnosis and decide on proper treatment.

Characteristics of Disease

Any disturbance of structure or function of the body may be regarded as **disease**. A disease is often associated with well-defined, characteristic structural changes called **lesions** that are present in various organs and tissues. One can recognize lesions by examining the diseased tissue with the naked eye, which is called a gross examination, or with the aid of a microscope, which is called a histologic examination. Sometimes histologic examinations are supplemented by specialized studies that evaluate the properties of the cell membranes and the proteins within the cells. A disease associated with structural changes is called an **organic disease**.

Disease
Any disturbance of the structure or function of the body.

Lesion (lē'shun)
Any structural abnormality or pathologic change.

Organic disease
A disease associated with structural changes in the affected tissue or organ.

Functional disease
A disease that is not associated with any recognizable structural changes in the body.

Pathology
The study of the structural and functional changes in the body caused by disease.

In contrast, a **functional disease** is one in which no morphologic abnormalities (*morphe* = structure or shape) can be identified even though body functions may be profoundly disturbed. However, as we develop new methods for studying cells, we can sometimes identify previously unrecognized abnormalities that disturb cell functions. Consequently, many of the traditional distinctions between organic and functional disease are no longer as sharply defined as in the past.

Pathology is the study of disease, and a pathologist is a physician who specializes in diagnosing and classifying diseases primarily by examining the morphology of cells and tissues. A clinician is any physician or other health practitioner who cares for patients.

A disease may cause various subjective manifestations, such as weakness or pain, in an affected individual: These are called symptoms. A disease may also produce objective manifestations, detectable by the clinician, which are called signs or physical findings. In many diseases, the quantity of blood cells in the circulation may change and so may the biochemical constituents in the body fluids. These alterations are reflected as abnormal laboratory test results.

A disease that causes the affected individual no discomfort or disability is called an asymptomatic disease or illness. A disease is often asymptomatic in its early stages. If the disease is not treated, however, it may progress to the stage where it causes subjective symptoms and abnormal physical findings. Therefore, the distinction between asymptomatic and symptomatic disease is one of degree, depending primarily on the extent of the disease.

Etiology
(ē-tē-ol′ō-jē)
The cause, especially the cause of a disease.

Pathogenesis
(path-ō-jen′e-sis)
Manner in which a disease develops.

The term **etiology** means cause. A disease of unknown etiology is one for which the cause is not yet known. Unfortunately, many diseases fall into this category. If the cause of a disease is known, the agent responsible is called the etiologic agent. The term **pathogenesis** refers to the manner by which a disease develops, and a pathogen is any microorganism, such as a bacterium or virus, that can cause disease.

Classifications of Disease

Diseases tend to fall into several large categories, although the diseases in a specific category are not necessarily closely related. Rather, the lesions produced by the various diseases in a category are morphologically similar or have a similar pathogenesis. Diseases are conveniently classified in the following large groups:

1. Congenital and hereditary diseases
2. Inflammatory diseases
3. Degenerative diseases
4. Metabolic diseases
5. Neoplastic diseases

CONGENITAL AND HEREDITARY DISEASES

Congenital and hereditary diseases are the result of developmental disturbances. They may be caused by genetic abnormalities, abnormalities in the numbers and distribution of chromosomes, intrauterine injury as a result of various agents, or an interaction of genetic and environmental factors. Hemophilia—the well-known hereditary disease in which blood does not clot properly—and congenital heart disease induced by the German measles virus are examples of diseases in this category.

INFLAMMATORY DISEASES

Inflammatory diseases are those in which the body reacts to an injurious agent by means of inflammation. Many of the diseases characterized by inflammation, such as a sore throat or pneumonia, are caused by bacteria or other microbiologic agents. Others, such as "hay fever," are a manifestation of an allergic reaction or a hypersensitivity state in the patient. Some diseases in this category appear to be caused by antibodies formed against the patient's own tissues, as occurs in some uncommon diseases classified as autoimmune diseases. The etiology of still other inflammatory diseases has not been determined.

DEGENERATIVE DISEASES

In degenerative diseases, the primary abnormality is degeneration of various parts of the body. In some cases, this may be a manifestation of the aging process. In many cases, however, the degenerative lesions are more advanced or occur sooner than would be expected if they were age related and are distinctly abnormal. Certain types of arthritis and "hardening of the arteries" (arteriosclerosis) are common examples of degenerative diseases.

METABOLIC DISEASES

The chief abnormality seen in metabolic diseases is a disturbance in some important metabolic process in the body. For example, the cells may not be utilizing glucose normally, or the thyroid gland may not properly regulate the rate of cell metabolism. Diabetes, disturbances of endocrine glands, and disturbances of fluid and electrolyte balance are common examples of metabolic diseases.

NEOPLASTIC DISEASES

Neoplastic diseases are characterized by abnormal cell growth that leads to the formation of various types of benign and malignant tumors.

Health and Disease: A Continuum

Health and disease may be considered two extremes of a continuum. At one extreme is severe, life-threatening, disabling illness with its corresponding major effect on the physical and emotional well-being of the patient. At the other extreme is ideal good health, which may be defined as a state of complete physical and mental well-being. The healthy person is emotionally and physically capable of leading a full, happy, and productive life that is free of anxiety, turmoil, and physical disabilities that limit activities. Between these two extremes are many gradations of health and disease, ranging from mild or short-term illness that limits activities to some extent to moderate good health that falls short of the ideal state. The midpoint in this continuum may be considered a "neutral" position in which one is neither ill nor in ideal good health. In this continuum, most of us are somewhere between midposition and the ideal state.

The goal of traditional medicine is to cure or ameliorate disease. This is accomplished by various means, ranging from administering an antibiotic to cure an infection to very complex "high-technology" treatments such as kidney transplants and heart surgery. The advances of modern medicine have done much to relieve suffering and advance human welfare, but modern medicine does not guarantee good health. Health is more than an absence of disease; it is a condition in which body and mind function efficiently and harmoniously as an integrated unit. Consequently, we must take an active part in achieving good health by assuming some responsibility for our own physical and emotional well-being. This means practicing such common sense measures as eating properly, exercising moderately, and avoiding harmful excesses such as overeating, smoking, heavy drinking, or using drugs, which can disrupt physical or emotional well-being. Taking responsibility for one's health also requires using one's mind constructively, expressing emotions, and feeling good about oneself. Positive mental attitudes are essential for good health because negative feelings may be reflected in disturbed bodily functions that are manifested as disease.

Principles of Diagnosis

Diagnosis
The determination of the nature and cause of a patient's illness.

Prognosis
The probable outcome of a disease or a disorder; the outlook for recovery.

The determination of the nature and cause of a patient's illness by a physician or other health practitioner is called a **diagnosis**. It is based on the practitioner's evaluation of the patient's subjective symptoms, the physical findings, and the results of various laboratory tests, together with other appropriate diagnostic procedures. When the practitioner has reached a diagnosis, he or she can then offer a **prognosis**: an opinion concerning the eventual outcome of the disease. Then a course of treatment is instituted.

THE HISTORY

The clinical history is a very important part of the evaluation. It consists of several parts:

1. The history of the patient's current illness
2. The past medical history
3. The family history
4. The social history
5. The review of systems

The history of the present illness elicits details concerning the severity, time of onset, and character of the patient's symptoms. Many diseases have characteristic symptoms. The patient's description of the oppressive substernal pain of a heart attack or the pain and urinary disturbances associated with a bladder infection, for example, may provide very helpful information that suggests the correct diagnosis. The past medical history provides details of the patient's general health and previous illnesses. These data may shed light on the patient's current problems as well. The family history provides information about the health of the patient's parents and other family members. Some diseases, such as diabetes and some types of heart disease, tend to run in families. The social history deals with the patient's occupation, habits, alcohol and tobacco consumption, and similar data. This information may also relate to the patient's general health and current problems. The review of systems inquires as to the presence of symptoms other than those disclosed in the history of the present illness; such symptoms might suggest disease affecting other parts of the body. For example, the practitioner inquires about such symptoms as pain or burning on urination, which suggest an abnormality of the urinary tract and coughing, shortness of breath, or chest pain, which may indicate disease of the respiratory system. In this way, possible dysfunctions of other organ systems are evaluated by systematic inquiry.

THE PHYSICAL EXAMINATION

The physical examination is a systematic examination of the patient. The practitioner places particular emphasis on the part of the body affected by the illness, such as the ears, throat, chest, and lungs in the case of a respiratory infection. Any abnormalities detected on the physical examination are correlated with the clinical history. At this point, the practitioner begins to consider the various diseases or conditions that would fit with the clinical findings. Sometimes, more than one possible diagnosis need to be considered. In a differential diagnosis, the practitioner considers a number of diseases that are characterized by the patient's symptoms. For example, if a patient complains of shortness of breath and abnormalities are detected when the lungs are examined with a stethoscope, the practitioner may consider both chronic lung disease and chronic heart failure in the differential diagnosis.

Often, the practitioner can narrow the list of diagnostic possibilities and arrive at a correct diagnosis by using selected laboratory tests or other specialized diagnostic procedures. In difficult cases, the clinician may also wish to obtain the opinion of a medical consultant who is a physician with special training and experience in the type of medical problem presented by the patient.

When dealing with patients who have long-standing chronic diseases such as chronic heart, kidney, or lung disease, or some types of cancer, the physician may be assisted by a disease-management team composed of a group of persons with special skills that are useful in the care and treatment of patients with these diseases. The management team may include persons who can explain to patients the nature of their disease, the goals of treatment, and how patients can contribute to their own care. Other health care team members such as dieticians, nurse clinicians, physician assistants, respiratory therapists, physiotherapists, and pharmacists can bring their own special skills to help physicians care for patients with chronic illnesses who require long-term care and who have special needs. Often, the team approach to management of patients with chronic diseases reduces the long-term cost of medical care, improves the patients' satisfaction with the quality of their medical care, and contributes to a more favorable response to treatment.

TREATMENT

After the diagnosis has been established, a course of treatment is initiated. There are two different types of treatment: specific treatment and symptomatic treatment.

A specific treatment is one that exerts a highly specific and favorable effect on the basic cause of the disease. For example, an antibiotic may be given to a patient who has an infection that is responsive to the antibiotic, or insulin may be given to a patient with diabetes. Symptomatic treatment, as the name implies, makes the patient more comfortable by alleviating symptoms but does not influence the course of the underlying disease. Examples are the treatment of fever, pain, and cough by means of appropriate medications. Unfortunately, there are no specific treatments for some diseases. Consequently, the clinician must be content with treating the manifestations of the disease, without being able to influence its ultimate course.

Screening Tests for Disease

PURPOSE AND REQUIREMENTS FOR EFFECTIVE SCREENING

Many diseases that respond to treatment are asymptomatic initially. If untreated, however, the disease often progresses slowly, causing gradual but progressive organ damage until eventually the person is seriously ill with far advanced organ damage caused by the disease. Unfortunately, treatment of late-stage disease is often much less effective and may not be able to restore the function of the organs that have been damaged. Had the disease been identified and treated in its early asymptomatic stage, the disease-related organ damage could have been prevented or minimized, and the affected person would have been spared the discomfort, disability, and shortened survival associated with late-stage disease.

A successful screening program should fulfill the following requirements:

1. A significant number of persons in the group being screened must be at risk for the disease.
2. A relatively inexpensive noninvasive test that does not yield an excessively high number of false-positive or false-negative results must be available to screen for the disease.
3. Early identification and treatment of the disease will favorably influence the health or welfare of the person with the disease.

GROUPS SUITABLE FOR SCREENING

Screening tests should target a group of persons in whom there is a relatively high frequency of disease, and tests should also target the age group in whom the disease is likely to be present. If the disease, for example, has its onset in middle age, then screening adolescents and children in the target group would not be productive.

SUITABLE SCREENING TESTS

Screening a group of persons for a disease in its early asymptomatic stage requires some type of test that can identify some characteristic manifestation of the disease, such as high blood sugar in the case of diabetes or the presence of blood in the stool in the case of a colon tumor. A test used for screening should be reasonably inexpensive and should have few false-positive results (test is positive when no disease is present) and few false-negative results (test is negative when disease is present). If the test produced a large number of false-positive results in the group being screened, many persons with false-positive test results would have to undergo more extensive and sometimes invasive testing, as well as a comprehensive medical evaluation, only to find that the test result was a "false alarm" and that they did not have the disease. On the other hand, less sensitive screening tests would yield an excess of false-negative tests, and many persons who actually had the disease would not be detected.

BENEFITS OF SCREENING

Screening test results should provide some benefit to the person being screened. Generally, there is no point in screening for a disease if no treatment is available to arrest the progression of the disease.

Examples of widely used cost-effective screening tests for disease include urine tests to detect glucose in the urine as a screening test for diabetes, tests to detect blood in the stools to screen for colon tumors, Papanicolaou smears (Pap tests) to screen for abnormalities in the epithelium of the uterine cervix that predispose to cancer, and breast x-ray examinations (mammograms) to screen for very early breast cancer at a stage when it can be treated most effectively.

SCREENING FOR GENETIC DISEASE

Screening tests can also be used to screen for carriers of some genetic diseases that are transmitted from parent to child as either dominant or recessive traits. When many persons in a population carry a recessive gene that can be detected by relatively simple screening tests, identifying carriers allows the affected persons to make decisions regarding future childbearing or management of a future pregnancy. One high-incidence recessive gene for which screening is available is the sickle hemoglobin gene, which occurs in about 8% of the black population. A child born to two carriers of the sickle hemoglobin gene who receives the sickle hemoglobin gene from each parent will develop a severe anemia called sickle cell anemia. The sickle hemoglobin gene and its clinical manifestations are considered in the hematopoietic and lymphatic systems discussion. Other examples of genetic diseases for which screening is available are described in the discussion on congenital and hereditary diseases.

Diagnostic Tests and Procedures

A wide array of diagnostic tests and procedures are available to help the practitioner diagnose and treat the patient properly. They fall into two classifications: invasive procedures and noninvasive procedures. Invasive procedures are so-named because the patient's body is actually "invaded" in some way in order to obtain diagnostic information. Such procedures involve introducing needles, catheters, or other instruments into the patient's body. Noninvasive procedures are those that entail no risk or minimal risk or discomfort to the patient, such as a chest x-ray or an examination of the urine.

Many diagnostic procedures entail some degree of risk or discomfort to the patient. The risk is greater with invasive procedures, but even some noninvasive procedures are not completely harmless. A chest x-ray, for example, exposes the patient to radiation. Even a relatively simple procedure such as the collection of a blood sample for a laboratory test may be complicated by bleeding around the vein or by formation of a blood clot in the vein at the site of puncture. Therefore, with any diagnostic procedure, the practitioner must balance the possible disadvantages to the patient against the benefits that may be derived from the information obtained by the procedure. Patients also must be fully informed about the possible risks and benefits so that they can make informed decisions as to whether or not to consent to the procedure. It would be unwise to perform a potentially risky diagnostic procedure if the information gained would not contribute significantly to the diagnosis or would not greatly influence the course of treatment. The physician would be much more likely to employ a diagnostic procedure that could provide much useful information at little or no risk to the patient.

Diagnostic tests and procedures can be classified in several major categories:

1. Clinical laboratory tests
2. Tests that measure the electrical activity of the body
3. Tests using radioisotopes (also called radionuclides)
4. Endoscopy
5. Ultrasound procedures
6. X-ray examinations
7. Magnetic resonance imaging (MRI)
8. Positron emission tomography (PET scans)
9. Cytologic and histologic examination of cells and tissues removed from the patient

CLINICAL LABORATORY TESTS

Clinical laboratory tests have many uses. They can be used to determine the concentration of various constituents in the blood and urine, which are frequently altered by disease. For example, the concentration of a substance in the blood called urea is elevated if the kidneys are not functioning properly because this constituent is normally excreted by the kidneys. The concentrations of hemoglobin and the quantity of red cells are reduced in patients with anemia. One also can determine the concentration (activity) of enzymes in the blood. Sometimes, the enzyme level is elevated because (a) enzymes are leaking from diseased or injured organs, (b) enzyme synthesis is increased as a result of disease, or (c) excretion of enzymes is impaired because disease has caused blockage of normal excretory pathways.

Clinical laboratory tests are also used to evaluate the functions of organs. Clearance tests measure the rate at which a substance such as urea or creatinine is removed from blood and excreted in the urine. This provides a measure of renal (kidney) function. Pulmonary function tests measure the rate at which air moves in and out of the lungs. Determinations of the concentration of oxygen and carbon dioxide in the blood also can indicate pulmonary function by evaluating how efficiently the lungs can oxygenate the blood and eliminate carbon dioxide, and a simple device applied to the finger can calculate rapidly the amount of oxygen carried by hemoglobin as another measure of pulmonary function. Tests that measure the uptake and excretion of various substances by the liver are used as a measure of liver function. One also can detect substances that are likely to be produced by tumors growing within the body and measure their concentration. Serial analyses of these substances can be used to monitor the response of certain tumors to treatment. Microbiologic tests detect the presence of disease-producing organisms in urine, blood, and feces. They also determine the responsiveness of the organisms to antibiotics. Serologic tests detect and measure the presence of antibodies as an indication of response to infectious agents.

TESTS OF ELECTRICAL ACTIVITY

Several different tests measure the electrical impulses associated with various bodily functions and activities. These include the electrocardiogram (ECG), the electroencephalogram (EEG), and the electromyogram (EMG). The most widely used of these tests is the ECG. Electrodes attached to the arms, legs, and chest are used to measure the serial changes in the electrical activity of the heart during the various phases of the cardiac cycle. The ECG also identifies disturbances in the heart rate or rhythm and identifies abnormal conduction of impulses through the heart. Heart muscle injury, such as occurs after a heart attack, also can be recognized by means of characteristic abnormalities in the cardiogram. The EEG measures the electrical activity of the brain, often called brain waves, by means of small electrodes attached to different areas in the scalp. Brain tumors, strokes, and many other abnormalities of cerebral structure or function may cause altered brain wave patterns that are detected by this examination. The EMG measures the electrical activity of skeletal muscle during contraction and at rest. Abnormal electrical activity is often encountered in various inflammatory or degenerative diseases involving the skeletal muscles. The test is performed by inserting a needle into the muscle that is being studied. The speed at which a nerve conducts impulses also can be measured by means of electrodes taped to the surface of the skin over the nerve being tested. Abnormal conduction of nerve impulses, encountered in some diseases, can be identified by such studies.

RADIOISOTOPE (RADIONUCLIDE) STUDIES

The function of various organs can be evaluated by administering a substance labeled with a radioactive material called a radioisotope. Specially designed radiation detectors then measure the uptake and excretion of the labeled substance. For example, in certain types of anemia, one measures the absorption and excretion of radioisotope-labeled vitamin B_{12}, which is a vitamin required for normal blood formation. The ability of the thyroid gland to concentrate and utilize radioactive iodine is used as a measure of thyroid function and also can be used to detect tumors within the thyroid gland. One may administer a radioactive material that is filtered out or concentrated in a tissue or organ and then measure the radioactivity by radiation detectors applied to the exterior of the body and connected to a computer. For example, specially processed albumin labeled with a radioisotope may be administered intravenously as a measure of pulmonary blood flow. The material is filtered out and retained in the lungs as the blood flows through them. If blood flow to a part of the lung is inadequate for any reason, less radioactivity is recorded in that area. This technique is frequently used to detect the presence of blood clots in the lung that impede blood flow to parts of the lung. Phosphorus-containing isotopes are concentrated in the skeletal system. If there are deposits of tumor in bone, the isotopes are concentrated around the tumor deposits and can be easily identified (FIGURE 1). Radioactive materials injected intravenously also can be used to evaluate blood flow to heart muscle and to identify areas of damaged heart muscle.

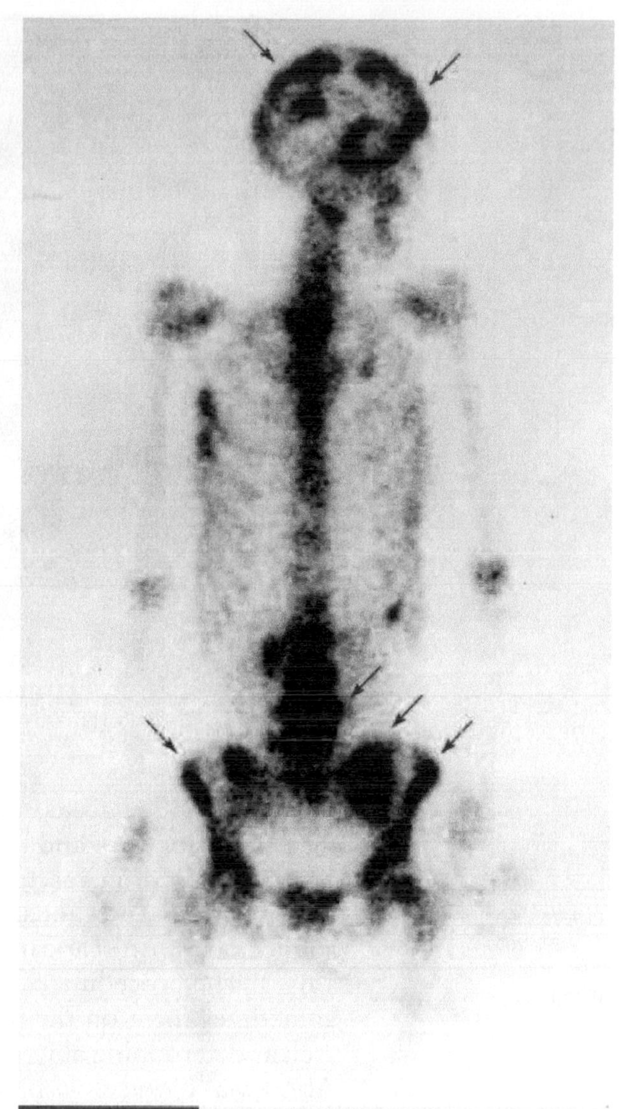

FIGURE 1 Radioisotope bone scan of head, chest, and pelvis. Dark areas (*arrows*) indicate the concentration of radioisotope around tumor deposits in bone.

ENDOSCOPY AND LAPAROSCOPY

An **endoscopy**, or endoscopic examination (*endo* = within + *skopeo* = examine), is an examination of the interior of the body by means of various types of rigid or flexible tubular instruments that are named according to the part of the body they are designed to examine. These instruments have a system of lenses for viewing and a light source to illuminate the region being examined. An esophagoscope, for example, is used to examine the interior of the esophagus; a gastroscope to examine the stomach; and a bronchoscope to examine the trachea and major bronchi. An instrument for viewing the interior of the bladder is called a cystoscope. A sigmoidoscope is a rigid tube used to examine the rectum and the sigmoid colon, and a colonoscope is a flexible tube that can be used to examine the entire length of the colon. An instrument called a **laparoscope** is used to visualize the abdominal and pelvic organs, and the procedure is called laparoscopy, which can be used not only to examine abdominal and pelvic organs but also to perform various surgical procedures, such as removal of the gallbladder (cholecystectomy), appendix (appendectomy), ovary (oophorectomy), and other surgical procedures that formerly were removed through much larger abdominal incisions. To perform a laparoscopic procedure, the peritoneal cavity is inflated first with carbon dioxide, which separates the organs within the peritoneal cavity so that they can be visualized more easily. Then the laparoscope is inserted through a small incision in the abdominal wall, often in or near the umbilicus. If a surgical procedure is to be performed, such as an appendectomy or cholecystectomy, one or two additional small incisions are needed in order to insert the instruments used to perform the surgical procedure and remove the organ from the abdominal cavity.

Endoscopy
(en-däs′kō-pē)
An examination of the interior of the body by means of various lighted tubular instruments.

Laparoscope
(lap′-ă-rō-skōp)
A long tubular telescope-like instrument passed through the abdominal wall to examine structures within the peritoneal cavity.

ULTRASOUND

Ultrasound is a technique for mapping the echoes produced by high-frequency sound waves transmitted into the body. Echoes are reflected wherever there is a change in the density of the tissue. The reflected waves are recorded on sensitive detectors, and images are produced. This method is widely used to study the uterus during pregnancy because it does not require the use of potentially harmful radiation and poses no risk to the fetus (FIGURE 2). The technique can be used to determine the

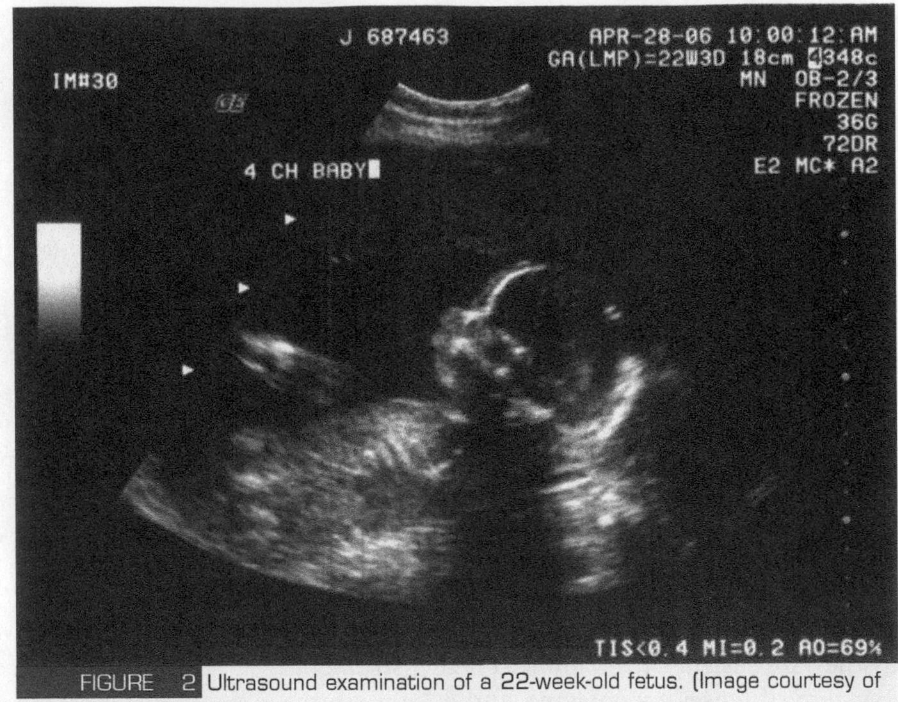

FIGURE 2 Ultrasound examination of a 22-week-old fetus. (Image courtesy of Belinda Thresher.)

position of the placenta and the fetus within the uterus; it also can identify some fetal abnormalities and detect twin pregnancies. Ultrasound is also often used to examine the cardiovascular system. When used for this purpose, the procedure is usually called an **echocardiogram**. The prefix term "echo" refers to the reflected sound waves. An echocardiogram can detect the structure and function of the heart valves. The procedure can detect valve abnormalities and identify blood clots that sometimes form on the heart valves in association with infection of the valve as well as determining abnormal communications between adjacent cardiac chambers. Abnormal blood flow patterns—characteristic of congenital or acquired valvular heart disease—can also be detected. An ultrasound examination can distinguish a significant heart murmur caused by a valve or chamber abnormality from a murmur caused by turbulent blood flow within a structurally normal heart, which is clinically significant. In many cases, ultrasound has replaced some radiology procedures because ultrasound avoids radiation, is not an invasive procedure, and is usually less expensive. Ultrasound can determine the thickness of the ventricular walls and septum and the size of the ventricular chambers during systole and diastole. It can also identify gallstones in the gallbladder and abnormalities in the prostate suspicious for prostate cancer. The technique has many other applications in medicine.

Echocardiogram
An examination of the heart by means of an ultrasound procedure.

X-RAY EXAMINATION

X-ray examinations are conducted in many ways, but the basic principle is the same for all types of x-ray studies. X-rays are passed through the part of the body to be examined, and the rays leaving the body expose an x-ray film. The extent to which the rays are absorbed by the tissues as they pass through the body depends on the density of the tissues. Tissues of low density, such as the air-filled lungs, transmit most of the rays, and thus, the film exposed to x-rays passing through them appears black. Tissues of high density, such as bone, absorb most of the rays; the film remains unexposed and appears white. Tissues of intermediate densities appear as varying shades of gray. The x-ray image produced on the film is called a radiograph or **roentgenogram**. The same basic principle is used to obtain x-ray films of the

Roentgenogram
(rent′gen-ō-gram)
A photograph taken with x-rays.

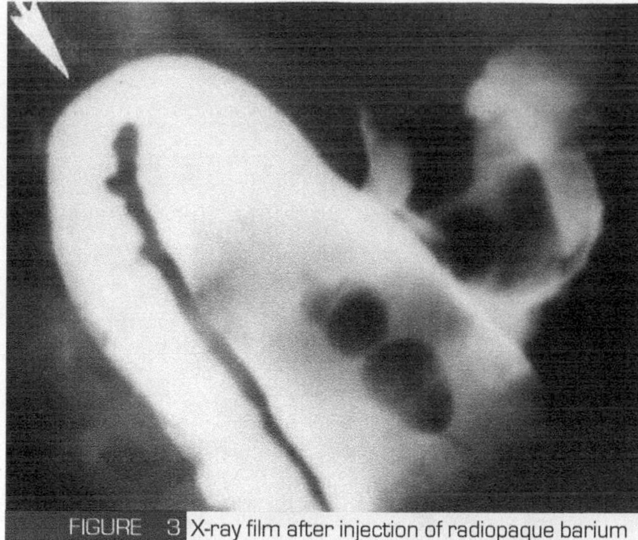

FIGURE 3 X-ray film after injection of radiopaque barium sulfate suspension into colon (barium enema), illustrating narrowed area (*arrow*) that impedes passage of bowel contents.

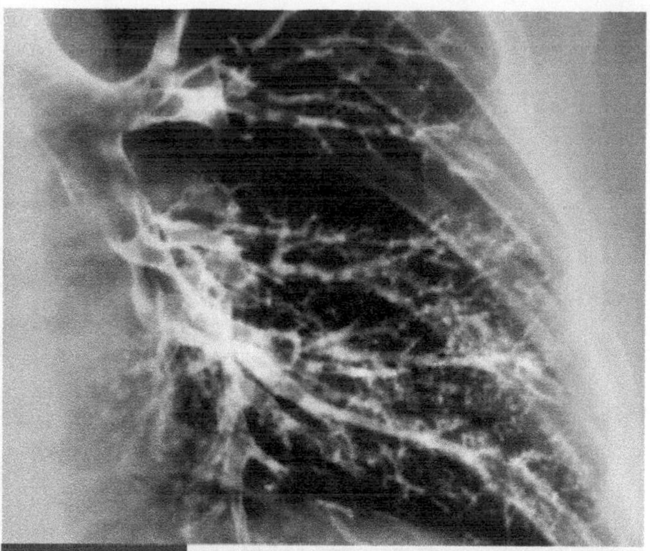

FIGURE 4 Bronchogram illustrating normal branching of bronchi and bronchioles that are normal in caliber and appearance.

breast. This procedure is called **mammogram**. The applications and limitations of the mammogram procedure are considered in diseases of the breast.

Although the linings of internal organs such as the intestinal tract, urinary tract, bronchi, fallopian tubes, and biliary tract have little contrast, they can be examined by administering a dense radiopaque substance called contrast medium. It coats and adheres to the lining of the structure being examined and enhances its visibility. To examine the interior of the gastrointestinal tract, for example, one gives the patient a suspension of barium sulfate to swallow or administers it as an enema. The opaque barium coats the lining of the intestinal tract, and an abnormality in the lining shows on the film as an irregularity in the column of barium (FIGURE 3). The lining of the bronchi can be visualized by instilling a radiopaque oil into the bronchi. The oil forms a thin film on the bronchial mucosa and delineates the contours of the bronchi. This procedure is called a bronchogram (FIGURE 4).

One uses the same principle to visualize the urinary tract. A radiopaque substance is injected into a vein and is excreted in the urine as the blood flows through the kidney, outlining the contour of the urinary tract. This is called an intravenous pyelogram (IVP) (FIGURE 5). Another method is to introduce the dye directly into both ureters through tubes that are inserted into both ureters by means of a cystoscope introduced into the bladder. This procedure is called a retrograde pyelogram. To visualize the gallbladder, the patient ingests tablets of radiopaque material that is absorbed into the circulation, excreted by the liver in the bile, and concentrated in the gallbladder. Gallstones can be identified because they occupy space in the gallbladder and cause irregularities in the radiopaque material concentrated there (FIGURE 6).

One can also use contrast material to study the flow of blood in large arteries and to identify areas of narrowing or obstruction. This procedure is called an **arteriogram** or **angiogram** (*angio* = blood vessel). A small flexible catheter is inserted into a large artery in the arm or leg and advanced into the aorta until it is positioned at the opening of the artery that is to be examined. Radiopaque material is then injected through the catheter. It mixes with the blood, and its flow through the vessel is followed by means of a series of x-ray films. If the vessel is narrowed by disease, the film will show areas in which the column of opaque material is narrowed. A complete obstruction of the vessel appears as an interruption of the column. Arteriography

Mammogram
(mam′ō-gram)
An x-ray of the breast, used to detect tumors and other abnormalities within the breast.

Arteriogram
(är-tēr′ē-ō-gram)
An x-ray technique for studying the caliber of blood vessels by injection of radiopaque material into the vessel.

Angiogram
(an′jē-ō-gram)
Same as arteriogram.

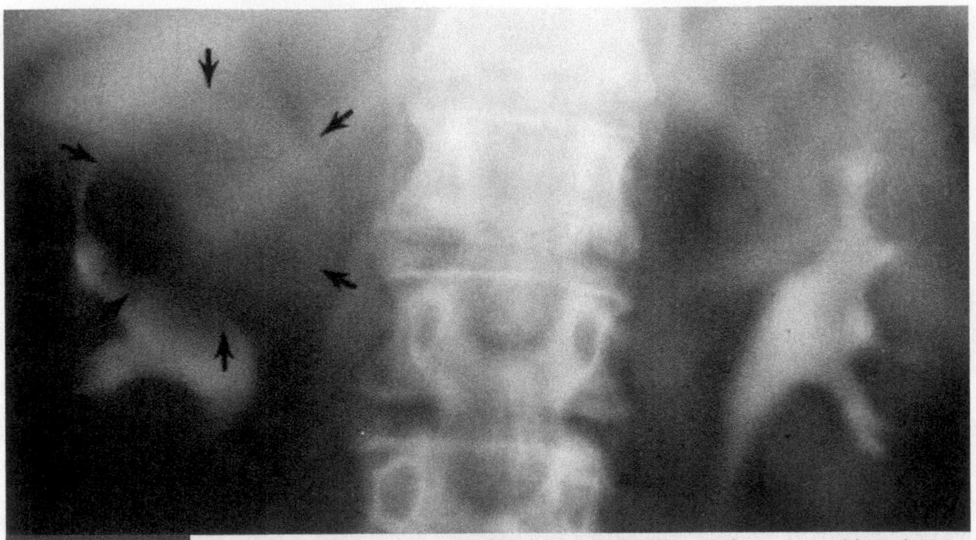

FIGURE 5 Intravenous pyelogram (IVP). *Arrows* outline filling defect caused by a large cyst in kidney that distorts renal pelvis and calyces. The opposite kidney appears normal.

Cardiac catheterization
A specialized technique to determine the blood flow through the chambers of the heart and to detect abnormal communications between cardiac chambers.

Computed tomographic (CT) scan
(tō-mo-graf′ik)
An x-ray technique producing detailed cross-sectional images of the body by means of x-ray tube and detectors connected to a computer. Sometimes called a CAT scan.

is often used to detect narrowing or obstruction of the coronary arteries or of the carotid arteries in the neck, which carry blood to the brain (FIGURE 7). Obstruction of the pulmonary arteries by blood clots also can be identified by arteriography. In this case, the catheter used to inject the radiopague material is inserted into a large vein in the arm, threaded up the vein and through the right side of the heart, and positioned in the pulmonary artery.

This same basic method can be used to study the flow of blood through the heart and can detect abnormal communications between cardiac chambers. This type of study is called **cardiac catheterization.**

Computed Tomographic Scans

A **computed tomographic scan** (**CT scan**) is performed by a highly sophisticated x-ray machine that produces images of the body in cross section by rotating the x-ray tube around the patient at various levels. The x-ray tube is mounted on a movable frame opposite an array of sensitive radiation detectors that encircle the

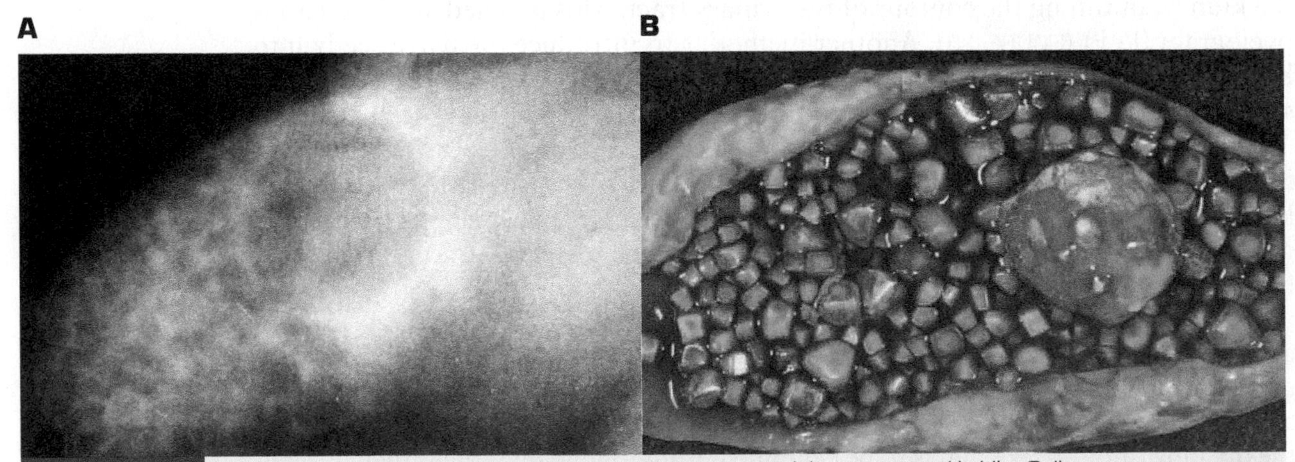

FIGURE 6 **A**, Gallstones demonstrated by means of radiopaque material concentrated in bile. Gallstones occupy space and appear as radiolucent (dark) areas within radiopaque (white) bile. Note the large radiolucent area, indicating a large gallstone, surrounded by smaller radiolucent areas, representing multiple smaller stones. **B**, Opened gallbladder removed surgically from the same patient. Compare appearance and location of stones with x-ray appearance.

patient. As the x-ray tube moves around the patient, the radiation detectors record the amount of radiation passing through the body (FIGURE 8). In computerized scanning, the amount of radiation absorbed is not read directly on an x-ray film. Instead, the data from the radiation detectors are fed into a computer, which reconstructs the data into an image that reproduces the patient's anatomy as a cross-section picture. The image is displayed on a television monitor and can be recorded on film (FIGURE 9). As with conventional x-rays, dense substances are white, and less dense substances appear darker in proportion to the amount of radiation they transmit. The individual organs appear sharply separated from one another because the various parts of the body are separated by planes of fat, which have very low density. These separations increase contrast between adjacent organs. Abnormalities of internal organs that cannot be identified by means of standard x-ray examinations can often be discovered with CT scans. FIGURE 10 shows a renal cyst located by CT scan.

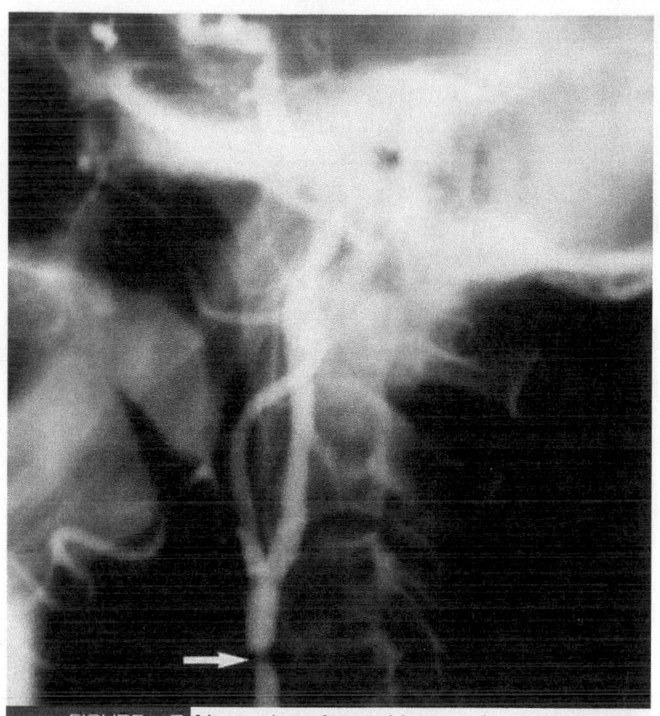

FIGURE 7 Narrowing of carotid artery in neck (*arrow*) demonstrated by carotid angiogram.

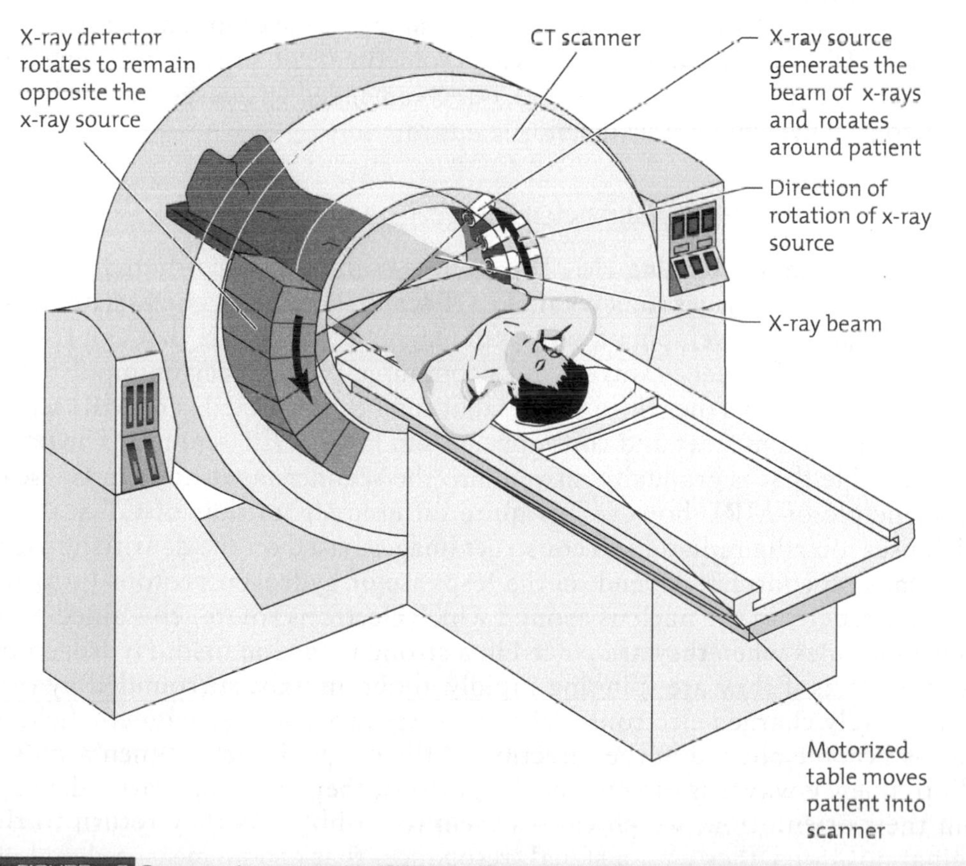

FIGURE 8 Computed tomographic (CT) scan. The patient lies on a table that is gradually advanced into the scanner. X-ray tube mounted in scanner rotates around patient, and radiation detectors also rotate so that detectors remain opposite the x-ray source. Data from radiation detectors generate computer-reconstructed images of the patient's body at multiple levels.

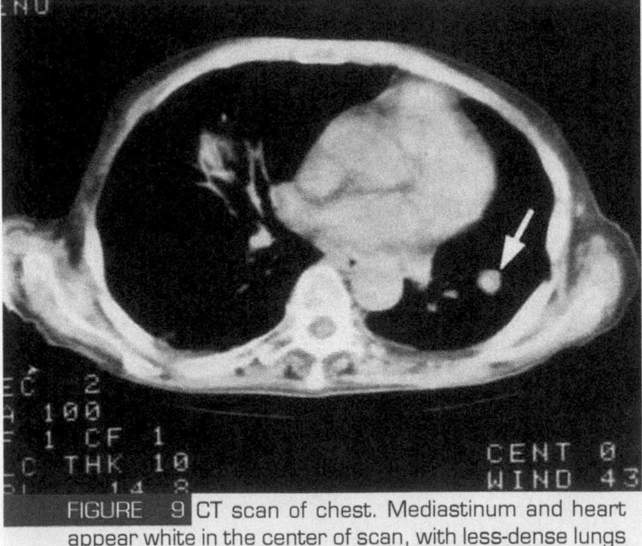

FIGURE 9 CT scan of chest. Mediastinum and heart appear white in the center of scan, with less-dense lungs on either side. The *arrow* indicates a lung tumor, which appears as white nodule in lung.

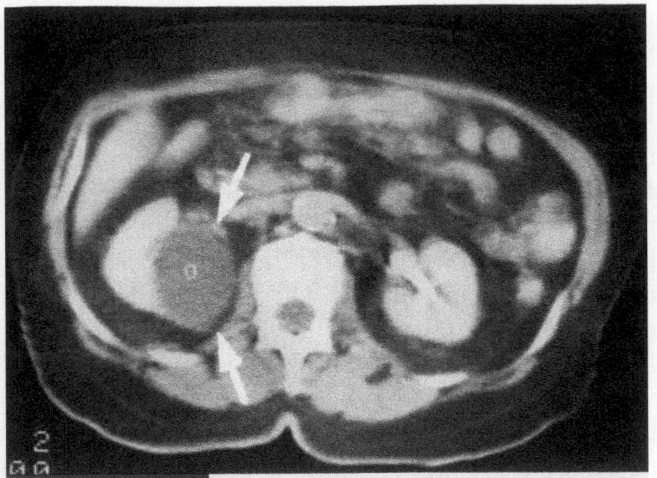

FIGURE 10 CT views of the abdomen at the level of kidneys, illustrating a fluid-filled cyst in the kidney (*arrow*). The cyst appears less dense than surrounding renal tissue. The opposite kidney (*right* side of photograph) appears normal.

Use of CT has increased greatly in recent years and provides much useful information. Much of the increased use has been for screening asymptomatic persons for unsuspected lung or colon tumors and for some screening studies in children. However, CT delivers a much greater dose of radiation than a standard x-ray examination, such as a chest x-ray, and some physicians are concerned that repeated CT examinations may deliver a significant and possibly excessive amount of radiation to the patient. Ultrasound examination, which sometimes can provide the same information without any radiation exposure, is recommended whenever it can substitute for CT to provide comparable diagnostic information.

MAGNETIC RESONANCE IMAGING

Magnetic resonance imaging (MRI)
A diagnostic procedure that yields computer-generated images based on the movement of hydrogen atoms in tissues subjected to a strong magnetic field.

Magnetic resonance imaging (MRI) produces computer-constructed images of various organs and tissues somewhat like CT scans. The device consists of a strong magnet capable of developing a powerful magnetic field; coils that can transmit and receive radiofrequency waves; and a computer, which receives impulses from the scanner and forms them into images that can be interpreted. The MRI scanner with the enclosed magnet and coils appears similar to a CT scanner. The patient lies on a table that is gradually moved into the scanner, as is done in CT scans. The principle of MRI, however, is quite different from that of CT scanning, which uses ionizing radiation to construct images based on the density of tissues. MRI scans, in contrast, depend on the response of hydrogen protons (positively charged particles in the nucleus around which electrons rotate) contained within water molecules when they are placed in a strong magnetic field. Hydrogen protons behave as if they are spinning rapidly about an axis, surrounded by orbiting negatively charged electrons. When subjected to a strong magnetic field, the protons become aligned in the direction of the magnetic field. When a pulse of radiofrequency waves is directed at the protons, they are temporarily dislodged from their orientation, which causes them to wobble. As they return to their original positions, they emit a signal (resonance) that can be measured and used to produce the computer-constructed images. Body tissues, which have a high water content, are a rich source of protons capable of excitation. The intensity of the signals produced is related to the varying water content of body tissues and

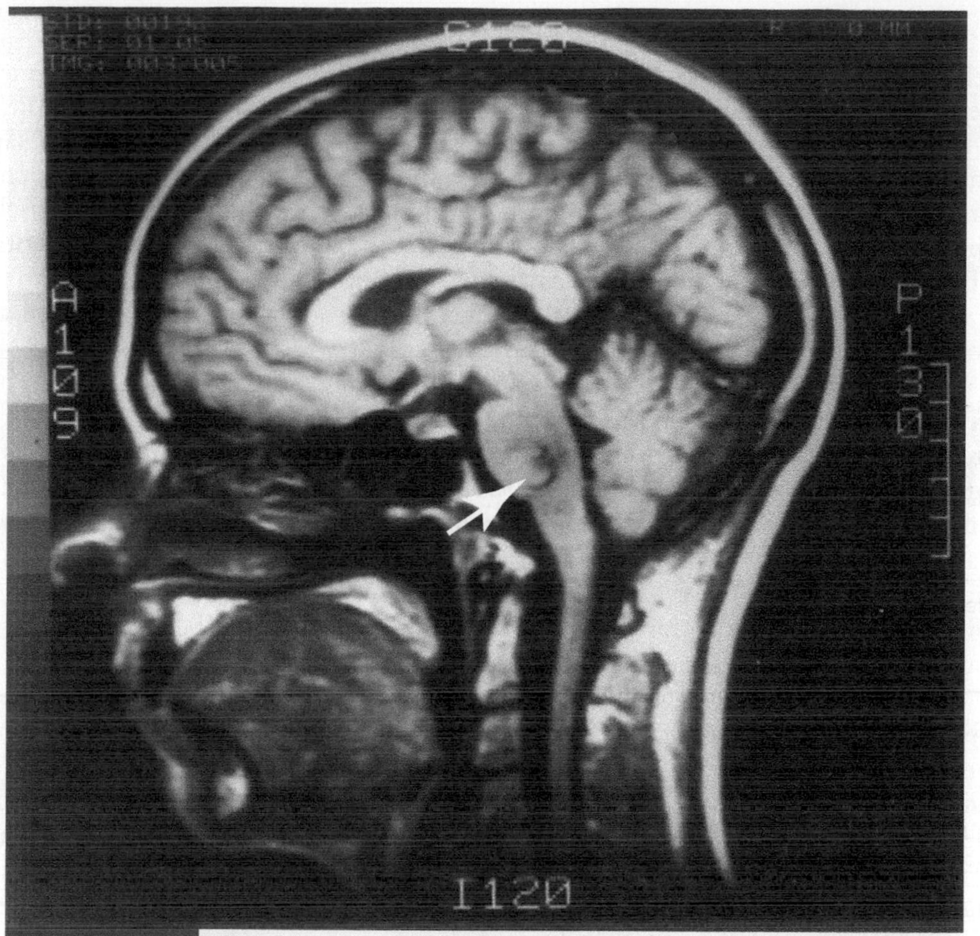

FIGURE 11 MRI view of brain, which is clearly visible because skull bones are not visualized by MRI. The white line surrounding the brain represents scalp tissue. The *arrow* indicates a malformation composed of blood vessels within the brain stem.

to the strength and duration of the radiofrequency pulse. Because an MRI does not use ionizing radiation, the patient does not receive radiation exposure. An MRI does expose the patient to strong magnetic fields and radiowaves, but this appears relatively safe on the basis of current knowledge.

Applications

An MRI detects many of the same types of abnormalities detected by a CT, and a CT is superior to an MRI for many applications. An MRI, however, offers distinct advantages over CT in special situations, as, for example, when attempting to detect abnormalities in tissues surrounded by bone, such as lesions in the spinal cord, orbits or near the base of the skull (FIGURE 11). In these locations, bone interferes with scanning because of its density, but it does not produce an image in MRI because the water content of bone is low. MRI also provides a sharp contrast between gray and white matter within the brain and spinal cord, which differ in their water content. For this reason, the technique is useful for demonstrating areas where myelin sheaths of nerve fibers have been damaged, as in a neurologic disease called multiple sclerosis (described in the discussion on the nervous system). MRI may also be superior to mammography for detecting breast carcinoma in a selected group of women who have a higher than normal risk of breast carcinoma (described in the discussion about breast disease). Further improvements in equipment will undoubtedly increase the usefulness of this diagnostic procedure.

POSITRON EMISSION TOMOGRAPHY

Related to radioisotope studies but much more complex and sophisticated is one of the newest of the diagnostic imaging tests called positron emission tomography (PET), or simply PET scans. Positrons are unique subatomic particles that have the same mass as electrons but carry a positive charge. They are formed when atoms such as carbon, oxygen, or nitrogen are bombarded in a cyclotron with high-energy particles, which breaks down the atomic nuclei and releases the positrons along with other subatomic particles. The positrons escaping from the nuclei collide with negatively charged electrons circling the nuclei, producing radiation that can be detected and measured by means of sensitive radiation detectors.

One uses PET scans to study body functions by injecting into the subject a biochemical compound, such as glucose, that is labeled with a positron-emitting isotope and then assessing the distribution and metabolism of the compound by measuring the radiation produced within the body by the isotope-labeled compound. The radiation output, measured by sensitive radiation detectors, is fed into a computer that constructs computer-generated images similar to those obtained with CT scans. Such studies provide information on the metabolic activities of the organ or tissue being studied, the site within an organ where the compound is being metabolized, and the blood flow to the organ being studied.

Although originally developed for research studies, PET scans have moved from the research laboratory into medical practice. A major application is to assess biochemical functions within the brain. One can detect and measure changes in brain functions associated with various neurologic diseases such as strokes, brain tumors, Alzheimer disease, Parkinson disease, and some hereditary degenerative diseases of the nervous system. The method has also been used to some extent to evaluate changes in blood flow and metabolism in heart muscle after a heart attack. PET scans following intravenous infusion of a labeled glucose compound have also been used to distinguish a benign from a malignant tumor growing within the body, based on the greater glucose uptake and metabolic activity within a malignant tumor, in contrast to the much lower labeled glucose uptake in a benign tumor. This same approach is also used to identify deposits of malignant tumor that have spread throughout the body by demonstrating the increased glucose uptake within the tumor deposits. When PET scans are used to determine how widely a malignant tumor has spread throughout the body, the initial PET scan is often followed by a follow-up scan after a course of treatment in order to evaluate the response to treatment. Because a PET scan is usually performed along with a CT scan, repeated PET–CT scans subject the patient to significant amounts of radiation. In addition, when a PET scan is used to aid in tumor diagnosis and to evaluate response to treatment, false-positive results may be obtained. Areas of inflammation are also associated with increased glucose uptake, which may be very difficult to distinguish from a tumor.

Although PET scans provide useful information, there are some drawbacks to their widespread application. They are very expensive procedures and may not be widely available. Because positron-emitting isotopes must be produced in a cyclotron, the isotopes produced have a very short duration of activity (half-life), and one must have facilities for incorporating the isotope into the biochemical compound required for the PET scan procedure.

CYTOLOGIC AND HISTOLOGIC EXAMINATIONS

Cells covering the surfaces of the body are continually cast off and replaced by new cells. Abnormal cells can often be identified in the fluids or secretions that come in

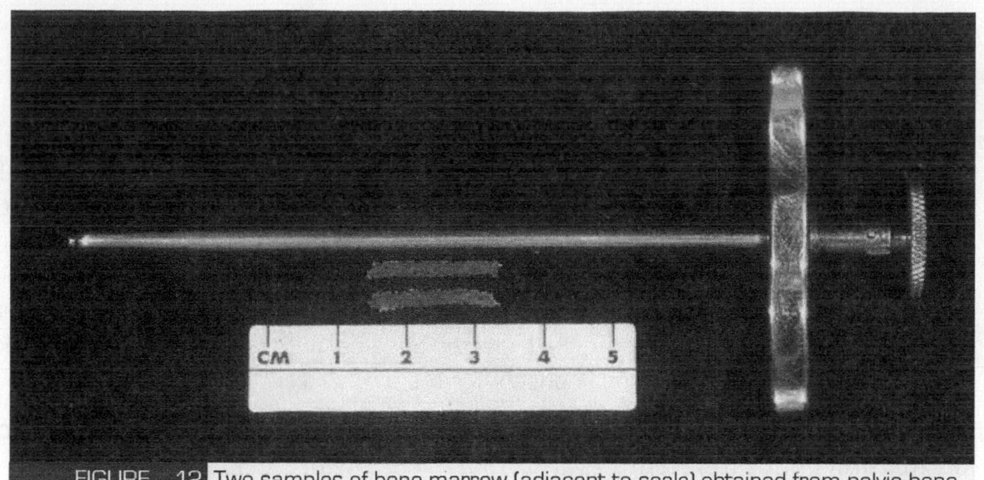

FIGURE 12 Two samples of bone marrow (adjacent to scale) obtained from pelvic bone by means of a specially designed needle, shown in the upper part of the photograph.

contact with the epithelial surface. This type of examination is called a Papanicolaou smear, or simply **Pap smear**, after the physician who developed the procedure. It is widely used as a screening test for recognizing early cancer of the uterus and can be used to detect cancers in other locations as well. The Pap smear is discussed in the section on neoplasms.

Pap smear
A study of cells from various sources, commonly used as a screening test for cancer.

Diseased tissues have abnormal structural and cellular patterns that can be recognized by the pathologist. Consequently, it is often possible to determine the cause of a patient's disease by histologic examination of a small sample of tissue removed from the affected tissue or organ. This procedure is called a **biopsy**. Samples of tissue can be obtained from any part of the body. Gastroscopes, bronchoscopes, and other instruments used for endoscopic examination, for example, are constructed so that specimens for biopsy can be obtained while the internal organs are being examined. Biopsy specimens can also be taken directly from internal organs such as the liver or kidney by inserting a thin needle through the skin directly into the organ. Samples of bone marrow are obtained in this way, and bone-marrow biopsy is often performed to diagnose blood disease (FIGURE 12).

Biopsy
(bī′op-sē)
Removal of a small sample of tissue for examination and diagnosis by a pathologist.

QUESTIONS FOR REVIEW

1. What are the five major categories of disease?
2. What are the definitions of the following terms: *etiology*, *symptom of disease*, *sign of disease*, *diagnosis*, and *prognosis*?
3. How does an organic disease differ from a functional disease?
4. What principal factors does the physician evaluate in arriving at a diagnosis?
5. What is the difference between specific and symptomatic treatment?
6. What are the major categories of diagnostic tests and procedures that can help the practitioner make a diagnosis? Give some examples.
7. What is the difference between an invasive and a noninvasive procedure?
8. What are the basic concepts on which the following procedures are based: Pap smear, x-ray examinations, ultrasound, electrocardiogram, and CT scans?

Baerlocher, M. O., and Detsky, A. S. 2010. Discussing radiation risks associated with CT scans in patients. *Journal of the American Medical Association* 304:2170–71.

- Use of CT has doubled every 2 years since the 1980s, as have concerns about the associated radiation risks and radiation-related cancers. Most patients are not informed of radiation risks associated with CT scans, and many patients with cardiovascular disease have multiple CT examinations. Physicians should explain to patients the reason for the procedures, the expected benefits, and the radiation-related risks and should obtain an informed consent for the procedure.

Brenner, D. J., and Hall, E. J. 2007. Computed tomography—an increasing source of radiation exposure. *New England Journal of Medicine* 357:2277–84.

- CT has revolutionized diagnostic radiology, and its use has increased greatly in recent years. It is used now for screening procedures on healthy patients to identify unsuspected colon or lung tumors and for total body screening; its use has also increased in pediatric patients. CT delivers a much greater radiation exposure than a standard x-ray examination, such as a chest x-ray. Too many CT exams are being performed and many may not be justified by medical need. In order to reduce radiation exposure to the patient, ultrasound examinations or MRI should substitute for CT whenever possible.

Dinan, M. A., Curtis, L. H., Hammill, B. G., et al. 2010. Changes in the use and costs of diagnostic imaging among Medicare beneficiaries with cancer, 1999–2006. *Journal of the American Medical Association* 303:1625–31.

- Imaging costs among Medicare patients with cancer increased from 1999 to 2006, which outpaced the rate of increase in the total costs among Medicare beneficiaries with cancer. In each cancer type, the number of PET scans increased at a mean annual rate of 35.9–53.6%. Patients with lung cancer or lymphoma had the largest increase in PET use.

Einstein, A. J., Weiner, S. D., Bernheim, A., et al. 2010. Multiple testing, cumulative radiation dose, and clinical indications in patients undergoing myocardial perfusion imaging. *Journal of the American Medical Association* 304:2137–44.

- The US Food and Drug Administration proposes reducing unnecessary radiation exposure. CT scans associated with perfusion of coronary arteries account for a large proportion of the radiation exposures. Many patients with suspected coronary artery disease have multiple tests, which lead to very high cumulative doses of radiation. Ways to reduce unnecessary repeat testing are described.

Figley, N. M., ed. 1983. Diagnostic imaging and related sciences. *American Journal of Roentgenology* (special section: NMR) 141:1101–353.

- A detailed reference on the various applications and limitations of nuclear magnetic resonance in medical diagnosis.

Guttmacher, A. E., Collins, F. S., and Carmona, R. H. 2004. The family history: More important than ever. *New England Journal of Medicine* 351:2333–6.

- We do patients a disservice if we fail to realize the value of the family history in pinpointing some of the more common diseases that have a hereditary or genetic component. A government-sponsored website is available that allows people to collect, organize, and maintain their family history in their own computers (www.hhs.gov/familyhistory). Patients are encouraged to bring their family history to their healthcare provider for further discussion, evaluation, and use.

Jacobson, H. G. 1987. Fundamentals of magnetic resonance imaging. Council on Scientific Affairs. *Journal of the American Medical Association* 258:3417–23.

► Describes principles and applications of this powerful diagnostic tool.

Juweid, M. E., and Cheson, B. D. 2006. Positron-emission tomography and assessment of cancer therapy. *New England Journal of Medicine* 354:496–507.

► A comprehensive, well-illustrated article dealing with the applications and limitations of PET scans used for the evaluation and treatment of malignant tumors.

Khoury, M. J., McCabe, L., and McCabe, E. R. 2003. Population screening in the age of genomic medicine. *New England Journal of Medicine* 348:50–8.

► Newborn infants are routinely screened for several inherited diseases so that early diagnosis can allow prompt treatment, thereby preventing the long-term adverse effects caused by the disease. Screening of adults for selected diseases can also provide benefits to the affected persons.

Matchar, D. B. 1990. Decision making in the face of uncertainty: The case of carotid endarterectomy. *Mayo Clinic Proceedings* 65:756–60.

► Excellent discussion of risks and benefits of therapeutic procedures, as well as biases. The wish to do everything possible for the patient must not lead to misguided actions.

McNutt, R. A. 2004. Shared medical decision making: Problems, process, progress. *Journal of the American Medical Association* 292:2516–8.

► Decisions about options for treatment of a disease should be a joint effort on the part of both the physician and the patient, and the patient needs to understand that every decision is influenced by uncertainty and risk. The physician can explain the possible risks and benefits of various methods of treatment, but the patient must make the final decision.

OUTLINE SUMMARY

Characteristics of Disease

DISTURBANCE OF STRUCTURE OR FUNCTION

Lesions: structural changes identified by gross or microscopic examination.
Symptoms: subjective manifestations.
Signs: objective findings.
Terminology:
Asymptomatic disease: not associated with symptoms or discomfort.
Symptomatic disease: associated with symptoms and abnormal physical findings.
Etiology: cause of disease.
Pathogenesis: manner in which disease develops.

Classifications of Disease

Congenital and hereditary disease: caused by genetic or chromosomal abnormality, intrauterine injury, or interaction of genetic and environmental factors.
Inflammatory disease: associated with inflammation.
Degenerative disease: associated with degeneration of tissues or organs.
Metabolic disease: associated with disturbed metabolic processes.
Neoplastic disease: characterized by various benign and malignant tumors.

Health and Disease: A Continuum

BASIC CONCEPTS

Health and disease are two extremes of a continuous spectrum.
Good health is more than absence of disease.
Modern medicine can cure disease but cannot guarantee good health.
Each individual must assume responsibility for achieving good health.

Principles of Diagnosis

DIAGNOSIS

Clinical history: information obtained from patient.
Physical examination: objective findings obtained by clinician.
Differential diagnosis: consideration of possible diseases that could be responsible for clinical manifestations.

TREATMENT

Specific treatment: produces specific curative effect.

Symptomatic treatment: alleviates symptoms but does not alter course of disease.

Screening Tests for Disease

Purpose is to detect early asymptomatic disease amenable to treatment, thereby preventing or minimizing late-stage organ damage.

Requirements for effective screening:

Significant population at risk for disease.

Inexpensive noninvasive test available to detect the disease.

Early identification and treatment favorably influences outcome.

Screening for genetic disease useful in selected cases.

Diagnostic Tests and Procedures

CATEGORIES OF DIAGNOSTIC PROCEDURES

Invasive procedure: "invades" patient's body to obtain diagnostic information.

Noninvasive procedure: not associated with significant risk or discomfort.

TYPES OF PROCEDURES

Clinical laboratory tests: chemical, serologic, microbiologic tests on blood and body fluids.

Tests that measure electrical activity: ECG, EEG, EMG.

Radioisotope studies: determine uptake and excretion of radioactive materials.

Endoscopy: examines interior of body with specially designed instruments.

Ultrasound: high-frequency sound waves directed into the body creates echoes based on differing densities of body organs. Used to evaluate body structure and functions.

X-ray examination: *x-rays absorbed in proportion to density of tissue.*

X-rays using contrast media: outline structures that cannot be visualized on standard films.

CT scans: x-rays transmitted to the computer produce cross-section views through various levels of the body.

MRI: detects same type of abnormalities as CT, but based on movement of protons in magnetic field; has advantages over CT in special situations.

PET scans: measure metabolism of biochemical compounds labeled with positron-emitting isotopes as measure of organ function.

Very expensive procedure; applications and limitations still being explored.

Major current application is assessment of brain functions in health and disease.

Cytologic and histologic examinations: smears and biopsy samples taken from patient's body have characteristic patterns that permit recognition of disease.

http://health.jbpub.com/humandisease/9e

Human Disease Online is a great source for supplementary human disease information for both students and instructors. Visit this website to find a variety of useful tools for learning, thinking, and teaching.

Cells and Tissues: Their Structure and Function in Health and Disease

LEARNING OBJECTIVES

1. Make a sketch of the general structure of a typical cell.
2. Explain how cells are organized to form tissues. Diagram the fundamental structure of the four basic types of tissues.
3. Explain how tissues are organized to form organ systems.
4. Write a general description of the three germ layers and their derivatives.
5. Describe how cells utilize the genetic code within DNA chains to convey genetic information to daughter cells during cell division.
6. Explain the process by which the DNA in the nucleus directs the synthesis of enzymes and other proteins in the cytoplasm.
7. Illustrate how materials move in and out of cells. List five processes by which cells adapt to changing conditions.
8. Explain three ways in which an aging cell becomes increasingly vulnerable to injury.

Organization of Cells

The cell is the basic structural and functional unit of the body. Groups of similar cells arranged to perform a common function form **tissues.** Tissues in turn are grouped together in different proportions to form **organs,** and groups of organs functioning together form **organ systems.** Finally, the various organ systems are integrated to form a functioning organism. Dysfunction at any of these levels of organization can cause disease.

Tissue *A group of similar cells joined to perform a specific function.*

Organs *A group of different tissues organized to perform a specific function.*

Organ systems *A group of organs that function together as a unit, such as the various organs of the gastrointestinal tract.*

The Cell

Cells having different functions differ somewhat in structure, but all have certain features in common (FIGURE 1). Each cell consists of a nucleus surrounded by the cytoplasm. The nucleus, which contains the genetic information stored in the cell, directs the metabolic functions of the cell, and structures in the cytoplasm carry out these directions. Within the cytoplasm are numerous small structures called **organelles**, which play an important part in the functions of the cell. The cytoplasm also contains filaments of structural protein that form the framework (cytoskeleton) of the cell. Some cells also contain filaments of contractile protein. The cytoplasm, nucleus, and organelles are surrounded by membranes composed of lipid and protein molecules, which separate these structures from one another.

Organelle
A small structure present in the cytoplasm of the cell, such as a mitochondrion.

Deoxyribonucleic acid (DNA)
The nucleic acid present in the chromosomes of the nuclei of cells that carries genetic information.

Ribonucleic acid (RNA)
A type of nucleic acid contained in the nucleoli of cells. A component of messenger, transfer, and ribosomal RNA.

THE NUCLEUS

The nucleus contains two different types of nucleic acid combined with protein. **Deoxyribonucleic acid (DNA)** is contained in the chromosomes, which are long and thin in the nondividing cell and cannot be identified as distinct structures. Instead, they appear as a network of granules called nuclear chromatin. **Ribonucleic acid (RNA)** is contained in spherical intranuclear structures called nucleoli (singular, nucleolus). The nucleus is separated from the cytoplasm by a double-layered nuclear membrane. Small pores in the nuclear membrane permit the nucleus and cytoplasm to communicate.

THE CYTOPLASM

The cytoplasm of the cell consists of a mass of protoplasm surrounded by a cell membrane, which acts selectively to allow some materials to pass into and out of the cell while it restricts the passage of others. It contains various organelles and may also contain products that accumulate within the cell, such as glycogen and fat. The most important organelles are the mitochondria, endoplasmic reticulum, Golgi apparatus, lysosomes, centrioles, and the tubules and filaments comprising the cytoskeleton of the cell. Some diseases are associated with characteristic abnormalities in cytoplasmic

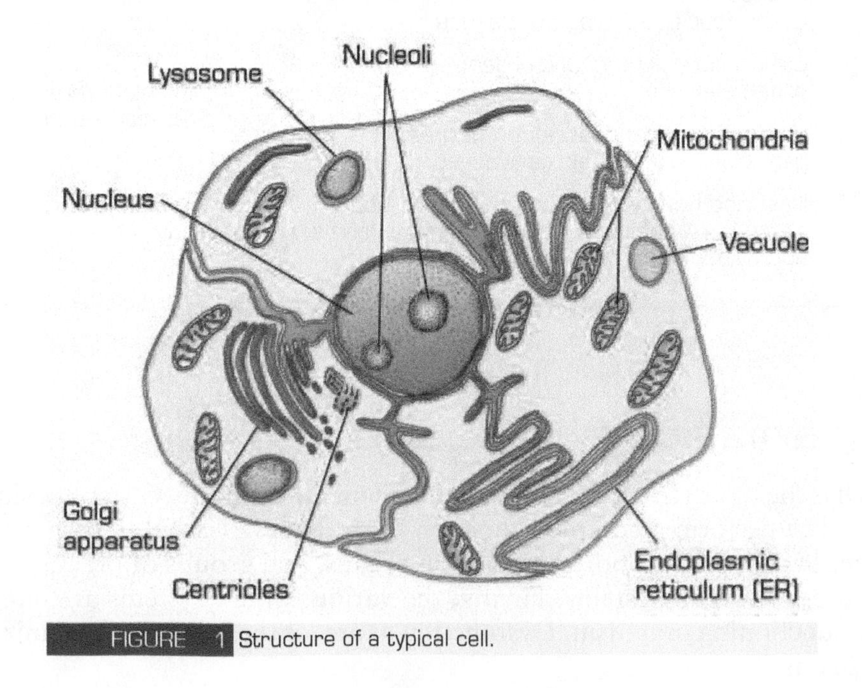

FIGURE 1 Structure of a typical cell.

organelles. The functions of the organelles are described in the following section and summarized in TABLE 1.

Mitochondria are sausage-shaped structures that contain enzymes capable of converting food materials into energy by oxidizing them. The cell uses this energy to manufacture a high-energy compound called **adenosine triphosphate (ATP)**, the fuel that powers the chemical reactions in the cell.

The **endoplasmic reticulum** is an interconnected network of tubular channels enclosed by membranes. This network communicates with both the nuclear membrane and the cell membrane. Rough endoplasmic reticulum (RER) has numerous small nucleoprotein particles called **ribosomes** attached to the external surfaces of its membranes. Its name derives from the knobby appearance that the attached ribosomes give the membranes, and its function is to synthesize protein that will be secreted by the cell. The attached ribosomes synthesize protein molecules that accumulate within the tubules of the RER and are eventually secreted. Digestive enzymes and antibody proteins, for example, are produced in this way. The second type of endoplasmic reticulum lacks ribosomes and is called the smooth endoplasmic reticulum (SER). Its membranes contain enzymes that synthesize lipids and some other substances.

The **Golgi apparatus** consists of groups of flattened membranelike sacs located near the nucleus. These sacs are connected with the tubules of the RER. The proteins produced by the ribosomes attached to the RER pass through the RER tubules into the Golgi apparatus, where large carbohydrate molecules are synthesized and

Mitochondria (mīt-o-kon'drē-uh) *Rod-shaped structures in the cell capable of converting foods into energy to power the cell.*

Adenosine triphosphate (ATP) *A high-energy phosphate compound that liberates energy to power numerous cellular metabolic processes.*

Endoplasmic reticulum *A mass of hollow tubular channels within the cytoplasm of the cell, frequently bordered by ribosomes.*

Ribosome *A small cytoplasmic organelle that serves as the site of protein synthesis. Ribosomes are usually attached to the endoplasmic reticulum but may be free in the cytoplasm.*

Golgi apparatus (gol'jē) *A group of membrane-lined sacs found in the cytoplasm of the cell near the nucleus.*

TABLE 1

Major cell organelles and their functions

Organelle	Function
Mitochondria	Convert food materials into energy to make adenosine triphosphate (ATP) used to power the chemical reactions in the cell
Rough endoplasmic reticulum (RER)	Tubular ribosome-containing channels that synthesize protein to be secreted by cells
Smooth endoplasmic reticulum (SER)	Tubular channels containing enzymes that synthesize lipids and some other compounds within the cells
Golgi apparatus	Flat sacs located near nucleus attach carbohydrate molecules to the proteins synthesized by RER
Lysosomes	Spherical organelles in cytoplasm containing digestive enzymes that break down worn-out cell organelles and material brought into cell by phagocytosis
Centrioles	Short cylinders that form the mitotic spindle that separates chromosomes during cell division
Cytoskeleton	Protein tubules and filaments that form structural framework of cells and promote cell functions such as motility and phagocytosis

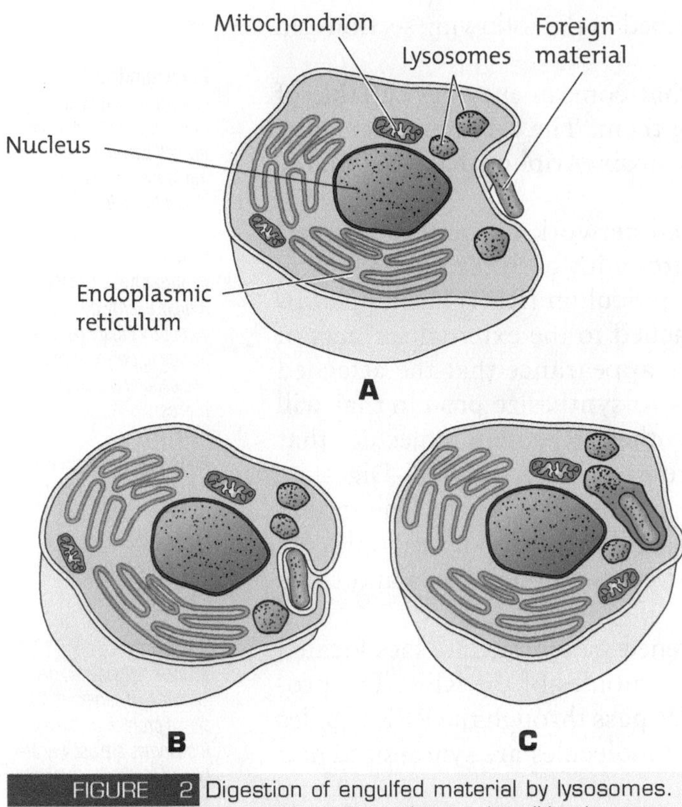

FIGURE 2 Digestion of engulfed material by lysosomes. **A**, Extensions of cytoplasm from phagocytic cell begin to surround particulate material. **B**, Cytoplasmic extensions engulf material and form phagocytic vacuole containing the engulfed material. **C**, Lysosome and phagocytic vacuole merge, and enzymes from lysosome digest the engulfed material.

combined with the proteins. Then they are formed into secretory granules and eventually discharged from the cell.

Lysosomes (*lysis* = dissolving + *soma* = body) are cytoplasmic organelles made by the Golgi apparatus that are filled with potent digestive enzymes. They function as the "digestive system" of the cell. Lysosomes break down material brought into the cell by phagocytosis; they also degrade worn-out intracellular components such as mitochondria and other organelles, making the breakdown products available to be recycled or excreted from the cells. When particulate material is ingested by **phagocytosis**, the particle becomes enclosed within a membrane-lined vacuole called a phagocytic vacuole. A lysosome then merges with the phagocytic vacuole, and their cell membranes fuse, allowing the digestive enzymes contained in the lysosome to flow into the phagocytic vacuole and digest the engulfed material. Digestion is accomplished entirely within the phagocytic vacuole, which prevents digestive enzymes from leaking into the cytoplasm of the cell and causing injury to the cell (FIGURE 2). The same type of digestive process is involved when worn-out components are broken down within cells. Unfortunately, in some diseases, the lysosomal enzymes are unable to function properly, and incompletely digested material accumulates within lysosomes, disrupting cell functions.

Lysosome
A small cytoplasmic vacuole containing digestive enzymes.

Phagocytosis
(fag-o-sī-tō′sis)
Ingestion of particulate of foreign material by cells.

Peroxisome
(per-ok′-si-sōm)
A cytoplasmic organelle containing various enzymes, including those that decompose potentially toxic hydrogen peroxide.

Centrioles
Short cylindrical structures located adjacent to the nucleus that participate in the formation of spindle fibers during cell division.

Cytoskeleton
(sigh′-toe-skeleton)
Protein tubules and filaments that form the structural framework of cells.

Closely related to lysosomes are smaller structures called **peroxisomes**, which contain enzymes that break down various potentially toxic intracellular molecules. The name of this organelle (*peroxi* = peroxide + *soma* = body) comes from hydrogen peroxide (H_2O_2), a potentially toxic by-product of enzyme action that is promptly decomposed by one of the enzymes in the peroxisome.

Centrioles are short cylindrical structures located adjacent to the nucleus. In cell division, they move to opposite poles of the cell and form the mitotic spindle. The spindle fibers attach to the chromosomes and cause them to separate in the course of cell division.

The **cytoskeleton** of the cell consists of three different types of protein tubules and filaments that form the structural framework of the cell and also are responsible for cell movements, such as phagocytosis. Microtubules are the largest cytoskeletal components, and microfilaments are the smallest. Intermediate filaments are small tough protein filaments that reinforce the interior of the cell, hold the organelles in proper position within the cell, and along with the other cytoskeletal structures are responsible for the characteristic shape of each specific type of cell. There are five different types of intermediate filaments that can be identified in cells by specific histologic techniques. Each type of intermediate filament is characteristic of a specific type of cell.

Identification and characterization of intermediate filaments in cells often provide both diagnostic and prognostic information. In some diseases, such as the degenerative disease of the nervous system called Alzheimer disease (described in the discussion on the nervous system), the intermediate filaments exhibit characteristic abnormalities that establish the diagnosis of the disease. Identification of the type of intermediate filaments in cells is also useful in the diagnosis of tumors (described in neoplastic disease discussion). Sometimes, when a pathologist is examining a biopsy of a malignant tumor, the tumor cells may be so immature and abnormal that it may be very difficult to determine the type of cell that gave rise to the tumor. Identifying a specific type of intermediate filament in the tumor cells helps determine the type of cell from which the tumor arose, which allows the pathologist to make a more precise diagnosis and provide a more reliable prognosis.

Tissues

A tissue is a group of similar cells joined together to perform a specific function. Tissues are classified into four major groups:

1. Epithelium
2. Connective and supporting tissues
3. Muscle tissue
4. Nerve tissue

EPITHELIUM

Epithelium consists of groups of cells closely joined together (FIGURE 3). Epithelial cells cover the exterior of the body and line the interior body surfaces that communicate with the outside, such as the gastrointestinal tract, urinary tract, and vagina. Epithelium

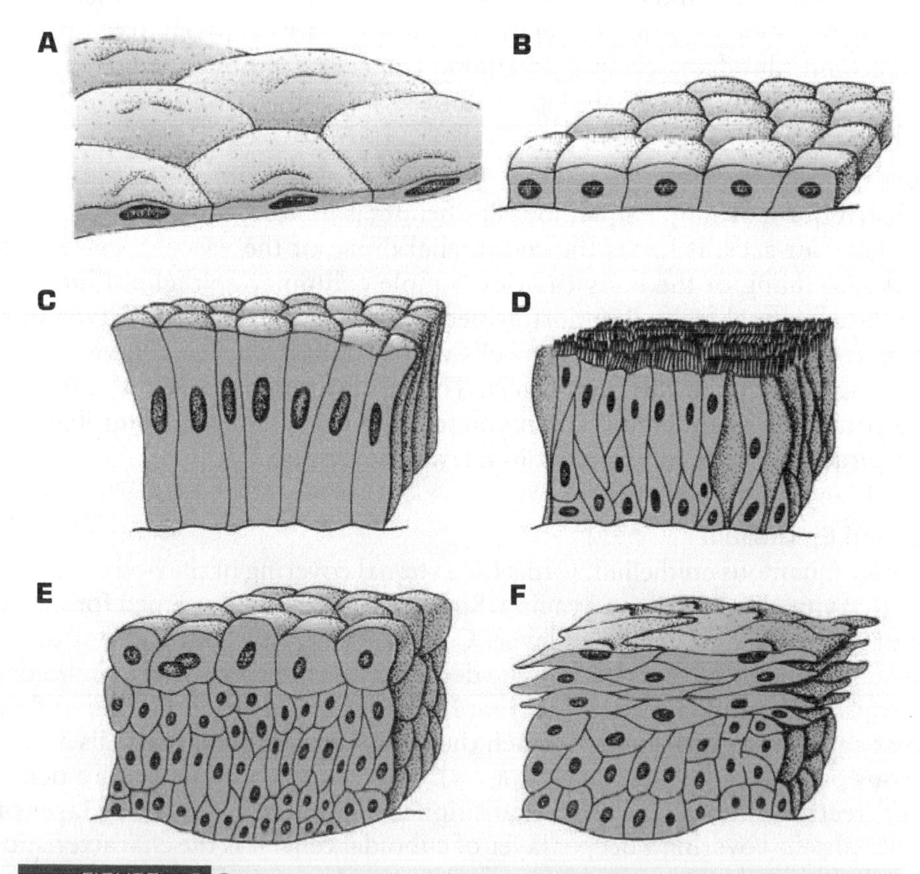

FIGURE 3 Common types of epithelium. **A**, Simple squamous. **B**, Cuboidal. **C**, Columnar. **D**, Pseudostratified columnar (ciliated). **E**, Transitional. **F**, Stratified squamous.

Parenchymal cell
(par-en′ki-mul)
The functional cell of an organ or tissue.

Parenchyma
(par-en′ki-muh)
The functional cells of an organ, as contrasted with the connective and supporting tissue that forms its framework.

Endothelium
(en-dō-thē′lē-um)
The internal lining of blood vessels and interior of the heart.

Mesothelium
(me-sō-thē′li-um)
A layer of flat squamous epithelial cells that covers the surfaces of the pleural, pericardial, and peritoneal cavities.

Mesoderm
(me′zō-derm)
The middle germ layer of the embryo, which gives rise to specific organs and tissues.

Keratin
An insoluble sulfur-containing protein that is the principal constituent of the hair and nails.

forms glands such as the thyroid and pancreas and also makes up the functional cells (often called **parenchymal cells** or **parenchyma**) of organs that have excretory or secretory functions, such as the liver and the kidneys. The individual cells may be flat and platelike (squamous cells), cube-shaped (cuboidal cells), or tall and narrow (columnar cells). Many columnar epithelial cells have become specialized to absorb or secrete, and some contain hairlike processes called cilia. Epithelial cells may be arranged in a single layer (simple epithelium) or may be several layers thick (stratified epithelium).

Endothelium and Mesothelium

The interiors of the heart, blood vessels, and lymphatic vessels are lined by a layer of simple squamous epithelium called **endothelium** (*endo* = within). A similar type of epithelium lining the pleural, pericardial, and peritoneal cavities is called **mesothelium** (*meso* = middle). Although these linings are classified as types of epithelium, they arise along with the connective tissues from the embryonic germ layer called the **mesoderm** and are therefore much more closely related to connective tissue than to other types of epithelium. Consequently, they are considered separately and are given distinct names. Moreover, tumors arising from endothelium or mesothelium behave more like tumors originating from connective tissue. They are classified with the connective tissue tumors rather than with tumors arising from surface, glandular, or parenchymal epithelium. This subject is considered in the discussion on neoplastic disease.

The Structure of Epithelium

Epithelial cells are supported by a thin basement membrane. The cells are firmly joined to each other, and the deeper layers of epithelium are firmly anchored to the basement membrane so that the epithelial cells remain relatively fixed in position. There are no blood vessels in epithelium. The cells are nourished by diffusion of material from capillaries located in the underlying connective tissue.

Simple Epithelium

The distribution of simple squamous epithelium is limited. It forms the lining of the pulmonary air sacs. It forms the endothelial lining of the vascular system and the mesothelial lining of the body cavities. Simple columnar epithelium lines most of the gastrointestinal tract. Pseudostratified columnar epithelium is a type of simple columnar epithelium in which the cells are so tightly packed together that their nuclei appear to lie at different levels. This gives an appearance of stratification. Pseudostratified epithelium is often ciliated. This type of epithelium lines most of the respiratory tract and is present in a few other areas.

Stratified Epithelium

Stratified squamous epithelium forms the external covering of the body and also lines the oral cavity, esophagus, and vagina. Stratified epithelium is named for the appearance of the most superficial cell layer. Consequently, this epithelium is designated "stratified squamous" even though the deeper layers are composed of cuboidal cells. The stratified squamous epithelium that forms the top layer of the skin undergoes a process called keratinization, in which the top layers of squamous cells accumulate a fibrous protein called **keratin** (FIGURE 4). This fibrous protein forms a dense layer that protects the underlying cells. Transitional epithelium consists of a layer of large superficial cells covering a deeper layer of cuboidal cells. It is the characteristic lining of the bladder and other parts of the urinary tract. The superficial cells of transitional epithelium become flattened when the bladder is distended and resume their original shape when the bladder is empty.

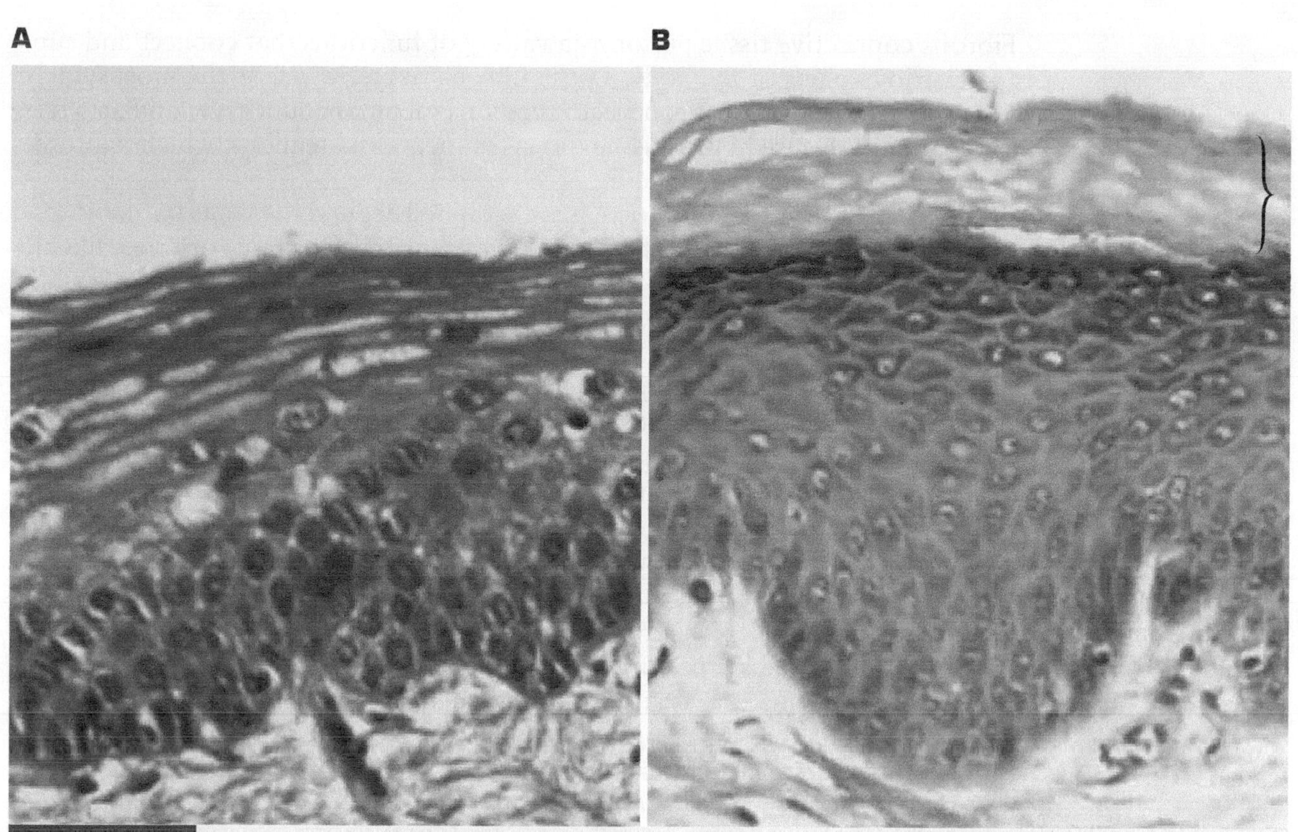

FIGURE 4 **A**, Nonkeratinized stratified squamous epithelium. **B**, Keratinized stratified squamous epithelium. The keratin layer (*bracket*) forms a dense acellular covering that protects the underlying epithelial cells (original magnification × 400).

Functions of Epithelium

Epithelium performs many different functions. All types of epithelium perform a protective function. Columnar epithelium, such as that lining the intestinal tract, is specialized to absorb and secrete. Other types of epithelium form glands that secrete mucus, sweat, oil, enzymes, hormones, or other products. Glands, such as the pancreas, that discharge their secretions through a duct onto an epithelial surface are called **exocrine glands** (*exo* = out). **Endocrine glands** (*endo* = within), such as the thyroid and adrenals, discharge their secretions directly into the bloodstream.

Exocrine glands
A gland that discharges its secretions through a duct onto a mucosal surface, in contrast to an endocrine gland that delivers its secretions directly into the bloodstream.

Endocrine glands
A gland that discharges its secretions directly into the bloodstream, in contrast to an exocrine gland that discharges its secretion through a duct onto a mucosal surface.

CONNECTIVE AND SUPPORTING TISSUES

Connective and supporting tissues consist of relatively small numbers of cells incorporated in a large amount of extracellular material called **matrix** in which are embedded various types of fibers. The proportions of cells, fibers, and matrix vary greatly in different types of connective tissue. Connective tissue fibers are of three types. Collagen fibers are long, flexible fibers composed of a protein called collagen. They are strong but do not stretch. Elastic fibers are composed of a protein called elastin. They are not as strong as collagen but stretch readily and return to their former shape when the stretching force is released. Reticulin fibers are very similar to collagen but are quite thin and delicate.

Matrix (mā′trix)
Material in which connective tissue cells are embedded.

Connective and supporting tissues include various types of loose and dense fibrous tissue, elastic tissue, reticular tissue, adipose tissue, cartilage, and bone. Hematopoietic (blood-forming) tissue and lymphatic (lymphocyte-forming) tissue also are classified as types of connective tissue, primarily because, like other types of connective tissue, they originate from the mesoderm.

Fibrous connective tissue performs a variety of functions that connect and support the various parts of the body. Loose fibrous tissue, which is the most widely distributed, forms the tissue just beneath the skin (subcutaneous tissue) and also fills in around organs. Dense fibrous tissue forms ligaments and tendons, which reinforce joints and attach muscles to bone.

Elastic tissue forms membranes that are wrapped around the walls of blood vessels and are responsible for the characteristic distensibility of large arteries. Elastic membranes also form part of the walls of the trachea and bronchi.

Reticular tissue is a special type of connective tissue characterized by a fine meshwork of reticulin fibers that form the supporting framework of various organs such as the liver, spleen, and lymph nodes.

Adipose tissue is a variety of loose fibrous tissue containing large numbers of fat cells. Fat is a stored form of energy and also functions as padding and insulation.

Cartilage is a type of supporting tissue in which the cells are dispersed in a dense matrix. There are three types of cartilage. Hyaline cartilage is the most common. It is blue and translucent and contains only a few fine collagen fibers suspended in the abundant matrix. Hyaline cartilage covers the ends of bones where they form movable joints, forms the greater part of the laryngeal and tracheal cartilages, and connects the ribs to the sternum. Elastic cartilage contains yellow elastic fibers in the matrix and is found in only few locations, such as the cartilaginous portions of the ears. The elastic fibers impart a flexibility to the cartilage that is lacking in other types of cartilage. Fibrocartilage contains many dense collagen bundles embedded in the matrix. It is found in areas where cartilage is subjected to marked weight-bearing stresses. It forms the disks between the vertebral bodies and some of the cartilages in the knee joints; it is also present in few other locations.

Bone is a highly specialized, rigid supporting tissue in which the matrix containing the bone-forming cells is impregnated with calcium salts.

MUSCLE TISSUE

Muscle cells contain filaments of specialized intracellular contractile proteins called actin and myosin. These are arranged in parallel bundles. During contraction of a muscle fiber, actin filaments slide inward on the myosin filaments, somewhat like pistons, causing the fiber to shorten. There are three types of muscle fibers. Smooth muscle is located primarily in the walls of hollow internal organs such as the gastrointestinal tract, biliary tract, and reproductive tract, and in the walls of the blood vessels where the muscle regulates the caliber of the vessels to control blood flow to the tissues; and in the skin where they attach to hair follicles and control elevation of the hairs. Smooth muscle functions automatically and is not under conscious control. Striated muscle moves the skeleton and is under voluntary control. Cardiac muscle is found only in the heart. It resembles striated muscle but has some features common to both smooth and voluntary muscle.

Neuron (nū'ron)
A nerve cell, including the nerve cell body and its processes.

Neuroglia (noo-rog′-lē-ah)
Supporting cells of tissue of the nervous system.

Astrocyte
A large stellate cell having highly branched processes. Forms the structural framework of the nervous system. One of the neuroglial cells.

Oligodendroglia (ol'ig-ō-den-drog'li-ah)
One type of neuroglia that surrounds nerve fibers within the central nervous system.

Microglia (mī-krog′-lē-ă)
Phagocytic cells of the nervous system comparable to macrophages in other tissues.

NERVE TISSUE

Nerve tissue is composed of nerve cells called **neurons**, which transmit nerve impulses, and supporting cells called **neuroglia**. Neuroglial cells are more numerous than neurons. They are of three different types. **Astrocytes** are long, star-shaped cells having numerous highly branched processes that interlace to form a meshwork. Astrocytes form the structural framework of the central nervous system in the way that the connective tissue fibers form the framework of internal organs. **Oligodendroglia** are small cells with scanty cytoplasm that surround individual nerve cells in the central nervous system. **Microglia** are phagocytic cells comparable to the macrophages found in other tissues.

Organs and Organ Systems

An **organ** is a group of different tissues that is integrated to perform a specific function. Generally, one tissue performs the primary function characteristic of the organ, and the other tissues perform a supporting function, such as providing the vascular and connective tissue framework for the organ. The functional cells of an organ are often called the **parenchymal cells**, and the total mass of functional tissue is called the **parenchyma.** The supporting framework of the organ is called the **stroma.** In the liver, for example, the parenchymal cells are formed by cords of epithelial cells that perform the many metabolic functions characteristic of the liver, such as the synthesis of protein and the excretion of bile. The cord cells are supported by a framework of connective tissue fibers. Numerous thin-walled blood vessels are interspersed between the cell cords, and the entire liver is surrounded by a capsule composed of dense fibrous tissue.

An organ system is a group of organs that is organized to perform complementary functions, such as the reproductive system, the respiratory system, and the digestive system. Finally, the various organ systems are integrated into a functioning individual.

Organ
A group of different tissues organized to perform a specific function.

Parenchymal cell
(par-en′ki-mul)
The functional cell of an organ or tissue.

Parenchyma
(par-en′ki-muh)
The functional cells of an organ, as contrasted with the connective and supporting tissue that forms its framework.

Stroma (strō′muh)
The tissue that forms the framework of an organ.

Trophoblast
Cell derived from the fertilized ovum that gives rise to the fetal membranes and contributes to the formation of the placenta.

Inner cell mass
A group of cells that are derived from the fertilized ovum and are destined to form the embryo.

Germ layers
The three layers of cells derived from the inner cell mass, each layer destined to form specific organs and tissues in the embryo.

The Germ Layers and Their Derivatives

The highly complex structure of the entire body evolves from a single cell, the fertilized ovum, by a complex process that includes periods of cell multiplication, differentiation, and organization to form organs and organ systems. (Prenatal development is considered in the discussion on prenatal development and diseases associated with pregnancy.) As the fertilized ovum grows, its cells differentiate into two groups. The peripheral group of cells is called the **trophoblast.** This forms the placenta and other structures that will support and nourish the embryo. The inner group of cells is called the **inner cell mass.** These are the cells that will give rise to the embryo, and they soon become arranged into three distinct layers called the **germ layers.** Each layer will form certain specialized tissues and organs (FIGURE 5). The outer layer,

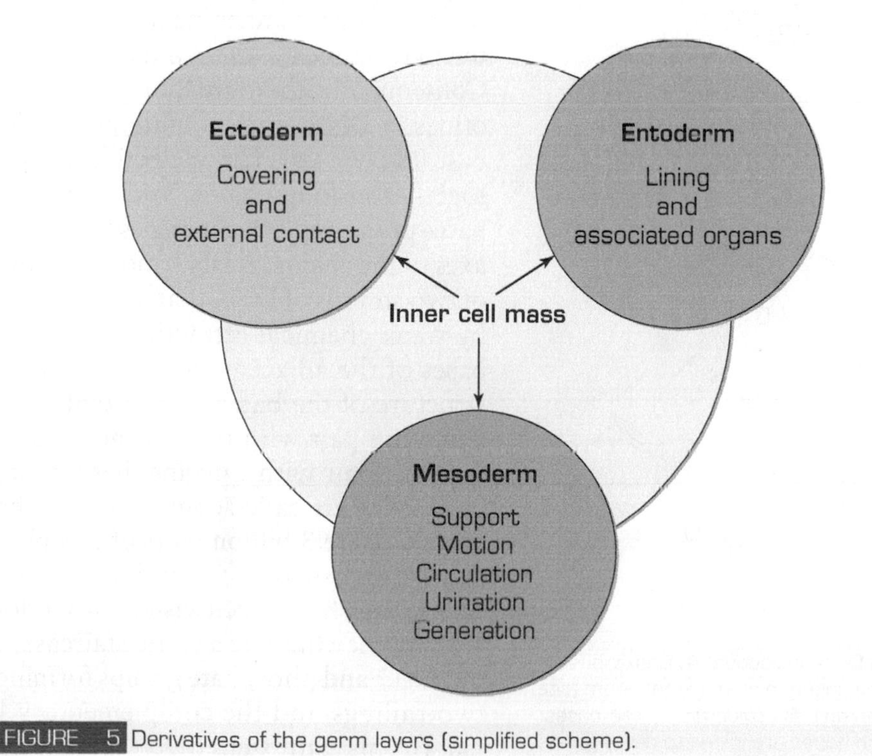

FIGURE 5 Derivatives of the germ layers (simplified scheme).

Ectoderm (ek′tō-derm) *The outer germ layer in the embryo that gives rise to specific organs and tissues.*

Entoderm (en′tō-derm) *The inner germ layer of the embryo that gives rise to specific organs and tissues.*

Mesoderm (me′zō-derm) *The middle germ layer of the embryo, which gives rise to specific organs and tissues.*

Genetic code (jen-et′ik kōd) *The information carried by the codons of DNA molecules in chromosomes.*

Base *A solution containing an excess of hydroxyl ions and having a pH greater than 7.0.*

called the **ectoderm** (*ecto* = outer + *derm* = skin), forms the external covering of the body and the various organs that bring the individual into contact with the external environment: the nervous system, eyes, and ears. The inner layer, called the **entoderm** (*ento* = within), forms the internal "lining": the epithelium of the pharynx, the respiratory tract, the gastrointestinal tract and the organs closely associated with it (the liver, biliary tract, and pancreas), and some parts of the urogenital tract. The **mesoderm** (*meso* = middle) is the layer of cells sandwiched between the other two layers. From these cells are derived the various supporting tissues (connective tissues, cartilage, and bone), muscle, the circulatory system (heart, blood, and blood vessels), and major portions of the urogenital system. Each normal cell in the body is part of a community of cells and is integrated with its neighbors so that it functions along with other cells to meet the body's needs.

Cell Function and the Genetic Code

The chromosomes contain a series of messages called the **genetic code.** It is this code that regulates the various functions of the cell. The genetic code is contained within the structure of DNA and is transmitted to each newly formed cell in cell division.

THE STRUCTURE OF DNA

The chromosomes are composed of DNA combined with protein. The basic structural unit of DNA, called a nucleotide, consists of a phosphate group linked to a five-carbon sugar, deoxyribose, which in turn is joined to a nitrogen-containing compound called a **base** (FIGURE 6A). There are two different types of DNA bases: a purine base, which contains a fused double ring of carbon and nitrogen atoms, and a pyrimidine base, which contains only a single ring. There are four different bases in DNA: the purine bases adenine and guanine and the pyrimidine bases thymine and cytosine. Consequently, there are four different nucleotides in DNA, each containing a different base (FIGURE 6B). The nucleotides are joined together in long chains, with the nitrogen bases projecting at right angles from the long axes of the chains. A DNA molecule consists of two strands of DNA that are held together by weak chemical attractions between the bases of the adjacent chains. The chemical structure of the bases is such that only adenine can pair with thymine and only guanine can pair with cytosine. Bases that pair in this way are called complementary bases, and there are 3 billion pairs of complementary bases (base pairs) in the human genome. The DNA chains are twisted into a double spiral somewhat like a spiral staircase, with the sugar and phosphate groups forming the two railings and the complementary base pairs forming the steps (FIGURE 7A, B, AND C).

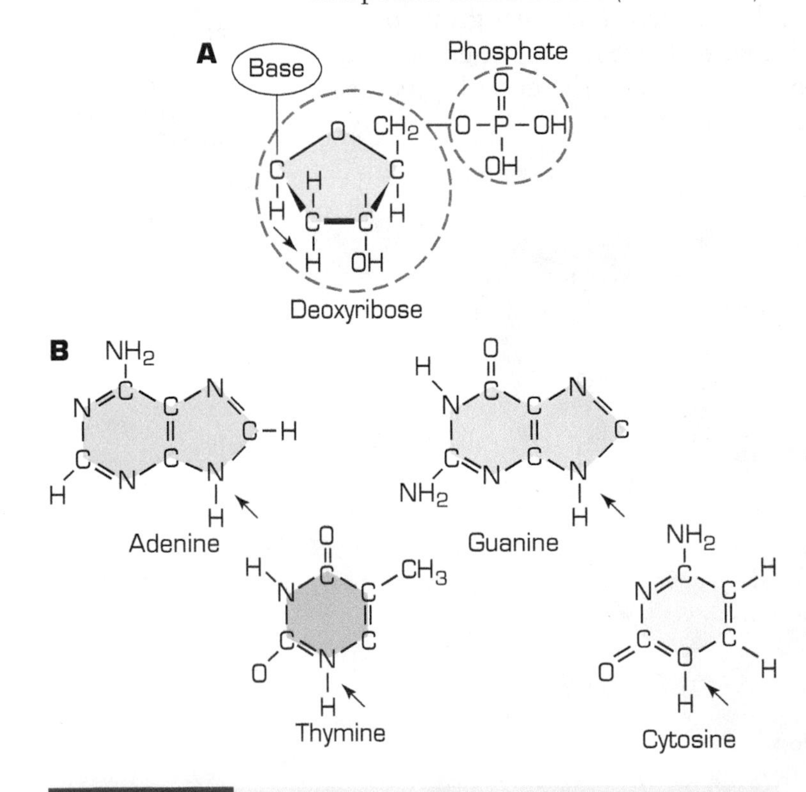

FIGURE 6 General structure of DNA nucleotide. **A**, Deoxyribose is identical with ribose except for the absence of an oxygen atom (site of missing oxygen indicated by *arrow*). **B**, Structure of the bases. The *arrows* indicate sites at which bases are joined to deoxyribose.

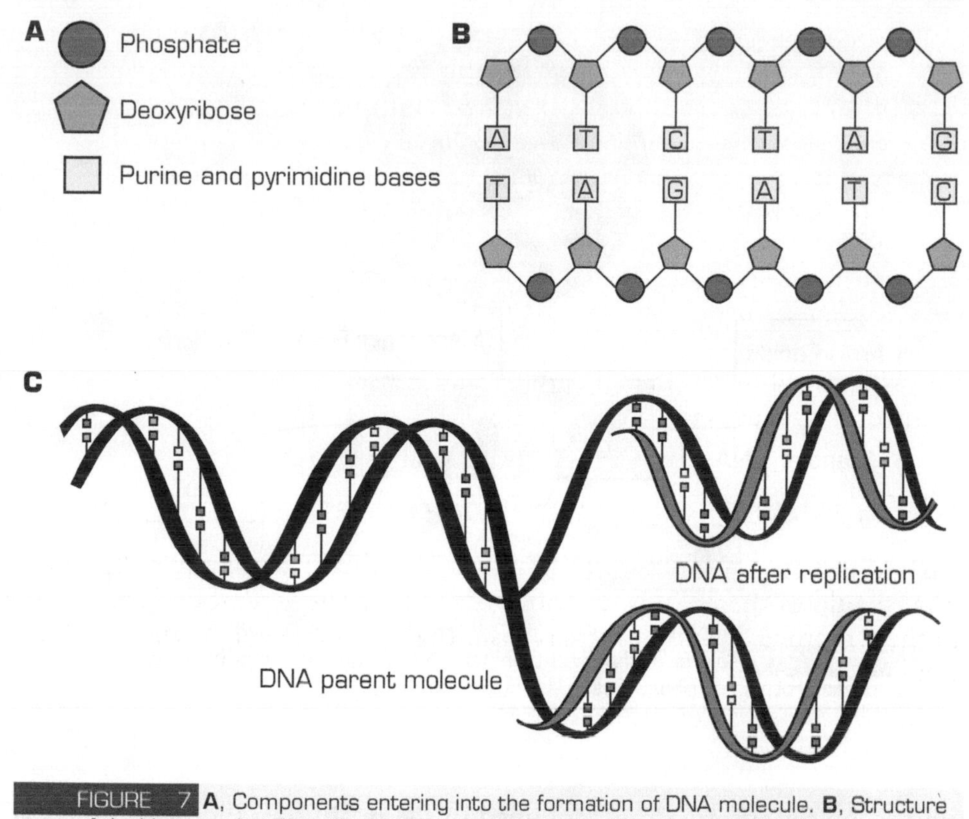

FIGURE 7 **A**, Components entering into the formation of DNA molecule. **B**, Structure of double stranded DNA. **C**, Duplication (replication) of DNA molecule.

DUPLICATION (REPLICATION) OF DNA

As a cell prepares to divide, the double strands of DNA duplicate themselves. The two chains separate, and each chain serves as the model for the synthesis of a new chain (FIGURE 7C). Because adenine always pairs with thymine and guanine with cytosine, the arrangement of the nucleotides in the original chains determines how the nucleotides will reassemble to form the new chains. The process of duplication forms two double strands, each containing one of the original strands plus a newly formed strand. In this way, each of the two daughter cells produced by cell division receives an exact duplicate of the genetic information possessed by the chromosomes of the parent cell.

THE GENETIC CODE

The DNA in the nucleus "tells the cell what to do" by directing the synthesis of enzymes and other proteins by the ribosomes located in the cytoplasm. The "instructions" are carried by messenger RNA (mRNA), so named because it carries the message encoded in the DNA to the ribosomes in the cytoplasm. mRNA is quite similar to DNA but consists of only a single rather than a double strand. It also differs by containing the five-carbon sugar ribose instead of deoxyribose and a base called uracil instead of thymine. During synthesis of mRNA, the DNA chains partially separate, and the DNA serves as the model on which the mRNA is assembled. Therefore, the information transported on the mRNA strand is an exact copy of the genetic information possessed by the nuclear DNA.

The mRNA strand leaves the nucleus through the pores in the nuclear membrane and becomes attached to the ribosomes in the cytoplasm, which are small nucleoprotein particles where enzymes and other proteins are constructed from individual amino acids. The combination of amino acids required to assemble the protein is

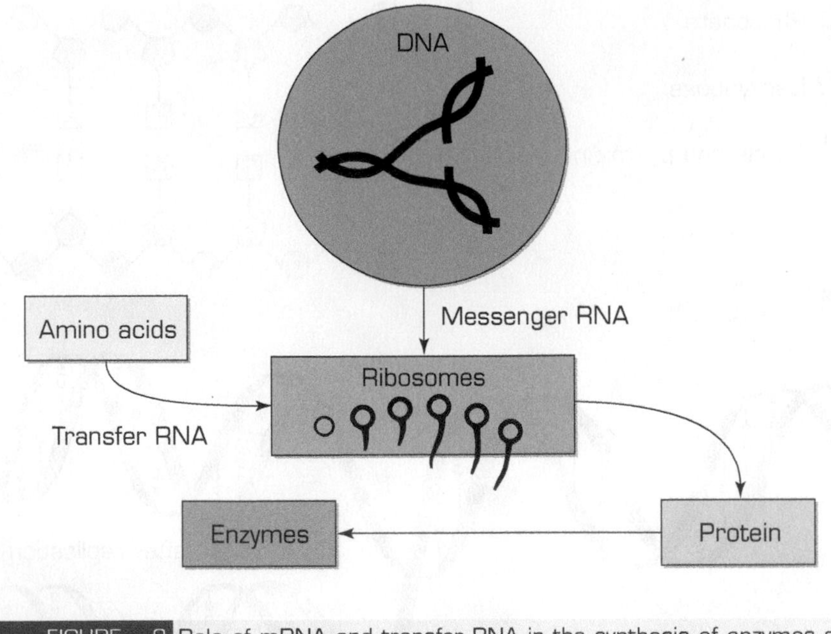

FIGURE 8 Role of mRNA and transfer RNA in the synthesis of enzymes and other proteins by ribosomes in the cytoplasm.

determined by the information contained in the mRNA strand. The amino acids are transported to the ribosomes by means of another type of RNA called transfer RNA (tRNA), so named because it "picks up" the required amino acids from the cytoplasm and transfers them to the ribosomes where they are assembled in proper order, as specified by the mRNA (FIGURE 8).

MicroRNA
Small RNA molecules that regulate the activity of individual genes.

Recently, another type of RNA has been described, which does not function like messenger, ribosomal, and transfer RNA. It is called **microRNA** (miRNA) because it is a smaller molecule than other RNA molecules, and its unique function is to regulate the activity of individual genes. About 1,000 different miRNA molecules have been described, each regulating the activity of a specific gene that it controls. This subject is considered in the section dealing with the human genome and its functions.

Movement of Materials Into and Out of Cells

In order for the cell to function properly, oxygen and nutrients must enter the cell, and waste products must be eliminated. Materials entering and leaving the cell must cross the cell membrane, which limits the passage of some molecules and is freely permeable to others. Materials cross the cell membrane in three ways:

1. Diffusion and osmosis
2. Active transport
3. Phagocytosis and pinocytosis

DIFFUSION AND OSMOSIS

Diffusion is the movement of dissolved particles (solute) from a more concentrated to a more dilute solution. Osmosis is the movement of water molecules from a dilute solution to a more concentrated solution (FIGURE 9). Both are passive processes that

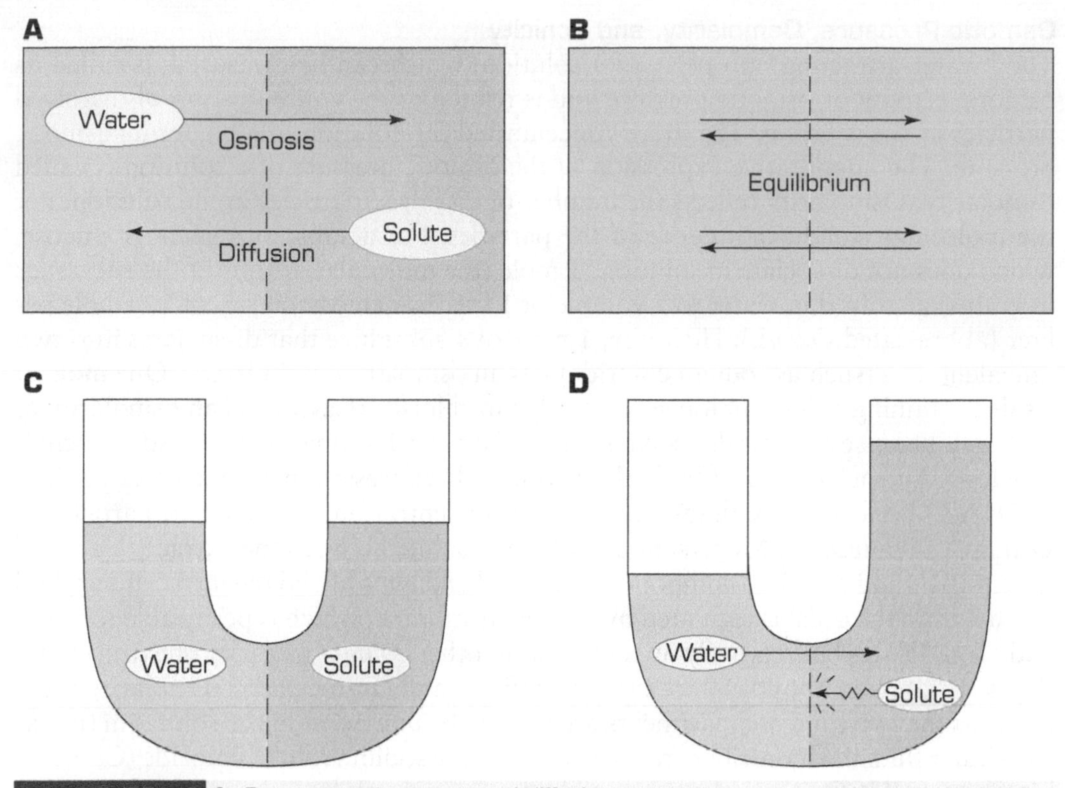

FIGURE 9 **A**, Processes of osmosis and diffusion across a porous membrane indicated by *dashed line*. **B**, At equilibrium, the concentrations of water and solute molecules are equal on both sides of membrane. **C**, The left compartment of U tube contains water. The right compartment contains solute impermeable to membrane. **D**, Water molecules diffuse freely across membrane, but solute molecules are unable to diffuse. The volume of solute increased by diffusion of water molecules into the solute. The volume of water in left limb of the U tube falls as water moves into the solute in the right limb of the U tube.

do not require the cell to expend energy. If the membrane is freely permeable to both water and solute particles (FIGURE 9A, B), the solute particles diffuse from the higher solute concentration on the right side of the membrane into the lower solute concentration on the left side. At the same time, water molecules diffuse in the opposite direction, from the more dilute solution on the right side of the membrane into the more concentrated solution on the left side. At equilibrium, the concentrations of solute particles and water molecules are the same on both sides of the membrane. Solute and water molecules continue to move in both directions across the membrane after equilibrium is attained, but the movements are equal in both directions, which does not change in the equilibrium volume and concentration of the solutions on the two sides of the membrane.

The situation is quite different if the membrane is not permeable to the solute particles in the solution on one side of the membrane (FIGURE 9C, D). Water molecules move by osmosis from the left side of the membrane into the more concentrated solution on the right side (containing fewer water molecules). Because diffusion of solute is restricted by the membrane but movement of water molecules across the membrane is not, the volume of the solution on the right side of the membrane increases, and its solute concentration falls as the water molecules move by osmosis across the membrane. Eventually, the solutions on both sides of the membrane have the same concentration of water molecules, but their volumes are quite different.

Osmolarity
A measure of the osmotic pressure exerted by a solution.

Isotonic solution
A solution having essentially the same osmolarity as body fluids so that cells neither shrink nor swell when exposed to the solution.

Hypertonic solution
A solution having a greater osmolarity than body fluids, which causes cells to shrink in such a solution because water moves by osmosis from the cells into the hypertonic solution.

Hypotonic solution
A solution having a lower osmolarity than body fluids, causing cells in the solution to swell because water moves by osmosis from the hypotonic solution into the cells.

Osmotic Pressure, Osmolarity, and Tonicity

The "water-attracting" property of a solution, which can be measured, is called its osmotic activity or osmotic pressure and is related to the concentration of dissolved particles in the solution. The more concentrated the solution, the higher its osmotic pressure. The quantitative expression of the osmotic pressure of a solution is called **osmolarity**. Osmolarity reflects the number of dissolved particles in the solution, not the molecular weight or valence of the particles. For a substance such as glucose, which does not dissociate in solution, 1 mole (the molecular weight of the substance in grams) dissolved in water to a volume of 1 liter has an osmolarity of 1 osmole per liter (abbreviated Osm/L). However, 1 mole of a substance that dissociates into two univalent ions (such as sodium chloride) has an osmolarity of 2 Osm/L. One mole of a salt containing a divalent ion such as calcium chloride ($CaCl_2$) has an osmolarity of 3 Osm/L because the salt dissociates into three particles: one calcium and two chloride ions. The osmolarity of body fluids is usually expressed in milliosmoles per liter (mOsm/L) because body fluids contain low concentrations of dissolved particles (1 Osm = 1,000 mOsm). Movement of water and solute between the extracellular fluid (interstitial fluid and fluid components of blood and lymph) and the intracellular fluid (fluid within the cells) is regulated by the cell membrane, which is permeable to water and some solutes but relatively impermeable to others. The osmolarity of extracellular fluids varies from about 280 to 295 mOsm/L, and the intracellular osmolarity is the same, as the two fluid compartments are in equilibrium. Most of the solutes in the extracellular fluid that contribute to its osmolarity are sodium (Na^+), chloride (Cl^-), and bicarbonate (HCO_3^-) ions. In contrast, the major intracellular ions are potassium (K^+) and phosphate (PO_4^{-3}). The sodium–potassium ion differences on the two sides of the cell membrane, which are essential for normal cell functions, are controlled by the cell.

The term tonicity, which is sometimes used to refer to the osmotic effects produced by a solution, is not quite the same as osmolarity. For practical purposes, however, we can consider that an **isotonic solution** (*iso* = equal) is osmotically equivalent to the patient's own body fluids and can safely be administered intravenously to patients. Generally, only isotonic solutions are used for intravenous administration. A **hypertonic solution** (*hyper* = above) is more concentrated. Cells exposed to a hypertonic solution shrink because water moves by osmosis from the cells into the hypertonic fluid. In contrast, a **hypotonic solution** (*hypo* = below) is a dilute solution, and cells exposed to a hypotonic solution swell as water moves by osmosis from the hypotonic fluid into the cells where the osmolarity is higher. The osmotic flow of water into cells, such as red cells, may be so great that the cell membranes of the overdistended cells may rupture, causing the cells to collapse and the hemoglobin to leak from the cells.

Osmotic Pressure Differences Between Cells and Extracellular Fluids

If the osmolarity of the extracellular fluid (ECF) is higher than that within the cells, water flows by osmosis from the cell into the ECF, causing the cell to shrink. Conversely, if the osmolarity of the ECF is lower than that of the cells, water moves by osmosis into the cells, causing the cells to swell. Normally, the osmotic pressures within the cell and in the ECF are equal; therefore, the shape and water content of the cells do not change. In disease, the osmolarity of the ECF may be abnormally low or high, which will lead to secondary changes in the water content of the cells and will impair their function. For example, a person with severe uncontrolled diabetes may have a very high blood glucose concentration that increases the ECF osmolarity because the glucose is unable to enter the cell. Consequently, the cells shrink because water moves by osmosis from the cells into the extracellular fluid. Conversely, cells swell in patients with kidney disease who consume excess water because the diseased kidneys are unable to excrete the water efficiently. The excess water dilutes the ECF, which lowers its osmolarity, and water moves by osmosis from the diluted body fluids into the cells.

ACTIVE TRANSPORT

Active transport is the transfer of a substance across the cell membrane from a region of low concentration to one of higher concentration. The process requires the cell to expend energy because the substance must move against a concentration gradient. Many metabolic processes depend on active transport of ions or molecules. For example, in order for the cell to function normally, the intracellular potassium concentration must be higher than the concentration in the ECF, and the intracellular sodium concentration must be much lower. This is accomplished by a mechanism that actively transports potassium into the cell and simultaneously moves sodium out.

PHAGOCYTOSIS AND PINOCYTOSIS

Phagocytosis is the ingestion of particles that are too large to pass across the cell membrane. The cytoplasm flows around the particle, and the cytoplasmic processes fuse, engulfing the particle within a vacuole in the cytoplasm of the cell. A similar process called **pinocytosis** consists of the ingestion of fluid rather than solid material.

Phagocytosis
(fag-o-sī-tō′sis)
Ingestion of particulate of foreign material by cells.

Pinocytosis
(pīn′o-sī-tō′sis)
Liquid absorption by cells in which a segment of cell membrane forms small pockets and engulfs the liquid. Similar to phagocytosis, except that liquids rather than particulate material are ingested.

Adaptations of Cells to Changing Conditions

Cells respond to changing conditions in various ways. Common adaptive mechanisms are:

1. Atrophy
2. Hypertrophy and hyperplasia
3. Metaplasia
4. Dysplasia
5. Increased enzyme synthesis

In many instances, the adaptation enables the cells to function more efficiently. Sometimes, however, the adaptive change may be detrimental to the cell, as occurs in dysplasia.

ATROPHY

Atrophy is a reduction in the size of cells in response to diminished function, inadequate hormonal stimulation, or reduced blood supply. The cell decreases in size in order to "get by" under the less favorable conditions. For example, skeletal muscles are reduced in size when an extremity is immobilized in a cast for long periods, and the breasts and genital organs shrink after menopause as a result of inadequate estrogen stimulation. A kidney becomes smaller if its blood supply becomes insufficient because of narrowing of the renal artery.

HYPERTROPHY AND HYPERPLASIA

If cells are required to do more work, they may increase either their size or their number in order to accomplish their task. **Hypertrophy** is an increase in the size of

Hypertrophy
An enlargement or overgrowth of an organ caused by an increase in size of its constituent cells.

individual cells without an actual increase in their numbers. The large muscles of a weight lifter, for example, result from hypertrophy of individual muscle fibers. The number of fibers is not increased. Similarly, the heart of a person with high blood pressure often enlarges as a result of hypertrophy of the individual cardiac muscle fibers. This occurs because the heart must work harder in order to pump blood at a higher than normal pressure.

Hyperplasia
(hī-per-plā′sēē-uh)
An increase in the number of cells.

Hyperplasia is an increase in the size of a tissue or organ caused by an increase in the number of cells. Hyperplasia occurs in response to increased demand. For example, the glandular tissue of the breast becomes hyperplastic during pregnancy in preparation for lactation. Endocrine glands such as the thyroid may enlarge in order to increase their output of hormones.

METAPLASIA

Metaplasia
(met-uh-plā′sē-yuh)
A change from one type of cell to a more resistant cell type.

Metaplasia is a change from one type of cell to another type that is better able to tolerate some adverse environmental condition. For example, if the lining of the bladder is chronically irritated and inflamed, the normal transitional epithelial lining may assume the characteristic structure of a thick layer of squamous epithelium. The metaplastic epithelium is more resistant to irritation and is better able to protect the bladder wall in the presence of chronic infection.

DYSPLASIA

Dysplasia
(dis-plā′sē-yuh)
Abnormal maturation of cells.

Dysplasia (*dys* = bad + *plasia* = formation) is a condition in which the development and maturation of cells are disturbed and abnormal. The individual cells vary in size and shape, and their relationship to one another is also abnormal (FIGURE 10). Dysplasia of epithelial cells may result from chronic irritation or inflammation. In some cases,

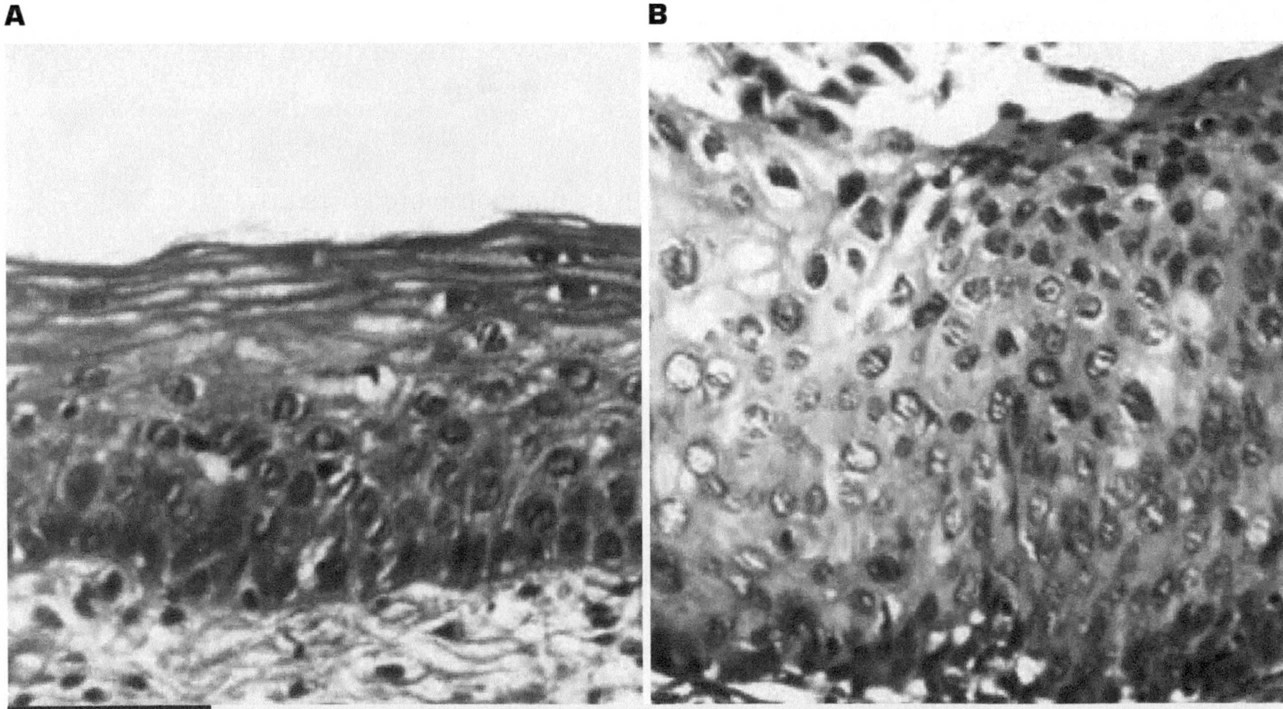

FIGURE 10 Comparison of normal, nonkeratinized stratified squamous epithelium. **A**, with dysplastic epithelium. **B**, Note the variation in nuclear size, polarity, and staining reaction (original magnification × 400).

dysplasia may progress to formation of a tumor; this is called **neoplasia.** The epithelium covering the uterine cervix is a common site of dysplasia, and cervical epithelial dysplasia sometimes progresses to cervical cancer. This subject is discussed in the female reproductive system.

Neoplasia (nē-ō-plā′se-yuh) *The pathologic process that results in the formation and growth of a tumor.*

INCREASED ENZYME SYNTHESIS

Increased synthesis of enzymes is another adaptive change that occurs in cells. Sometimes, cells are called on to inactivate or detoxify drugs or chemicals by means of the enzymes present in the smooth endoplasmic reticulum (SER). If increased demands are placed on the cells, they respond by synthesizing more SER enzymes so that drugs or chemicals can be processed more efficiently. After the cells increase their ability to handle such chemicals or drugs, they can rapidly eliminate other substances that are handled by means of the same enzyme systems. A person accustomed to heavy consumption of alcohol, for example, is able to metabolize the alcohol more efficiently because of this adaptive change. Such an individual may also metabolize and eliminate other drugs at a greatly accelerated rate. Consequently, if a physician administers a medication that is metabolized by the same enzyme systems, the usual therapeutic doses of the medications may be ineffective.

Cell Injury, Cell Death, and Cell Necrosis

CELL INJURY

An injured cell may exhibit various morphologic abnormalities. The two most common changes are cell swelling and fatty change.

Cell Swelling

A normally functioning cell actively transports potassium into the cell and moves sodium out. This process requires the cell to expend energy. If the cell is injured and unable to function normally, the transport mechanism begins to fail. Sodium diffuses into the cell, and water moves into the cell along with the sodium, causing the cell to swell. If the swelling continues, fluid-filled vacuoles may accumulate within the cell, and eventually, it may rupture.

Fatty Change

If the enzyme systems that metabolize fat are impaired, leading to accumulation of fat droplets within the cytoplasm, fatty change may occur. This condition is a common manifestation of liver cell injury because liver cells are actively involved in fat metabolism.

CELL DEATH AND CELL NECROSIS

A cell dies if it has been irreparably damaged. Several hours after the cell dies, various structural changes begin to take place within the nucleus and cytoplasm. Lysosomal enzymes are released and begin to digest the cell. The nucleus shrinks and either dissolves or breaks into fragments. Sometimes, calcium is deposited in the dead cells and tissues. These structural changes are termed cell **necrosis.** All necrotic cells are dead, but a dead cell is not necessarily necrotic because

Necrosis (nek-rō′sis) *Structural changes associated with cell death.*

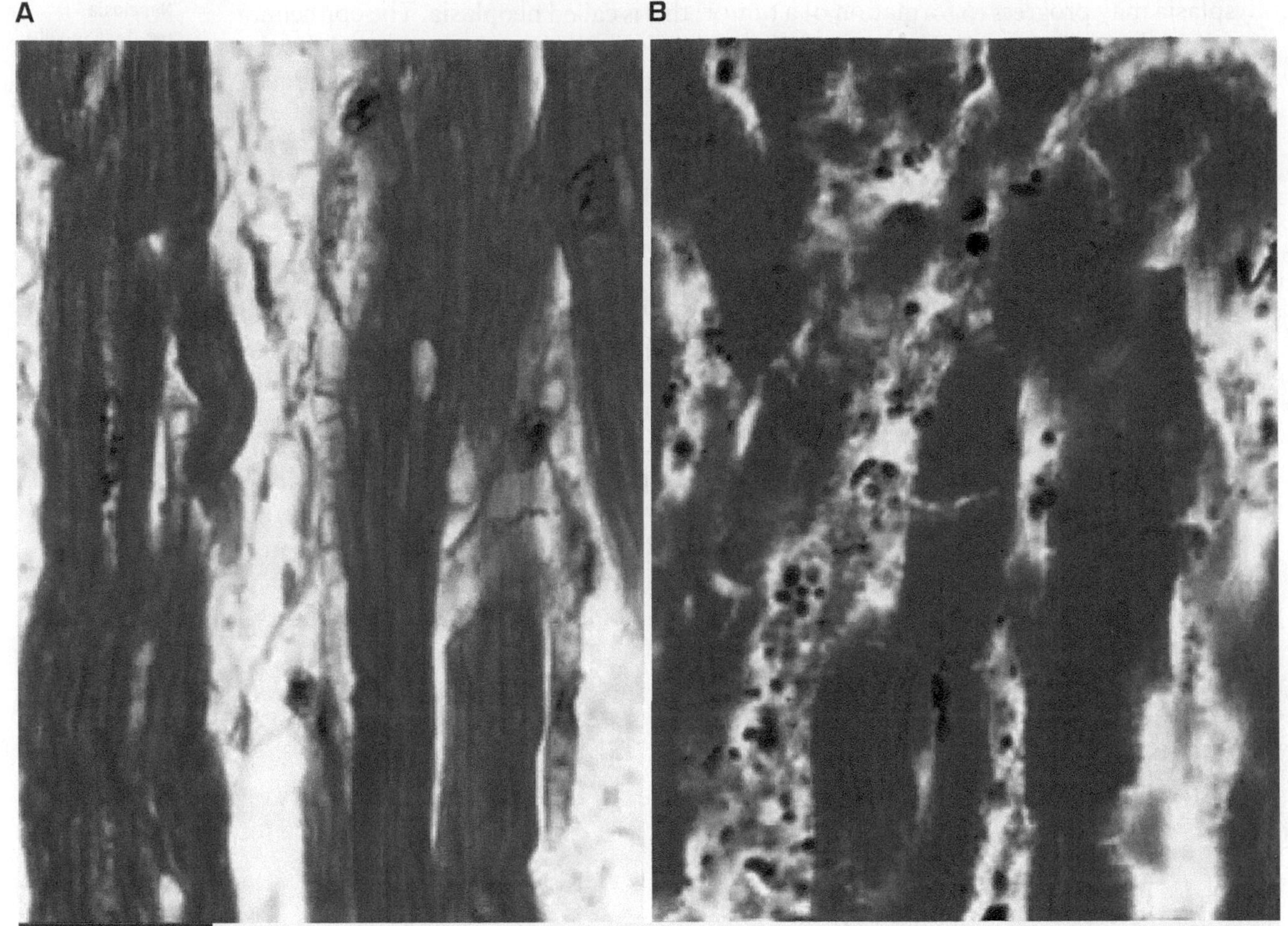

FIGURE 11 Comparison of normal cardiac muscle fibers **A**, with necrotic fibers. **B**, Note the fragmentation of fibers, the loss of nuclear staining, and the fragmented bits of nuclear debris (original magnification × 400).

the structural changes that characterize cell death take several hours to develop. Necrotic cells are easily recognized on histologic examination because they appear quite different from normal cells in both their structural and their staining characteristics (FIGURE 11).

PROGRAMMED CELL DEATH: APOPTOSIS

Not all cell death results from cell injury. All normal cells have a predetermined life span and are programmed to die after a specific period of time. The number of functional cells in all our body tissues is determined by a balance between proliferation of new cells and death of older "worn-out" cells. The older cells die because they are genetically programmed to "shut down" when they have reached the end of their predetermined life span. This form of programmed self-destruction is called **apoptosis.** The rates of cell proliferation and cell death vary in different body tissues. If the genes that regulate apoptosis become deranged and cease to function properly, cells may continue to proliferate instead of dying as they should. Excessive numbers of cells may accumulate in organs or tissues, which disrupts their functions and leads to disease. Some tumors appear to result from failure of the normal mechanisms regulating apoptosis.

Apoptosis
(ah-pop-toe′-sis, or ah-po-toe′-sis)
Programmed cell death that occurs after a cell has lived its normal life span.

Aging and the Cell

All organisms grow old and eventually die, and each species has a predetermined life span. Although human life expectancy has increased over the years, the increase is chiefly because early deaths from infectious diseases, accidents, and other conditions have been greatly reduced. The causes of aging are not well understood but appear to reside in the cell. Although each type of cell has a definite life span, under normal circumstances, cell longevity is also influenced by environmental factors. The life span of an individual in turn reflects the survival of the various populations of cells that together form the individual.

Many investigators believe that aging of cells is genetically programmed and is an inherent property of the cell itself. Examples can be seen in the graying of the hair, which is the result of an eventual failure of the hair cells to produce pigment, and in menopause, which is a predetermined failure of reproductive function. Aging changes in the brain appear to be caused by the wearing out and eventual death of neurons, which are not capable of cell division. The degenerative changes in the walls of arteries, called arteriosclerosis, are thought to be caused partially by a gradual failure of the endothelial cells lining the blood vessels to prevent fatty substances from seeping into the arterial walls. The common type of arthritis seen in older persons begins as an aging change in the cartilage covering the ends of the bones.

As a cell ages, many of its enzyme systems become less active, and the cell becomes less efficient in carrying out its functions. The cell also becomes more susceptible to harmful environmental influences that may shorten its life. For example, the life span of a red cell is 4 months, and therefore the red cells circulating in the bloodstream vary greatly in age, ranging from newly produced cells to those nearing the end of their life span. Each red cell contains enzyme systems that generate its energy, enable it to perform its varied metabolic functions, and maintain the hemoglobin in a condition suitable for transporting oxygen. As the red cell ages and its enzyme systems gradually decline, the cell is less able to protect itself from injury than is a young, "vigorous" cell. If the red cells are exposed to harmful drugs or antibodies that damage the cell membranes, it is the older cells that bear the brunt of the damage and die. The younger cells are able to survive and continue to function.

An example of aging change in cells that affects the organism as a whole can be seen in the lymphocytes of which our immune system is composed. These cells help eliminate pathogenic organisms and also eliminate any of our own cells that become abnormal and have the potential of forming tumors. The cells of the immune system become less efficient as they age. Consequently, the aging individual becomes more susceptible to various infectious diseases, which can shorten the life span. The aging immune system also becomes less able to eliminate abnormal cells that arise sporadically within the body. This may predispose to the formation of malignant tumors, which occur with increasing frequency in older persons.

Aging of cells may also be caused by damage to cellular DNA, RNA, and cytoplasmic organelles that occurs at a pace more rapid than the cell's ability to repair itself. According to this concept, these components become damaged by radiation or other environmental factors or by accumulation of metabolic products within cells. Eventually, the cells begin to malfunction. Some cells can repair the damage and continue to function. Others cannot and die. The more efficient the repair process within the cell, the more likely the cell is to survive.

In summary, cells have a finite life span. However, the less they are exposed to harmful environmental influences and the more efficient they are in repairing their own malfunctions, the greater their chances for survival to a "ripe old age."

QUESTIONS FOR REVIEW

1. How does the nucleus direct the activities of the cell? What is the genetic code, and what is its role in directing the functions of the cell?
2. What are the functions of the following organelles: rough endoplasmic reticulum, ribosomes, lysosomes, and centrosomes?
3. How is epithelium classified, and what are its functions? Why are mesothelium and endothelium considered separately from other types of epithelium?
4. What are the germ layers, and what are their functions?
5. What is the difference between atrophy and hypertrophy, between metaplasia and dysplasia, and between cell death and cell necrosis?
6. What morphologic abnormalities are manifested by an injured cell? Why do they develop?
7. What factors cause a cell to age?

SUPPLEMENTARY READINGS

Guyton, A. C., and Hall, J. E. 2006. *Textbook of medical physiology*. 11th ed. Philadelphia: Elsevier Saunders.

- Good sections on cell biology.

Hetts, S. W. 1998. To die or not to die: An overview of apoptosis and its role in disease. *Journal of the American Medical Association* 279:300–7.

- A review of programmed cell death and how derangement of the process can lead to various diseases.

Levine, A. J. 1995. The genetic origins of neoplasia (Editorial). *Journal of the American Medical Association* 273:592.

- Mutations in three groups of genes contribute to the origins and progression of neoplasms: oncogenes, tumor suppressor genes, and DNA repair genes. Mutations that convert proto-oncogenes into oncogenes include amplifications, translocations, and point mutations, and they act as dominant mutations. Mutations of tumor suppressor genes are the basis of inherited predisposition to cancer and are inherited in the heterozygous state. A random mutation of the remaining normally functioning allele leads to loss of regulator function that results in malignancy. DNA repair genes correct errors in DNA duplication, and loss of gene function increases the mutation rate.

OUTLINE SUMMARY

Organization of Cells

Basic structural and functional unit.
Forms tissues, organs, and organ systems.

The Cell

COMPOSITION

Nucleus: contains genetic information and directs activities.
Cytoplasm: carries out metabolic activities directed by nucleus.
Mitochondria: oxidize food to form ATP, energy source of cell.
Endoplasmic reticulum: two types of hollow tubes in cytoplasm. RER has ribosomes and synthesizes protein. SER has enzymes and synthesizes lipids and other materials.
Golgi apparatus: functions with endoplasmic reticulum to synthesize and package secretory granules, which are eventually discharged.
Lysosomes: vacuoles containing digestive enzymes.
Centrioles: short cylinders that form mitotic spindle during cell division.

Tissues

EPITHELIUM

Structure:

Forms coverings and linings.

Simple: one layer thick.

Stratified: multiple layers.

Endothelium and mesothelium: separate category.

Forms parenchymal cells of excretory or secretory organs.

Function:

Protection.

Absorption.

Secretion.

Forms glands: exocrine and endocrine.

CONNECTIVE AND SUPPORTING TISSUES

Structure and function:

Fibrous connective tissue: connection and support.

Elastic tissue: stretches. Wrapped around blood vessels.

Reticular tissue: framework of liver, spleen, lymph nodes.

Adipose tissue: energy storage, padding, insulation.

Cartilage and bone: support.

MUSCLE TISSUE

Structure and function:

Smooth: in walls of hollow organs and blood vessels. Regulatory.

Striated: moves skeleton under voluntary control

Cardiac: found only in heart. Properties intermediate between smooth and skeletal muscle.

NERVE TISSUE

Structure and function:

Impulse transmission.

Composed of nerve cells and supporting cells: neuroglia.

Organs and Organ Systems

ORGANS

A group of different tissues integrated to perform a specific function.

Composed of parenchymal (functional) cells and stromal (supporting) cells.

ORGAN SYSTEMS

A group of organs that perform related functions; for example, reproductive system.

The Germ Layers and Their Derivatives

FUNCTION

Embryonic cell layers that give rise to specific tissues and organs.

Ectoderm: external coverings, nervous system, eyes, ears.

Entoderm: lining of body and associated organs.

Mesoderm: supporting tissue, muscle, circulatory system, urogenital system.

Cell Function and the Genetic Code

FUNCTION

DNA composed of chains of nucleotides containing genetic information.

In cell division, original chain serves as model for building new chain.

GENETIC CODE

Nucleus directs activities of cytoplasm by means of mRNA, which attaches to ribosomes and directs protein synthesis.

Transfer RNA brings amino acids to ribosomes for assembly as specified by nucleotides in mRNA.

MicroRNA: a unique RNA that regulates the activity of individual genes.

Movement of Materials Into and Out of Cells

DIFFUSION AND OSMOSIS

Diffusion: movement of solute from concentrated to dilute solution.

Osmosis: movement of water from dilute to more concentrated solution.

Osmotic pressure: a measure of concentration.

Depends on number of dissolved particles.

Tonicity often used interchangeably with osmolarity.

ACTIVE TRANSPORT

Transfer of materials against a concentration gradient.

Necessary to maintain proper concentration of intracellular and extracellular ions.

PHAGOCYTOSIS AND PINOCYTOSIS

Phagocytosis: ingestion of particulate material.

Pinocytosis: ingestion of water.

Adaptations of Cells to Changing Conditions

NATURE OF ADAPTATIONS

Atrophy: reduction in size in response to unfavorable conditions.

Hypertrophy: increase in cell size for more efficient function.

Hyperplasia: increase in number of cells to increase functional capabilities.

Metaplasia: change from one type of cell to a more resistant type.

Dysplasia: disturbed development. May proceed to neoplasia.

Increased enzyme synthesis: adaptation in order to inactivate or detoxify materials more efficiently.

Cell Injury, Cell Death, and Cell Necrosis

CELL INJURY

Cell swelling: mechanism for transporting sodium out of cell begins to fail when cell is injured. Sodium diffuses into cell along with water, causing cell to swell.

Fatty change: fat metabolism impaired; fat accumulates in cell.

CELL DEATH AND NECROSIS

Cell death follows irreparable injury.

Structural changes that follow called cell necrosis.

PROGRAMMED CELL DEATH: APOPTOSIS

Cells have predetermined life span and are genetically programmed to die eventually.

If regulatory mechanisms fail, cells continue to proliferate.

Accumulation of excessive numbers of cells disrupts organ functions.

Some tumors result from failure of regulatory mechanisms controlling cell longevity.

Aging and the Cell

BASIC CONCEPTS

Cells and organisms have predetermined life span.

Harmful environmental factors damage DNA, RNA, and organelles. This shortens life span.

Cells are capable of repairing damage. The more efficient the repair process, the greater the likelihood of cell survival.

http://health.jbpub.com/humandisease/9e

Human Disease Online is a great source for supplementary human disease information for both students and instructors. Visit this website to find a variety of useful tools for learning, thinking, and teaching.

Inflammation and Repair

LEARNING OBJECTIVES

1. List the characteristics and clinical manifestations of an acute inflammation. Differentiate inflammations on the basis of their component of fluid and inflammatory cells (serous, purulent, fibrinous, and hemorrhagic inflammations).
2. Describe the possible outcomes of an inflammatory reaction.
3. Name the chemical mediators of inflammation. Explain how they interact to intensify the inflammatory process.
4. Describe the harmful effects of inflammation. Explain why it is sometimes necessary to suppress the inflammatory process.
5. Compare inflammation and infection. Name some of the terms used to describe infections.

The Inflammatory Reaction

The inflammatory reaction is a nonspecific response to any agent that causes cell injury. The agent may be physical (such as heat or cold), chemical (such as a concentrated acid or alkali or another caustic chemical), or microbiologic (such as a bacterium or virus). The inflammatory reaction is characterized by both local and systemic effects, as indicated diagrammatically in FIGURE 1.

Local effects consist of dilatation (expansion) of blood vessels and increased vascular permeability. Leukocytes (white blood cells) are attracted to the site of injury. They adhere to the endothelium of the small blood vessels, force their way

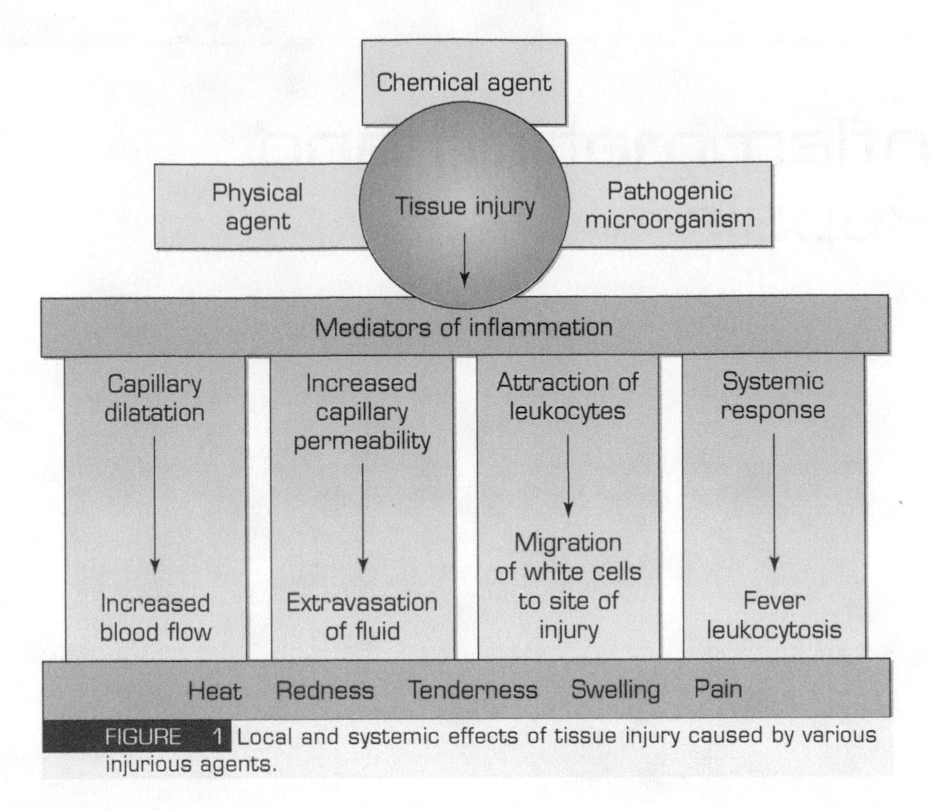

FIGURE 1 Local and systemic effects of tissue injury caused by various injurious agents.

through the walls, and migrate to the area of tissue damage (FIGURE 2). The characteristic signs of inflammation are heat, redness, tenderness, swelling, and pain. The increased warmth and redness of the inflamed tissues are caused by dilatation of capillaries and slowing of blood flow through the vessels. Swelling occurs because the extravasation (leakage) of plasma from the dilated and more permeable vessels causes the volume of fluid in the inflamed tissue to increase (FIGURE 3). The tenderness and pain are secondary to irritation of sensory nerve endings at the site of the inflammatory process.

Exudate
(ex′yū-dāt)
The fluid, leukocytes, and debris that accumulate as a result of an inflammation.

The polymorphonuclear leukocyte is the most important cell in the acute inflammatory response. It is an actively phagocytic cell that is attracted to the area by the cell injury. Mononuclear cells (monocytes, macrophages) appear later in the inflammation reaction. One of their major functions is to clean up the debris produced by the inflammatory process. These cells are also active in chronic inflammatory reactions.

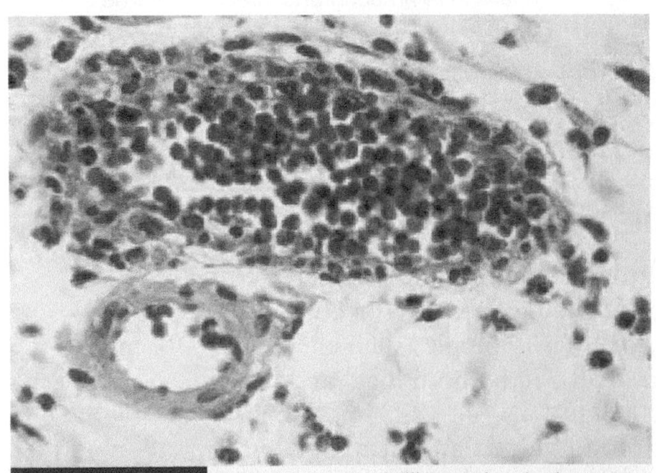

FIGURE 2 Photomicrograph illustrating leukocytes adherent to capillary endothelium and migrating through wall to site of tissue injury (original magnification × 160).

The fluid mixture of protein, leukocytes, and debris that forms during the inflammatory process is called **exudate**. Its proportions of protein and inflammatory cells vary in different exudates, and the appearance of the exudate will also vary. It is convenient to describe an exudate as serous, purulent, fibrinous, or hemorrhagic based on its appearance. If the exudate consists primarily of fluid containing very little protein, the term serous exudate is used. If a large amount of serous fluid accumulates in injured tissues—as, for example, after a severe burn of the skin—blisters may form (FIGURE 4). An exudate consisting largely of inflammatory cells is called a purulent exudate, and the creamy yellow exudate is called pus. The term fibrinous exudate is used if the fluid in the exudate is rich in a blood protein called fibrinogen, which coagulates and forms fibrin, producing a sticky film on the surface of the inflamed tissue (FIGURE 5). (The proteins concerned in the coagulation of the blood are considered in the discussion on abnormalities of blood coagulation.) A hemorrhagic exudate occurs when the inflammatory process had ruptured many small capillaries, allowing red blood cells to escape into the tissues so that the exudate appears bloody.

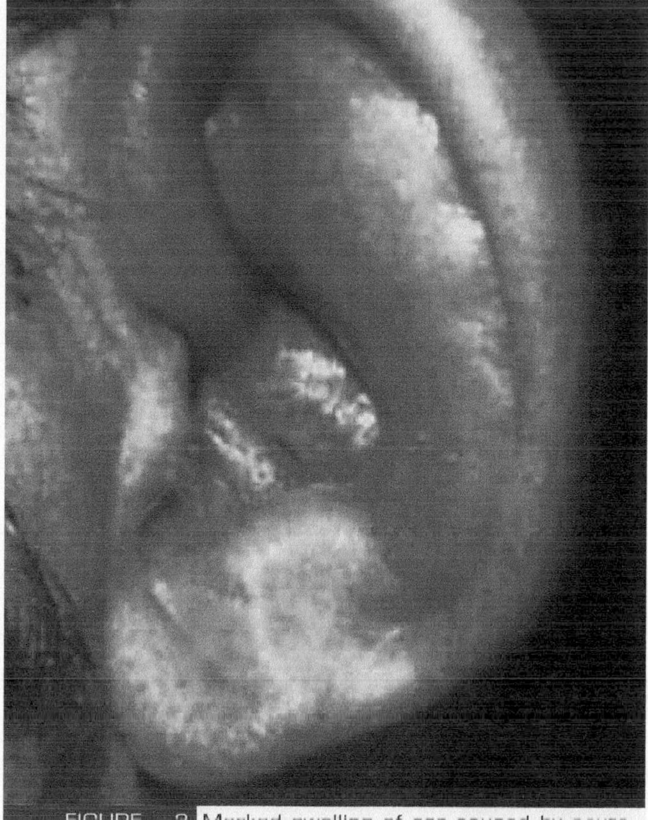

FIGURE 3 Marked swelling of ear caused by acute inflammation.

If a fibrinous exudate involves two surfaces in close proximity, such as adjacent loops of small intestine, the surfaces may stick together. This type of inflammation often heals by ingrowth of fibrous tissue, which binds the adjacent surfaces together by means of fibrous bands called **adhesions** (FIGURE 6).

If the inflammatory process is severe, systemic effects become evident. The individual feels ill, and the temperature is elevated. The bone marrow accelerates its production of leukocytes so that the number of leukocytes circulating in the bloodstream increases. The liver produces several proteins called acute phase proteins that are released into the bloodstream in response to tissue injury or inflammation, which help protect the body from the tissue injury caused by the inflammation. The best known of these proteins is called C reactive protein, which is often measured to monitor the activity of diseases characterized by tissue inflammation.

Adhesions
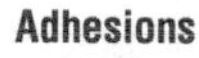
(ad-hē′shuns)
Bands of fibrous tissue that form subsequent to an inflammation and bind adjacent tissues together.

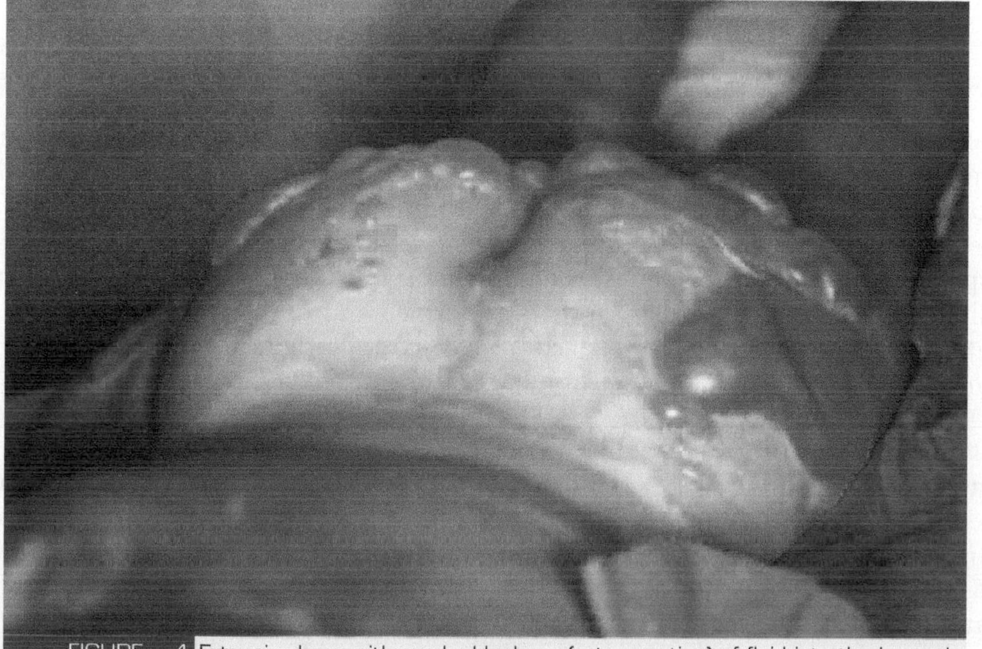

FIGURE 4 Extensive burn with marked leakage (extravasation) of fluid into the burned area leading to formation of large blisters.

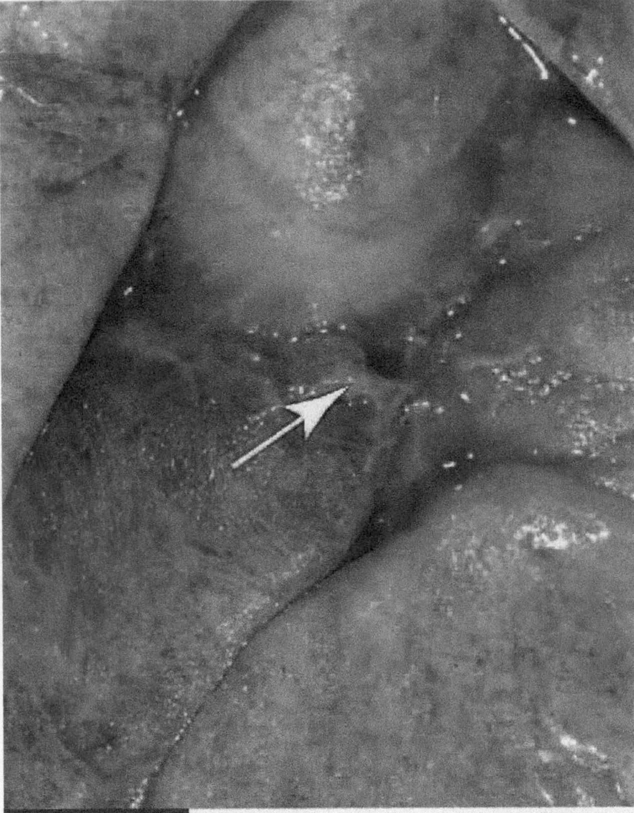

FIGURE 5 Fibrinous inflammation involving the surface of the heart (epicardium) and pericardium. The pericardial sac has been opened to expose the surface of the heart, which appears rough because fibrin has accumulated on the epicardium. The *arrow* indicates a large aggregate of fibrin adjacent to the right atrial appendage.

FIGURE 6 Multiple fibrous adhesions (*arrows*) between loops of small intestine resulting from previous abdominal inflammation.

The outcome of an inflammation depends on how much tissue damage has resulted from the inflammation. If the inflammation is mild, it soon subsides, and the tissues return to normal. This process is called **resolution**. If the inflammatory process is more severe, tissue is destroyed to some extent and must be repaired (FIGURE 7). During healing, damaged cells are replaced, and the framework of the injured tissue is repaired as an ingrowth of cells produces connective tissue fibers and new blood vessels. Scar tissue replaces large areas of tissue destruction (FIGURE 8). Sometimes, the scarring subsequent to a severe inflammation is so severe that function is seriously disturbed (FIGURE 9).

Resolution
A regression of an inflammatory process without significant tissue destruction and with return of the tissues to normal.

CHEMICAL MEDIATORS OF INFLAMMATION

The inflammatory reaction is a nonspecific, stereotyped response to tissue injury and is much the same no matter what caused the injury. For example, an injury caused by dropping a book on your foot produces the same type of inflammatory response as does a severe sunburn in the same region. The reason is because the inflammatory response is not directly caused by the tissue injury. It is caused by chemical agents called mediators of inflammation that are formed and released when the tissue is damaged. Some mediators are derived from cells, and others are formed from proteins in the blood plasma that accumulate in the injured area.

Cell-Derived Mediators

Mast cells, a major source of cell-derived mediators, are specialized cells that are widely distributed throughout the connective tissues of the body. Their cytoplasm is filled with granules containing histamine and other chemicals. If tissue is injured, the mast cells discharge their granules, liberating the chemicals to initiate the inflammatory process. Histamine is a potent **vasodilator** (*vas* = blood vessel + *dilate* = expand) and also greatly increases vascular permeability. Blood platelets also contain histamine and another mediator called **serotonin**, which are released when platelets

Mast cell
A specialized connective tissue cell containing granules filled with histamine and other chemical mediators.

Vasodilator
A substance that dilates blood vessels.

Serotonin
(sēr-o-tō′-nin)
A vasoconstrictor mediator of inflammation released from platelets.

adhere to collagen fragments at the site of tissue injury. Other important cell-derived mediators are a group called **prostaglandins** (so named because compounds of this type were first isolated from the prostate gland) and a group of similar compounds called **leukotrienes**. These biologically active compounds are synthesized by cells from arachidonic acid present in cell membranes in response to stimuli that induce inflammation, and they function as mediators that intensify the inflammatory process.

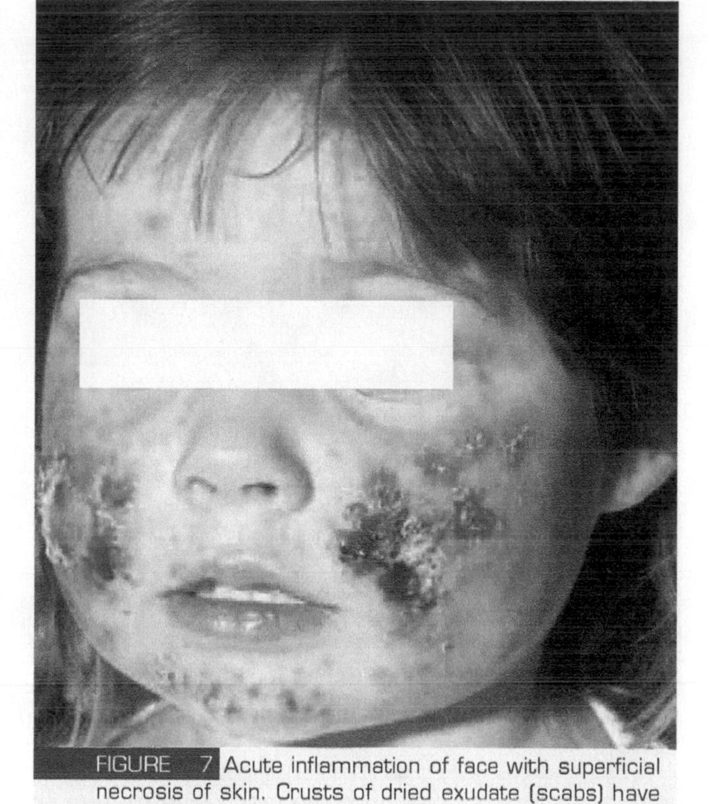

FIGURE 7 Acute inflammation of face with superficial necrosis of skin. Crusts of dried exudate (scabs) have formed on skin surface.

Mediators from Blood Plasma

Blood plasma contains various protein substances that circulate as inactive compounds and leak from the permeable capillaries into the area of tissue damage where they become transformed (activated) by a complex process into chemical mediators. One important group of mediators formed in this way is called **bradykinins** (or simply kinins). The series of reactions that leads to the formation of bradykinins is triggered by one of the proteins concerned with blood coagulation, which is activated by the tissue injury.

Mediators of inflammation are also formed from another group of blood proteins called complement. Complement consists of several separate protein components, designated C_1 through C_9, that interact in a regular sequence to yield a series of by-products, some of which function as mediators of inflammation. Complement is activated when an antigen combines with an antibody but may also be activated in other ways that do not require an antigen–antibody interaction. The various functions of the complement system are considered in connection with immunity, hypersensitivity, allergy, and autoimmune diseases.

FIGURE 10 illustrates how the various mediators interact. The release of mediators from any source not only initiates the inflammatory process but also induces release of more mediators from other sources, setting off a "chain reaction" that intensifies the inflammatory process.

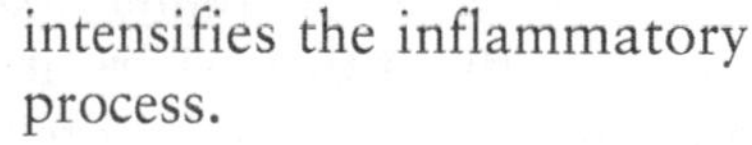

Prostaglandin
(pros-ta-glan′din)
A complex derivative of a fatty acid (prostanoic acid) that has widespread physiologic effects.

Leukotriene
(lōō-kō-try′-ēn)
A prostaglandin-like mediator of inflammation.

Bradykinin
(brā-dē-kī′nin)
A chemical mediator of inflammation derived from components in the blood plasma.

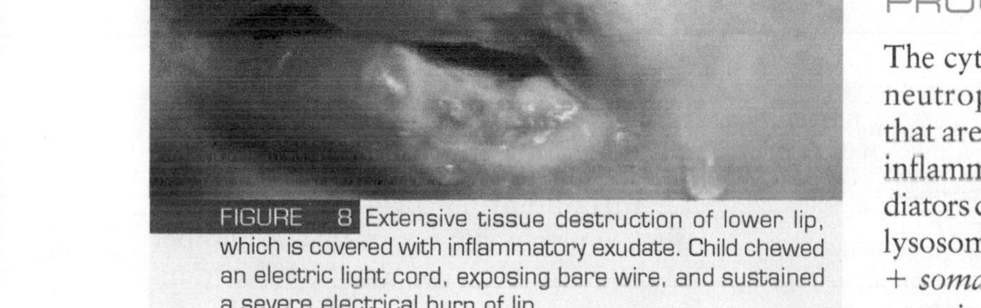

FIGURE 8 Extensive tissue destruction of lower lip, which is covered with inflammatory exudate. Child chewed an electric light cord, exposing bare wire, and sustained a severe electrical burn of lip.

THE ROLE OF LYSOSOMAL ENZYMES IN THE INFLAMMATORY PROCESS

The cytoplasm of phagocytic neutrophils and monocytes that are attracted to the site of inflammation by chemical mediators contains granules called lysosomes (*lysis* = dissolving + *soma* = body). Lysosomes contain potent enzymes that

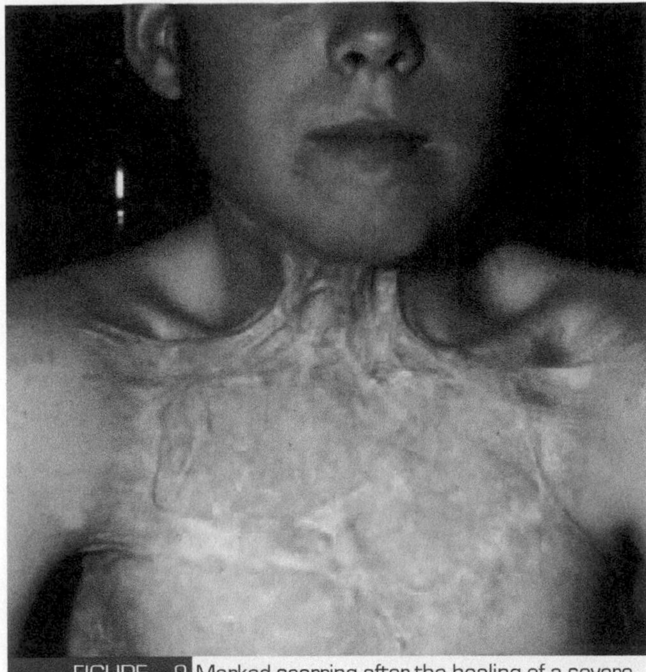

FIGURE 9 Marked scarring after the healing of a severe burn, which has restricted motion of neck and arms. Skin grafting was required to improve function.

are capable of digesting the material brought into the cytoplasm of the cells by phagocytosis. During phagocytosis, bacteria or other foreign materials become enclosed within vacuoles in the cell cytoplasm, and the lysosomes dissolve the material by discharging their enzymes into the vacuoles, as described in the discussion on cells and tissues (FIGURE 2).

In the course of any inflammatory reaction, many neutrophils and monocytes are damaged or destroyed, and their lysosomal enzymes are released. Some lysosomal enzymes also escape from intact leukocytes during phagocytosis. Much of the tissue injury in an area of inflammation is a result of the destructive effect of the lysosomal enzymes released from leukocytes. The tissue injury in turn generates more mediators, and this induces further inflammatory changes.

INFLAMMATION CAUSED BY ANTIGEN-ANTIBODY INTERACTION

Antibodies are one of the body's defense mechanisms. This is discussed in immunity, hypersensitivity, allergy, and autoimmune diseases. When antigen and antibody interact, an intense inflammatory reaction with marked tissue necrosis often follows. The interaction of antigen and antibody activates complement, and the mediators generated from complement activation induce the inflammatory reaction. Large numbers of leukocytes are attracted to the site, and the release of potent lysosomal enzymes from the leukocytes is the chief cause of the tissue damage.

HARMFUL EFFECTS OF INFLAMMATION

The tissue injury that results from an inflammation is due in part to the injurious agent and in part to the inflammatory reaction itself. In most cases, the inflammatory process is self-limited and subsides when the harmful agent has been eliminated. At times, however, an inflammatory process may persist and cause extensive, progressive tissue injury. If this occurs, it is sometimes necessary to suppress the inflammatory process by administering adrenal corticosteroid hormones to reduce the tissue damage that would result if the inflammatory process were not restrained. (Suppression of the immune response is considered in the discussion on immunity, hypersensitivity, allergy, and autoimmune diseases.)

Infection
Inflammation caused by a disease-producing organism.

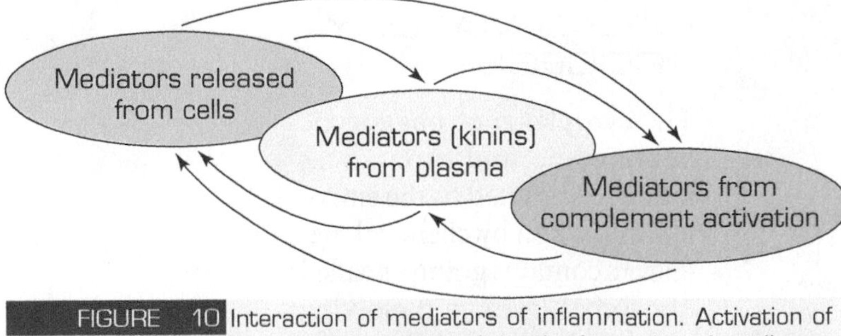

FIGURE 10 Interaction of mediators of inflammation. Activation of mediators from any source also leads to the formation of mediators from other sources, which intensifies the inflammatory reaction.

Infection

TERMINOLOGY OF INFECTION

The term **infection** is used to denote an inflammatory process caused by disease-producing organisms. A number of different terms are used to refer to infections in various sites. Generally, the

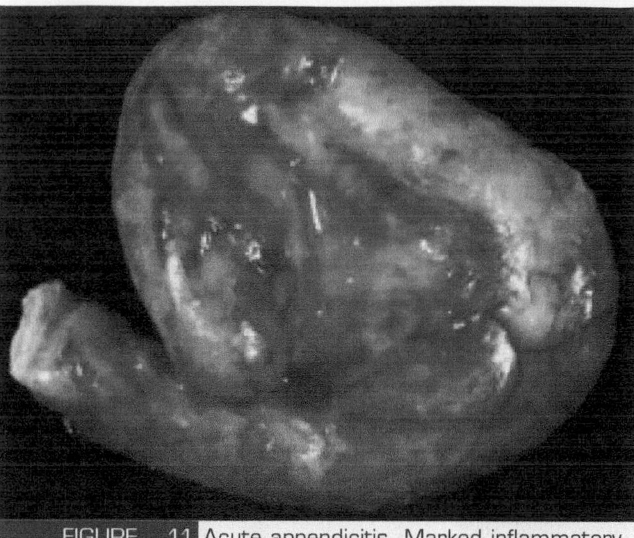

FIGURE 11 Acute appendicitis. Marked inflammatory exudate on the surface of the appendix.

ending *-itis* is appended to the name of the tissue or organ in order to indicate an infection or inflammatory process. For example, the terms appendicitis (FIGURE 11), hepatitis, colitis, and pneumonitis refer to inflammation of the appendix, liver, colon, and lung, respectively. An acute spreading infection at any site is called **cellulitis** (FIGURE 12). Usually, this term is used to refer to an acute infection of the skin and deeper tissues. The term **abscess** is used when an infection is associated with breakdown of the tissues and the formation of a localized mass of pus (FIGURE 13). If a localized infection spreads into the lymphatic channels draining the site of inflammation, the term **lymphangitis** is used. **Lymphadenitis** refers to infection in the regional lymph nodes draining the primary site of infection. The term **septicemia** is used to refer to an overwhelming infection in which pathogenic bacteria gain access to the bloodstream.

Cellulitis (sell-ū-lī′tis)
An acute spreading inflammation affecting the skin or deeper tissues.

Abscess (ab′sess)
A localized accumulation of pus in tissues.

Lymphangitis (limf′an-jī′tis)
An inflammation of lymph vessels draining a site of infection.

Lymphadenitis (limf-a-den-ī′tis)
An inflammation of lymph nodes draining a site of infection.

Septicemia (sep-ti-sē′mē-yuh)
An infection in which large numbers of pathogenic bacteria are present in the bloodstream.

Pathogenic (path-ō-jen′ik)
Capable of producing disease.

Virulence (vir′u-lenz)
The ability of an organism to cause disease.

FACTORS INFLUENCING THE OUTCOME OF AN INFECTION

In any infection, the invading organism is pitted against the defenses of the body. Bacteria and other microbiologic agents vary in their ability to cause disease. Many are not harmful to humans. Others, capable of causing human disease, are called **pathogenic** (*pathos* = disease + *genic* = producing) organisms. The term **virulence**

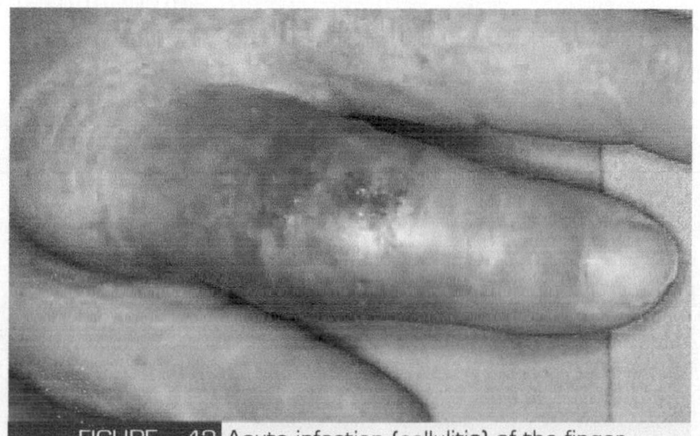

FIGURE 12 Acute infection (cellulitis) of the finger.

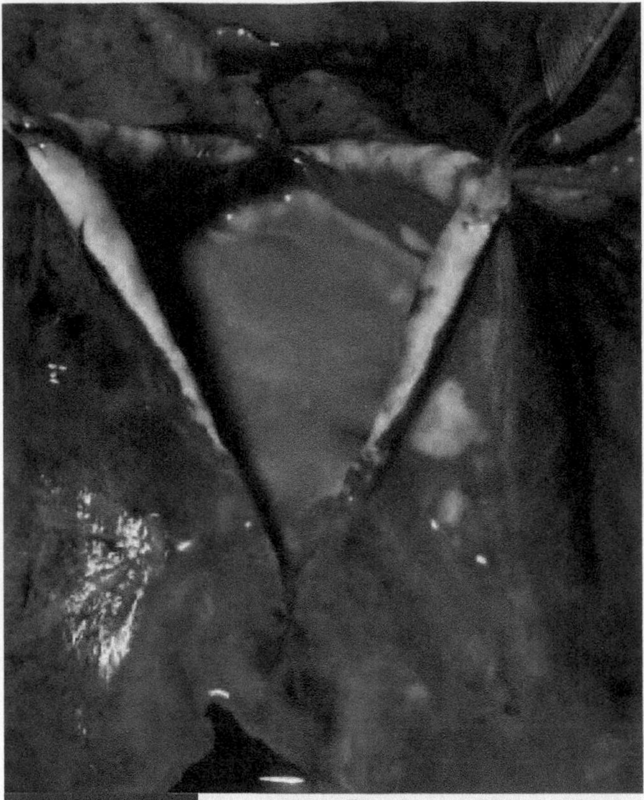
FIGURE 13 Lung abscess. The pleural surface has been incised to expose a large abscess cavity filled with pus.

refers to the ease with which a pathogenic organism can overcome the defenses of the body. A highly virulent organism is one that is likely to produce progressive disease in the majority of susceptible individuals. In contrast, an organism of low virulence is capable only of producing disease in a highly susceptible individual under favorable circumstances.

The outcome of any infection depends on two factors: the virulence of the organism combined with the numbers ("dosage") of the invading organisms and the resistance of the infected individual (often called the **host**). These may be considered balanced against one another, as indicated diagrammatically in FIGURE 14. When large numbers of organisms of high virulence are introduced into the body, especially when host resistance is lowered, the balance is tipped in favor of the invader, and progressive or fatal disease develops. When the virulence or dosage of the organism is low or the body's resistance is high, the balance is tipped in favor of the host. The infection is then overcome and healing occurs.

Chronic Infection

Sometimes, the organism and host are evenly matched. Neither can gain the advantage; the result is a stalemate. Clinically, this results in a chronic infection, characterized by a relatively quiet, smoldering inflammation that is usually associated with vigorous attempts at healing on the part of the host. The balance between the host and the invader is precarious. The infection may flare up at times when the pathogen obtains a temporary advantage, or it may become quiescent at other times when the defenses of the host gain the upper hand. Lymphocytes, plasma cells, and monocytes are the predominant cells in chronic inflammatory processes.

Host
Individual infected with a disease-producing organism.

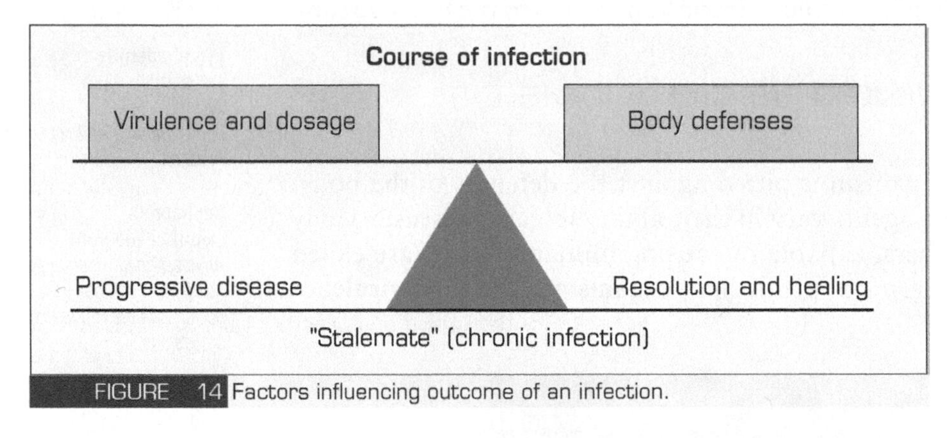

FIGURE 14 Factors influencing outcome of an infection.

QUESTIONS FOR REVIEW

1. What is the inflammatory reaction? What are its clinical manifestations?
2. What factors influence the outcome of an infection?
3. What are mediators of inflammation? How do they function?
4. What is meant by the following terms: *chronic infection*, *pathogenic*, *complement*?

SUPPLEMENTARY READINGS

Charo, I. F., and Ransohoff, R. M. 2006. The many roles of chemokines and chemokine receptors in inflammation. *New England Journal of Medicine* 354:610–21.

- Chemokines are small protein molecules (cytokines) that attract neutrophils and monocytes to sites of inflammation. Several research projects are underway to explore ways to minimize leukocyte-mediated tissue damage in persons with long-standing chronic diseases by drugs that block the cytokines that attract leukocytes.

Hotchkiss, R. S., and Karl, I. E. 2003. The pathophysiology and treatment of sepsis. *New England Journal of Medicine* 348:138–50.

- Sepsis is the inflammatory response to an infection. Many factors contribute to mortality, and ways to improve survival are considered.

Johnston, R. B., Jr. 1988. Current concepts: Immunology. Monocytes and macrophages. *New England Journal of Medicine* 318:747–52.

- Describes the structure and function of the mononuclear phagocyte system. Monocytes form in the marrow, have a half-life of about 3 days in the blood, and then migrate to the tissues where they live for several months. They are activated by lymphokines from T lymphocytes.

Kumar, V., Abbas, A. K., Fausto, N., et al. 2010. *Robbins and Cotran pathologic basis of disease*, 8th ed. Philadelphia: Elsevier Saunders.

- A standard textbook with detailed treatment of the inflammatory reaction in all of its aspects.

OUTLINE SUMMARY

The Inflammatory Reaction

CHARACTERISTICS OF THE INFLAMMATORY REACTION

Dilatation of blood vessels.

Migration of leukocytes through vessel walls to the site of inflammation.

Increased capillary permeability.

Extravasation of fluids.

CLINICAL MANIFESTATIONS OF INFLAMMATION

Heat and redness: dilated blood vessels.

Swelling: accumulation of fluid and exudate.

Tenderness and pain: irritation of nerve endings.

TYPES OF INFLAMMATION REACTIONS

Serous inflammation: chiefly fluid exudate.

Purulent inflammation: chiefly inflammatory cells.

Fibrinous inflammation: exudate rich in protein, which coagulates.

Hemorrhagic inflammation: many capillaries ruptured, allowing escape of red cells.

SYSTEMIC EFFECTS OF INFLAMMATION

Patient feels ill.

Elevated temperature.

Leukocytosis.

OUTCOME OF INFLAMMATION

Resolution: inflammation subsides and tissues return to normal.

Repair: replacement of damaged cells and tissues.

Large areas of destruction replaced by scar tissue.

Mediators intensify inflammatory process and generate more mediators.

CHEMICAL MEDIATORS OF INFLAMMATION

Mast cells: discharge granules containing mediators.

Kinins form from blood proteins leaking into inflamed area.

Activation of complement generates mediators.

THE ROLE OF LYSOSOMAL ENZYMES IN THE INFLAMMATORY PROCESS

Lysosomal enzymes released from leukocytes cause tissue injury.

Injury generates more mediators, which promotes further inflammation and tissue injury.

INFLAMMATION CAUSED BY ANTIGEN ANTIBODY INTERACTION

Interaction activates complement, leading to formation of mediators. This attracts leukocytes.

Lysosomal enzymes from leukocytes cause tissue injury.

HARMFUL EFFECTS OF INFLAMMATION

Inflammation usually subsides.

Persisting inflammation may cause severe tissue injury.

It may be necessary to suppress inflammatory reaction by corticosteroids to reduce tissue damage.

Infection

AN INFLAMMATION CAUSED BY A PATHOGENIC ORGANISM

Terms used to name infections:

Named by adding -itis to name of affected organ.

Cellulitis: acute spreading infection.

Abscess: tissue breakdown forming pus pockets.

Lymphadenitis: inflammation of draining lymph nodes.

Septicemia: bloodstream infection.

Factors influencing outcome:

Virulence of organism.

Dosage.

Resistance of host's body.

CHRONIC INFECTION

Organisms and host evenly balanced.

Lymphocytes and plasma cells predominate.

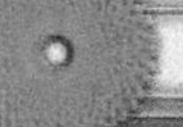

http://health.jbpub.com/humandisease/9e

Human Disease Online is a great source for supplementary human disease information for both students and instructors. Visit this website to find a variety of useful tools for learning, thinking, and teaching.

Neoplastic Disease

LEARNING OBJECTIVES

1. Compare the general characteristics of benign and malignant tumors. Explain how tumors are named. List the common exceptions to standard terminology.
2. Summarize the features of the principal types of lymphoma.
3. Differentiate between infiltrating and in situ carcinoma. Explain the role of the Pap smear in early diagnosis of neoplasm.
4. Explain how leukemias are classified. Describe the clinical manifestations of each type and its response to treatment.
5. Differentiate myeloma from leukemia. Describe its clinical manifestations, and explain how it is diagnosed.
6. Explain the mechanisms of the body's immunologic defenses against tumor.
7. Summarize the principal modalities of tumor treatment, including advantages, disadvantages, and common side effects of each technique.
8. Describe the applications and limitations of tumor-associated antigens in the diagnosis and treatment of patients with tumors.
9. Compare the incidence and survival rates for various types of malignant tumors. Explain the mechanisms of late recurrence. Define the role of adjuvant therapy in preventing late recurrence.
10. Understand the role of activated oncogenes and disturbance in suppressor gene function on the pathogenesis of tumors.

Tumors: Disturbed Cell Growth

Normal life processes are characterized by continuous growth and maturation of cells, and all cells are subject to control mechanisms that regulate their growth rate. This ongoing growth process serves the purpose of replacing cells that have been injured or have undergone degenerative changes. In contrast, a neoplasm (*neo* = new + *plasm* = growth) is an overgrowth of cells that serves no useful purpose. Neoplasms appear not to be subject to the control mechanisms that normally regulate cell growth and differentiation.

Tumors

CLASSIFICATION AND NOMENCLATURE

Tumor
A benign or malignant overgrowth of tissues that serves no normal function.

The terms neoplasm and **tumor** have essentially the same meaning and may be used interchangeably. There are two large classes of neoplasms:

1. Benign tumors
2. Malignant tumors

TABLE 1 compares the major characteristics of the two classes.

COMPARISON OF BENIGN AND MALIGNANT TUMORS

Generally, a benign tumor grows slowly and remains localized. Although it pushes surrounding normal tissue aside, it does not infiltrate surrounding tissues or spread by blood and lymphatic channels to distant sites. Usually, a benign tumor can be completely removed surgically without difficulty (FIGURES 1, 2, and 3). Histologically, the cells in a benign tumor appear mature and closely resemble the normal cells from which the tumor was derived.

In contrast to a benign tumor, a malignant neoplasm is composed of less well-differentiated cells (FIGURE 4), grows more rapidly, and infiltrates the surrounding tissues rather than growing by expansion (FIGURE 5). Frequently, the infiltrating strands of tumor find their way into the vascular and lymphatic channels. Bits of tumor may be carried in the lymphatics to reach the lymph nodes, where they establish secondary sites of tumor growth not connected with the original tumor (FIGURE 6). Eventually, the tumor may spread widely throughout the lymphatic channels. Tumor cells may also gain access to the bloodstream and be carried to distant sites, leading to secondary tumor deposits throughout the body. The process by which a tumor spreads some

TABLE 1

Comparison of benign and malignant tumors

	Benign tumor	Malignant tumor
Growth rate	Slow	Rapid
Character of growth	Expansion	Infiltration
Tumor spread	Remains localized	Metastasis by bloodstream and lymphatics
Cell differentiation	Well differentiated	Poorly differentiated

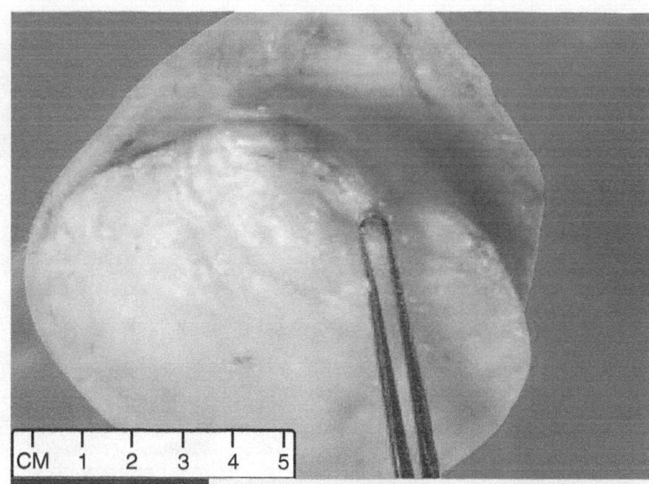

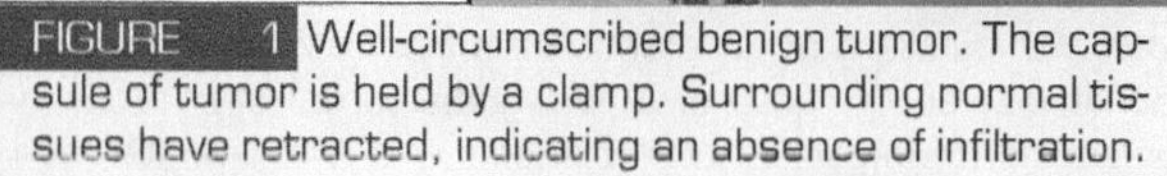
FIGURE 1 Well-circumscribed benign tumor. The capsule of tumor is held by a clamp. Surrounding normal tissues have retracted, indicating an absence of infiltration.

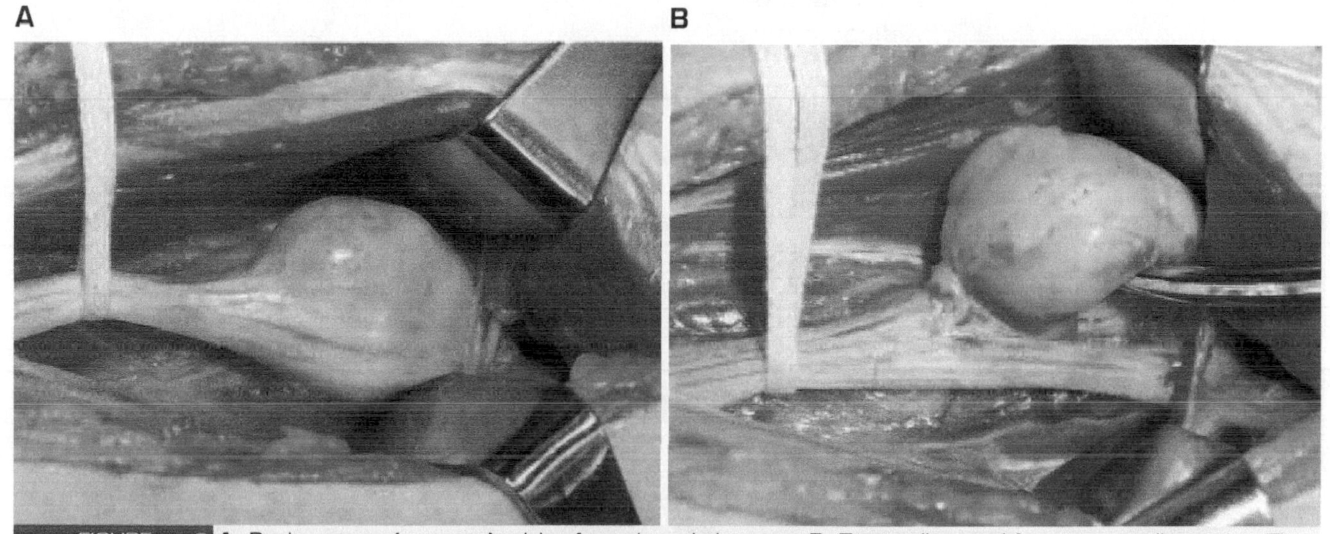

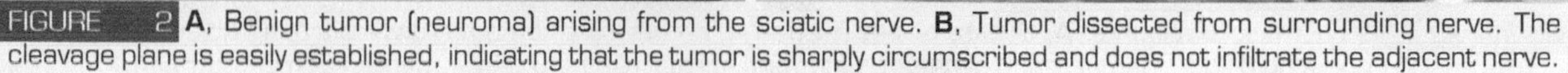
FIGURE 2 **A**, Benign tumor (neuroma) arising from the sciatic nerve. **B**, Tumor dissected from surrounding nerve. The cleavage plane is easily established, indicating that the tumor is sharply circumscribed and does not infiltrate the adjacent nerve.

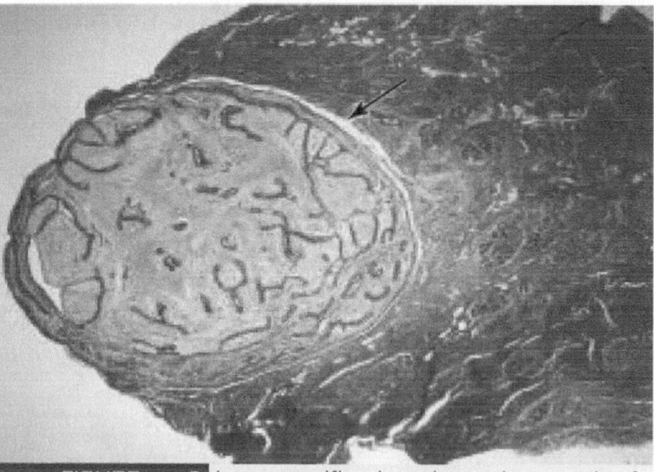
FIGURE 3 Low-magnification photomicrograph of benign breast tumor (fibroadenoma). Note the sharp demarcation between the tumor and surrounding breast tissue (*arrow*).

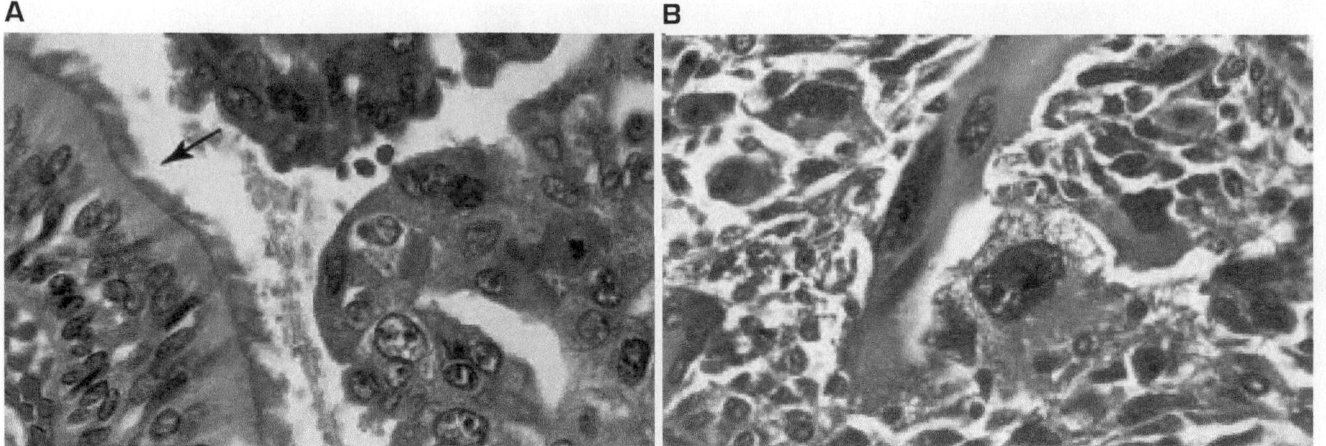

FIGURE 4 Cellular abnormalities in malignant tumors. **A**, Biopsy of a bronchus from a patient with lung carcinoma, comparing normal respiratory epithelium (*arrow*) with clusters of neoplastic cells from a lung carcinoma. Cancer cells grow in a haphazard pattern and exhibit great variation in size and structure. **B**, Malignant tumor of smooth muscle (leiomyosarcoma), illustrating large, bizarre, elongated tumor cells showing little resemblance to normal smooth muscle cells from which the tumor arose.

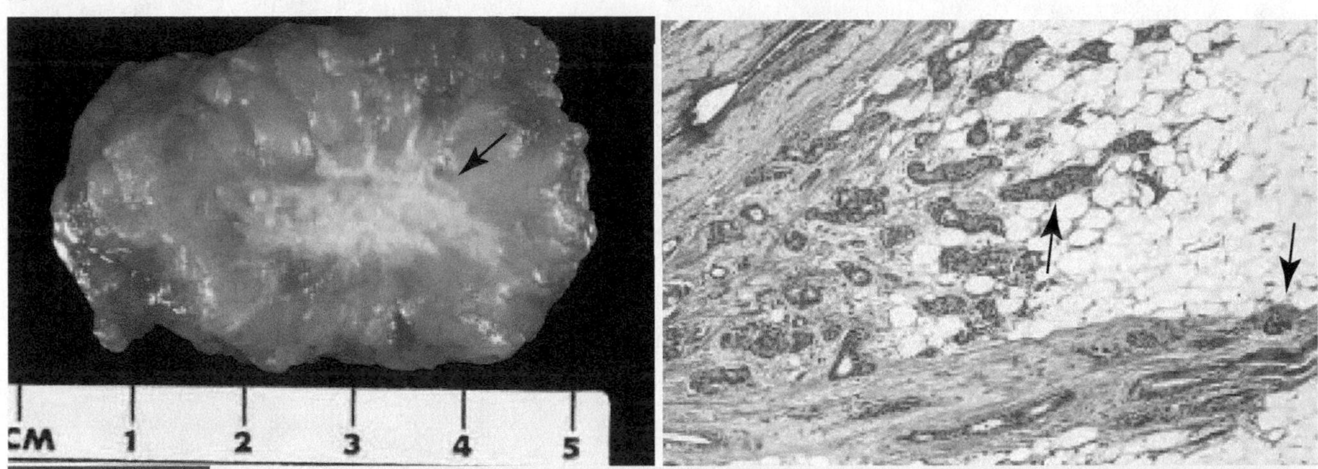

FIGURE 5 Breast carcinoma. **A**, Breast biopsy illustrating breast carcinoma (*arrow*) infiltrating adjacent fatty tissue of breast. There is no distinct demarcation between tumor and normal tissue. **B**, Low-magnification photograph illustrating the margin of infiltrating breast carcinoma. Small clusters of tumor cells (*arrows*) infiltrate adipose tissues of breast (original magnification × 20).

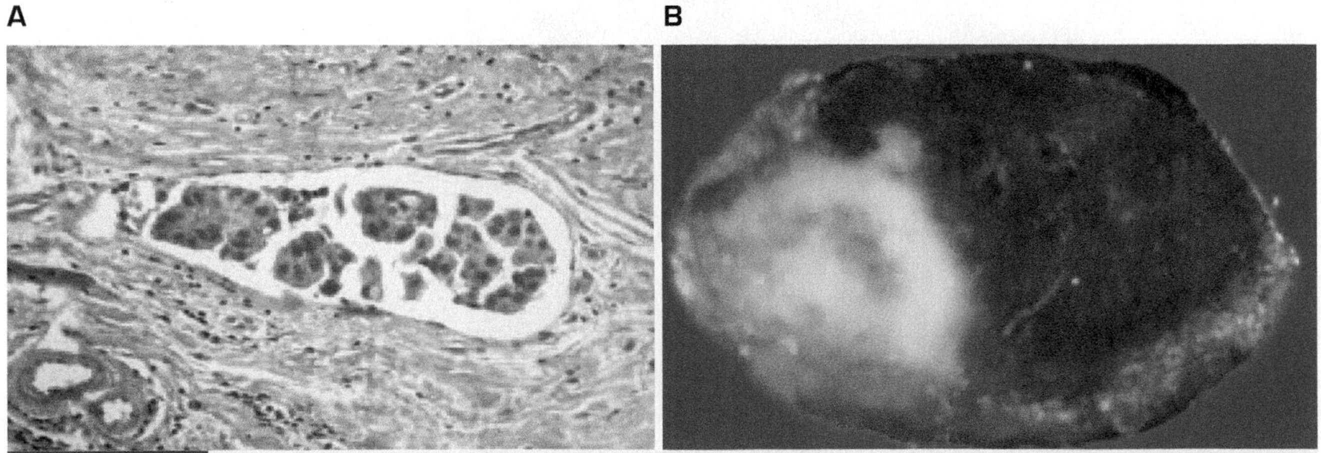

FIGURE 6 Lymphatic spread of carcinoma. **A**, Cluster of tumor cells in lymphatic vessel (original magnification × 400). **B**, Deposit of metastatic carcinoma (white mass within node) that has spread via lymphatic channels into a small regional lymph node.

distance from the primary site is called **metastasis** (*meta* = beyond + *stasis* = standing), and the secondary deposits are called metastatic tumors (FIGURE 7). If a malignant tumor is not eradicated promptly, it may eventually become widely disseminated throughout the body and may kill the patient. Benign tumors do not metastasize.

Tumors are named and classified according to the cells and tissues from which they originate. Therefore, understanding the primary tissue classifications explained in the discussion on cells and tissues: their structure and function in health and disease is helpful in understanding the names of tumors. Tumor nomenclature is not completely uniform, but certain generalizations are possible.

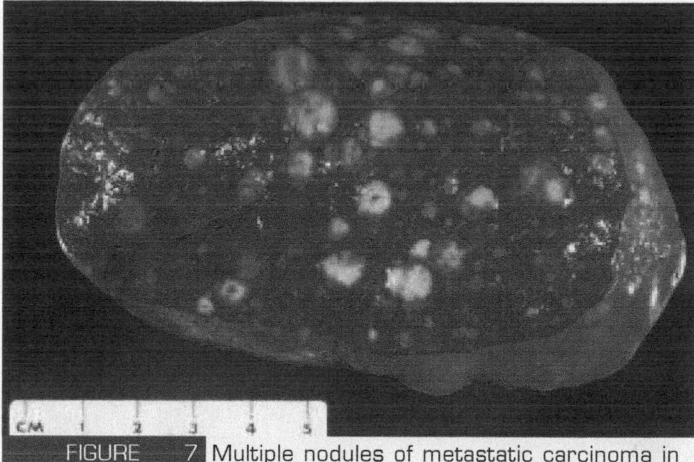

FIGURE 7 Multiple nodules of metastatic carcinoma in spleen.

BENIGN TUMORS

A benign tumor that projects from an epithelial surface is usually called a **polyp** or **papilloma** (FIGURE 8). Most other benign tumors are named by adding the suffix *-oma* to the prefix that designates the cell of origin, as shown in TABLE 2. For example, a benign tumor arising from glandular epithelium is called an adenoma. A benign tumor of blood vessels is an angioma (FIGURE 9), and one arising from cartilage is designated a chondroma.

MALIGNANT TUMORS

There are many types of malignant tumors, but all can be classified into three groups: (1) carcinomas, (2) sarcomas, or (3) leukemias. The term cancer is a word used to indicate any type of malignant tumor.

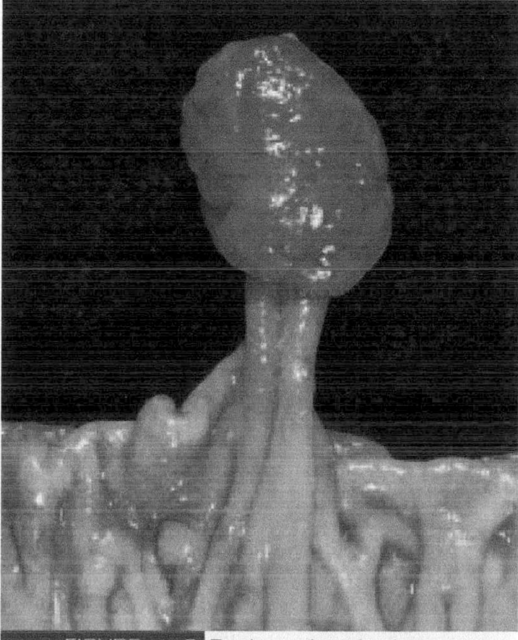
FIGURE 8 Benign polyp of colon.

TABLE 2

Common prefixes used to name tumors

Prefix	Meaning
Adeno-	Gland
Angio-	Vessels (type not specified)
Chondro-	Cartilage
Fibro-	Fibrous tissue
Hemangio-	Blood vessels
Lymphangio-	Lymph vessels
Lipo-	Fat
Myo-	Muscle
Neuro-	Nerve
Osteo-	Bone

Metastasis
The spread of cancer cells from the primary site of origin to a distant site within the body.

Polyp
A descriptive term for a benign tumor projecting from an epithelial surface.

Papilloma
(pap-pil-ō′muh)
A descriptive term for a benign tumor projecting from an epithelial surface.

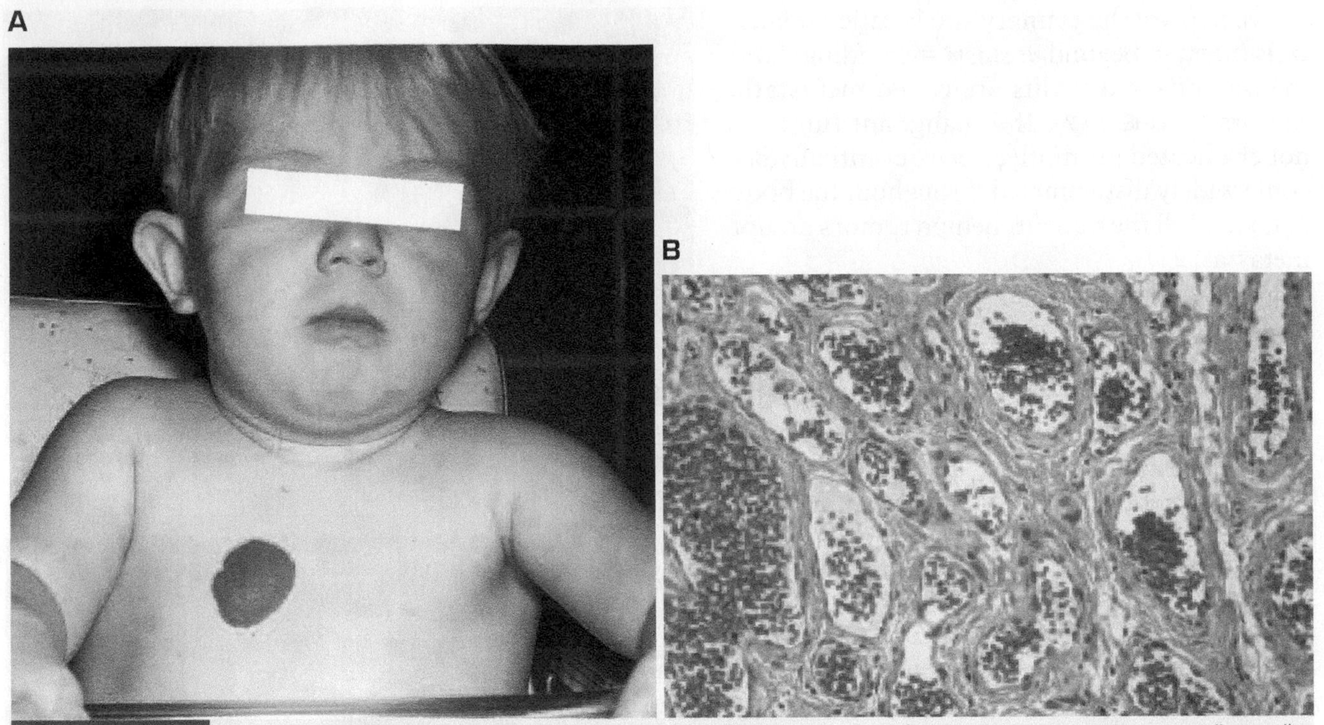

FIGURE 9 Benign blood vessel tumor (angioma) of skin. **A**, Clinical appearance. **B**, Histologic appearance revealing well-formed mature blood vessels (original magnification × 400).

It is generally agreed that a malignant tumor starts from a single cell that has sustained some type of damage to its genome that causes it to proliferate abnormally, forming first a clone of identical cells and, if unchecked, eventually developing into a distinct tumor. Cells of malignant tumors exhibit behavior that is quite different from that of normal cells. They do not respond to normal growth regulatory signals from other cells, and they continue to proliferate when there is no need to do so. Indeed, some cancer cells actually secrete growth factors to stimulate their own growth. As they grow, they acquire properties that allow them to flourish at the expense of the surrounding normal cells. They secrete enzymes that break down normal cell and tissue barriers, which allows them to infiltrate into adjacent tissues, invade lymphatic channels and blood vessels, and eventually spread throughout the body. Moreover, the proliferating tumor cells do not "wear out" and die after a specific number of cell divisions, as normal cells do. They become "immortal" and can proliferate indefinitely.

Carcinoma
(kär-sin-ō′-mah)
A malignant tumor derived from epithelial cells.

A **carcinoma** is any malignant tumor arising from surface, glandular, or parenchymal (organ) epithelium. (The term is not applied, however, to malignant tumors of endothelium or mesothelium, which behave more like malignant connective tissue tumors.) A carcinoma is classified further by designating the type of epithelium from which it arose. For example, a malignant tumor arising from the transitional epithelium of the urinary bladder is called a transitional cell carcinoma of the bladder. A carcinoma arising from the glandular epithelium of the pancreas is termed an adenocarcinoma of the pancreas (*aden* = gland), and a tumor arising from the squamous epithelium of the esophagus is called a squamous cell carcinoma of the esophagus.

Sarcoma
(sar-kō′muh)
A malignant tumor arising from connective and supporting tissues.

Sarcoma is a general term referring to a malignant tumor arising from primary tissues other than surface, glandular, or parenchymal epithelium. The exact type of sarcoma is specified by prefixing the term designating the cell of origin. For example, a malignant tumor of cartilage is designated as a chondrosarcoma. Fibrosarcoma, liposarcoma, myosarcoma, osteosarcoma, and angiosarcoma indicate, respectively, malignant tumors of fibroblasts, fat cells, muscle cells, bone-forming cells, and blood vessels.

The term **leukemia** is applied to any neoplasm of blood-forming tissues. Neoplasms arising from the precursors of white blood cells usually do not form solid tumors. Instead, the abnormal cells proliferate diffusely within the bone marrow, where they overgrow and crowd out the normal blood-forming cells. The neoplastic cells also "spill over" into the bloodstream, and large numbers of abnormal cells circulate in the peripheral blood.

Leukemia
(lōō-kē′mē-yuh)
A neoplastic proliferation of leukocytes.

TABLE 3 summarizes the general principles used to name both benign and malignant tumors.

VARIATIONS IN TERMINOLOGY

There are some inconsistencies and exceptions to the general principles of nomenclature. Exceptions are encountered in the naming of lymphoid tumors, skin tumors arising from pigment-producing cells within the epidermis, certain tumors of mixed cellular components, and certain types of tumors composed of primitive cells seen in children. In other cases, names of tumors seem to follow no rules or general principles. The student should not be unduly concerned about the exceptions or unusual situations but should attempt to grasp the general principles of naming tumors.

Lymphoid Tumors

All neoplasms of lymphoid tissue are called **lymphomas.** With extremely rare exceptions, these tumors are malignant (FIGURE 10). Therefore, the term lymphoma without qualification refers to a malignant, not a benign, tumor. Often, to avoid confusion, the term malignant lymphoma, rather than simply lymphoma, is used.

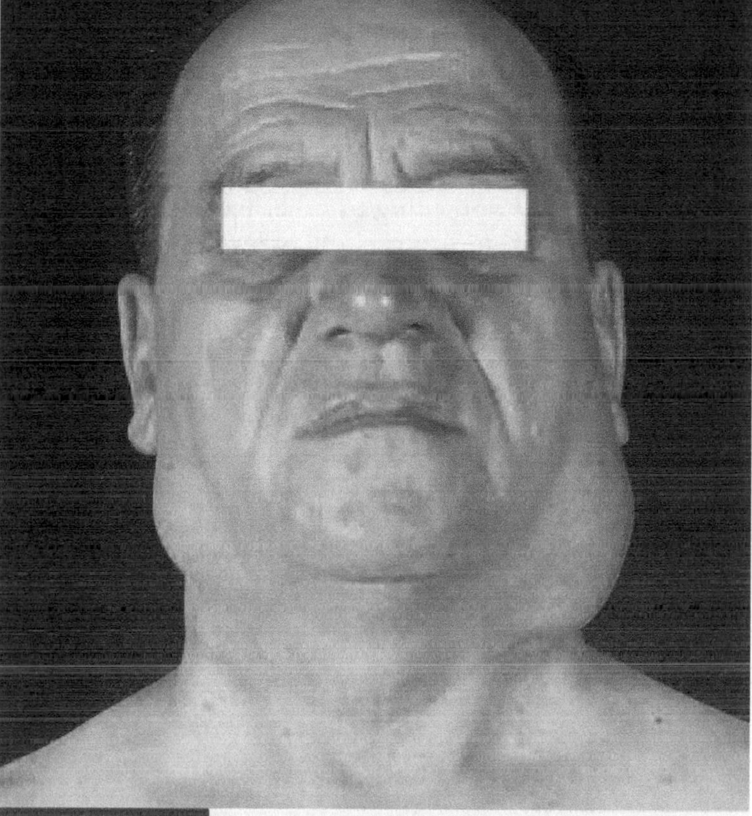

FIGURE 10 Marked enlargement of cervical lymph nodes as a result of malignant lymphoma.

Lymphoma
(limf-ō′muh)
A neoplasm of lymphoid cells.

TABLE 3

General principles of naming tumors

General term	Meaning
Polyp, papilloma	Any benign tumor projecting from surface epithelium.
____ + oma (suffix)	A benign tumor. The prefix designates primary tissue of origin.
Carcinoma	Malignant tumor arising from surface, glandular, or parenchymal epithelium (but not endothelium or mesothelium).
Sarcoma	Malignant tumor of any primary tissue other than surface, glandular, and parenchymal epithelium.
Leukemia	Neoplasm of blood cells.

Over 80% of lymphomas arise from B cells. Most of the rest come from T cells, and a few originate from NK cells (natural killer cells) or histiocytes. The neoplastic cells of most lymphomas arise from early precursor stages in the development of mature B and T cells, and the tumors sometimes resemble masses of neoplastic precursor B or T cells that have failed to mature normally. The abnormal proliferation of lymphoid cells may also disrupt the normal functions of the immune system, which may be manifested either as an impairment of the body's immune defenses resulting in increased susceptibility to infection or as an abnormal immune response manifested as some type of autoimmune disease.

Hodgkin's disease
One type of lymphoma.

Reed-Sternberg cell
The characteristic cell of Hodgkin's disease, containing two "mirror image" nuclei with prominent nucleoli.

Lymphomas are subdivided into two major groups: Hodgkin's lymphoma, more often called **Hodgkin's disease**, and non-Hodgkin's lymphoma. Hodgkin's lymphoma has several features that are quite different from other lymphomas. The disease frequently occurs in young adults, in contrast to non-Hodgkin's lymphoma, which usually affects much older persons. The disease usually starts in a single lymph node or small group of nodes and then spreads to adjacent nodes before eventually spreading to other parts of the body. The tumor has a variable histologic appearance consisting of large atypical B cells called **Reed-Sternberg cells** intermixed with lymphocytes, plasma cells, eosinophils, and fibrous tissue. The Reed-Sternberg cells make up only a small proportion of the total cells in the tumor, but they secrete cytokines that attract the other cells, which become intermixed with the Reed-Sternberg cells. The typical Reed-Sternberg cell is a large cell that characteristically contains either a single nucleus or two nuclei that appear as mirror images of each other. Each nucleus contains a large nucleolus surrounded by a clear halo (FIGURE 11). Several different histologic types of Hodgkin's disease are recognized that differ somewhat in their clinical behavior and prognosis. A person with Hodgkin's lymphoma usually first becomes aware of a painless enlargement of a single lymph node or group of nodes. In more advanced cases, several groups of nodes may be involved. Previously, patients with early stage Hodgkin's disease were treated with radiation therapy to the enlarged lymph nodes which was quite successful in most patients, but unfortunately the disease recurred in some radiotherapy-treated patients. Now most patients are treated with courses of chemotherapy consisting of four drugs (doxorubicin, bleomyxin, vinblastine, and dacarbazine) as well as radiotherapy to the involved areas and the combined therapy approach has been very successful.

All other lymphomas are grouped together under the general term of non-Hodgkin's lymphomas. Most are B-cell lymphomas that are quite variable in their

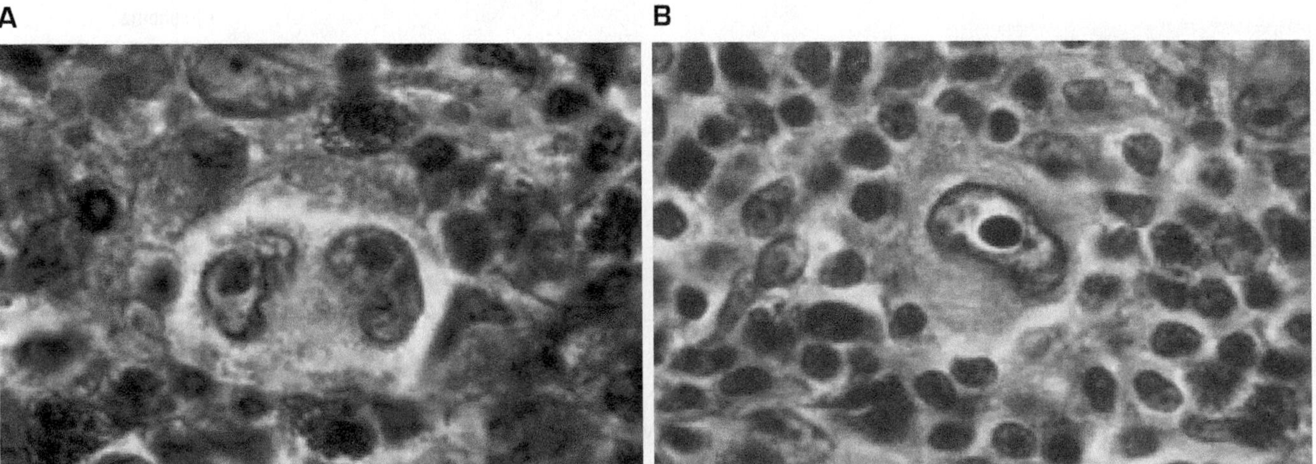

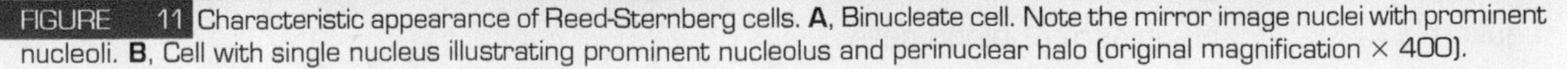
FIGURE 11 Characteristic appearance of Reed-Sternberg cells. **A**, Binucleate cell. Note the mirror image nuclei with prominent nucleoli. **B**, Cell with single nucleus illustrating prominent nucleolus and perinuclear halo (original magnification × 400).

appearance, behavior, and prognosis. Most patients have widespread disease by the time the lymphoma is diagnosed, and it is difficult to cure the lymphoma because the tumor cells have already spread throughout the body. Some tumors are very aggressive and grow rapidly, whereas other tumors that appear somewhat similar grow more slowly. Some lymphomas respond reasonably well to specific anticancer drugs, whereas others do not. Moreover, some lymphomas, which initially were composed of mature, slowly growing cells, may transform abruptly into aggressive rapidly growing tumors composed of very immature cells.

The variable appearance and sometimes poor correlation between histologic appearance and biologic behavior have created difficulties when attempting to classify lymphomas. Various classifications have been proposed to provide a better guide to prognosis and treatment. One classification is based on the size, shape, and growth pattern of the neoplastic cells. Lymphomas can also be classified into prognostic groups based on their histologic appearance. The most recent classification divides lymphomas into four large groups based on the type of cells giving rise to the tumor (T cells, B cells, NK cells, or histiocytes) and the maturity of the cells, with many subgroups within each of the four major groups. This classification system helps the physician determine the specific type of non-Hodgkin's lymphoma affecting the patient, which also helps determine the prognosis and the appropriate type of treatment.

Keratinocyte (ker-u-tin′ō-cyte) *A keratin-forming cell in the epidermis.*

Melanocyte (me-lan′o-cyte) *Melanin-producing cell in the epidermis.*

Melanin *Dark pigment found in the skin, in the middle coat of the eye, and in some other regions.*

Nevus (nē′vus) *A benign tumor of pigment-producing cells.*

Melanoma (mel-uh-nō′muh) *A malignant tumor of pigment-producing cells.*

Skin Tumors

Most skin tumors arise either from the keratin-forming cells or from the pigment-producing cells of the epidermis. The keratin-forming cells are called **keratinocytes.** The deepest layer of keratinocytes adjacent to the dermis consists of cuboidal cells called basal cells that proliferate and give rise to the upper layers of cells, which are called squamous cells. Interspersed among the keratinocytes are the skin cells that normally produce pigment and are responsible for normal skin color. These are called **melanocytes**, and the black pigment that they produce is called **melanin**. The common benign pigmented skin lesion that is derived from melanin-producing cells is called a **nevus**, a Latin word that means "birthmark" (FIGURE 12). The malignant counterpart is called a **melanoma** (or malignant melanoma), the name being derived from the pigment elaborated by the cells.

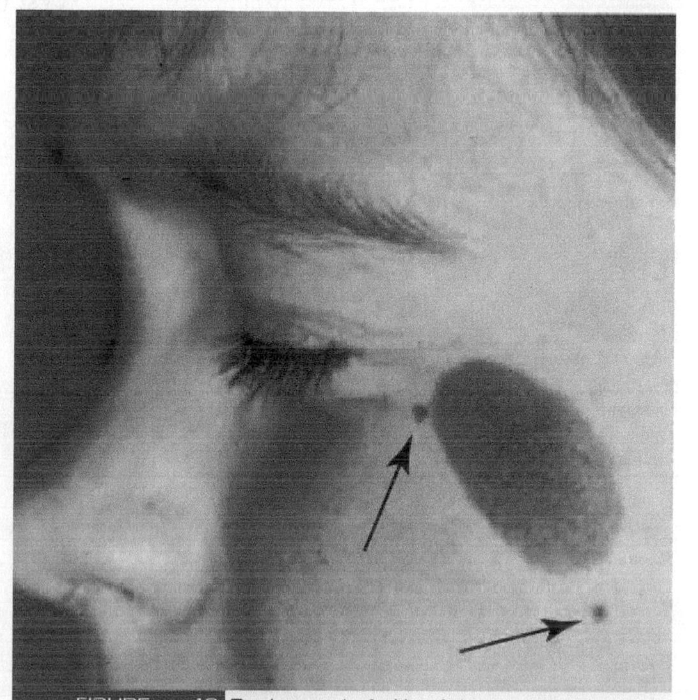

FIGURE 12 Benign nevi of skin. A large nevus is near the eye, and two smaller adjacent nevi are shown (*arrows*).

Keratinocytes can give rise to benign proliferations, called keratoses, and two types of skin carcinomas. One type, called a basal cell carcinoma, is composed of clusters of infiltrating cells that resemble the normal basal cells of the epidermis. It is a rather indolent, slowly growing tumor that can be locally destructive but rarely metastasizes. The other type, composed of abnormal infiltrating squamous cells, is called a squamous cell carcinoma and is a more aggressive tumor that sometimes metastasizes. Both types generally can be cured by complete surgical excision and carry a very good prognosis. Excessive sunlight exposure predisposes to the development of all types of skin cancer, including the potentially lethal melanoma, and also predisposes to the development of some types of keratoses, as well as causing skin damage and premature aging of the skin (FIGURE 13).

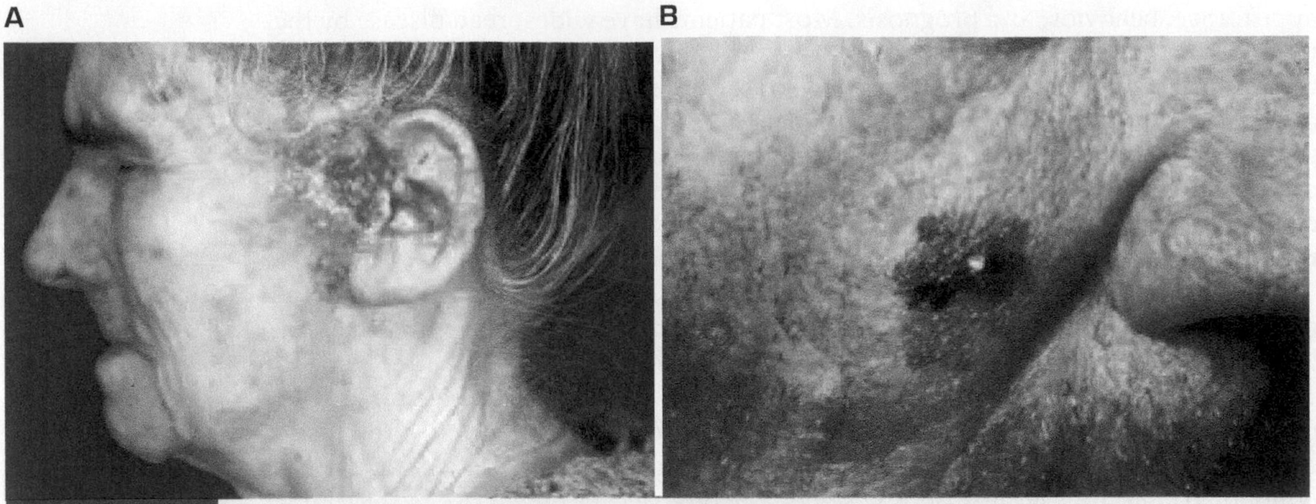

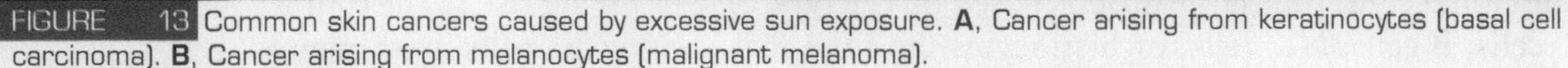

FIGURE 13 Common skin cancers caused by excessive sun exposure. **A**, Cancer arising from keratinocytes (basal cell carcinoma). **B**, Cancer arising from melanocytes (malignant melanoma).

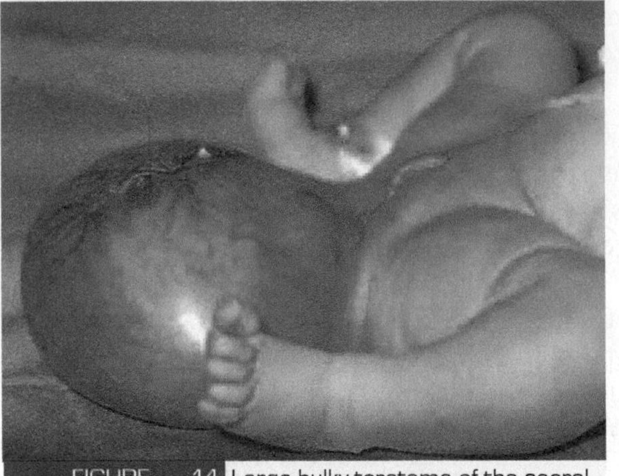

FIGURE 14 Large bulky teratoma of the sacral region in a female infant.

Tumors of Mixed Components (Teratomas)

A **teratoma** is a tumor derived from cells that have the potential of differentiating into many different types of tissue (bone, muscle, glands, epithelium, brain tissue, and hair). Frequently, such tumors consist of poorly organized mixtures of many tissues. Teratomas often arise in the reproductive tract but may also develop in some other locations. Because a teratoma may be either benign or malignant, one must specify the type, calling the tumor either a benign teratoma or a malignant teratoma (FIGURE 14). A common type of cystic benign teratoma arising in the ovary is usually called a **dermoid cyst** (FIGURE 15).

Teratoma
(tăr-uh-tō′muh)
A tumor of mixed cell components.

Dermoid cyst
(derm′oyd)
A common type of benign cystic teratoma that commonly arises in the ovary.

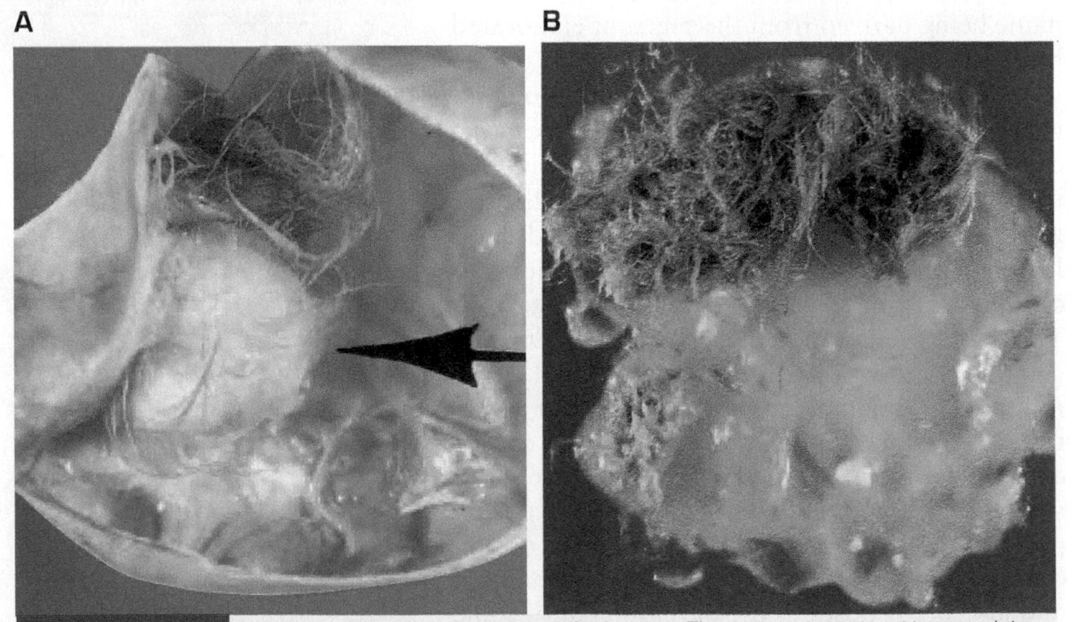

FIGURE 15 **A**, Cystic teratoma (dermoid cyst) of ovary. The cyst is lined by skin containing sweat and sebaceous (oil secreting) glands, and the skin surface is covered by hair. The *arrow* indicates a nodule in the cyst wall containing fat, muscle, and bone. **B**, Contents of cyst, consisting of matted hair and oil derived from skin lining the cyst.

Childhood Primitive Cell Tumors

Certain unusual and relatively rare tumors encountered in children may arise in the brain, retina of the eye, adrenal gland, kidney, liver, or genital tract. Primitive cell tumors of this type are named from the site of origin, with the suffix *-blastoma* added (*blast* = a primitive cell + *oma* = tumor). Thus, a primitive cell tumor arising from the retina of the eye is a retinoblastoma (FIGURE 16) and one of hepatic origin is called a hepatoblastoma. A primitive cell tumor of the kidney, however, is usually called a **Wilms tumor** rather than a nephroblastoma.

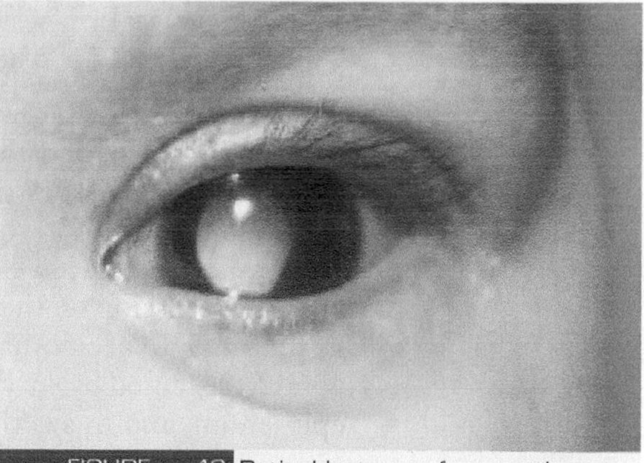

FIGURE 16 Retinoblastoma of an eye that appears as a pale mass of tissue seen through the dilated pupil.

Wilms tumor
A malignant renal tumor of infants and children.

NECROSIS IN TUMORS

Tumors derive their blood supply from the tissues they invade. Malignant tumors frequently induce new blood vessels to proliferate in the adjacent normal tissues to supply the demands of the growing tumor. However, a malignant tumor may outgrow its blood supply. When this occurs, the parts of the tumor with the poorest blood supply undergo necrosis (FIGURE 17). If the tumor is growing within an organ such as the lung or kidney and is surrounded by normal tissue, the blood supply is best at the junction of tumor and adjacent normal tissue and poorest in the center of the tumor, which often degenerates. In contrast, if the malignant tumor is growing outward from an epithelial surface, such as the colon, the best blood supply is at the base of the tumor. The poorest blood supply is at the surface, which frequently becomes necrotic and sloughs, leaving a shallow crater covered with degenerated tissue and inflammatory exudate (FIGURE 18). Often, small blood vessels are exposed in the ulcerated base of the tumor. Blood may ooze continuously from these vessels, eventually leading to anemia from chronic blood loss. Sometimes the ulcerated tumor may be the source of a severe hemorrhage.

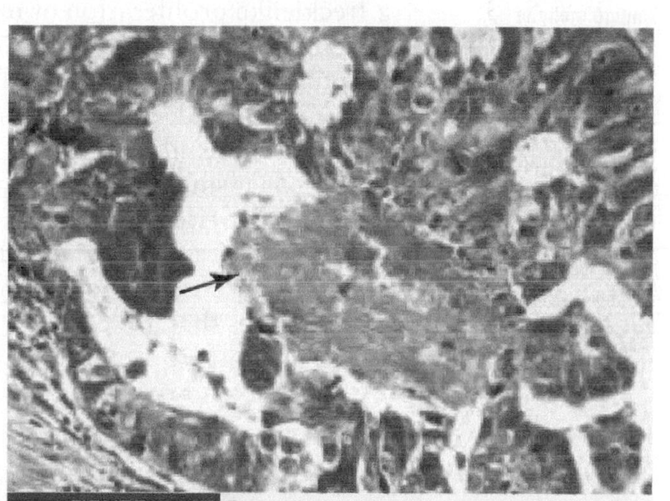

FIGURE 17 Central necrosis (*arrow*) within cells of a breast carcinoma arising from duct epithelium.

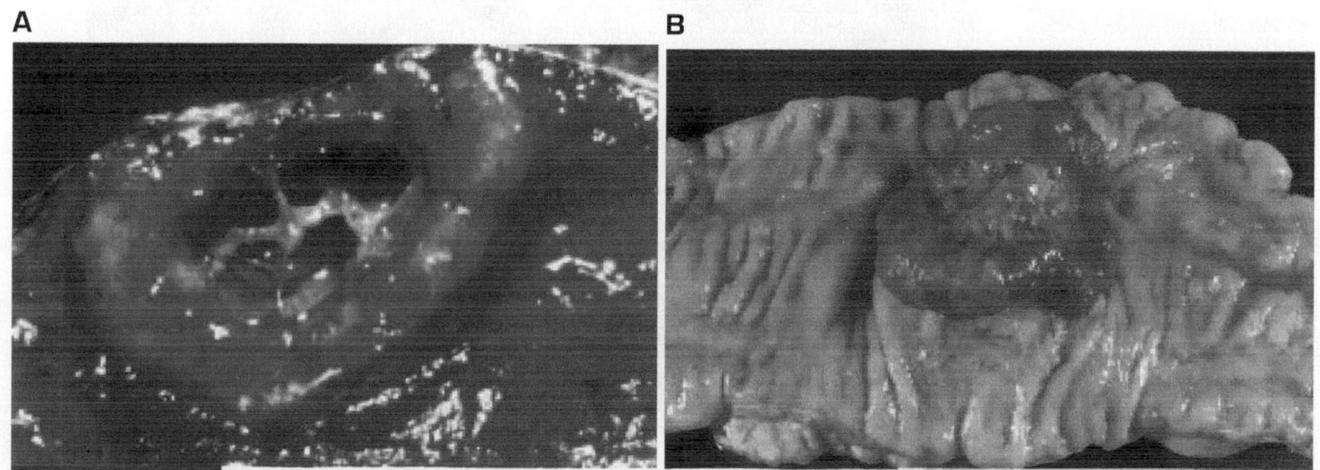

FIGURE 18 **A**, Carcinoma of lung with central necrosis. **B**, Carcinoma of colon exhibiting superficial ulceration.

NONINFILTRATING (IN SITU) CARCINOMA

Infiltration and metastasis are two characteristic features of malignant tumors. However, we now know that many carcinomas arising from surface epithelium remain localized within the epithelium for many years before evidence of infiltration into the deeper tissues or spread to distant sites becomes apparent. This has been well documented for squamous cell carcinoma of the cervix (FIGURE 19). Noninfiltrating tumors have also been recognized in many other locations, including the breast (discussion on the breast), urinary tract, colon, and skin. The term carcinoma in situ (in-site carcinoma) is used for this type of neoplasm. In situ carcinoma can be completely cured by surgical excision or other treatment that eradicates the abnormal epithelium, and this is the stage most favorable to successful treatment.

PRECANCEROUS CONDITIONS

Actinic keratosis
(ak-ti′-nik ke-rä-tō′sis)
A precancerous warty proliferation of squamous epithelial cells in sun-damaged skin of older persons.

Lentigo maligna
A precancerous, pigmented skin lesion arising from proliferation of atypical melanin-producing epithelial cells (melanocytes).

Leukoplakia
A white patch of hyperplastic and usually atypical squamous epithelium on the oral mucosa or genital tract mucosa.

Sometimes the term precancerous is used when referring to conditions that have a high likelihood of eventually developing into cancer. Prolonged exposure to sunlight, for example, not only causes premature aging of the skin, but also causes small, crusted, scaly patches to develop on sun-exposed skin called **actinic keratoses** ("actinic" refers to sun rays). Untreated, many keratoses eventually develop into skin cancers. Another precancerous condition resulting from prolonged sun exposure is a frecklelike proliferation of melanin-producing cells in the skin called **lentigo maligna** (a Latin term meaning "malignant freckle"). They are so named because many eventually become transformed into melanomas. Precancerous, thick white patches descriptively called **leukoplakia** (*leuko* = white + *plakia* = patch) may develop in the mucous membranes of the mouth as a result of exposure to tobacco tars from pipe or cigar smoking or from use of smokeless tobacco (snuff and chewing tobacco) and may give rise to squamous cell cancers of the oral cavity. Somewhat similar precancerous changes may take place in the epithelium of the vulva (discussion on the female reproductive system) and may eventuate into vulvar cancer. Some types of colon polyps that are prone to malignant change also are considered precancerous. There are many precancerous conditions, of which these are only a few examples.

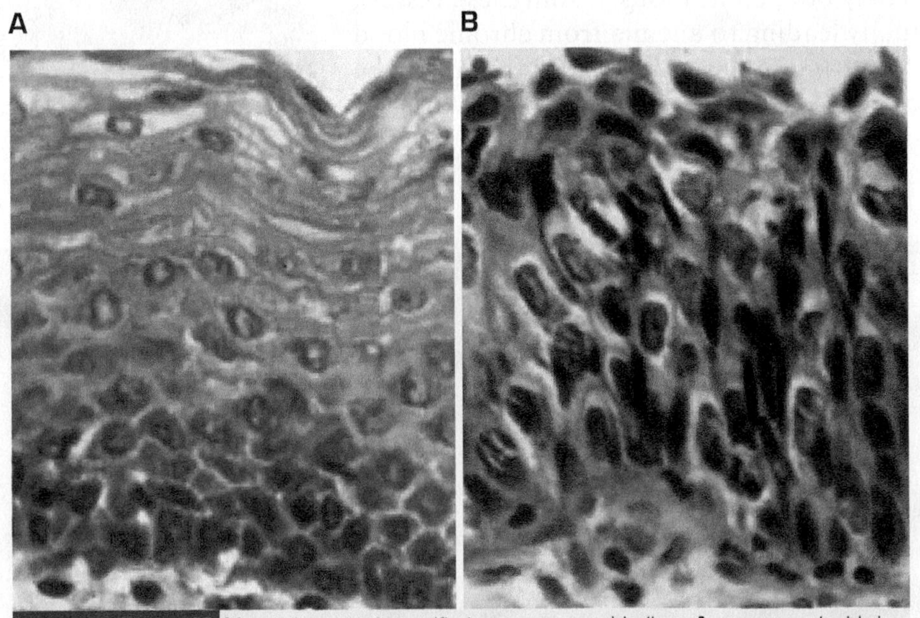

FIGURE 19 Normal cervical stratified squamous epithelium **A**, compared with in situ carcinoma of cervix **B**. Note the nuclear abnormalities characteristic of carcinoma. The tumor has not yet infiltrated the underlying tissues (original magnification × 400).

Precancerous conditions should always be treated appropriately in order to prevent malignant change, which occurs in many, but not all, cases.

Etiologic Factors in Neoplastic Disease

VIRUSES

Many types of tumors in animals are caused by viruses and can be readily transmitted by appropriate methods to animals of the same or a different species. In some instances, a single type of virus is capable of producing many different types of tumors in various species of animals. At least some of the cancers in humans also appear to be caused by viruses. Some unusual types of leukemia and lymphoma are caused by a virus called the human T cell leukemia–lymphoma virus (HTLV-1), which is related to the virus that causes the acquired immune deficiency syndrome (AIDS). Kaposi's sarcoma in AIDS patients is caused by a herpes virus, designated human herpesvirus 8 (HHV-8). Some strains of the papilloma virus that cause genital condylomas (discussion on the female reproductive system) appear to predispose to cervical carcinoma and are also responsible for some squamous cell carcinomas of the mouth, throat, and larynx (oropharyngeal carcinomas). Chronic viral hepatitis (discussion on the liver and the biliary system) predisposes to primary carcinoma of the liver. Some types of nasophyngeal carcinoma and some types of lymphoma appear to be related to Epstein-Barr virus infections, the virus that causes infectious mononucleosis.

GENE AND CHROMOSOMAL ABNORMALITIES

The basic process common to all neoplasms is an alteration of the genes on the chromosomes of a cell so that the cell no longer responds to normal control mechanisms and proceeds to proliferate without regard for the needs of the body. In the body, many billions of cells are dividing all the time. They are also continually subjected to radiation, various chemical carcinogens (cancer-producing substances), or other agents that can alter the structure of genes. A change in the gene's structure is called a **mutation** (*muto* = change), and the mutated gene may function differently from a normal gene.

Three large groups of genes play important roles in regulating cell functions, and derangements of these genes are associated with formation of tumors. The first group comprises **proto-oncogenes.** The second group consists of **tumor suppressor genes**, and the third group is the **DNA repair genes** (TABLE 4).

Mutation
(mū-tā′shun)
An alteration in a base sequence in DNA; may alter cell function. Transmitted from parents to offspring only if mutation is in gametes.

Proto-oncogene
(pro-to-on′-koh-jēn)
A normal gene that regulates some aspect of cell growth, maturation, or division.

Tumor suppressor gene
A gene that suppresses cell proliferation.

DNA repair genes
Genes that monitor and correct errors in DNA replication during cell division.

TABLE 4

Gene mutations that disrupt cell function

Gene	Normal function	Malfunction
Proto-oncogene	Promotes normal cell growth	Point mutation, amplification, or translocation forms an oncogene, resulting in unrestrained cell growth
Paired tumor suppressor genes	Inhibit cell proliferation	Both genes inactivated in same cell promotes cell proliferation
Paired DNA repair genes	Correct errors in DNA duplication	Gene inactivation increases mutation rate

Proto-Oncogenes

Human chromosomes contain a number of normal "growth genes" that promote some aspect of cell growth, differentiation, or mitotic activity. They are called proto-oncogenes; they are closely related to genes carried by viruses that cause tumors in experimental animals, and they are named from the tumor viruses that they resemble. A proto-oncogene is a normal gene that regulates some normal growth function in a cell, but a proto-oncogene can undergo a mutation or become translocated to another chromosome where its functions are deranged. Either event can convert a normally functioning proto-oncogene into an **oncogene** (*onkos* = tumor), an abnormally functioning gene that stimulates cell growth excessively and leads to unrestrained cell proliferation. An oncogene is a "gene that causes cancer."

Oncogene
(on′-koh-jēn)
An abnormally functioning gene that causes unrestrained cell growth leading to formation of a tumor. Results from mutation or translocation of a proto-oncogene.

Conversion of a proto-oncogene into an oncogene (activation of an oncogene) may consist of a change in only a single nucleotide in the DNA of the gene, which is called a point mutation, or the mutation may generate multiple copies of the same gene, called gene amplification, which greatly increases the activity of the gene. Translocation to another chromosome activates an oncogene because of the way in which genes are related on individual chromosomes. A specific gene, such as one that regulates some aspect of cell growth or mitotic activity, is influenced by other nearby genes that either suppress or stimulate its activities. Cell growth and differentiation are normal when the proto-oncogene ("growth gene") and its neighbors function together in an orderly manner, but may be deranged if this relation is disturbed. For example, the translocation may bring the proto-oncogene to a new location on another chromosome where it is freed from the inhibitory genes that formerly controlled its activities. Alternatively, the translocation may bring the proto-oncogene to a new location on another chromosome adjacent to another gene that stimulates its functions.

Tumor Suppressor Genes

These are groups of different genes that function to suppress cell proliferation. Loss of suppressor gene function by mutation or another event disrupts cell functions and can lead to unrestrained cell growth. Suppressor genes exist in pairs at corresponding gene loci on homologous chromosomes, and both suppressor genes must cease to function before the cell malfunctions.

Tumor suppressor genes may also play a role in determining how many times a cell can divide before it involutes and dies. In some cases, loss of a tumor suppressor gene function may allow the cell to proliferate indefinitely rather than dying after a predetermined number of cell divisions, as normal cells do.

Loss of function of specific tumor suppressor genes has been correlated with specific tumors, and the suppressor genes are often named from the tumors with which they have been associated.

DNA Repair Genes

DNA repair genes are part of the cell's "quality control" and repair system. These genes regulate the processes that monitor and repair any errors in DNA duplication that may occur when the cell's chromosomes are duplicated in the course of cell division; they are also concerned with the repair of DNA that has been damaged by radiation, chemicals, or other environmental agents. Any change in the normal arrangement of DNA nucleotides on the DNA chain constitutes a DNA mutation. Consequently, failure of DNA repair gene function increases the likelihood of DNA mutations within the affected cell. A high mutation rate within cells predisposes to tumors because some mutations may affect cell functions that promote unrestrained cell growth.

Like tumor suppressor genes, DNA repair genes also exist in pairs in homologous chromosomes, and both must become nonfunctional before the repair functions regulated by the genes are compromised. Persons with an inherited mutation of a DNA repair gene are at increased risk of some tumors because if a spontaneous mutation of the other gene occurs, the affected cell is no longer able to regulate cell growth properly. Uncontrolled cell proliferation results and gives rise to a tumor.

Genes Regulating Apoptosis

Another group of genes plays a more limited role in regulating cell functions by influencing the survival time of cells. Normal cells live for a variable period of time, depending on the cell type. Then the cell dies and is replaced by a new cell. The predetermined death of a cell is regulated by genes within the cell and is called programmed cell death or **apoptosis**. If the genes regulating programmed cell death fail to function properly, the cells don't die as they should and continue to accumulate, eventually forming a tumor. Some lymphoid tumors, for example, appear to result primarily from an accumulation of long-surviving lymphocytes within lymph nodes rather than excessively rapid proliferation of lymphocytes.

Apoptosis
(ah-pop-toe′-sis, or ah-po-toe′-sis)
Programmed cell death that occurs after a cell has lived its normal life span.

Multistep Progression of Genetic Changes Leading to Cancer In most cases, cancers do not result from mutation of a single gene, but rather are the result of multiple genetic "insults" to the genome characterized by activation of oncogenes along with loss of function of one or more tumor suppressor genes. The transition, for example, from a benign polyp of the colon to an invasive colon cancer requires activation of an oncogene (called ras) and inactivation of three distinct tumor suppressor genes (designated *APC*, *DCC*, and *p53*).

After a cell has been deregulated and has formed a tumor, additional random genetic changes may take place in the tumor cells, which is indicative of the instability of the tumor cell genome. Often, individual genes may undergo additional mutations or they may reduplicate themselves by gene amplification, forming multiple copies of a single gene. Chromosomes may fragment; pieces of chromosomes may be lost from the cells or be translocated to other chromosomes. Some of these mutations in the unstable tumor cell genome may produce new mutant cells that exhibit more aggressive growth than the original tumor cells, and the new mutant may eventually outgrow the other cells in the tumor. Clinically, this event may be manifested by more rapid growth and aggressive behavior of the tumor, and often the tumor may become less responsive to the anticancer drugs that formerly could control it.

Chromosomal Abnormalities Not all gene alterations that activate oncogenes or inactivate tumor suppressor genes can be identified from examination of the tumor cell chromosomes. Point mutations do not change chromosome structure, but translocations relocate large pieces of chromosomes and change their structure, as do deletions of chromosome material and amplification of individual genes. Some chromosomal abnormalities occur quite frequently in specific tumors and may be of diagnostic value. Others may give some indication of how aggressively a tumor may behave. The best-known neoplasm-associated chromosomal abnormality, which is called Philadelphia or Ph1 chromosome (named after the city where it was discovered), can be demonstrated in the white cells of patients with chronic granulocytic leukemia (described in the section on leukemia). The abnormality is a reciprocal translocation of broken end pieces between chromosomes 9 and 22. In this translocation, a proto-oncogene (designed *abl*) on chromosome 9 is moved to a position on chromosome 22. There it becomes fused with another gene (called *bcr*) to form

Tyrosine kinase
Enzyme that produces multiple effects concerned with cell growth and cell division.

a composite gene (*bcr/abl*) that directs the synthesis of an uncontrolled extremely active **tyrosine kinase** enzyme that produces multiple effects concerned with cell growth and cell division. It is the excessive unregulated activity of this enzyme that stimulates the unrestrained proliferation of white blood cells characteristic of chronic granulocytic leukemia (FIGURE 20). The same type of translocation also occurs in some patients with acute lymphocytic leukemia, but the composite gene *bcr/abl* resulting from the translocation is slightly different, which leads to a different and more aggressive type of lymphoma.

FAILURE OF IMMUNOLOGIC DEFENSES

The basic processes common to all neoplasms are gene mutations within a cell that deregulate the cell, causing it to proliferate abnormally. Many environmental factors can induce mutations. A mutant cell often produces different cell proteins not present in a normal cell. These mutant-gene–encoded proteins are recognized as abnormal by the immune system, which attempts to destroy the abnormal cell by means of various cell-mediated and humoral mechanisms. Apparently, mutations leading to neoplastic transformation of cells are relatively common, but the body recognizes the altered cells as abnormal and destroys them as soon as they are formed. Only a tiny percentage of abnormal cells ever develop into clinically apparent tumors. Therefore, one may consider a tumor to manifest in part a failure of the body's immune defenses. This concept is supported by evidence that individuals with congenital deficiencies of immunologic defense mechanisms have a higher than expected incidence of tumors. Tumors also occur frequently in persons whose immune responses have been deliberately suppressed by drugs or other substances.

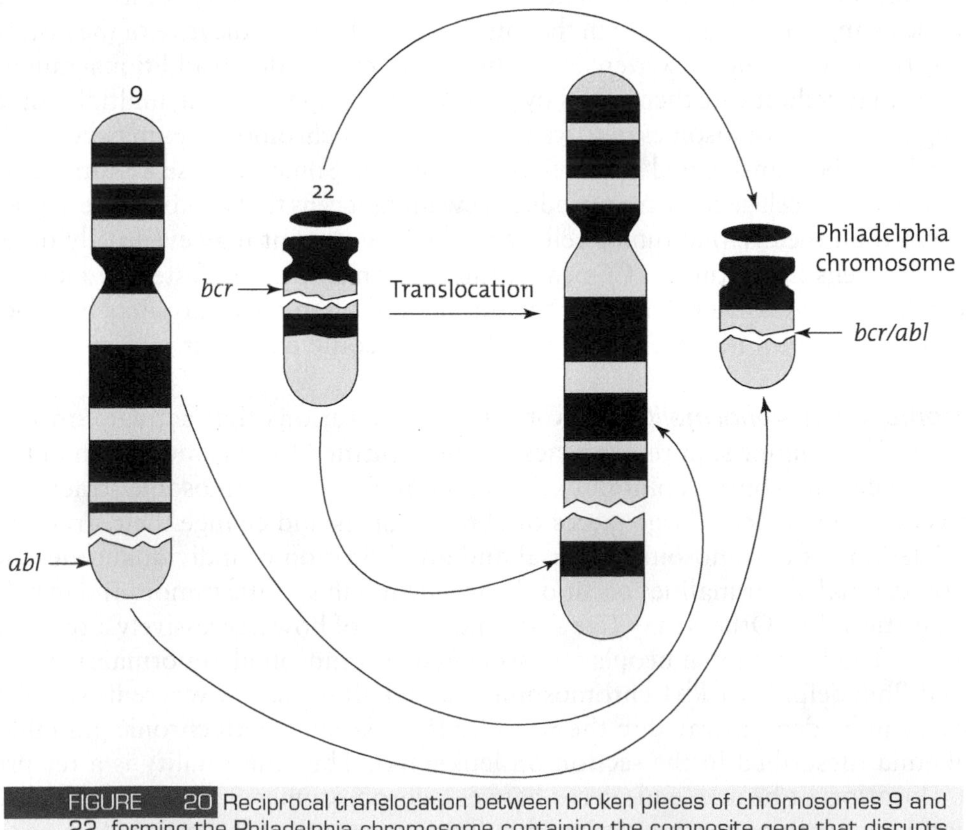

FIGURE 20 Reciprocal translocation between broken pieces of chromosomes 9 and 22, forming the Philadelphia chromosome containing the composite gene that disrupts normal cell functions.

FIGURE 21 illustrates the interrelation of the factors concerned with the defense against tumors. On one hand, abnormal cells arise and tend to proliferate, leading to tumors. On the other hand, the immune–defense mechanisms destroy these abnormal cells before they can prove hazardous to the body. Tumors result when the defense mechanisms fail. Fortunately, in most instances, the immune surveillance system eliminates the "bad" cells as soon as they appear. Although the immune-defense mechanisms are quite efficient in eliminating abnormal cells before they develop into a tumor, they are much less effective in eliminating an established tumor.

HEREDITY AND TUMORS

Although there is no strong hereditary predisposition to most common malignant tumors, hereditary factors do play a small role in some common tumors. A person whose parent or sibling has been afflicted with a breast, colon, or lung carcinoma has about a three times greater risk of developing a similar tumor than do other people. The predisposition is apparently the result of a multifactorial inheritance pattern in which the individual at risk has inherited sets of genes that influence some hormonal- or enzyme-regulated biochemical process within the body that slightly increases the susceptibility to a specific cancer. The increased risk may be caused by genetic

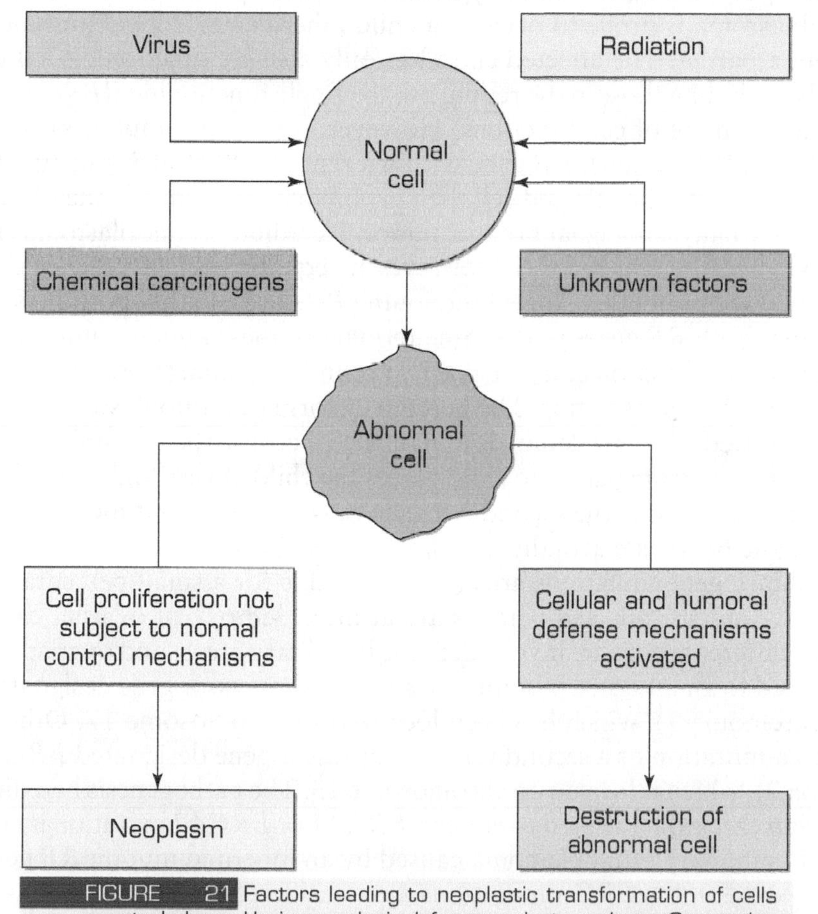

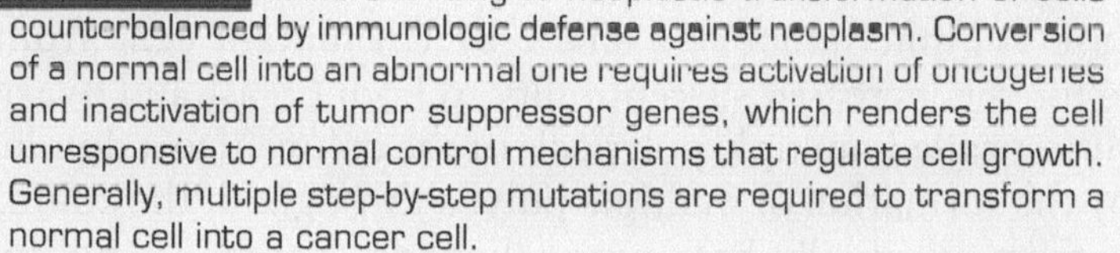

FIGURE 21 Factors leading to neoplastic transformation of cells counterbalanced by immunologic defense against neoplasm. Conversion of a normal cell into an abnormal one requires activation of oncogenes and inactivation of tumor suppressor genes, which renders the cell unresponsive to normal control mechanisms that regulate cell growth. Generally, multiple step-by-step mutations are required to transform a normal cell into a cancer cell.

differences in various biochemical or physiologic activities that influence cell functions, such as

1. Differences in circulating hormone levels that could influence cell growth rates
2. Variations in the rate at which the cell can metabolize and inactivate cancer-causing chemicals to which the cells are exposed
3. Variations in the ability to repair DNA that has been damaged by injurious agents
4. Variations in the efficiency of the immune system in eliminating abnormal cells as they arise

Heredity does play an important role in some tumors. The classic example is retinoblastoma, an uncommon childhood tumor illustrated in Figure 16. This tumor is also a typical example of how tumor suppressor genes control cell function and how loss of control can cause a tumor. Retinoblastoma is a malignant tumor of primitive retinal cells occurring in infants and children that is caused by loss of function of tumor suppressor genes called *RB* genes. Normal *RB* genes exist in pairs, one on each of the homologous pair of chromosome 13, and both *RB* genes must be nonfunctional in a retinal cell before a tumor arises. About half the retinoblastomas are hereditary; the rest occur sporadically, without any hereditary predisposition. The hereditary form of retinoblastoma is prone to occur if a child inherits a defective nonfunctional *RB* gene from a parent. The affected child has only a single functioning *RB* gene in all body cells, including those in the retina, but the single functioning *RB* gene is sufficient to maintain control of cell functions. However, if a chance mutation occurs in the remaining single functional *RB* gene within a retinal cell, all *RB* gene function in the affected cell is lost. The affected cell then proliferates to form a clone of unregulated cells and eventually a malignant retinal tumor. Hereditary retinoblastomas may occur in both eyes because retinal cells in both eyes are equally vulnerable to similar random *RB* gene mutations in other single functioning *RB* genes. In the sporadic form of retinoblastoma, both *RB* genes in the same retinal cell must undergo mutation in order to deregulate cell function and give rise to a retinoblastoma. FIGURE 22 summarizes the pathogenesis of this tumor. The hereditary form of retinoblastoma is considered to be transmitted as a Mendelian dominant trait because the transmission of a single defective *RB* gene from parent to child places the child at very high risk of developing this tumor, even though the second *RB* gene must become nonfunctional in a retinal cell before the neoplasm actually arises.

Hereditary gene mutations are also responsible for a small percentage of breast carcinomas, and the affected persons are at increased risk of ovarian carcinoma as well. Two different genes are involved. Some hereditary breast and ovarian carcinomas can be traced to an inherited mutation of a tumor suppressor gene designated *BRCA1* (breast carcinoma 1), which has been localized to chromosome 17. Other cases are related to a mutation of a second tumor suppressor gene designated *BRCA2* (breast carcinoma 2), which is located on chromosome 13. The pathogenesis hereditary breast and ovarian carcinoma related to either a *BRCA1* or *BRCA2* mutation is comparable to that of hereditary retinoblastoma caused by an inherited mutant *RB* gene as illustrated in FIGURE 22. *BRCA* mutations are considered to be inherited as dominant traits because the inheritance of a single *BRCA* mutant gene from either parent is responsible for the increased susceptibility to both breast and ovarian carcinomas.

A condition called multiple polyposis of the colon, also a dominant trait, is characterized by the formation of multiple polyps throughout the colon, and usually one or more of them eventually becomes malignant. Another condition transmitted as

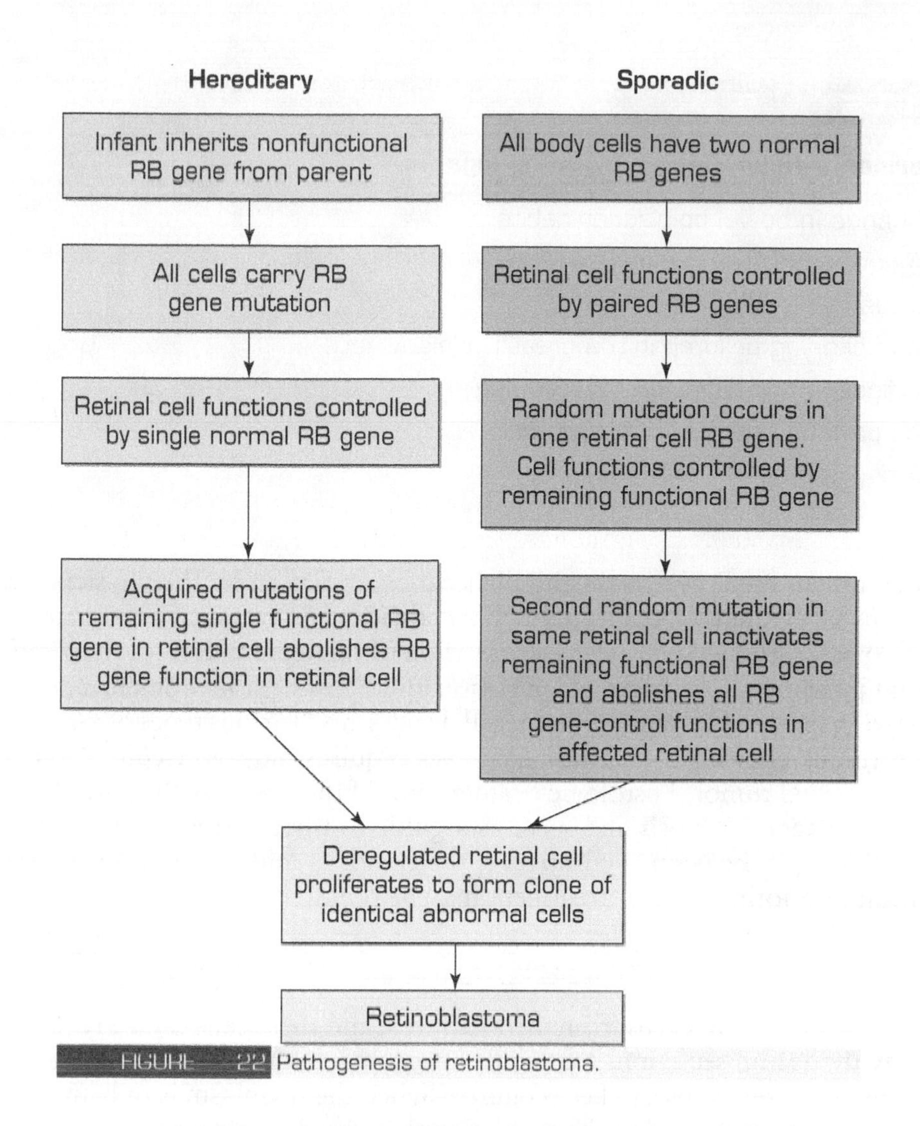

FIGURE 22 Pathogenesis of retinoblastoma.

an autosomal dominant trait is called multiple neurofibromatosis (discussion on the nervous system). Many of the nerves throughout the body give rise to benign tumors called neurofibromas, and often one of these tumors eventually undergoes malignant change. Still, another hereditary tumor syndrome, also an autosomal dominant transmission, is called multiple endocrine adenomatosis and is characterized by the formation of adenomas arising in several different endocrine glands, as the name indicates.

There are many other examples of tumors related to hereditary gene mutations, but it is important to remember that they make up only a small fraction of the benign and malignant tumors afflicting humans.

Diagnosis of Tumors

EARLY RECOGNITION OF NEOPLASMS

The American Cancer Society publicizes a number of signs and symptoms that should arouse suspicion of cancer (TABLE 5). In general, any abnormality of form or function may be an early symptom of a neoplasm and should be investigated by a physician. For example, a lump in the breast, an ulcer on the lip, or a change in the character of a wart or mole may be considered an abnormality of form. Menstrual bleeding in a postmenopausal woman or a change in bowel habits manifested by constipation or diarrhea is an abnormality of function.

TABLE 5

American Cancer Society warning signals

1.	Change in bowel or bladder habits
2.	A sore that does not heal
3.	Unusual bleeding or discharge
4.	A thickening or lump in the breast or elsewhere
5.	Indigestion or difficulty in swallowing
6.	An obvious change in wart or mole
7.	A nagging cough or hoarseness

A complete medical history and physical examination by the physician are the next steps in evaluating suspected abnormalities. The physical examination may include special studies such as an examination of the rectum and colon by means of a special instrument, a vaginal examination and Pap smear in women, examination of the esophagus and stomach with special devices, and various types of x-ray studies.

If a tumor is discovered, exact diagnosis requires biopsy or complete excision of the suspected tumor. Histologic examination of the tissue by the pathologist will provide an exact diagnosis and serve as a guide to further treatment. If the tumor is benign, simple excision is curative. If the tumor is malignant, a more extensive operation or another kind of treatment may be required.

CYTOLOGIC DIAGNOSIS OF NEOPLASMS

Tumors shed abnormal cells from their surfaces, and these cells can be recognized in the body fluids and secretions that come into contact with the tumor (FIGURE 23). Often the abnormal cells can be recognized when the neoplasm is only microscopic in size and is still confined to the surface epithelium. These observations have been applied to the cytologic diagnosis of tumors. The method is named after the physician who played a large part in developing and applying cytologic methods, Dr. George Papanicolaou. The microscopic slides of the material prepared for cytologic examination are called Papanicolaou smears or, simply, **Pap smears.**

Pap smear
A study of cells from various sources, commonly used as a screening test for cancer.

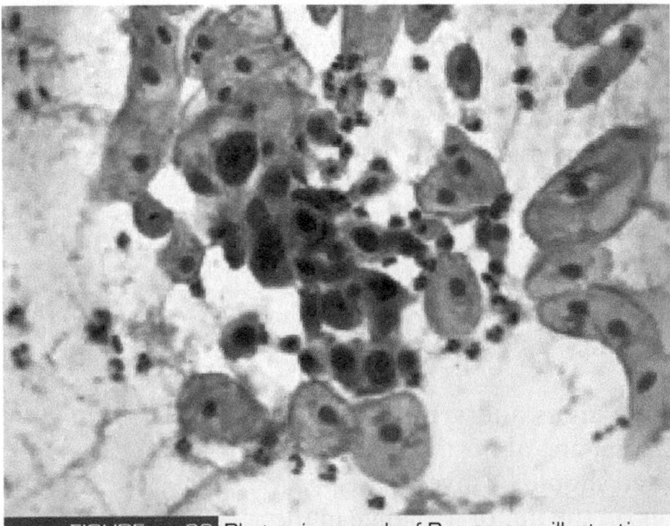

FIGURE 23 Photomicrograph of Pap smear, illustrating cluster of abnormal cells from in situ carcinoma of cervix. Cells appear much different from adjacent normal squamous epithelial cells (original magnification × 160).

In carcinoma of the uterine cervix, abnormal cells can often be found in the vaginal secretions. They are more readily identified, however, in smears prepared from material that has been gently scraped from the epithelium of the cervix surrounding the cervical opening (external os) by means of a small, disposable wooden spatula. Usually, secretions for study are also obtained from the cervical canal at the same time. Widespread application of cytologic methods has led to much earlier detection of cervical carcinoma than had previously been possible and has played a significant role in reducing mortality from carcinoma of the uterine cervix. Cytologic methods can also be applied to the diagnosis of neoplasms in other locations by examining sputum, urine, breast secretions, and fluids obtained from the pleural or peritoneal cavities. However, cytology has been most valuable in the early diagnosis of cervical cancer. It should be emphasized, however, that an abnormal cervical Pap smear indicates only that the cervical epithelium is shedding atypical or abnormal cells. It does not necessarily indicate a diagnosis of cancer because some benign diseases are occasionally associated with desquamation of atypical cells. A Pap smear should be considered as a screening procedure, and an atypical or abnormal smear should be followed by further studies, which may include a biopsy and histologic examination of the tissue to establish an exact diagnosis. This subject is considered further in the discussion on the female reproductive system.

Cytologic Diagnosis by Fine-Needle Aspiration

Cells for cytologic study can also be obtained by aspirating material from organs or tissues by means of a fine needle attached to a syringe and preparing slides from the aspirated material. This technique is often used to evaluate nodules in the thyroid or breast, and often one can determine whether the nodule is benign or malignant from the appearance of the aspirated cells, avoiding the need for a biopsy. Suspected tumors in the lung, liver, pancreas, kidney, and other internal organs also can be examined by fine-needle aspiration. When attempting aspiration from internal organs, one must precisely determine the location of the suspected tumor by means of a CT scan or other x-ray examination or by ultrasound and insert the needle into the suspected tumor under x-ray guidance. In general, the diagnostic accuracy of fine-needle aspiration is not as good as an actual biopsy but often is adequate for diagnosis and avoids a major surgical operation, which would be required to obtain tissue for biopsy.

FROZEN-SECTION DIAGNOSIS OF NEOPLASMS

Many times, it is important that a surgeon learn immediately whether a tumor discovered in the course of an operation is benign or malignant because the extent of resection performed may depend on the nature of the neoplasm. Often, the surgeon must also find out during the operation whether a tumor has been excised completely or whether it has spread to lymph nodes or distant sites. A pathologist can provide the surgeon with a rapid histologic diagnosis and other information by means of a special technique called a **frozen section**. In this method, a portion of the tumor or other tissue to be examined histologically is frozen solid at a subzero temperature. A thin section of the frozen tissue is cut by means of a special instrument called a microtome, and slides are prepared and stained. The slides can then be examined by the pathologist, and a rapid histologic diagnosis can be made. The entire procedure takes only a few minutes.

Frozen section
A method of rapid diagnosis of tumors used by the pathologist; tissue is frozen solid, cut into thin sections, stained, and examined microscopically.

TUMOR-ASSOCIATED ANTIGEN TESTS

Some cancers secrete substances called **tumor-associated antigens**. These are either absent from normal mature tissues or present only in trace amounts. Most tumor-associated antigens are carbohydrate–protein complexes (glycoproteins) that are secreted as a coating on the surface of the cancer cells. Some of the glycoprotein gains access to the circulation, where it can be detected by means of specialized laboratory tests performed on the blood of patients with cancer.

A well-known tumor-associated antigen is a substance called **carcinoembryonic antigen (CEA)**, so named because it resembles a glycoprotein antigen secreted by the cells lining the fetal intestinal tract. It has been postulated that cancer cells elaborate CEA because they are immature and have acquired some properties of fetal cells that adult cells do not have (FIGURE 24).

Tumor-associated antigen
An antigen associated with growing tumor cells, which serves as an indicator of tumor growth in the body.

Carcinoembryonic antigen (CEA)
(kär′sin-ō-em-bry-on′ik)
A tumor-associated antigen that resembles the antigen secreted by the cells of the fetal gastrointestinal tract.

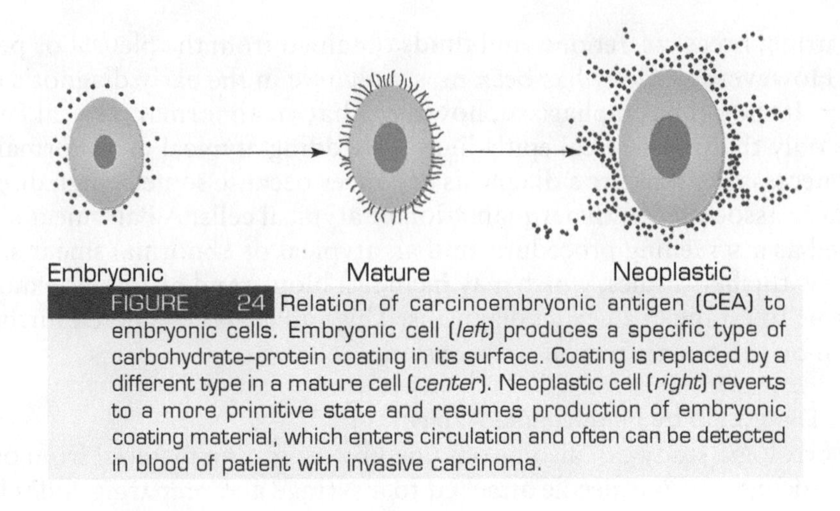

FIGURE 24 Relation of carcinoembryonic antigen (CEA) to embryonic cells. Embryonic cell (*left*) produces a specific type of carbohydrate–protein coating in its surface. Coating is replaced by a different type in a mature cell (*center*). Neoplastic cell (*right*) reverts to a more primitive state and resumes production of embryonic coating material, which enters circulation and often can be detected in blood of patient with invasive carcinoma.

Alpha fetoprotein (al′fuh fē′tō-prō′tēn) *Protein produced by fetal liver early in gestation. Sometimes produced by tumor cells. Level is elevated in amnionic fluid when fetus has neural tube defect.*

Human chorionic gonadotropin (HGC) (kōr-ō-on′ik gō-na-dō-trō′pin) *A hormone made by the placenta in pregnancy having actions similar to pituitary gonadotropins. Same hormone is made by neoplastic cells in some types of malignant testicular tumors.*

Not all malignant tumors secrete CEA. Moreover, elevation of CEA levels is not specific for any one type of cancer. CEA is produced by most malignant tumors of the gastrointestinal tract and pancreas, but it is also secreted by many cancers of the breast and lung and by other cancers as well. The amount of CEA secreted is related to the size of the tumor. CEA is usually not elevated in the blood of persons with small, early cancers, but the levels are often quite high in persons with large tumors or tumors that have metastasized. When CEA is elevated in a patient with cancer, the level falls after the tumor has been removed and often rises again if the tumor recurs or metastasizes (FIGURE 25). One can perform serial determinations of CEA to monitor the course of patients with CEA-secreting tumors. If CEA falls after removal of the tumor and later becomes elevated, this usually means that the tumor has recurred and indicates that additional treatment is needed. Slight elevations of CEA are sometimes detected in patients with diseases other than cancer. This does not detract from the usefulness of the CEA test, however, because the CEA levels are usually much lower than in patients with malignant tumors.

Other products secreted by tumor cells that can be used to monitor tumor growth are discussed in the discussion on the male reproductive system. They include **alpha fetoprotein**, a protein produced by fetal tissues but not normally produced by adult cells, and **human chorionic gonadotropin**, the hormone normally produced by the

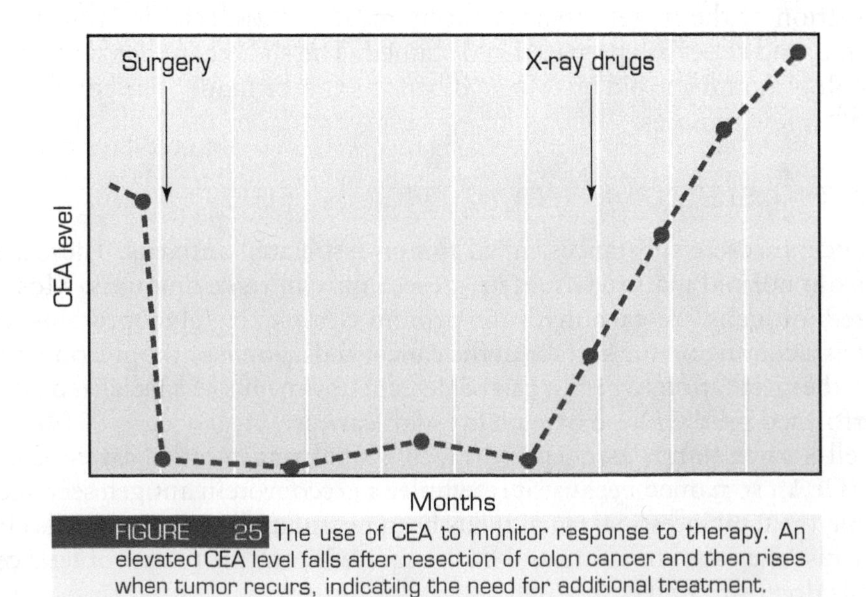

FIGURE 25 The use of CEA to monitor response to therapy. An elevated CEA level falls after resection of colon cancer and then rises when tumor recurs, indicating the need for additional treatment.

placenta in pregnancy, which are often elevated in patients with testicular carcinoma. Alpha fetoprotein is also frequently elevated in patients with primary carcinoma of the liver. Prostatic-specific antigen (PSA), produced by prostatic epithelial cells, often is elevated in the bloodstream of men with prostatic carcinoma. The PSA test often is used as a screening test to detect early prostate carcinoma before symptoms develop and also to monitor the response to treatment. Many other tumor-associated substances have been described (sometimes called tumor markers), which are used to monitor patients with various types of lung, breast, and ovarian carcinoma.

Treatment of Tumors

Benign tumors are completely cured by surgical excision. Malignant tumors are much more difficult to treat. Four major forms of treatment are directed against malignant tumors:

1. Surgery
2. Radiotherapy
3. Hormones
4. Anticancer drugs (chemotherapy)

The method of treatment depends on the type of tumor and its extent, and sometimes several methods are combined. In many cases, treatment eradicates the cancer, and the patient is cured. In less favorable cases, cure is no longer possible, but the growth of the cancer is arrested and life is prolonged. Before a course of treatment is selected, usually further information is needed, which is obtained by grading and staging the tumor, as described in the following section.

GRADING AND STAGING MALIGNANT TUMORS

After a biopsy has established the diagnosis of a malignant tumor, the selection of the appropriate treatment is based on the characteristics of the tumor cells and the extent of the tumor. Grading the tumor is attempting to predict the behavior of the tumor from the biopsy material based on the differentiation of the tumor cells, their growth rate based on the number of mitoses, and any characteristics of the tumor cells that would influence the type of treatment selected, such as the response of the tumor cells to estrogen in the case of a breast carcinoma (as described in the discussion on the breast). Staging the tumor is determining whether the tumor is still localized or has spread to regional lymph nodes or distant sites, which is very useful additional information to guide selection of the best treatment. For example, a small well-differentiated breast carcinoma that responds to estrogen and has not spread to the regional lymph nodes would be treated differently from a large, poorly differentiated carcinoma that does not respond to estrogen and has already spread to distant sites. Often, the various characteristics of a tumor identified by grading and staging are expressed in a classification called the TNM system. The *T* refers to the characteristics of the tumor, which is graded in terms of tumor size and differentiation as T1 through T4, with T0 used to indicate a noninvasive (in situ) carcinoma. *N* refers to the spread of tumor to regional lymph nodes, with N0 indicating no spread, and N1 through N3 indicating progressively greater lymph node spread. *M* refers to distant metastasis, with M0 indicating no distant spread and M1 and M2 indicating progressively more extensive distant metastases.

Grading and staging are useful not only for selecting treatment, but also as an indication of prognosis as well as being useful in clinical research studies. For example, if a study were evaluating the effectiveness of a new anticancer chemotherapy treatment in one group of patients compared with the response to the current treatment method in another group, both groups of patients should have the same TNM classification to ensure that any difference in response to treatment was based on the treatment and not on differences in the stage of disease between the two patient groups.

SURGERY

Many malignant tumors are treated by wide surgical excision of the tumor and the surrounding tissues, usually with removal of the regional lymph nodes that drain the tumor site. This treatment is successful if the tumor has not already spread to distant sites. Unfortunately, many cancers have already metastasized when first detected and may no longer be curable by surgery alone. Other methods of treatment must be used—frequently in combination with surgery.

RADIOTHERAPY

Malignant lymphomas and some epithelial tumors are quite radiosensitive and can be destroyed by radiotherapy rather than by surgical excision. In some cases, antibodies can be used to deliver radiotherapy to the tumor cells. Antibodies can be prepared in animals then can attach to specific cells, such as B lymphocytes, and can be labeled with radioactive iodine and administered to patients with B cell lymphomas that have spread throughout the body. The isotope-labeled antibody can seek out the B cells, attach to them, and destroy them wherever they are located. In other cases, radiation and surgery are combined. For example, radiation may be administered preoperatively to reduce the size of a tumor, thereby facilitating its surgical resection; in other instances, radiotherapy is given after a malignant tumor has been resected (cut out) in order to destroy any cancer cells that may have been left behind. Radiotherapy is also used to control the growth of widespread tumors and to treat deposits of metastatic tumor that cause pain and disability. The treatment relieves symptoms and makes the patient more comfortable, even though the cancer is not curable.

HORMONE THERAPY

Some malignant tumors require hormones for their growth and are called hormone responsive. They regress temporarily if deprived of the required hormone. For example, many prostate tumors require testosterone and are inhibited by removal of the testes (eliminating the source of testosterone) or by administration of estrogens (which suppresses testosterone secretion). Many breast carcinomas in postmenopausal women are estrogen responsive and can be controlled by drugs that block estrogen so that the tumor cells are no longer stimulated by estrogen.

Adrenal cortical hormones (corticosteroids) also inhibit the growth of many malignant tumors. Corticosteroids inhibit protein synthesis, thereby suppressing the growth and division of the tumor cells. Tumors of the lymphatic tissues are especially susceptible to the effects of corticosteroids.

ANTICANCER DRUGS

Cancer cells, like normal cells, synthesize deoxyribonucleic acid (DNA) from various precursors. The DNA directs the production of the various forms of ribonucleic acid (messenger RNA, transfer RNA, and ribosomal RNA), and the RNA in turn takes part in the synthesis of enzymes and other proteins that are necessary for cell function. Anticancer drugs impede the growth and division of cells by disrupting some phase of this complex process.

The various drugs differ in their mechanisms of action. Some inhibit the synthesis of either DNA or RNA. Others alter the structure of DNA or disturb its function. Still, others inhibit protein synthesis or prevent the mitotic spindle from forming, and thus, the cell cannot divide. Frequently, several different anticancer drugs are administered simultaneously, each drug blocking a different phase in the cell's metabolic processes. Another group of anticancer drugs act by suppressing the proliferation of the blood vessels that nourish the tumor, thereby inhibiting tumor growth by interfering with its blood supply.

Most anticancer drugs work best against fast-growing tumors that contain large numbers of actively growing and dividing cells. They are usually less effective against slowly growing tumors because only relatively small numbers of the tumor cells are in the stages of cell growth or division that are susceptible to the injurious effects of the drugs.

One important group of anticancer drugs is called **alkylating agents**. These drugs interact with both strands of the paired DNA chains in the nucleus and bind them together so that they cannot separate. This reaction is called cross-linking of the DNA chains. It disrupts the function of DNA because the chains must separate for duplication of the DNA chains and for synthesis of RNA. Alkylating agents also disturb cell function by altering the structure of the DNA chains. In contrast to most anticancer drugs, these agents are effective against nondividing ("resting") cells as well as actively growing cells.

Alkylating agent
(al'kil-ā-ting)
An anticancer drug that disrupts cell function by binding DNA chains together so that they cannot separate.

Another large group of anticancer drugs is called **antimetabolites**. They resemble essential compounds required for cell growth and multiplication, but they cannot be used by the cell. Therefore, they disrupt the cell's metabolic processes. (Some antimicrobial agents inhibit bacterial growth in this way, as described in the section on competitive inhibition in the discussion on pathogenic microorganisms.)

Antimetabolite
(an-ti-met-ab'o-līte)
A substance that competes with or replaces another substance (metabolite) required for cell growth or multiplication.

Most anticancer drugs are quite toxic. They injure normal cells as well as cancer cells and must be administered very carefully in order to assure maximum damage to tumor cells without irreparable injury to normal cells. Lymphoid tissue is quite susceptible to the destructive effects of these potent drugs, and consequently, one unavoidable side effect of anticancer drugs is impairment of cell-mediated and humoral immunity.

Recently, several less toxic and more cell-specific anticancer drugs have been developed that function by blocking the action of specific cell components that stimulate the tumor cells. Some of these drugs suppress tumor growth by blocking growth factor receptors on the surface of the tumor cells so that growth factors produced by normal cells cannot attach to the receptors and stimulate the tumor cells. Other drugs inhibit the functions of important intracellular proteins, such as the enzyme tyrosine kinase, that in various ways stimulate cell proliferation.

ADJUVANT CHEMOTHERAPY

Sometimes surgical resection of a cancer appears to be successful, but metastases appear several years later and eventually prove fatal. The operation fails to eradicate the tumor because small, unrecognized metastases have already spread throughout the body. Even though the main tumor has been removed, the minute metastases continue to grow until eventually they form many large, bulky deposits of metastatic tumor that kill the patient.

In order to forestall the development of late metastases, a current trend is to administer a course of anticancer drugs after surgical resection of some tumors. This is called **adjuvant chemotherapy** (*adjuvare* = to assist). The drugs destroy any small, undetected foci of metastatic tumor before they become large enough to produce clinical manifestations. In some cases, adjuvant chemotherapy combined with surgery appears to achieve better results than surgery alone. Many anticancer drugs are quite toxic, however, and the potential benefits of adjuvant chemotherapy must be weighed against the harmful effects of the drugs on normal tissues.

Adjuvant chemotherapy
(ad'joo-vent)
Anticancer chemotherapy administered after surgical resection of a tumor in an attempt to destroy any small undetected foci of metastatic tumor before they become clinically detectable.

IMMUNOTHERAPY

The immune system has evolved a number of ways to deal with abnormal cells that can proliferate and form tumors and to deal with established tumors.

1. Cytotoxic T cells recognize antigens on tumor cells that are displayed along with the cells' own MHC Class I proteins and can damage the tumor cells by secreting destructive lymphokines.
2. Natural-killer lymphocytes can attack and destroy tumor cells without prior antigenic stimulation, and some killer lymphocytes specialize in attacking antibody-coated tumor cells.
3. Activated macrophages can destroy tumor cells by phagocytosis and by secreting tumor necrosis factor along with other cytokines that stimulate lymphocytes to attack tumor cells.
4. Antibodies formed against tumor cell antigens can affix to tumor cells and activate complement; products of complement activation attract lymphocytes and macrophages and form destructive attack complexes that damage the cell membranes of the tumor cells.

Despite the array of immunologic defenses, many tumors circumvent or overwhelm the body's immune defenses, and thus, they become ineffective and no longer retard the growth of the tumor. Some tumor cells produce little or no MHC Class I protein. Because cytotoxic T cells can recognize tumor cell antigens only if they are displayed along with MHC Class I proteins, the lymphocytes cannot attack the tumor cells because they cannot recognize the tumor antigens without the associated MHC Class I proteins. Some tumor cells thwart the immune system because the tumor cells release large amounts of soluble tumor-specific antigens that saturate the body to such an extent that the lymphocytes are no longer capable of responding to the tumor-specific antigens on the surface of the tumor cells. In addition, the chemotherapy and irradiation used to treat tumors also suppress the body's immune responses. When the patient's immune capacity is impaired for any reason, attempts have been made to stimulate the body's immune system so that it can deal more effectively with the tumor in order to improve the patient's prognosis. Treatment of tumors by stimulating the body's immune defenses is called **immunotherapy**. Nonspecific immunotherapy is directed toward bolstering the patient's own immune defenses so that the patient can deal more effectively with the tumor. Specific immunotherapy directs the immune system against the specific antigens present in the patient's own tumor.

Immunotherapy
(im′mū-nō-ther′uh-pē)
Treatment given to retard growth of a disseminated malignant tumor by stimulating to body's own immune defenses.

Nonspecific Immunotherapy

Initially, attempts were made to stimulate the immune system nonspecifically by immunizing the patient with vaccines prepared from various types of bacteria or bacterial products, but this approach had very limited success and was associated with serious complications.

More recent approaches have consisted of the administration of various cytokines that either stimulate cells of the immune system or act against the tumor cells. The two cytokines that have been used with greatest success against tumors are **interferon** and **interleukin-2**.

Interferon
(in-tur-fēr′on)
A broad-spectrum antiviral agent manufactured by various cells in the body.

Interleukin-2
(inter-lōō′kin)
A lymphokine that stimulates growth of lymphocytes.

Interferon Interferon is the name given to a group of carbohydrate-containing, "broad-spectrum" antiviral protein substances produced by cells in response to viral infection (discussion on pathogenic microorganisms), but interferon has other functions. It regulates the functions of the immune system and regulates cell growth, inhibiting the growth of rapidly dividing cells. These latter properties have led to the use of interferon for treating tumors as well as viral infections. After methods for producing interferon commercially were developed, large quantities of interferon became available for clinical use, and studies were undertaken in patients with various tumors in order to evaluate the usefulness of this material. To date, the best results have been obtained in patients with a relatively rare type of leukemia called "hairy cell" leukemia (so named because of the hairlike processes projecting from the cytoplasm of the tumor cell). Interferon has also produced responses in some patients with other types of leukemia, multiple myeloma (described later in this chapter), some lymphomas, and some widely disseminated carcinomas that had not responded to other methods of treatment. Interferon has the advantage of being much less toxic than many anticancer drugs, and treatment by intramuscular injection several times per week is usually well tolerated.

Interleukin-2 Interleukin-2 is a lymphokine produced by T cells. It stimulates natural-killer cells and cytotoxic T cells that can destroy tumor cells, but it has no direct effects against the tumor cells. Interleukin-2 is administered in multiple courses and has produced beneficial effects in the treatment of metastatic melanoma and renal cell carcinoma. High doses of interleukin-2 produce a variety of toxic effects that limit its use to some extent.

Interleukin-2 has also been administered along with lymphocytes obtained from the patient, an approach called cell transfer immunotherapy. One method is to collect blood from the patient and incubate the blood with interleukin-2 in the laboratory, which stimulates the lymphocytes to proliferate and generates a large population of natural-killer lymphocytes. Then the lymphocytes (which are called lymphokine-activated killer cells) are infused into the patient to seek out and destroy the tumor.

Other Cytokines Various other cytokines have been produced by genetic engineering and are undergoing clinical evaluation. They include tumor necrosis factor and a cytokine produced by macrophages called interleukin-1, which has antitumor activity.

Specific Immunotherapy

Specific immunotherapy targets the patient's own tumor cells for attack. Three different approaches appear promising: (1) administration of cytotoxic T lymphocytes directed against the tumor, which are called tumor-infiltrating lymphocytes; (2) administration of tumor vaccines; and (3) administration of antitumor antibodies.

Tumor-Infiltrating Lymphocyte Therapy This is a specific type of cell transfer immunotherapy in which the lymphocytes infused back into the patient are obtained from the patient's own tumor. These lymphocytes are actually infiltrating the tumor and are trying to destroy it, and they are obtained when the tumor is biopsied or excised. The tumor-infiltrating lymphocytes contain a large concentration of cytotoxic T lymphocytes specifically targeted against the antigens in the patient's own tumor, as well as numbers of natural-killer lymphocytes that also can destroy tumor cells. The lymphocytes from the tumor are grown in the laboratory with interleukin-2 to stimulate growth of the lymphocytes and then infused back into the patient to attack and destroy the tumor. This approach has been used with some success to treat metastatic malignant melanoma.

Tumor Vaccines Tumor vaccines prepared from the patient's own tumor also have been used to immunize the patient against the tumor in an effort to reduce the likelihood that the tumor will recur or metastasize after it has been resected. Tumor cells are obtained from the resected tumor, grown in the laboratory, and then killed so that they cannot proliferate in the patient but can still generate an immune response. They are then used to prepare a vaccine that will stimulate an immune response to the resected tumor. Tumor vaccines have been used as an additional treatment after resection of a malignant melanoma or a colon carcinoma when the patient is considered at high risk of recurrence.

Tumor Antibody Therapy In this approach, antibodies are prepared against tumor cell antigens, and then the antibodies are linked to some antitumor drug or toxin that can kill tumor cells. The antibodies with attached drug or toxin are then infused back into the patient to seek out and destroy the tumor cells without damaging normal cells.

Results of Immunotherapy

Results of immunotherapy have been mixed. There have been some notable successes, as in the use of interferon therapy for one type of leukemia called hairy cell leukemia. Some types of immunotherapy have produced gratifying results in persons with specific types of widespread tumors when no other methods of treatment were available to control the tumor. No single method works against all types of tumors, and ongoing clinical trials continue to assess the applications and limitations of these various methods. Unfortunately, most patients treated with immunotherapy have advanced diseases, and often the body's immune defenses are incapable of dealing with such large amounts of tumor even when stimulated by immunotherapy.

Leukemia

Leukemia
(lōō-kē′mē-yuh)
A neoplastic proliferation of leukocytes.

The term **leukemia** refers to a neoplasm of hematopoietic tissue. In contrast to solid tumors, which form nodular deposits, leukemic cells diffusely infiltrate the bone marrow and lymphoid tissues, spill over into the bloodstream, and infiltrate throughout the various organs of the body. The leukemic cells may be mostly mature, or they may be extremely primitive. The overproduction of white cells in leukemia may be revealed in the peripheral blood by a very high white blood count. In some cases of leukemia, however, the proliferation of the white cells is largely confined to the bone marrow, and there is no significant increase in the number of white cells in the bloodstream.

CLASSIFICATION OF LEUKEMIA

Leukemia is classified on the basis of both the cell type and the maturity of the proliferating cells. Any type of hematopoietic cells can give rise to leukemia, but the most common types are granulocytic, monocytic, and lymphocytic. Leukemia developing from stem cells that would normally give rise to the leukocytes containing specific granules (neutrophils, eosinophils, and basophils) is called granulocytic leukemia. Monocytic leukemia develops from precursor cells that give rise to monocytes. Lymphocytic leukemia is derived from lymphoid precursor cells. Various subclassifications have been established within these major groups on the basis of the characteristics of the cell membranes and the enzymes present within the leukemic cells, as determined by highly specialized techniques.

If the leukemia cells are mostly primitive forms, the leukemia is classified as acute leukemia (FIGURE 26), and if the cells are mostly mature, the leukemia is classified as chronic leukemia. In chronic granulolcytic leukemia, most of the circulating cells are maturing granulocytes and neutrophils, and there are few primitive cells (FIGURE 27). In chronic lymphocytic leukemia, the circulating cells are mostly mature lymphocytes (FIGURE 28). Another type of leukemia also arises from lymphoid cells and has some unusual features. Cytoplasmic processes projecting from the cells give the cells a distinctive appearance, which is responsible for the descriptive term hairy cell leukemia, which is applied to this condition (FIGURE 29).

In most instances, the total number of white blood cells in the peripheral blood is significantly above normal. Occasionally, however, the marrow may be crowded

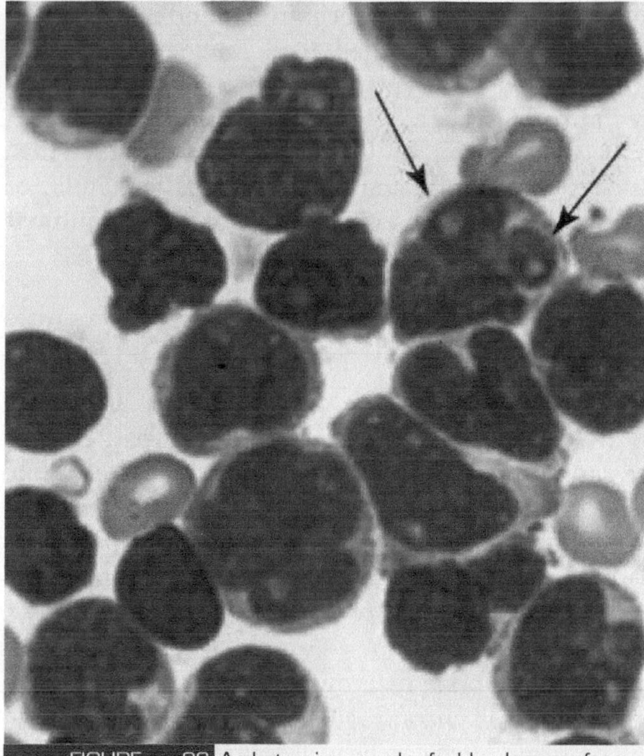

FIGURE 26 A photomicrograph of a blood smear from a patient with acute leukemia. The nuclei of the white cells have fine chromatin structure and prominent nucleoli indicating immaturity (*arrows*). Nuclei are irregular in size and configuration (original magnification × 1,000).

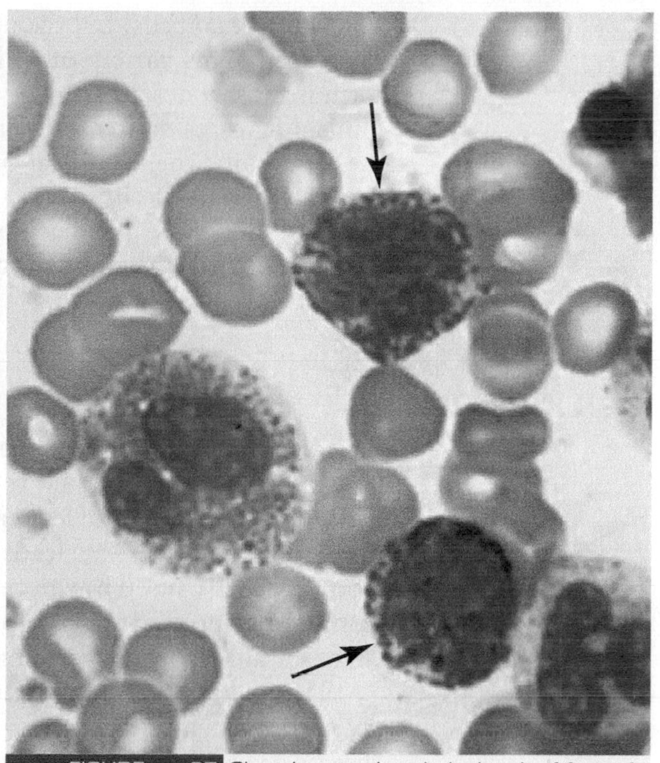

FIGURE 27 Chronic granulocytic leukemia. Most of the cells in the photomicrograph are mature. Note the basophils (*arrows*), the eosinophil (left of *arrows*), and the two neutrophils (right of *arrows*) (original magnification × 1,000).

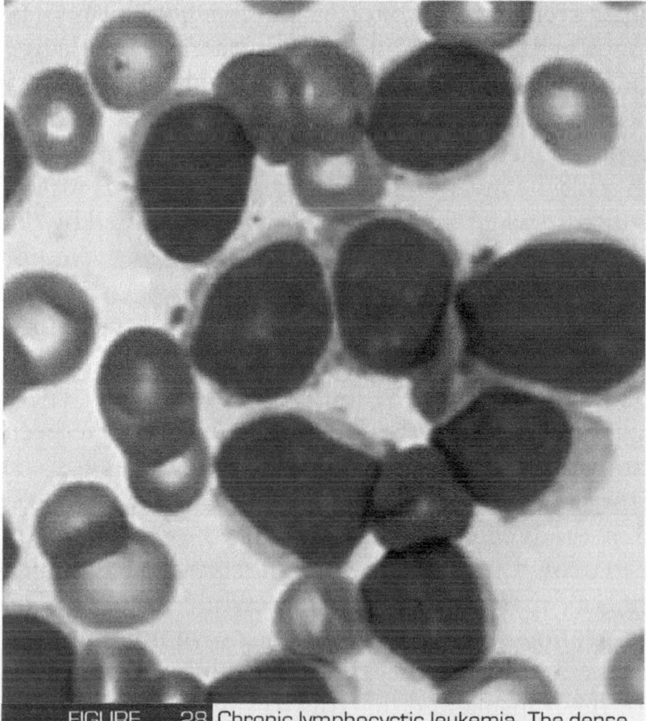

FIGURE 28 Chronic lymphocyctic leukemia. The dense nuclear chromatin structure indicates that the lymphocytes are mature (compare with Figure 26). The total white count is elevated (original magnification × 1,000).

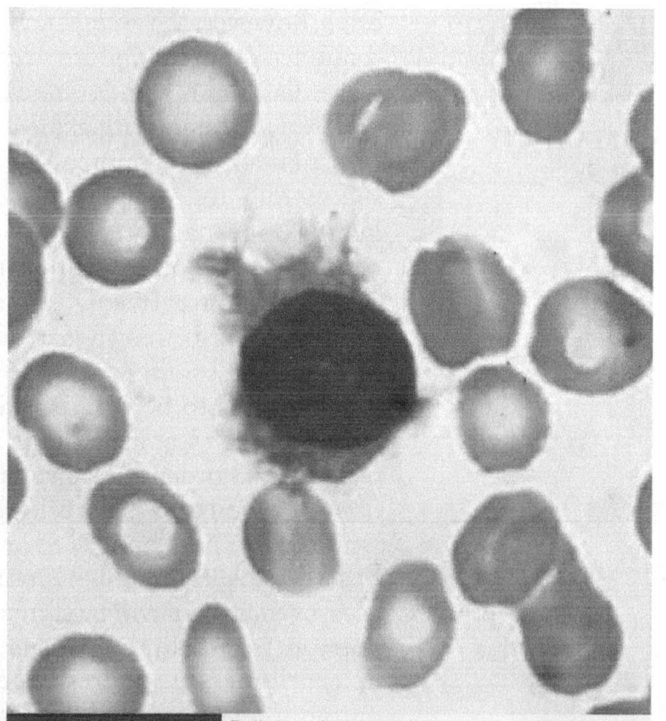

FIGURE 29 Cellular characteristics of neoplastic cell in "hairy cell" leukemia. Uniform nuclear chromatin and scanty cytoplasm with multiple cytoplasmic process (original magnification × 1,000).

with abnormal cells, but the number of white blood cells in the blood is normal or decreased. This variety of leukemia is sometimes called aleukemic leukemia. The term is merely descriptive and does not denote a type of leukemia with any special clinical features or any difference in prognosis.

Generally, the classifications by cell type and maturity are used together. Thus, one may speak of chronic granulocytic leukemia, acute lymphocytic leukemia, or acute monocytic leukemia. The term aleukemic is sometimes added if the number of white cells in the circulating blood is reduced.

CLINICAL FEATURES AND PRINCIPLES OF TREATMENT

The clinical features of leukemia are of two kinds: those caused by impairment of bone marrow function and those caused by infiltration of the viscera by leukemic cells. The overgrowth of leukemic cells in the bone marrow often crowds out normal bone marrow cells. This leads to anemia as a result of inadequate red cell production, bleeding caused by thrombocytopenia, and infection resulting from inadequate numbers of normal white blood cells, which are an important part of the body's defenses against pathogenic organisms.

The leukemic cells not only infiltrate the bone marrow, but also spread into the spleen, liver, lymph nodes, and other tissues. In chronic leukemia, the evolution of the disease proceeds at a relatively slow pace and often can be well controlled by treatment for long periods of time. Therefore, the patient with chronic leukemia may survive for many years in relatively good health. In contrast, acute leukemia is often a rapidly progressive disease. Symptoms of bone marrow infiltration and visceral infiltration make their appearance early and are quite conspicuous. In some patients with acute leukemia, the abnormal proliferation of the leukemic cells can be stopped for a variable period of time by various anticancer drugs, and the patient appears to have completely recovered. An arrest of the disease induced by therapy is called a remission. In many cases, however, the patient undergoes a relapse, and the disease ultimately proves fatal. Acute leukemia in children responds better to anticancer chemotherapy than acute leukemia in adults, and some children have been completely cured by intensive therapy.

Some patients with acute leukemia can be treated successfully by a bone marrow transplant from a compatible donor. Marrow transplantation has also been used successfully to treat patients with multiple myeloma, widespread lymphoma affecting the bone marrow, Hodgkin's disease when the bone marrow is infiltrated by the neoplasm, and other neoplastic diseases affecting the bone marrow that have not responded to treatment.

Before performing a marrow transplant, the patient's own bone marrow cells must be destroyed by anticancer (cytotoxic) drugs and radiation treatment. Then the bone marrow cells to be transplanted are injected into the patient's bloodstream where they become established in the patient's bone marrow whose own cells have been destroyed in order to receive the transplanted bone marrow. Within a few weeks, the donor's blood cells (stem cells) in their new location begin to produce mature red cells, white cells, and platelets. Several methods can be used to increase the concentration of stem cells in the donor's bone marrow before the transplant is performed, which assures that there will be sufficient bone marrow cells for a successful transplant. The marrow transplant is a foreign tissue, however, and the patient's own immunologic defenses must be suppressed (discussion on immunity, hypersensitivity, allergy, and autoimmune diseases) in order for the transplanted marrow to survive.

The transplant patient also faces another problem related to immunologic differences between the cells of the donor and those of the patient, which is called a graft-versus-host reaction. The donor lymphocytes in the transplanted marrow recognize the patient's cells as antigenically different and attempt to destroy them, leading to various clinical manifestations, including skin rash, liver injury, and gastrointestinal symptoms. This is the reverse of the usual situation in which the patient tries to reject the transplant. Here, the transplant tries to reject the patient! A less intense cytotoxic drug and irradiation treatment used successfully to perform bone marrow transplants on persons with sickle cell anemia can also be used to treat selected patients with myeloma and other hematopoietic diseases. The treatment modification has reduced the frequency of graft-versus-host disease and also increased the long-term survival of treated patients.

Although marrow transplantation is an important advance, it is not always successful. Patients may develop life-threatening infections related to the immunosuppression required to maintain the transplant, and in some patients, the leukemia recurs, arising from the patient's surviving leukemic cells that were not destroyed by the prior chemotherapy and radiation.

Newer transplantation methods are being developed in which the patient's own marrow is used for transplantation, which is called an autologous bone marrow transplant (*auto* = self). One approach comprises collecting the patient's own marrow while the patient is in remission, treating the marrow to destroy any surviving leukemic cells, and storing the marrow in liquid nitrogen for later use should the patient develop recurrent leukemia. If this occurs, the patient's leukemic marrow is destroyed by anticancer drugs and radiation, and the stored leukemic-free marrow is reinfused into the patient as a transplant. Because the transplant is the patient's own marrow, immunosuppression is not required, and complications related to immunosuppression are avoided. Autologous bone marrow transplants have also been used to treat patients with acute leukemia when no compatible marrow transplant donor is available. In this situation, the leukemic patient's marrow is collected in the same way as marrow is from a donor. Then the patient is treated with chemotherapy and radiation to destroy the diseased marrow. Meanwhile, the patient's previously collected marrow is treated with specific antibodies that destroy the leukemic cells without affecting the normal marrow cells. Then the treated marrow is returned to the patient, and if all goes well, the leukemia-free marrow becomes reestablished and functions normally.

Not all leukemic patients are suitable candidates for bone marrow transplantations, and many patients require some type of chemotherapy. The types of chemotherapy drugs used and the treatment schedules are being evaluated and adjusted continually. As new drugs become available, their effectiveness and side effects are compared with drugs currently used, and treatment schedules may be readjusted as required in order to provide the maximum benefit to the patient. Patients with Philadelphia chromosome-positive chronic granulocytic leukemia and those with Philadelphia chromosome-positive lymphocytic leukemia can often be treated successfully with a drug that inhibits the hyperactive tyrosine kinase enzyme produced by the composite *bcr/abl* gene. Blocking the activity of this dysfunctional enzyme suppresses the proliferation of the leukemic cells.

PRECURSORS OF LEUKEMIA: THE MYELODYSPLASTIC SYNDROMES

For many years, it has been recognized that acute leukemia in older patients may not have an abrupt onset but is preceded by a period lasting from several months to several years in which the affected patients have only a moderate anemia, sometimes associated with reduced white cells (leukopenia) and low blood platelets

Myelodysplastic syndrome (my′elo-dis-plas′tik) *A disturbance of bone marrow function that is characterized by anemia, leukopenia, and thrombocytopenia and that may be a precursor to leukemia in some patients.*

(thrombocytopenia). Examination of the bone marrow of these patients reveals variable degrees of disturbed growth and maturation of red cells, white cell precursors, and megakaryocytes but not leukemia. This condition has been called preleukemia, although it was realized that not all patients with bone marrow maturation disturbances of this type develop leukemia, and one could not reliably predict which patients would eventually become leukemic. Recently, these conditions have been grouped together under the general term **myelodysplastic syndromes** (*myelo* = marrow + *dysplasia* = disturbed growth). Several different types have been described that differ somewhat in their clinical and hematologic manifestations. In general, the more severe the maturation disturbance in the bone marrow, the greater the likelihood that leukemia would eventually occur. Unfortunately, there is no specific treatment available for most patients with these conditions, although some patients with severe "preleukemic" changes in their bone marrow have been treated successfully by bone marrow transplantation.

Multiple Myeloma

Multiple myeloma (my-el-ō′muh) *A malignant neoplasm of plasma cells.*

Immunoglobulin (im′mū-nō-glob′u-lin) *An antibody protein.*

Multiple myeloma is a neoplasm arising from plasma cells within the bone marrow (FIGURE 30). In many ways, it resembles leukemia, but the neoplastic plasma cell proliferation is generally confined to the bone marrow. Infiltration of the viscera by the abnormal plasma cells is unusual; outpouring of large numbers of plasma cells into the peripheral blood also is uncommon. The abnormal plasma cells either may infiltrate the bone marrow diffusely or may form discrete tumors that weaken the bone, leading to spontaneous fractures, pain, and disability (FIGURE 31).

Normal plasma cells produce antibody proteins (**immunoglobulins**), as described in the discussion on immunity, hypersensitivity, allergy, and autoimmune diseases. In myeloma, the neoplastic cells also often produce large amounts of protein. This greatly increases blood proteins and, correspondingly, blood viscosity. The protein produced by the myeloma cells is generally a single type of immunoglobulin, usually IgG. In some patients, the production of immunoglobulins also is abnormal, and an excess of light chains is produced. Any light chains that are not incorporated into

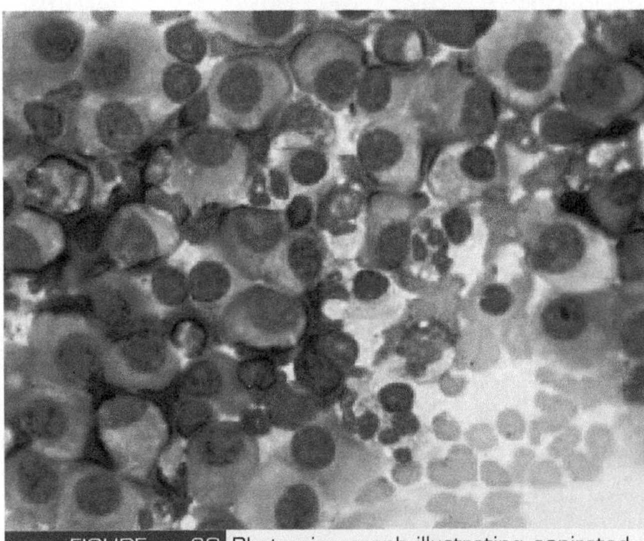

FIGURE 30 Photomicrograph illustrating aspirated bone marrow from a patient with multiple myeloma. Almost all cells are immature plasma cells containing large eccentric nuclei and abundant cytoplasm (original magnification × 400).

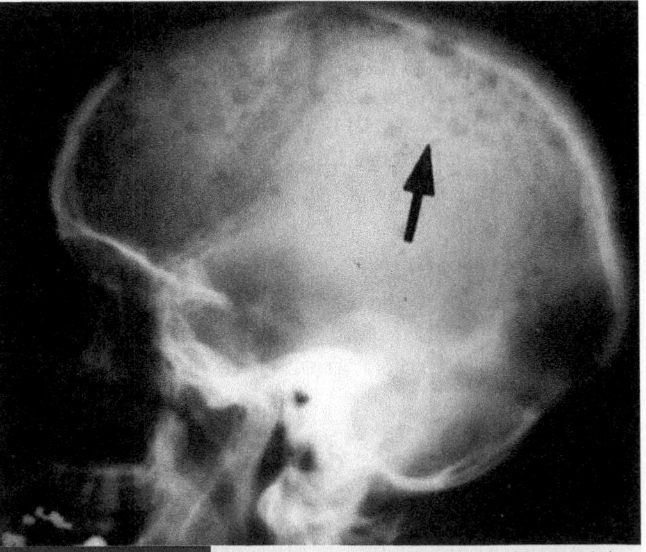

FIGURE 31 A skull x-ray from a patient with multiple myeloma. Multiple punched-out areas in skull bones (*arrow*) result from bone destruction caused by nodular masses of neoplastic plasma cells growing in bone marrow.

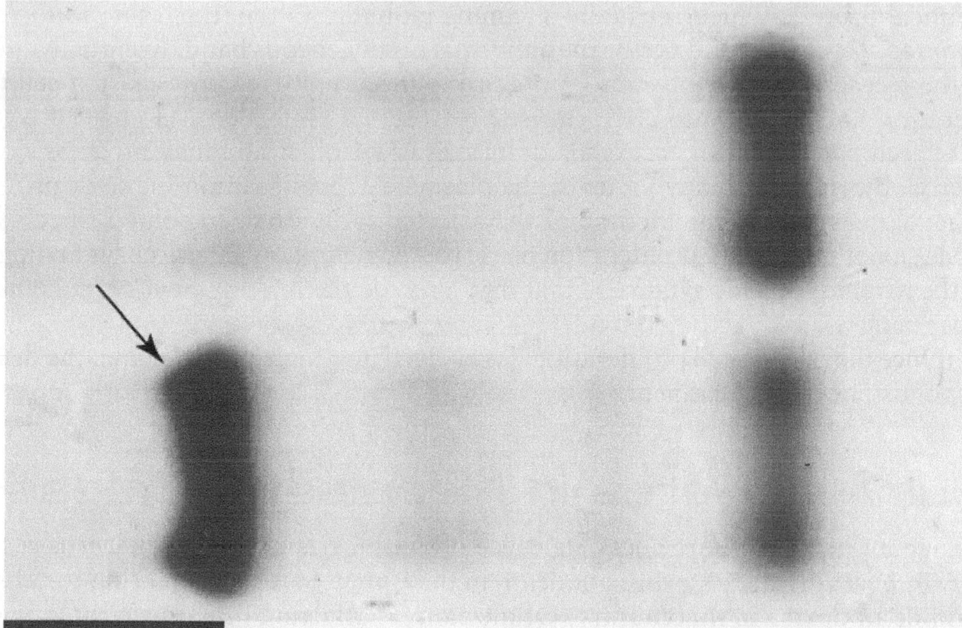

FIGURE 32 An examination of serum proteins by a special technique (*electrophoresis*) that separates serum proteins into various fractions. The upper pattern is from normal serum, with the dense albumin band at the *far right* in the photograph and the less intensely stained globulin bands to the left of the albumin band. The lower pattern is from a patient with multiple myeloma. The *arrow* indicates densely stained homogeneous globulin band representing large amounts of a single type of globulin protein produced by the abnormal plasma cells.

the immunoglobulin molecules are excreted in the urine. The myeloma protein can be identified in the blood (FIGURE 32), and the free light chains can be identified in the urine by special laboratory tests.

Masses of coagulated myeloma protein may accumulate within the patient's own tissues, and thus the function of the affected tissues is severely impaired. Some patients with myeloma die of kidney failure because masses of protein produced by the plasma cells infiltrate the kidneys and block the renal tubules.

A number of different drugs and treatment schedules are used to treat myeloma. Thalidomide and similar drugs derived from thalidomide have been quite effective, primarily by suppressing the proliferation of the blood vessels that support the growth of the myeloma cells. Radiotherapy may also be useful for treating localized areas of bone destruction caused by myeloma. In highly selected patients, a bone marrow transplant may improve the patient's survival but usually does not cure the patient.

PRECURSORS OF MULTIPLE MYELOMA

Increased Monoclonal Protein of Uncertain Significance

In many patients who eventually develop multiple myeloma, blood protein abnormalities can be demonstrated long before the characteristic features of the disease appear. The condition is an asymptomatic **premyeloma** phase of several years duration characterized by a relatively small number of plasma cells in the bone marrow and a single small but uniform (homogeneous) protein band identified by serum protein electrophoresis. There are no clinical manifestations of multiple myeloma. The condition may not be recognized unless routine blood chemistry tests reveal the protein abnormality, which is caused by a group (clone) of plasma cells derived from a single precursor plasma cell in which all the plasma cells in the group produce an

Premyeloma
An early stage of multiple myeloma in which plasma cell proliferation in the bone marrow is only slightly increased and only minor blood protein abnormalities are present.

identical protein, which is usually a gamma globulin. Often, the term *monoclonal gammopathy* is used to describe the abnormal homogeneous band. Eventually, many of these cases slowly evolve into more pronounced bone marrow plasma cell proliferation and finally into characteristic features of multiple myeloma. However, this precursor condition occurs in adults ages 65 or older and may progress slowly over many years. In many patients, the plasma cell proliferation may not progress to myelomas during the lifetime of the affected individual. In some respects, the monoclonal plasma cell proliferation phase preceding multiple myeloma is analogous to the myelodysplastic syndrome that may precede the development of leukemia in older persons.

Once the plasma cell proliferation has evolved into multiple myeloma, the disease responds poorly to treatment.

Survival Rates in Neoplastic Disease

Malignant neoplasms are a leading cause of disability and death. Cancer is second only to heart disease as a cause of death in the United States, accounting for almost 23% of all deaths in this country. Of the cancers affecting major organs, lung carcinoma is a common malignant tumor in men, and breast carcinoma is the most frequent in women. Carcinoma of the intestine is quite common in both sexes. The survival rate for patients with malignant tumors depends on whether the disease has been diagnosed and treated early, before it has spread. The chances for survival are significantly reduced if the tumor has metastasized to regional lymph nodes or to distant sites.

The curability of the various types of cancer can be assessed in terms of 5-year survival rates, which range from more than 95% for patients with thyroid cancer to a discouraging 5% for those with pancreatic carcinoma (TABLE 6). Attempts are being made continually to improve survival rates by means of earlier diagnosis and more effective therapy. Unfortunately, 5-year survival does not necessarily indicate

TABLE 6

Malignant neoplasms: 5-year survival rates

	5-Year survival (%)			5-Year survival (%)	
Type of neoplasm	White	Black	Type of neoplasm	White	Black
Thyroid	97	94	Kidney	65	66
Melanoma	93	75	Non-Hodgkin's lymphoma	64	54
Uterus, cervix	73	63	Ovary	45	39
Uterus, body	85	60	Multiple myeloma	33	32
Breast	90	77	Leukemia	49	47
Bladder	83	65	Stomach	22	23
Larynx	67	52	Lung	15	12
Prostate	100	98	Esophagus	16	11
Hodgkin's disease	87	81	Pancreas	5	5
Colon-rectum	65	55			

Cases diagnosed 1996–2002. Survival for all ages with survival for whites and blacks listed separately. Average survival for both sexes used when neoplasm occurs in both sexes.
Data from *CA: A Cancer Journal for Clinicians*. 2007. 57:43–66.

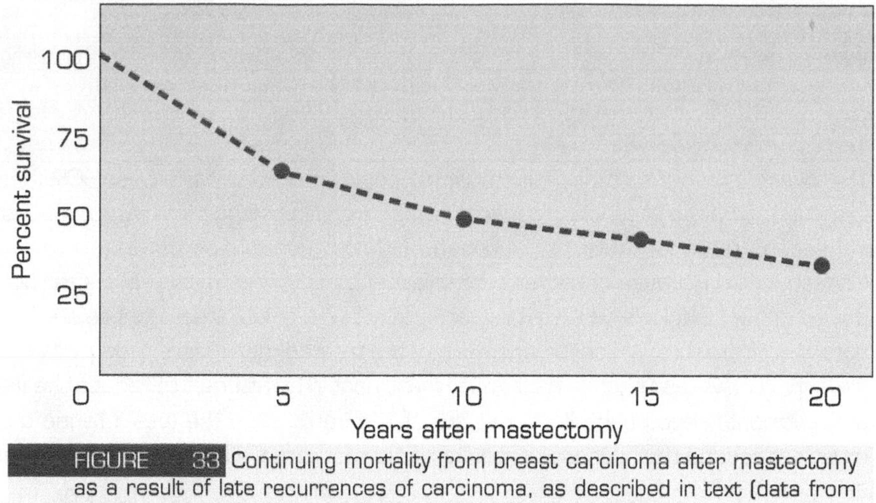

FIGURE 33 Continuing mortality from breast carcinoma after mastectomy as a result of late recurrences of carcinoma, as described in text (data from J. Berg and G. Robbins. *Surg Gynecol Obstet* June 1966).

that the patient is cured because some types of malignant tumors may recur and prove fatal many years after initial treatment. Breast carcinoma and malignant melanomas are two such tumors that are prone to late recurrence. For breast carcinoma, for example, the overall 5-year survival rate in one large group of patients followed for many years is approximately 65% (although more recent 5-year survival data indicated in Table 6 reveal higher survival rates). The 10-year rate in this group is only 50% because of late recurrences and metastases. Even after 10 years, a small proportion of patients eventually die of their original tumor (FIGURE 33). In such cases, the tumor had already spread by the time it was first recognized and treated, but the metastatic deposits were held in check by the body's immune defense mechanisms. The recurrence was caused by an eventual failure of the body's defenses, which allowed the tumor to become reactivated.

QUESTIONS FOR REVIEW

1. What are the major differences between a benign and a malignant tumor (see Table 1)?
2. How are tumors named? What are the common prefixes used in naming tumors? How would you name the following tumors: a benign tumor of fat, a malignant tumor of muscle, a malignant tumor of squamous epithelium, a benign tumor of glandular epithelium arising from the surface of the colon and projecting into the lumen, a malignant tumor of cartilage?
3. How does the body defend itself against abnormal cells that arise spontaneously in the course of cell division? What is the consequence of failure of these defense mechanisms (see Figure 21)?
4. What is a lymphoma? What is the difference between a nevus and a melanoma? What is a teratoma?
5. What is a Pap smear? How is it used in the early diagnosis of tumors? What is the significance of a Pap smear containing atypical cells?
6. What is a frozen section? How is it used in the diagnosis of tumors? How are neoplasms treated?
7. What is leukemia? What are its major clinical manifestations? How is leukemia classified? What is the difference between multiple myeloma and leukemia?

Armitage, J. O. 2010. Early-stage Hodgkin's lymphoma. *The New England Journal of Medicine* 363:653–62.

- The 5-year survival rate of patients with Hodgkin's lymphoma is over 90%. However, long-term follow-up of surviving patients reveals significant long-term complications, including second malignant tumors, leukemia, and radiation-related cardiovascular disease. Consequently, because of the late complications occurring many years after successful treatment of Hodgkin's lymphoma, more patients die of late treatment-related complications than from the disease for which they were treated many years previously. Now many patients receive less intense anticancer treatment in an attempt to reduce the frequency of treatment-related complications, but at the same time the less intense treatment must not reduce the successful results of chemotherapy and radiation treatment.

Artandi, S. E. 2006. Telomeres, telomerase, and human disease. *The New England Journal of Medicine* 355:1195–97.

- Telomeres (*telos* = end + *meros* = part) are repeating DNA segments on the ends of chromosomes. Telomeres shorten progressively with each cell division as the terminal repeating DNA segments are lost until eventually the telomeres become so short that they lose their ability to protect the ends of the chromosomes, and the telomere-depleted cell is recognized by the cell DNA repair system and is eliminated. Progressive telomere shortening limits the number of cell divisions that a normal cell can perform, which limits its longevity and, in turn, affects the survival of the various cell populations that make up an individual.
- Recently, an enzyme called telomerase has been identified that can restore telomeres, which greatly extends the life span of the cell by allowing the cell to divide repeatedly without "wearing out." Most human tumors contain telomerase enzyme, which allows them to proliferate indefinitely.

Black, W. C., and Baron, J. A. 2007. CT screening for lung cancer: Spiraling into confusion? *Journal of the American Medical Association* 297:995–97.

- A discussion of the different conclusions reached on the value of CT scans to detect early lung carcinoma. One study revealed a threefold increase in the number of lung cancer cases and a tenfold increase in lung cancer resections related to CT scans but no decrease in advanced lung cancer cases, which indicated that CT scanning has no effect on mortality. Another study revealed an 88% 10-year survival in early lung carcinoma detected by CT, which decreased mortality by 80%. The author indicates that early detection of disease does not necessarily reduce mortality; it only detects the tumor earlier, which leads to a longer interval between initial diagnosis and death from the tumor.

Connors, J. M. 2005. Radioimmunotherapy—Hot new treatment for lymphoma. *The New England Journal of Medicine* 352:496–98.

- Most patients with B-cell lymphomas have widespread disease by the time the lymphoma is diagnosed, and it is difficult to cure the lymphoma because the tumor cells have already spread throughout the body. Recently, antibodies directed against B cells and labeled with a radioisotope have been used to seek out and destroy the B-lymphoma cells wherever they are located in the body. Studies on a selected group of patients have yielded encouraging results.

Dantal, J., and Soulillou, J. P. 2005. Immunosuppressive drugs and the risk of cancer after organ transplantation. *The New England Journal of Medicine* 352:1371–73.

- Immunosuppressive therapy, which is essential for survival of organ transplants, has some important limitations: cardiovascular disease, infections, and cancer. Many of the cancers result from activation of oncogenic viruses: lymphomas related to EB virus, Kaposi's sarcoma caused by human herpesvirus 8, and skin cancer caused by human papilloma virus. Most immunosuppressive agents favor cancer development, but a few actually reduce cancer risk by suppressing cell proliferation. Hopefully, effective combinations of immunosuppressive drugs can prevent organ rejection and also reduce cancer risk.

D'Souza, G., Kreimer, A. R., Viscidi, R., et al. 2007. Case-control study of human papillomavirus and oropharyngeal cancer. *The New England Journal of Medicine* 356:1944–56.

► The association between some types of oropharyngeal cancer and HPV infections appears to be firmly established. HPV type 16 (one of the same types responsible for cervical HPV infections and cervical carcinoma) also occurs frequently associated with oropharyngeal carcinoma.

Geenen, M. M., Cardous-Ubbink, M. C., Kremer, L. C., et al. 2007. Medical assessment of adverse health outcomes in long-term survivors of childhood cancer. *Journal of the American Medical Association* 297:2705–15.

► Improved survival of children with cancer has been associated with multiple treatment-related complications. Long-term follow-up revealed a large number of late complications. Seventy-five percent had one or more late complications. Twenty-four point six percent had five or more complications. The highest complication rates occurred in radiotherapy-treated children.

Gooley, T. A., Chien, J. W., Pergam, S. A., et al. 2010. Reduced mortality after allogeneic hematopoietic-cell transplantation. *The New England Journal of Medicine* 363:2091–101.

► Over the past decade, advances have been made in the care of patients undergoing transplantation. We found that less intense cytotoxic chemotherapy and radiation treatment resulted in better results because of less organ damage, infection, and severe graft-versus-host disease.

Harousseau, J. L., and Moreau, P. 2009. Autologous hematopoietic stem-cell transplantation for multiple myeloma. *The New England Journal of Medicine* 360:2645–54.

► A description of the evolution of plasma cell proliferation into myeloma and various methods of treatment, including details of bone marrow transplantation and its effects on patient survival.

Hoagland, H. C. 1995. Myelodysplastic (preleukemia) syndromes: The bone marrow factory failure problem. *Mayo Clinic Proceedings* 70:673–77.

► A review of classification, clinical features, cytogenetic abnormalities, diagnosis, and management.

Jacobs, A. D., Champlin, R. E., and Golde, D. W. 1985. Recombinant alpha-2-interferon for hairy cell leukemia. *Blood* 65:1017–20.

► Interferon is a highly effective therapy for hairy cell leukemia.

Jemal, A., Siegel, R., Ward, E., et al. 2007. Cancer statistics, 2007. *CA: A Cancer Journal for Clinicians* 57:43–66.

► Extensive cancer data from the American Cancer Society, including most recent 5-year survival rates of cancers diagnosed 1996–2002.

Krause, D. S., and Van Etten, R. A. 2005. Tyrosine kinases as targets for cancer therapy. *The New England Journal of Medicine* 353:172–87.

► Tyrosine kinase (TK) enzymes perform many functions concerned with cell growth and differentiation, and unrestrained cell proliferation follows if TK malfunctions, as occurs in chronic myelogenous leukemia. Several other tumors result from disturbed

TK function. TK can also be inhibited by blocking its receptor using a monoclonal antibody. Some toxic effects related to TK-directed therapy may be related to inhibition of TK activity in normal tissues.

Landgren, O., and Waxman, A. J. 2010. Multiple myeloma precursor disease. *Journal of the American Medical Association* 304:2397–404.

- Myeloma is often preceded by blood protein abnormalities which may slowly evolve into the characteristic features of multiple myeloma.

OUTLINE SUMMARY

Tumors: Disturbed Cell Growth

Classification and Nomenclature

BENIGN TUMORS

Descriptive: polyp, papilloma.
Tissue of origin + *oma*.

MALIGNANT TUMORS

Cancer: general term.
Carcinoma: arising from surface, glandular, or parenchymal epithelium.
Sarcoma: solid tumor arising from other primary tissues.
Leukemia: neoplasm of blood-forming tissues.

Comparison of Benign and Malignant Tumors

BENIGN TUMORS

Grow slowly.
Grow by expansion.
Remain localized.
Cells well differentiated.

MALIGNANT TUMORS

Grow more rapidly.
Grow by infiltration.
Metastasize.
Cells not well differentiated.

Variations in Terminology

LYMPHOID TUMORS

Lymphoma: a malignant lymphoid tumor.
Classification:
Hodgkin's disease: characteristic Reed-Sternberg cells.
Non-Hodgkin's lymphoma: well-differentiated and poorly differentiated.

SKIN TUMORS

From melanocytes:
Benign: nevus.
Malignant: melanoma.
From keratinocytes:
Benign: keratoses.
Malignant: basal cell carcinoma, squamous cell carcinoma.
Sun exposure damages skin and predisposes to development of tumors.

TUMORS OF MIXED COMPONENTS (TERATOMAS)

Frequently occur in reproductive tract.
Must specify as either benign or malignant.

PRIMITIVE CELL TUMORS

Arise from persisting groups of primitive cells.
Named from tissue of origin + *blastoma*.

Necrosis in Tumors

PATHOGENESIS

Tumor outgrows blood supply.
Necrosis occurs in center of deeply placed tumor.
Necrosis occurs on the surface of tumors growing from epithelial surface.

Noninfiltrating (In Situ) Carcinoma

CHARACTERISTICS

Remains localized for many years.
Frequently occurs in cervix, but encountered in other locations as well.
Most favorable stage for cure.

PRECANCEROUS CONDITIONS

Characteristics:
Nonmalignant conditions with tendency to eventually become malignant.
Treatment prevents progression.
Common precancerous conditions:
Actinic keratosis: arises in sun-damaged skin and may form skin cancers.
Lentigo maligna: arises in sun-damaged skin and may lead to melanoma.
Leukoplakia: affects oral mucosa, usually caused by exposure to tobacco tars. May affect vulva
Some colon polyps.

Etiologic Factors in Neoplastic Disease

VIRUSES

Some animal tumors are caused by viruses.

Some human tumors also may be virus induced.

GENE AND CHROMOSOME ABNORMALITIES

Activation of oncogenes and inactivation of tumor suppressor genes deregulates cell, which proliferates to form tumor.

Translocation or deletion may change the relation of genes on the chromosome, disturbing cell regulation and growth functions.

Philadelphia chromosome is the best-known abnormality.

Reciprocal translocation of ends of chromosomes 9 and 22.

Oncogene on translocated piece of chromosome 9 exhibits increased activity.

FAILURE OF IMMUNOLOGIC DEFENSES

Body produces abnormal cells periodically.

Immune defenses eliminate abnormal cells.

Failure of elimination may allow overgrowth, forming malignant tumors.

HEREDITY AND TUMORS

No strong hereditary predisposition to most tumors.

Slightly increased susceptibility in relatives of cancer patients may be caused by multifactorial inheritance pattern.

Some breast carcinomas have strong hereditary background, owing to inheritance of mutant gene.

Rare tumors:

Autosomal dominant inheritance:

Some retinoblastomas.

Multiple polyposis of colon.

Neurofibromatosis.

Multiple endocrine adenomas.

Only small fraction of all tumors affecting humans.

Diagnosis of Tumors

EARLY RECOGNITION

An abnormality of form or function requires evaluation by physician.

If abnormality discovered, perform biopsy or excise.

Excision of benign tumor is curative; malignant tumor may require further treatment.

CYTOLOGIC DIAGNOSIS

Tumor cells shed from the surface or can be scraped from the epithelial surface.

Abnormal smear indicates need for further studies but not diagnostic of neoplasm.

FROZEN-SECTION DIAGNOSIS

Means of rapid evaluation of abnormal tissue obtained at surgery.

Permits immediate decision about proper course of treatment.

TUMOR-ASSOCIATED ANTIGEN TESTS

Carbohydrate–protein complexes secreted by tumor cells.

Can be detected in the blood.

Used to monitor response to treatment.

Treatment of Tumors

Pretreatment tumor grading and staging helps determine prognosis, helps select the most appropriate treatment, and provides useful information for future clinical research studies.

SURGERY

Extensive resection of tumor with draining lymph nodes.

Not curative if tumor has already metastasized to distant sites.

RADIOTHERAPY

Lymphomas and some epithelial tumors treated primarily by radiotherapy.

May be used in conjunction with surgery.

Useful for pain relief.

HORMONES

Hormone-dependent tumors undergo temporary regression when deprived of required hormones.

Some tumors inhibited by hormones, corticosteroids, estrogens.

ANTICANCER DRUGS

Impede processes concerned with cell growth and cell division.

Most effective against rapidly growing tumors.

Alkylating agents.

Antimetabolites.

Some drugs act by blocking cell growth factor receptors or inhibit intracellular enzymes that promote cell growth.

ADJUVANT CHEMOTHERAPY

Used after surgical resection of tumor.

Attempts to eradicate small metastases before they become apparent clinically.

IMMUNOTHERAPY

Nonspecific immunotherapy:

Interferon:

Interferon regulates cell growth and functions of immune system in addition to antiviral activity.

Large quantities available from commercial production.

Best results in hairy cell leukemia, but useful for causing regression of some other neoplasms.

Low toxicity.

Interleukin-2:

Stimulates production of natural killer cells that attack tumor.

Best results in metastatic melanoma and renal cell carcinoma.

Other cytokines under investigation.

Specific immunotherapy:

Tumor-infiltrating lymphocytes:

Cytotoxic T cells attack patient's own tumor.

Some success in treating metastatic melanoma.

Tumor vaccines:

Vaccine prepared from patient's own tumor induces immune response.

Used as additional treatment after melanoma or colon cancer if patient at high risk of recurrence.

Tumor antibody therapy:
Antibodies prepared against tumor antigens and coupled with antitumor drug or toxin.
Antibody infused into patient and damages tumor cells without injuring normal cells.

Leukemia

CLASSIFICATION

By cell type: granulocytic, lymphocytic, or monocytic.
By maturity of cells: acute (primitive cells) or chronic (mature cells).
By number of circulating white cells: descriptive term *aleukemic* indicates low white count in peripheral blood.

CLINICAL FEATURES/PRINCIPLES OF TREATMENT

As a result of impaired bone marrow function: anemia, thrombocytopenia, and infections caused by reduced numbers of mature functional leukocytes.
As a result of infiltration of organs: splenomegaly, hepatomegaly, lymphadenopathy.
Chronic leukemia well controlled by treatment; relatively long survival.
Acute leukemia difficult to treat and has poor prognosis in many cases; childhood leukemia has better prognosis and may be cured by treatment.
Bone marrow transplant available in selected patients.
Philadelphia chromosome positive subjects respond to drug that inhibits the hyperactive intracellular tyrosine kinase enzyme that promotes cell growth.

Preleukemia/Myelodysplasia

MANIFESTATIONS

Disturbed growth and maturation of marrow cells.
Anemia, leukopenia, thrombocytopenia.
May be precursor of leukemia in some patients.

Multiple Myeloma

CHARACTERISTICS

A neoplasm of plasma cells.
Differs somewhat from leukemia.
Nodular deposits of plasma cells in bone.
Plasma cells produce protein.
Usually no visceral infiltration.
May be preceded by "premyeloma"

Premyeloma

CHARACTERISTICS

An early stage of multiple myeloma characterized by only slightly increased plasma cell proliferation in bone marrow along with slightly increased but abnormal blood protein.

Survival Rates in Neoplastic Disease

NATURE OF PROBLEM

Cancer is leading cause of disability and mortality.
Survival rates vary from 4% to 95%, depending on tumor.
Early diagnosis and treatment may enhance survival.
Some tumors may recur many years after treatment.

Leonard Crowley, An Introduction to Human Disease: Pathology and Pathophysiology, Ninth Edition, 2013

Immunity, Hypersensitivity, Allergy, and Autoimmune Diseases

LEARNING OBJECTIVES

1. List the basic features of cell-mediated and humoral immunity. Explain the role of lymphocytes in the immune response.
2. Compare immunity and hypersensitivity. Explain why it is sometimes necessary to suppress the immune response and describe how this is accomplished.
3. List the five classes of antibodies and explain how they differ from one another.
4. Describe the pathogenesis of allergic manifestations and the role of IgA in allergy. Compare the methods of treatment.
5. Summarize the theories concerning the pathogenesis of autoimmune disease, the clinical manifestations, and the methods of treatment.

The Body's Defense Mechanisms

The body has two separate defense mechanisms for dealing with pathogenic microorganisms and other potentially harmful substances. One mechanism consists of the inflammatory reaction, which is a nonspecific response to any harmful agent and includes phagocytosis of the material by neutrophils and macrophages. The second, which depends on the immune system, consists of the development of an acquired immunity. The two mechanisms complement one another and function together to protect an individual from disease.

Acquired immunity, which develops after contact with a pathogenic microorganism, is only one manifestation of a person's capacity to react to a large number

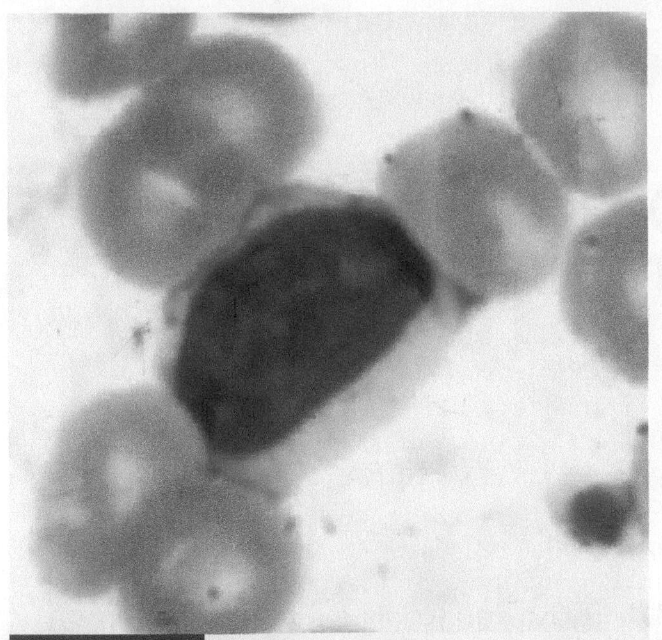

FIGURE 1 Structure of mature lymphocyte in the peripheral blood (original magnification × 1,000).

of foreign antigens. There are two different types of acquired immunity: humoral immunity and cell-mediated immunity.

Humoral immunity is associated with the production of antibodies that can combine with and eliminate the foreign material. Humoral immunity is the body's major defense against many bacteria and bacterial toxins. **Cell-mediated immunity** is characterized by the formation of a population of lymphocytes that can attack and destroy the foreign material. It is the main defense against viruses, fungi, parasites, and some bacteria. Cell-mediated immunity is the mechanism by which the body rejects transplanted organs and eliminates the abnormal cells that sometimes arise spontaneously in cell division.

Acquired immunity is often associated with a stage of altered reactivity to bacterial products or foreign material, leading to an intense inflammatory reaction at the site of contact with the foreign antigen. This increased responsiveness is called **hypersensitivity.** For example, contact with the tubercle bacillus leads to cell-mediated immunity and is also associated with the development of tissue hypersensitivity to antigens of the tubercle bacillus. An individual who displays hypersensitivity to an organism or its products usually possesses some degree of immunity as well. However, many diseases are associated with the development of an acquired immunity without demonstrable hypersensitivity.

Normally, a person develops an immune response not against cell proteins in his or her own cells and tissues (called self-antigens) but only against foreign antigens (called non–self-antigens) because the body has developed a tolerance to the self-antigens present within it. Any lymphocytes that are inadvertently programmed in the course of prenatal development to react against self-antigens are destroyed or inactivated or their functions are suppressed.

However, there are some diseases that result when our own immune system attacks us, producing groups of destructive lymphocytes and injurious antibodies directed against our own cells and tissues, which may cause considerable organ damage. Antibodies directed against us are called **autoantibodies** (*auto* = self), and the diseases resulting from tissue damage caused by our own immune system are called **autoimmune diseases.**

Humoral immunity
Immunity associated with formation of antibodies produced by plasma cells.

Cell-mediated immunity
Immunity associated with population of sensitized lymphocytes.

Hypersensitivity
A state of abnormal reactivity to a foreign material.

Autoantibody
(aw′tō-an′ti-bod-ē)
An antibody formed against one's own cells or tissue components.

Autoimmune disease
A disease associated with formation of cell-mediated or humoral immunity against the subject's own cells or tissue components.

Lymphokine
(limf′ō-kīn)
A soluble substance liberated by lymphocytes.

Cytokine
A general term for any protein secreted by cells that functions as an intercellular messenger and influences cells of the immune system. Cytokines are secreted by macrophages and monocytes (monokines), lymphocytes (lymphokines), and other cells.

Immunity

THE ROLE OF LYMPHOCYTES IN ACQUIRED IMMUNITY

The important cells of the immune system are the lymphocytes (FIGURE 1), which respond to foreign antigens, and the macrophages and related cells that process the antigen and "present" it to the lymphocytes.

The various cells of the immune system communicate with one another and produce many of their effects by secreting soluble protein (peptide) chemical messengers. Those secreted by lymphocytes are called **lymphokines.** The general term **cytokines** is used to designate any chemical messengers that take part in any function of the immune system, and some cytokines have specific names. Those that act by interfering with the multiplication of viruses within cells are called **interferons.** Those that send regulatory signals between cells of the immune system are called **interleukins.** Cytokines that can destroy foreign or abnormal cells are called **tumor necrosis factors**, so named because they can destroy tumor cells, although their destructive functions are not restricted to tumor cells.

Interferon
(in-tur-fēr′on)
A broad-spectrum antiviral agent manufactured by various cells in the body.

Interleukin-2
(inter-lōō′kin)
A lymphokine that stimulates growth of lymphocytes.

Tumor necrosis factor
A cytokine that can destroy foreign or abnormal cells.

T lymphocyte
A type of lymphocyte associated with cell-mediated immunity.

B lymphocyte
A lymphocyte that differentiates into plasma cells and is associated with humoral immunity.

DEVELOPMENT OF THE LYMPHATIC SYSTEM

Development of Immune Competence

The precursor cells of the lymphocytes are formed initially from stem cells in the bone marrow, and they eventually develop into either of two groups of lymphocytes, depending on where they undergo further development and "learn" their functions—a process called developing immune competence. In the fetus, some of these precursor cells migrate from the marrow into the thymus, where they undergo further maturation and develop into cells that are destined to form a specific type of lymphocyte called T (thymus-dependent) **lymphocytes.** Other lymphoid cells remain within the bone marrow, where they differentiate and develop into cells destined to form a second specific type of lymphocyte called B (bone marrow) **lymphocytes.**

The programming process by which lymphocytes acquire immune competence involves a rearrangement of genes within the developing B and T lymphocytes. Each programmed lymphocyte develops antigen receptors on its cell membrane that enable the lymphocyte to "recognize" and respond to a specific antigen. The antigen receptors of B lymphocytes are immunoglobulin (antibody) molecules, each a copy of the antibody that the B lymphocyte will eventually produce when stimulated by the appropriate antigen. T lymphocytes develop somewhat different types of receptors, but they serve the same functions as those on B cells. When the programming process has been completed, many millions of different T and B cells have formed, each programmed to recognize and respond to a different antigen. Although a single lymphocyte can respond to only a single antigen, there is such an enormous population of lymphocytes that some member of the "immunologic response team" can respond to any antigen the individual may ever encounter.

Migration and Circulation of Lymphocytes

Before birth, the precursor cells of both T and B lymphocytes migrate into the spleen, lymph nodes, and other sites. Here they proliferate to form the masses of mature lymphocytes that populate the various lymphoid organs.

T lymphocytes are usually classified into two major groups based on the type of protein molecules, called CD (cluster of differentiation) antigens, on their cell membranes. Lymphocytes containing CD4 antigens are usually called T4 lymphocytes, and those with CD8 antigens are called T8 lymphocytes. As described later, each group of T lymphocytes has different functions and responds somewhat differently when stimulated by an antigen.

Lymphocytes vary in their life span. Some have only a short survival time, but others live for many years. Lymphocytes do not remain localized within lymphoid organs. They continually recirculate between the bloodstream and the various lymphoid tissues. T and B lymphocytes are both present in the circulation and can be distinguished by special techniques.

About two-thirds of the circulating lymphocytes are T lymphocytes, and most of the rest are B lymphocytes. From about 10 to 15% of the circulating lymphocytes, however, have neither T nor B cell receptors. These cells are called **natural killer cells** or simply **NK cells.** Their major targets are virus-infected cells and cancer cells, which they can attack and destroy by secreting destructive lymphokines, even though they

Natural killer cells
Lymphocytes capable of destroying foreign or abnormal cells, although they have not had any prior antigenic contact with the cells.

NK cells
An abbreviation for natural killer cells.

have not been previously exposed to the foreign antigens that they are attacking. Furthermore, NK cells can destroy the target cells as soon as they are encountered, in contrast to T and B cells, which need time to become activated and function effectively. Although NK cells are not actually part of either the cell-mediated or the humoral immune defense systems, their functions are to some extent regulated by the immune system. NK cells are related to cell-mediated immunity because they are activated and function much more effectively when stimulated by lymphokines secreted by T lymphocytes. They are also related to humoral immunity because some types of NK cells possess cell membrane receptors for antibody molecules, which makes it easier for the NK lymphocytes to attach to and destroy target cells coated with antibodies.

RESPONSE OF LYMPHOCYTES TO FOREIGN ANTIGENS

Entry of a foreign antigen into the body triggers a chain of events that involves interactions between T and B lymphocytes and macrophages or similar antigen-processing cells. Macrophages are monocytes that have left the bloodstream and taken up permanent residence in the tissues throughout the body where they phagocytose and process antigens. Another important group of widely distributed antigen-processing cells is called dendritic cells, named from their long cytoplasmic processes that resemble the dendrites of a nerve cell. T and B lymphocytes respond differently to foreign antigens. T lymphocytes can only respond to processed antigens, but B lymphocytes can process intact antigens and display antigen fragments on their cell membranes. The interactions between antigen and antigen-processing cells involve three phases:

1. Recognition of the foreign antigen
2. Proliferation of the lymphocytes programmed to respond to the antigen, forming a large group (clone) of cells
3. Destruction of the foreign antigen by the lymphocytes that have responded to the antigen

FIGURE 2 summarizes the role of lymphocytes in acquired immunity. The first step in the immune defense reaction is the interaction of lymphocytes with the antigen that they have been programmed to recognize. The antigen must first be "processed" and displayed on the cell membrane of the antigen-processing cell before the immune response can be set in motion. Antigens are very large molecules. Only small fragments of the processed antigen called antigenic determinants or epitopes are displayed, not the entire molecule. When appropriately stimulated, B lymphocytes proliferate and mature into antibody-forming plasma cells, and T lymphocytes proliferate to form a diverse population of cells that both regulate the immune response and generate a cell-mediated immune reaction to eliminate the antigenic material.

Initial contact with a foreign antigen is followed by a lag phase of a week or more before an immune response is demonstrated. This lag corresponds to the time required for processing the antigen and for the lymphocytes to respond. After the body's immune mechanisms have reacted to a foreign antigen, however, some of the lymphoid cells retain a "memory" of the antigen that induced sensitization. They pass this information to succeeding generations of lymphocytes. Consequently, any later contact with the same antigen provokes a renewed proliferation of sensitized lymphocytes or antibody-forming plasma cells.

Role of Major Histocompatibility Proteins in Displaying Processed Antigen

The major histocompatibility (MHC) proteins play an essential role in "presenting" processed antigen to the responding cells of the immune system in order to generate

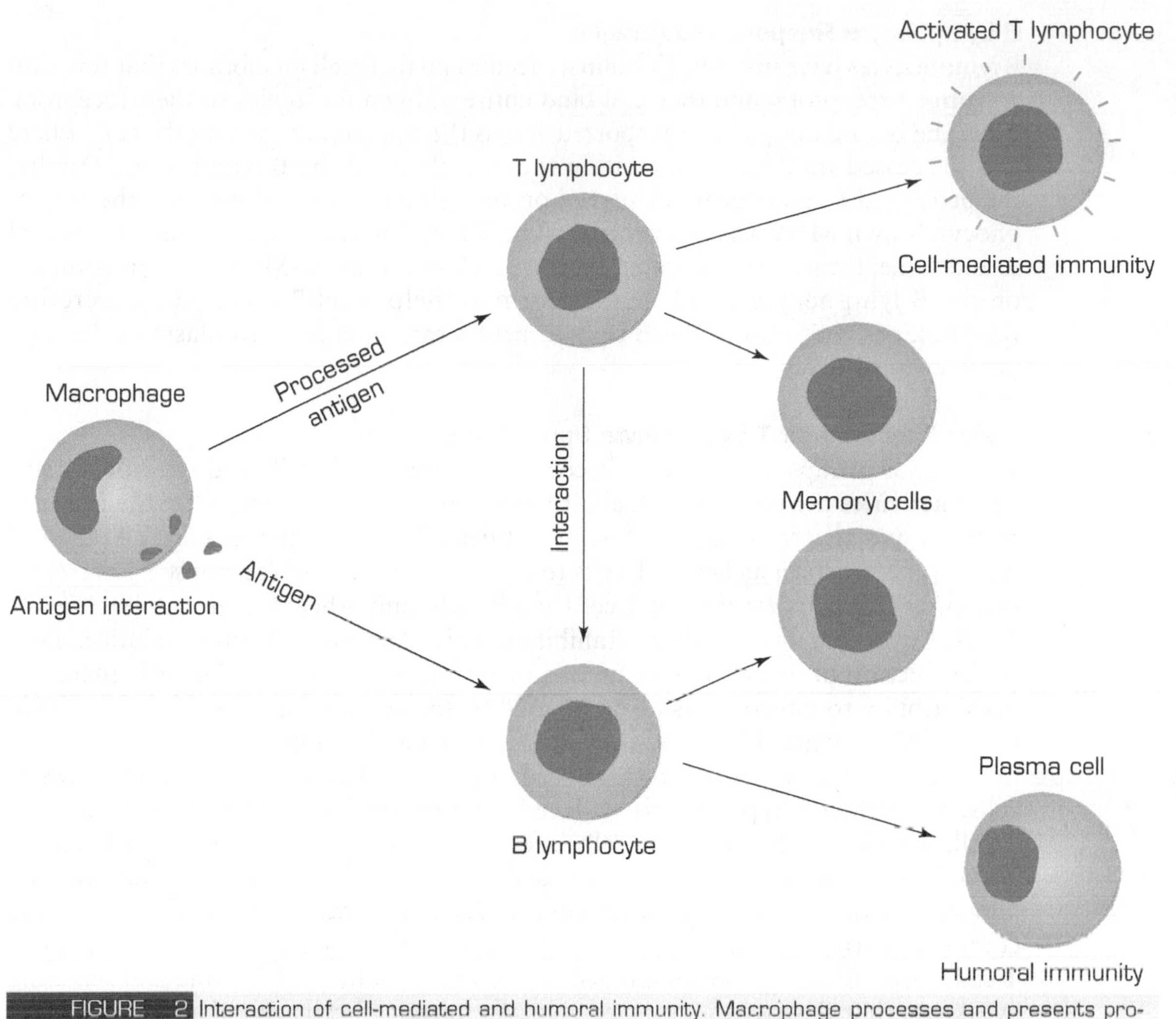

FIGURE 2 Interaction of cell-mediated and humoral immunity. Macrophage processes and presents processed antigen fragments to T lymphocyte; B lymphocyte processes intact antigen and displays fragments of the same antigen on its cell membrane. T lymphocyte, which has responded to the same antigen, stimulates the B lymphocyte to proliferate, mature into plasma cells, and make antibodies.

an immune response. The MHC proteins are carbohydrate–protein (glycoprotein) molecules on the surface of cells that distinguish the cells of one person from those of another. As described in the discussion on chromosomes, genes, and cell division, there are two major classes of MHC proteins: MHC Class I proteins are present on all nucleated cells; MHC Class II proteins are restricted to B lymphocytes, macrophages and related antigen-processing cells, and some activated T lymphocytes. The main function of the MHC proteins is to serve as a carrier for the processed foreign antigen fragments on the surface of cells to which the immune system can respond.

T Lymphocyte Response to Antigen

T lymphocytes are unable to respond to a foreign antigen until a macrophage or similar macrophagelike antigen-processing cell has phagocytosed the antigen, digested it, and displayed on its cell membrane the antigen fragments combined with its own MHC Class II proteins. In response to the displayed antigen-MHC Class II proteins, the T lymphocyte having the corresponding antigen receptors responds by proliferating and forms a group (clone) of identical T cells. The macrophages are also activated when they process and present antigen to T cells, and they secrete a cytokine that stimulates the T cells to proliferate.

B Lymphocyte Response to Antigen

B lymphocytes have immunoglobulin molecules on their cell membranes that function as antigen receptors, and they can bind entire antigen molecules to their receptors. Then the bound antigen is transported across the cell membrane into the cell, where it is processed into fragments within the cytoplasm of the B lymphocyte. Finally, the processed fragments are displayed on the cell membrane along with the B lymphocyte's own MHC Class II proteins. The T lymphocytes that have also responded to the same antigen are activated by the displayed antigen–MHC protein complex on the B lymphocytes, and they perform a "helper cell" function by secreting lymphokines that induce the B cells to proliferate, mature into plasma cells, and produce antibodies.

Major Functions of T Lymphocyte Populations

Two major groups of T cells are recognized: regulator T cells and effector T cells. Their activities are coordinated, and they function together to regulate the immune response and also to act against foreign antigens. The regulator cells are T4 (CD4+) cells. Some function as helper T cells to promote the immune response by secreting cytokines that activate effector T cells and B cells, and others function as suppressor T cells by producing cytokines to inhibit excessive immune system stimulation. Loss or destruction of helper T cells inhibits the immune response and greatly increases susceptibility to infection, as demonstrated by the acquired immune deficiency syndrome (AIDS) caused by a virus that destroys helper T lymphocytes.

Effector T cells
Cytotoxic and delayed hypersensitivity T cells that protect the body by attacking and destroying body cells infected with bacteria or viruses.

There are two types of **effector T cells**: cytotoxic T cells, which are T8 (CD8+) cells, and delayed hypersensitivity T cells, which are T4 (CD4+) cells. Cytotoxic T cells attack and destroy body cells infected with viruses or intracellular bacteria. The infected cells are marked for destruction because some of the viral or bacterial antigens are broken down within the infected cells and transported to the cell surface combined with MHC Class I proteins (present on all nucleated cells). The cytotoxic T cells respond to the foreign antigen–MHC complex by proliferating and secreting cytokines that destroy the infected cells. Cytotoxic T cells can also attack cancer cells, which display antigens different from normal cell antigens combined with MHC Class I proteins, and they are also responsible for the rejection of transplanted organs, which also contain foreign antigens.

Delayed hypersensitivity cells, also called sensitized T cells, are produced by a subgroup of helper T cells. The delayed hypersensitivity T cells respond to foreign antigens processed by macrophages or similar cells by accumulating at the site of the antigenic material, where they secrete a variety of lymphokines that attract macrophages, activate them, and stimulate them to secrete additional cytokines, including interferon and tumor necrosis factor. Some of the lymphokines also stimulate cytotoxic T cells and NK cells, both of which also secrete destructive cytokines. In this way, the delayed hypersensitivity reaction generates an intense inflammatory response directed against the antigens that stimulated the response.

In addition to regulator and effector T cells, a population of long-lived memory cells is also generated that can initiate a rapid cell-mediated immune response on later contact with the same antigen. TABLE 1 summarizes the classification and functions of the immune system cells.

Relation of MHC Proteins to Effector T Cell Responses

The two types of effector T cells are restricted in their ability to respond to processed antigens complexed and presented with MHC proteins. Cytotoxic T cells, which are T8 (CD8+) cells, can respond only to antigens complexed with MHC Class I proteins displayed on infected host cells, indicating to the immune system that some of the body's

TABLE 1

Classification and functions of immune system cells

Cell function	Cell type	Action of cell
Antigen processing	Macrophages, B lymphocytes, dendritic cells	Process antigen and present to lymphocytes
Regulate immune response	Regulator T cells (CD4+)	Cytokines regulate immune system activity
Promote cytotoxic immune response	Cytotoxic T cells (CD8+)	Produce cytokines that destroy foreign or abnormal cells displaying antigen fragments combined with MHC Class I antigens
Promote delayed hypersensitivity response	Delayed hypersensitivity T cells (CD4+)	Respond to antigen-processing cells presenting foreign antigen fragments combined with MHC Class II antigens; produce cytokines that activate and stimulate macrophages, cytotoxic T cells, and NK cells
Destroy virus-infected cells and cancer cells	NK cells	Cytokine-mediated cell destruction; no previous contact with antigen required
Produce antibodies	Plasma cells	Antigen processed by B lymphocytes and presented to responding T cells stimulates B lymphocytes to mature into plasma cells and make antibodies

own cells have been infected and should be destroyed. In contrast, delayed hypersensitivity cells, which are T4 (CD4+) cells, can respond only to processed antigen displayed on macrophages or related cells along with MHC Class II proteins, signaling the immune system cells to become activated in order to deal with the threat. Consequently, the manner in which the processed antigen is displayed determines which type of effector T cell will respond to the complexed antigen. Cytotoxic T cells are "designed" to attack and destroy infected host cells or other antigenically foreign or abnormal cells. Delayed hypersensitivity T cells function by orchestrating an intense inflammatory reaction to any type of foreign antigen, including micro-organisms such as the tubercle bacillus that are phagocytosed by macrophages. Activated macrophages, assisted by lymphoid cells, are the cells that play a major role in eliminating the antigenic material.

Immune-Response Genes

The ability to generate an immune response is under genetic control. Genes called **immune-response genes**, which are closely associated with the HLA complex on chromosome 6 in the discussion on chromosomes, genes, and cell division, control the

Immune-response genes
Genes on chromosome 6 that control the immune response to specific antigens.

immune response by regulating T cell and B cell proliferation. In this way, the genes regulate the intensity of the cell-mediated immune reaction and control the synthesis of antibody molecules. As a result, they influence resistance to infection and resistance to tumors. They also influence the likelihood of acquiring an autoimmune disease.

THE ROLE OF COMPLEMENT IN IMMUNE RESPONSES

Complement functions along with the immune system to destroy or inactivate all types of foreign antigens, including invading micro-organisms. As described in the discussion on inflammation and repair, complement can be activated in two ways: the classical pathway, which is triggered by antigen–antibody interactions, and the alternative pathway, in which complement is activated by bacterial cell wall material or products generated during the inflammatory reaction. When complement is activated, the complement components interact to accomplish several important functions. Some components function as mediators of inflammation. Other components coat the surface of invading bacteria, which makes them easier for macrophages and neutrophils to phagocytose. Finally, the interaction of the complement components generates a large molecule called an attack complex, which destroys the target micro-organism or abnormal cell by "punching holes" in its cell membrane (FIGURE 3).

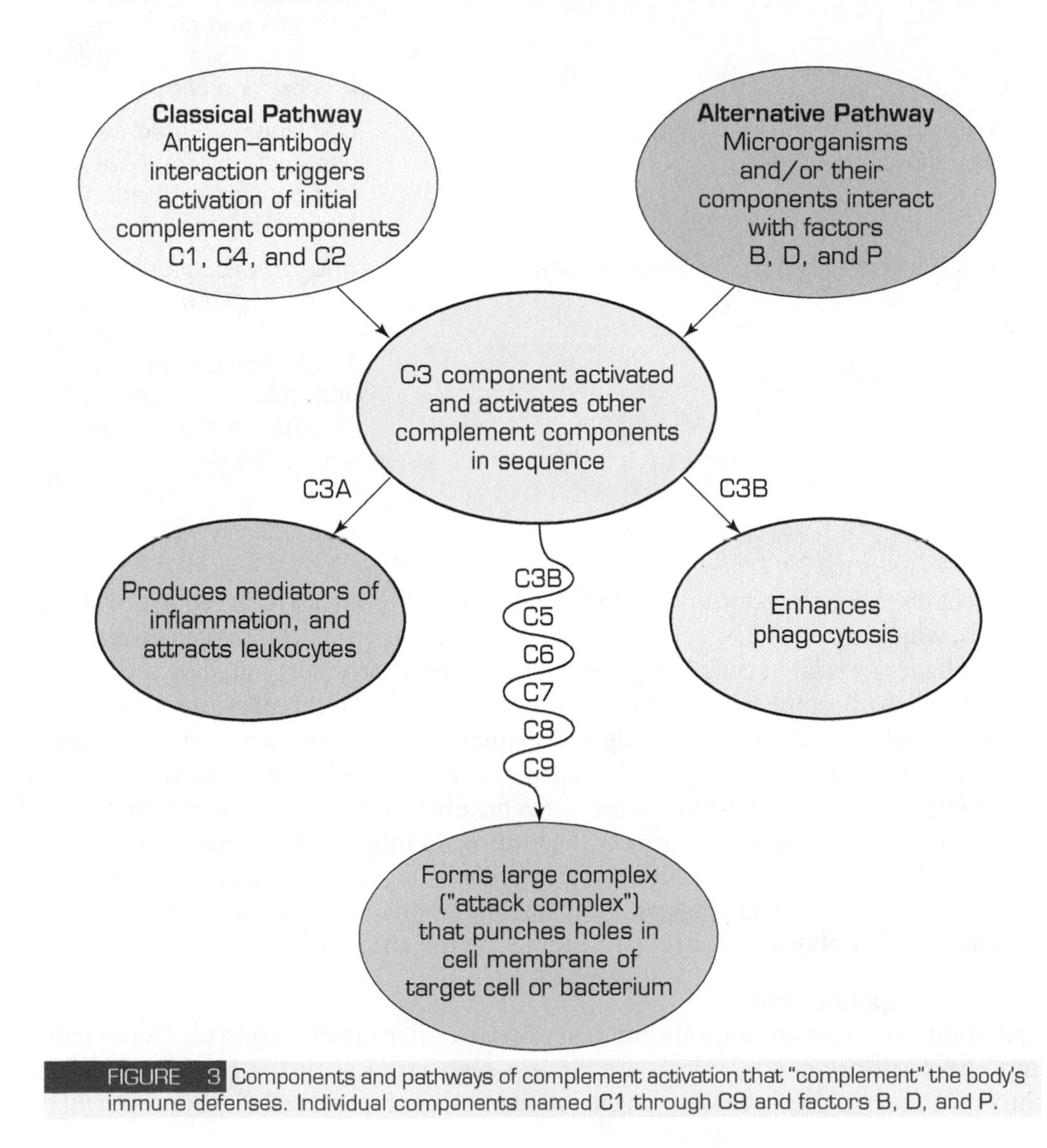

FIGURE 3 Components and pathways of complement activation that "complement" the body's immune defenses. Individual components named C1 through C9 and factors B, D, and P.

Antibodies (Immunoglobulins)

Antibodies are globulins produced by plasma cells and are usually called **immunoglobulins** to emphasize their role in immunity. There are five different classes of immunoglobulins:

Immunoglobulin (im′mū-nō-glob′u-lin) *An antibody protein.*

1. Immunoglobulin M (IgM)
2. Immunoglobulin G (IgG)
3. Immunoglobulin A (IgA)
4. Immunoglobulin D (IgD)
5. Immunoglobulin E (IgE)

Although the immunoglobulins differ somewhat from one another in their chemical composition, molecular weight, and size, they all have the same basic structure: two matched pairs of polypeptide (protein) chains joined by chemical bonds (FIGURE 4). One pair is called heavy chains. The second pair is only half as long as the heavy chains and is called light chains.

The arrangement of the Ig chains somewhat resembles the appearance of a fork. The ends of the Ig chains that combine with the antigen can be compared with its prongs. The "prong" end of the immunoglobulin molecule, which is different in each antibody, is called the variable part of the molecule. It is this part that imparts specificity to the molecule. Because of its structure, the antibody can react only with the specific antigen that induced its formation. The constant part of the chain, which can be compared with the handle of the fork, is the same for each major class of antibody. The "handle" end does not combine with antigen but determines other properties of the antibody, such as the ability to activate complement or fix to the surface of cell membranes.

All Ig molecules have the same basic four-chain unit structure, but some immunoglobulins characteristically aggregate to form clusters of two, three, or five individual units. For example, IgM is usually a cluster of five individual units, and IgA is usually a pair of units.

An antibody molecule is not a rigid structure. The junction of its constant and variable parts is quite flexible and is called the hinge region. This feature allows the variable end of the Y-shaped molecule to adapt to the configuration of the antigen that it is binding. Treatment with enzymes breaks an immunoglobulin molecule into three fragments. The variable region yields two fragments called the F_{ab} fragments (antibody-combining fragments), each consisting of a light chain and the associated part of the heavy chain. The other fragment is the constant region of the molecule and is called the F_c fragment (constant fragment).

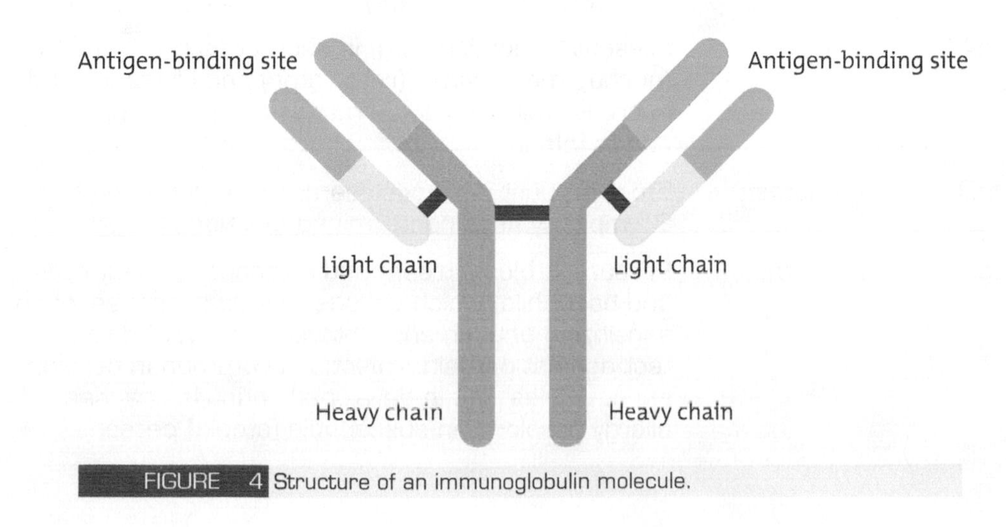

FIGURE 4 Structure of an immunoglobulin molecule.

IgM is present in the blood as a cluster of five individual molecules (a pentamer) joined together in a star-shaped configuration with the antigen-binding ends projecting outward and the opposite ends of the molecules directed toward the center of the cluster. As a pentamer, IgM forms a very large antibody cluster that is very efficient in combining with large particulate antigens such as fungi; it is often called a macroglobulin because of its large size and high molecular weight. IgM molecules are also found as single (monomeric) molecules attached, with their antigen-binding sites protruding, to the cell membranes of B lymphocytes, where they function as the antigen receptors on the surface of B lymphocytes. IgG is a much smaller antibody molecule and is the principal type of antibody molecule formed in response to the majority of infectious agents. IgA is produced by antibody-forming cells located in the respiratory and gastrointestinal mucosa. It is present in secretions of the respiratory and gastrointestinal tracts. IgA apparently functions by combining with potentially harmful ingested or inhaled antigens, forming antigen–antibody complexes that cannot be absorbed. In this way, IgA prevents the antigens from inducing sensitization. IgD is found on the cell membranes of B lymphocytes, along with the monomeric form of IgM and is present in only minute quantities in the blood. IgE is normally present in only small quantities in the blood of most persons, but its concentration is greatly increased in allergic individuals.

TABLE 2 summarizes the types and functions of the various immunoglobulins.

TABLE 2

Types and functions of immunoglobulins

Immunoglobulin	Usual type of secretion	Properties and functions
IgM	Pentamer	First Ig formed in response to foreign antigen (primary immune response). Present in bloodstream but not in tissues. Large pentamer antibody cluster very effective for combining with foreign antigen.
IgG	Monomer	Most prevalent Ig produced rapidly in large amounts (secondary immune response) to replace IgM. Found in blood and tissues. Crosses placenta to protect fetus until infant immune system can produce antibodies.
IgA	Dimer	Present in bloodstream, in secretions produced by mucous membranes (respiratory and GI tract), and in breast milk to provide maternal antibody protection to infant.
IgD	Monomer	Small amount in bloodstream and on surface of B lymphocytes. Undetermined functions.
IgE	Monomer	Present in bloodstream and attaches to mast cells and basophils, which causes allergic response when sensitizing antigen encountered. IgE evolved to protect against parasitic infections common in developing countries, but in developed countries causes allergy problems in susceptible (atopic) persons.

Hypersensitivity Reactions: Immune System-Related Tissue Injury

The immune system, while protecting us from foreign antigens that could harm us, may also damage the tissues where the immune response occurs. The desirable effect, which eliminates the foreign antigen, is called **immunity**. The undesirable effect, which is the associated tissue damage, is called **hypersensitivity**. Both are manifestations of the same process. The situation could be compared with the successful efforts of firefighters in putting out a potentially destructive house fire but at the same time breaking some windows and causing some water damage to the house and furniture.

Immunity
Resistance to disease.

Hypersensitivity
A state of abnormal reactivity to a foreign material.

It is conventional to classify the various types of hypersensitivity reactions based on how the immune system caused the injury (TABLE 3). Four different types of hypersensitivity reactions, usually designated by roman numerals, are recognized. The first three types are related to antibodies formed in response to antigenic material, and the fourth type is a cell-mediated hypersensitivity reaction. This section deals with the various mechanisms of immunologic injury. Specific examples of immune-mediated organ damage will be considered in connection with the disease of the various organ systems.

TABLE 3

Mechanisms of immunologic Injury

Type	Mechanism	Examples
I: Immediate hypersensitivity	IgE antibodies fix to mast cells and basophils. Later contact with sensitizing antigen triggers mediator release and clinical manifestations.	Localized response: hay fever, food allergy, etc. Systemic response: bee sting or penicillin anaphylaxis, etc.
II: Cytotoxic hypersensitivity reactions	Antibody binds to cell or tissue antigen, and complement is activated, which damages cell, causes inflammation, and promotes destruction of antibody-coated cell by phagocytosis.	Autoimmune hemolytic anemia Blood transfusion reactions Rh hemolytic disease Some types of glomerulonephritis
III: Immune complex disease	Circulating antigen–antibody complexes form, which activate complement and cause inflammatory reaction.	Some types of glomerulonephritis Lupus erythematosus Rheumatoid arthritis
IV: Delayed (cell-mediated) hypersensitivity	Sensitized (delayed hypersensitivity) T cells release lymphokines that attract macrophages and other inflammatory cells.	Tuberculosis Fungus and parasitic infections Contact dermatitis

TYPE I. IMMEDIATE HYPERSENSITIVITY REACTIONS: ALLERGY AND ANAPHYLAXIS

Type I hypersensitivity reactions follow contact with foreign antigens that induce formation of specific IgE antibodies in the sensitized person. IgE has the unusual property of attaching to the surface of mast cells and similar cells circulating in the blood called basophils. The IgE attaches itself to the cell membrane by means of the F_c end of the molecule (the "handle of the fork"). If the sensitized person is later exposed to the sensitizing antigen, the antigen attaches to the free antibody-combining sites (the "prongs of the fork") on the IgE molecules. The union of antigen and antibody causes the cells to release their cytoplasmic granules filled with histamine, prostaglandins, and other potent chemical mediators. Immediate hypersensitivity reactions either may be localized, called allergic reactions, or may evoke a widespread systemic reaction, called **anaphylaxis**.

Anaphylaxis
(a-nä-fil-aks′is)
A severe generalized IgE-mediated hypersensitivity reaction characterized by marked respiratory distress and fall in blood pressure.

Atopic
(ā-top′ik)
Having a genetic predisposition to certain allergic conditions such as hay fever and asthma.

Allergen
(al′ler-jen)
A substance capable of inducing an allergic reaction in a predisposed individual.

Desensitization
A method of inducing a diminished response to allergens by inducing the formation of specific IgG and IgA antibodies.

Allergy

Individuals who develop localized IgE-mediated reactions are predisposed to form specific IgE antibodies (become allergic) to ragweed, other plant pollens, and various other antigens that do not affect most persons. The allergy-prone individual is called an **atopic person**. The sensitizing antigen is called an **allergen**, and the allergic manifestations are localized to the tissues that are exposed to the allergens—for example, swollen itchy eyes, stuffy nose, and sneezing in a ragweed-sensitive person (FIGURE 5).

Because histamine is one of the mediators released from the IgE-coated cells, antihistamine drugs (which block the effects of histamine) often relieve many of the allergic symptoms. A more specific method of treating an allergic individual consists of immunizing the person to the offending allergen by repeated subcutaneous injections of the antigen that induced the allergy, such as an extract of ragweed pollen in a ragweed-sensitive person. This method of treatment, which is called **desensitization**, induces the formation of specific IgA and IgG antibodies against the offending allergen. The IgA and IgG act by combining with the allergen before it can affix to the cell-bound IgE and trigger the release of mediators. In a ragweed-sensitive person, for example, the ragweed-specific IgA present in the secretions of the respiratory tract combines with some of the inhaled ragweed antigen and helps prevent absorption of the allergen. At the same time, the ragweed-specific IgG circulating in the bloodstream combines with much of the absorbed ragweed antigen before it can interact with the IgE on the surface of the mast cells and basophils. Because less antigen is available to combine with cell-bound IgE and thereby trigger release of mediators, the allergic manifestations are minimized.

Anaphylaxis and Anaphylactoid Reactions

A severe generalized IgE-mediated hypersensitivity reaction may be life threatening and is called anaphylaxis. The condition results from an initial exposure to a substance (allergen) that induces the sensitization in a susceptible person. Commonly implicated allergens include penicillin, bee stings, peanuts, latex products, as well as various other sensitizing agents. Once sensitization has occurred, a later exposure to the sensitizing antigen triggers widespread mediator release from IgE-coated mast cells and basophils. This release may lead to a fall in blood pressure with circulatory collapse and is often accompanied by severe respiratory distress caused by mediator-induced spasm of smooth muscle in the walls of the bronchioles, which restricts air flow into and out of the lungs. Prompt treatment of this immunologic catastrophe with epinephrine and other appropriate agents is essential. A similar condition called an **anaphylactoid reaction** resembles an anaphylactic reaction but is not caused by IgE and occurs after the first contact with a foreign substance, possibly by stimulating mast cells directly or by activating complement. Aspirin, other nonsteroidal

Anaphylactoid reaction
(a-na-fil-ack-toyd)
A hypersensitivity reaction resembling anaphylaxis but not caused by IgE antibodies.

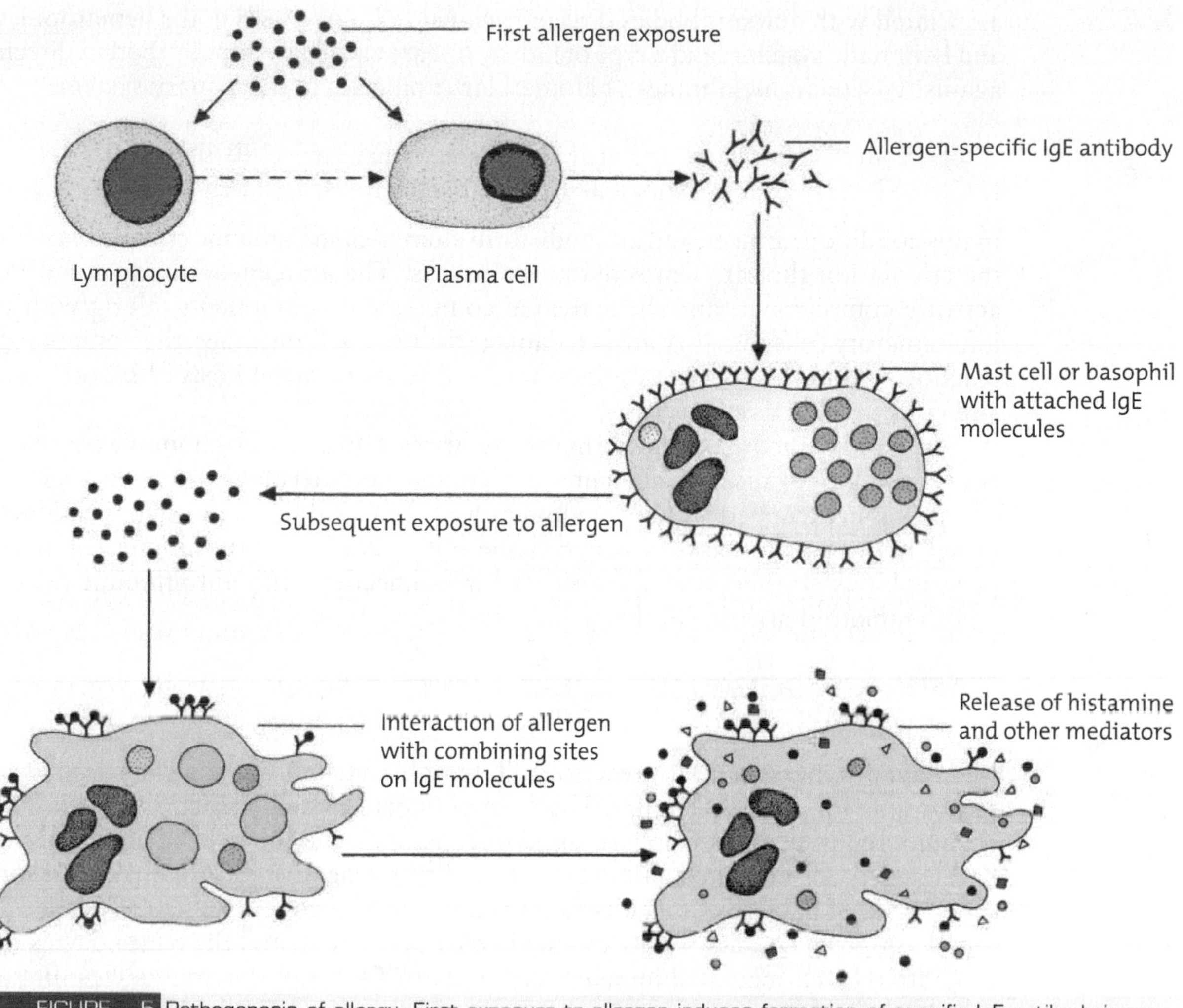

FIGURE 5 Pathogenesis of allergy. First exposure to allergen induces formation of specific IgE antibody in susceptible individual, which binds to mast cells and basophils by nonantigen receptor end of molecule. Subsequent exposure to allergen leads to an antigen–antibody interaction, liberating histamine and other mediators from mast cells and basophils. These mediators induce allergic manifestations.

anti-inflammatory drugs, some antibiotics, and radiopaque iodine-containing contrast material used for x-ray examinations may trigger an anaphylactoid reaction. The treatment is the same as for an anaphylactic reaction.

TYPE II. CYTOTOXIC HYPERSENSITIVITY REACTIONS

In this type of hypersensitivity reaction, antibody formed against a cell or tissue antigen binds to the surface of the target cell or tissue. The antigen–antibody reaction activates complement, and products of complement activation directly or indirectly damage the target. The complement components interact to form a large molecule called an attack complex that directly damages the target cell membrane. Inflammatory cells also are attracted and contribute to the tissue injury by releasing destructive enzymes; they may also destroy the antibody-coated target cells by phagocytosis.

Examples of Type II reactions include transfusion reactions caused by administration of incompatible blood, hemolytic disease of newborn infants caused by Rh incompatibility in prenatal development, some types of chronic hemolytic anemia associated with autoantibodies directed against red blood cells in the hematopoietic and lymphatic systems, and a type of kidney disease caused by autoantibodies directed against basement membranes of glomerular capillaries in the urinary system.

TYPE III. TISSUE INJURY CAUSED BY IMMUNE COMPLEXES ("IMMUNE COMPLEX DISEASE")

In this condition, antigen and antibody form clumps called immune complexes within the circulation that are deposited in the tissues. The antigen–antibody complexes activate complement, and the activated complement components, along with the inflammatory cells that they attract, damage the tissues. Sometimes, the immunologic reaction within the tissues is quite severe and leads to thrombosis of blood vessels and considerable tissue necrosis.

An example of organ damage in the urinary system caused by immune complexes is a type of kidney disease called immune-complex glomerulonephritis, in which the complexes are trapped within the glomeruli as the blood flows through the kidneys. Other important diseases in which tissue injury is related to immune complexes include lupus erythematosus, considered in connection with autoimmune disease, and rheumatoid arthritis in the musculoskeletal system.

TYPE IV. DELAYED (CELL-MEDIATED) HYPERSENSITIVITY REACTIONS

In delayed hypersensitivity reactions, T lymphocytes rather than antibodies are responsible for the tissue injury. This type of hypersensitivity reaction is commonly encountered in persons who have been infected with the tubercle bacillus and have developed a cell-mediated immune reaction directed against the organism, but some other types of bacteria, as well as fungi and parasites, evoke a similar response. The initial antigenic contact sensitizes the affected individual, and the lymphocytes that generate the cell-mediated immune response are T4 (CD4+) lymphocytes that are called delayed hypersensitivity T cells or, simply, sensitized T cells. After sensitization has occurred, any subsequent contact with the sensitizing antigen induces proliferation of T4 cells that accumulate at the site of antigen contact. The sensitized T cells secrete cytokines that attract and activate macrophages and other lymphocytes and incite an inflammatory reaction.

Delayed hypersensitivity reactions may also follow skin exposure to poison ivy, as well as various drugs, cosmetics, and chemicals. These agents combine with normal skin proteins to form a complex that induces sensitization. Any later skin contact with the offending agent that induced the initial sensitization provokes an intense cell-mediated inflammatory reaction in the skin, a condition called contact dermatitis.

Unlike immediate hypersensitivity reactions, which are mediated by antibodies, a cell-mediated inflammatory reaction requires from 24 to 48 hours to develop, the delay being the time necessary for sensitized T cells to accumulate at the site and generate an inflammatory reaction. Because this type of reaction takes place in persons who have been infected with the tubercle bacillus, a delayed hypersensitivity reaction is sometimes called tuberculin type hypersensitivity. The commonly used Mantoux skin test to detect infection with the tubercle bacillus is based on the presence or absence of a delayed hypersensitivity reaction to proteins of the tubercle bacillus. If an individual has had a previous contact with the tubercle bacillus, injection of a small test dose of proteins from the tubercle bacillus leads to an inflammatory reaction at the injection site. A positive test, however, only indicates a previous infection with the organism and development of cell-mediated immunity, along with associated hypersensitivity to the tubercle bacillus, but does not necessarily indicate that the person has active tuberculosis.

Suppression of the Immune Response

REASONS FOR SUPPRESSION

Cell-mediated and humoral immune responses protect against potentially harmful micro-organisms and other foreign substances. These same immunologic mechanisms may at times have undesirable effects:

1. They may be directed against the individual's own cells or tissue components, leading to autoimmune diseases.
2. They are responsible for the rejection of transplanted organs.
3. They lead to Rh hemolytic disease in newborn infants.

METHODS OF SUPPRESSION

It is sometimes necessary to suppress the immune response to treat certain autoimmune diseases, to perform organ transplants, and to prevent Rh hemolytic disease. There are many types of immunosuppressive agents that have found wide application in clinical medicine. The main types of immunosuppressive agents that are commonly used by physicians are as follows:

1. Radiation
2. Immunosuppressive drugs that impede cell division or cell function
3. Adrenal corticosteroid hormones
4. Immunoglobulin preparations

Radiation and Immunosuppressive Drugs

Radiation destroys normal cells. It exerts its immunosuppressive effect by destroying lymphoid tissue, which plays a key role in both cell-mediated and humoral immunity. There are several types of drugs that can suppress the immune response. **Cytotoxic drugs** (*cyto* = cell + *toxic* = poisonous) act by suppressing growth and division of lymphocytes. Lymphoid tissue is especially susceptible to the inhibitory effect of these drugs. **Antimetabolites**, as the name implies, inhibit important cellular metabolic functions, thereby inhibiting cell proliferation and suppressing the inflammatory reaction. Another important immunosuppressive drug called cyclosporine is often used to suppress the immune response in patients who have received organ transplants. The drug selectively inhibits T lymphocytes by interfering with the formation of a lymphokine called interleukin-2, which stimulates T lymphocyte proliferation. As a result, cell-mediated immune responses are suppressed with little effect on humoral immune responses or on the inflammatory reaction. (Cytotoxic drugs and antimetabolites are also used to treat some types of leukemia and malignant tumors, as described in the discussion on neoplastic disease.)

Cytotoxic drugs
(sī-tō-tok'sik)
Producing cell necrosis or destruction.

Antimetabolite
(an-ti-met-ab'o-līte)
A substance that competes with or replaces another substance (metabolite) required for cell growth or multiplication.

Corticosteroids

Adrenal corticosteroids act in several ways. They suppress the inflammatory response and impair phagocytosis. They also inhibit protein synthesis, thereby suppressing the growth and division of lymphocytes and inhibiting antibody formation by plasma cells.

Antibodies as Immunosuppressive Agents

Antibodies themselves may suppress or inhibit an immune response under certain circumstances. For example, injections of immunoglobulins appear to be a safe, effective treatment for many autoimmune neuromuscular diseases, although the optimal dose and frequency of administration are still being investigated. The immunoglobulins act by interfering with the generation of cytotoxic T cells, cytokines, and autoantibodies.

Eliminating a foreign antigen before the immune system can respond to the antigen is another effective way to suppress an immune response and is used routinely to prevent hemolytic disease of newborn infants caused by Rh incompatibility. Postdelivery administration of Rh immune globulin containing potent Rh antibodies to an Rh-negative mother who has given birth to an Rh-positive infant eliminates any antigenic Rh-positive fetal cells that may have entered the mother's bloodstream during delivery. Because the antigenic fetal cells are rapidly removed from the mother's circulation, the mother does not form Rh antibody, and Rh hemolytic disease is prevented in subsequent pregnancies. This application is described in connection with prenatal development and diseases associated with pregnancy.

TISSUE GRAFTS AND IMMUNITY

An individual will accept a graft of his or her own tissue or that of an identical twin, but not that of another person, because a graft from another person contains HLA antigens foreign to the recipient. The body "recognizes" the foreign antigens in the transplant, which becomes infiltrated by lymphocytes and macrophages and is eventually destroyed. This process is called **rejection** of the transplanted organ, and it is a manifestation of a cell-mediated immune reaction. Physicians who are treating kidney failure by transplantation can keep a foreign kidney from being rejected by inhibiting the recipient's immunologic defenses, using drugs that suppress the immune response. Transplantation of kidneys and other organs has been successful because it is usually possible to suppress the body's immune responses sufficiently to allow the transplanted organ to survive.

Rejection
An immunologic process characterized by destruction of a transplanted organ.

Autoimmune Diseases

The reasons why an individual forms an autoantibody to his or her own cells or tissue components are not well understood. Unfortunately, after an individual develops an autoimmune disease, it usually "doesn't go away." Although the affected person experiences periods when the disease is in remission or the manifestations are controlled by treatment, the disease persists and often progresses. Three major mechanisms have been postulated to explain the pathogenesis of autoimmune diseases:

1. Alteration of the patient's own (self) antigens that causes them to become antigenic and provoke an immune reaction
2. The formation of cross-reacting antibodies against foreign antigens that also attack the patient's own antigens
3. Defective regulation of the immune response by regulator T lymphocytes

The subject's own antigens may be altered by a viral infection or an infection with some other microbiologic agent in such a manner that the immune system no longer recognizes the antigen as a self-antigen, and an immune reaction is generated against the altered antigen (FIGURE 6A). Alternatively, some drug or medication ingested by the patient may change the structure of a self-antigen so that it is perceived as foreign and generates an immune response. Cross-reacting antibodies may induce organ damage when an antibody is formed against a foreign antigen, such as an invading bacterium, that shares antigenic determinants with some of the subject's

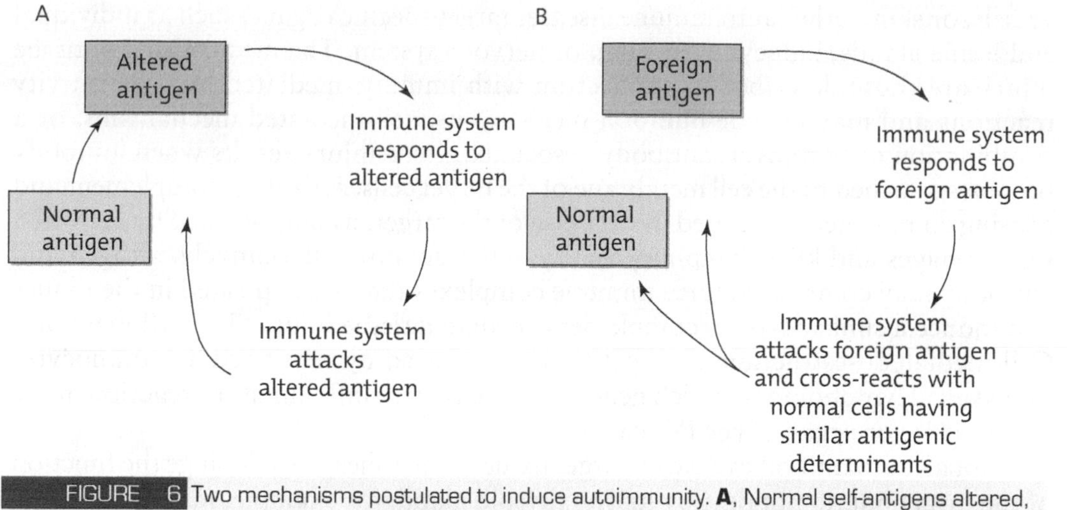

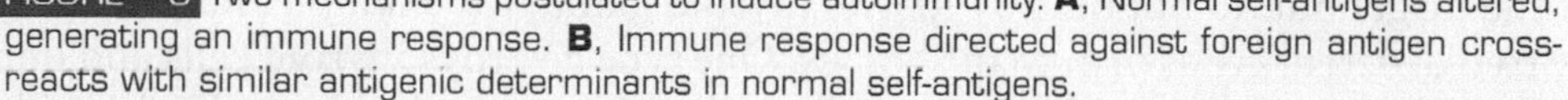
FIGURE 6 Two mechanisms postulated to induce autoimmunity. **A**, Normal self-antigens altered, generating an immune response. **B**, Immune response directed against foreign antigen cross-reacts with similar antigenic determinants in normal self-antigens.

own cell or tissue antigens. As a result, the antibody that formed against the antigenic determinants in the foreign antigen cross-reacts with similar antigenic determinants in the subjects own tissues, leading to tissue injury (FIGURE 6B). The harmful effects of a cross-reacting antibody are demonstrated clearly by a newly described nervous system disease called **progressive inflammatory neuropathy** that occurred in workers at some Midwestern pork-processing plants. The affected persons worked in an area of the plant where pig brains were removed from the animal cranial cavities by using a high-pressure, compressed-air system that sprayed aerosolized pig brain tissue and blood into the air. Some of the employees inhaled small bits of pig tissue. Their immune systems responded by forming antibodies against the pig tissues, which contain antigens similar to those in human tissues. As a result, the anti-pig antibodies also attacked the nerve tissue of the affected employees, leading to the pain, numbness, and weakness associated with the disease.

Progressive inflammatory neuropathy
An autoimmune neurologic disease caused by inhalation of pig brain tissue.

Three factors appear to predispose to autoimmune diseases:

1. A genetic component, which in part is related to the genes on chromosome 6, which code for our own unique self-antigens. These are the same antigens that are involved in presenting processed antigen to lymphocytes by macrophages or other antigen-processing cells. Certain HLA types appear to be associated with an increased susceptibility to specific autoimmune diseases.
2. A gender component, as many autoimmune diseases occur much more frequently in women than in men.
3. An infection component in a genetically predisposed individual, as the onset of many autoimmune diseases appears to be associated with a recent infection, often a viral infection. An infection in a person with a chronic autoimmune disease may also cause a flare-up of disease.

AUTOIMMUNE DISEASE MANIFESTATIONS AND MECHANISMS OF TISSUE INJURY

The manifestations of autoimmune disease depend on which cells or tissue components are targeted for attack by the immune system. Some autoimmune diseases attack specific tissues throughout the body, such as bone, cartilage, connective tissue, blood vessels, or skin. Other autoimmune diseases target specific organs, such as individual endocrine glands, kidney, liver, lung, or nervous system. The mechanisms of tissue injury are those described in connection with immune-mediated hypersensitivity reactions and may include humoral mechanisms, cell-mediated mechanisms, or a combination of both. Autoantibody-associated tissue injury results when antibody becomes attached to the cell membrane of the target cells, activating complement and causing complement-mediated destruction of the target, usually assisted by activated macrophages and killer lymphocytes (Type II reaction). Alternatively, antigen and antibody may combine to form immune complexes that are deposited in the tissues and induce a similar type of complement-mediated tissue injury (Type III reaction). Cell-mediated destruction of target tissues is caused by sensitized T lymphocytes that secrete lymphokines, which generate a destructive inflammatory reaction in the target tissue or organ (Type IV reaction).

Not all autoantibodies destroy target tissue. Sometimes, they derange the function of the target but do not destroy it. The thyroid gland, for example, may be attacked by two different types of autoantibodies. One type destroys thyroid cells and impairs thyroid function, causing hypothyroidism. Another type stimulates the thyroid cells and makes them hyperfunction, causing hyperthyroidism.

In general, treatment of autoimmune disease is not very satisfactory. Various methods of treatment have been used to minimize inflammation and tissue damage, to suppress the function of the immune system, and to block the destructive effects of cytokines produced by T lymphocytes and macrophages.

TABLE 4 summarizes the features of some of the more important diseases in which autoantibody formation appears to play a role. These diseases are considered in greater detail in subsequent chapters.

CONNECTIVE TISSUE (COLLAGEN) DISEASES

The fibrous connective tissue that forms the framework of all tissues in the body is called collagen. The term connective tissue disease, or collagen disease, is used to describe a group of diseases characterized by necrosis and degeneration of collagen fibers throughout the body. In many instances, autoantibodies directed against antigens present in various cells and tissues can be detected in the serum of affected individuals, and aggregates of antigen combined with antibody (termed antigen–antibody complexes) can be identified at the sites of tissue damage. Often, large numbers of lymphocytes and plasma cells accumulate in the affected tissues. These cells are presumed to be responsible for the tissue injury by means of cell-mediated immune reactions and formation of autoantibodies. Therefore, the connective tissue diseases are usually classified as autoimmune diseases.

The clinical features of a connective tissue disease depend on the organ system affected and the extent of the injury to the tissues. Involvement of the connective tissue of the joints and periarticular tissues is manifested by swelling, pain, and tenderness in the joints. FIGURE 7 compares the cellular structure of a normal joint lining with a diseased one. Connective tissue diseases that affect the cardiovascular system cause collagen fibers of the heart valves to swell and degenerate (leading to valve injury). The heart muscle becomes inflamed. The connective tissue in the myocardium becomes necrotic, and destructive lesions occur in the small- and medium-sized blood vessels. Renal manifestations include inflammation and scarring of the glomeruli, damage to the glomerular basement membrane, and consequent leakage of protein and red blood cells into the urine. Severe glomerular damage impairs renal function and may eventually lead to renal insufficiency. Injury to the connective tissue of the lungs, pleura, and pericardium leads to pleural and pericardial pain, sometimes with

TABLE 4

Etiology and clinical manifestations of common autoimmune diseases

	Probable pathogenesis	Major clinical manifestations
Rheumatic fever	Antistreptococcal antibodies cross-react with antigens in heart muscle, heart valves, and other tissues.	Inflammation of heart and joints
Glomerulonephritis	Some cases caused by antibodies formed against glomerular basement membrane; other cases caused by antigen–antibody complexes trapped in glomeruli.	Inflammation of renal glomeruli
Rheumatoid arthritis	Antibodies formed against serum gamma globulin.	Systemic disease with inflammation and degeneration of joints
Autoimmune blood diseases	Autoantibodies formed against platelets, white cells, or red cells; in some cases, antibody apparently is formed against altered cell antigens, and antibody reacts with both altered and normal cells.	Anemia, leukopenia, or thrombocytopenia, depending on nature of antibody
Lupus erythematosus, scleroderma, and related collagen diseases	Various autoantibodies cause widespread injury to tissues and organs.	Systemic disease with manifestations in several organs
Thyroiditis (Hashimoto thyroiditis)	Antithyroid antibody causes injury and inflammatory cell infiltration of thyroid gland.	Hypothyroidism
Diffuse toxic goiter (Graves disease)	Autoantibody mimicking thyroid-stimulating hormone (TSH) causes increased output of thyroid hormone.	Hyperthyroidism
Diabetes (Type 1)	Autoantibodies and activated T lymphocytes destroy pancreatic islet beta cells	Diabetes mellitus caused by insulin deficiency
Pernicious anemia	Autoantibodies destroy gastric mucosa cells	Macrocytic anemia and nervous system damage resulting from adequate absorption of vitamin B_{12}
Vasculitis (various types of blood vessel inflammation)	Autoantibody-mediated damage to small, medium, and large blood vessels	Blood vessel damage interferes with blood vessel function and blood supply to tissues
Various skin conditions and diseases causing loss of skin pigment or skin blisters	Some autoantibodies damage pigment-producing cells in skin; others attack intercellular connections between skin cells	Pigment cell loss causes areas of skin depigmentation (vitiligo); blisters result from loss of skin intercellular connections
Myasthenia gravis	Autoantibodies destroy acetylcholine receptors at muscle–nerve junctions	Muscle weakness resulting from inadequate transmission of impulses from nerves to muscles

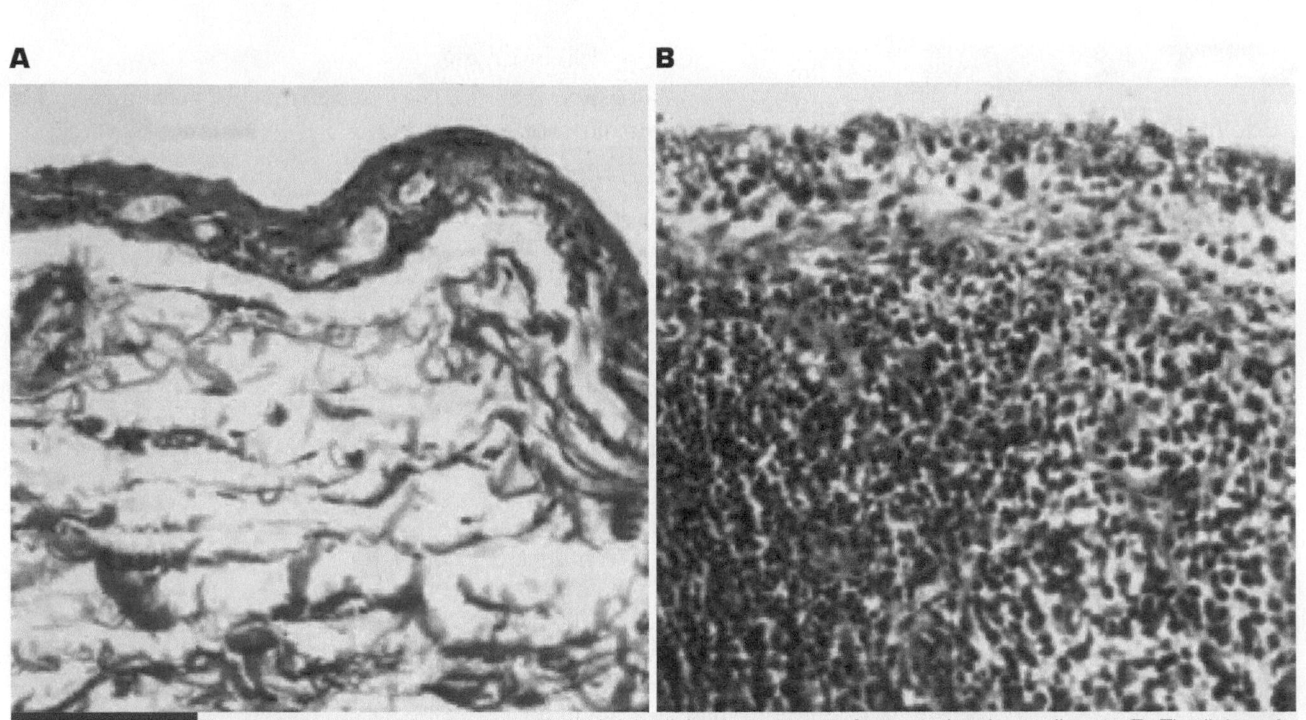

FIGURE 7 Comparison of normal joint lining **A**, with joint lining in one type of connective tissue disease **B**, The lining of the affected joint is heavily infiltrated with lymphocytes and plasma cells, and the joint injury is secondary to the inflammatory reaction (original magnification × 400).

Hemolytic anemia
An anemia caused by increased blood destruction.

Leukopenia
(lōō-kō-pē′ni-uh)
An abnormally small number of leukocytes in the peripheral blood.

accumulation of fluid in the serous cavities. Autoantibodies directed against one or more of the formed elements in the blood may cause anemia caused by destruction of red blood cells (**hemolytic anemia**), reduction in platelets (thrombocytopenia), or a decrease in the number of white blood cells (**leukopenia**).

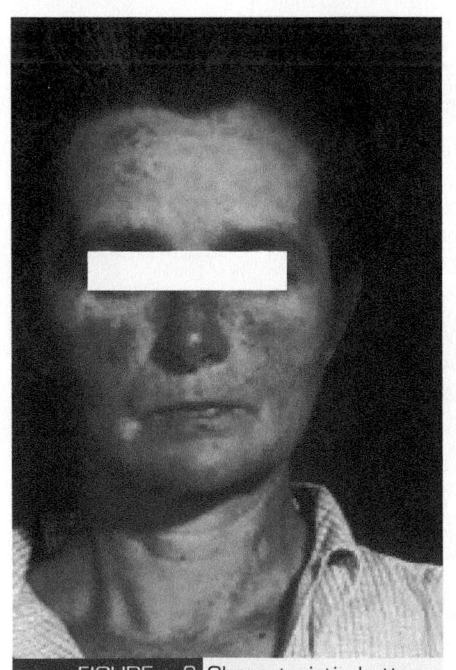

FIGURE 8 Characteristic butterfly rash in woman with lupus erythematosus.

LUPUS ERYTHEMATOSUS

One of the more common connective tissue diseases is called lupus erythematosus. This disease is seen most frequently in young women and is characterized by widespread damage to fibrous connective tissue in the skin, articular tissues, heart, serous membranes (pleura and pericardium), and kidneys. The skin rash often has a characteristic appearance and is called a *malar rash* because it affects both cheeks (*mala* = cheek) joined by an extension across the bridge of the nose. The rash is also sometimes called a *butterfly rash* from its fancied resemblance to a butterfly with spread wings (FIGURE 8). Hemolytic anemia, leukopenia, and thrombocytopenia are frequent hematologic manifestations of lupus; these are caused by autoantibodies. Many patients die of renal failure resulting from the severe renal glomerular injury.

Patients with lupus develop a variety of autoantibodies directed against cells and tissues, including antinucleoprotein antibodies and antibodies directed against red cells, white cells, platelets, and plasma proteins. Circulating antigen–autoantibody complexes (immune complexes) form and are deposited in kidney glomeruli, blood vessels, and other tissues. Complement is

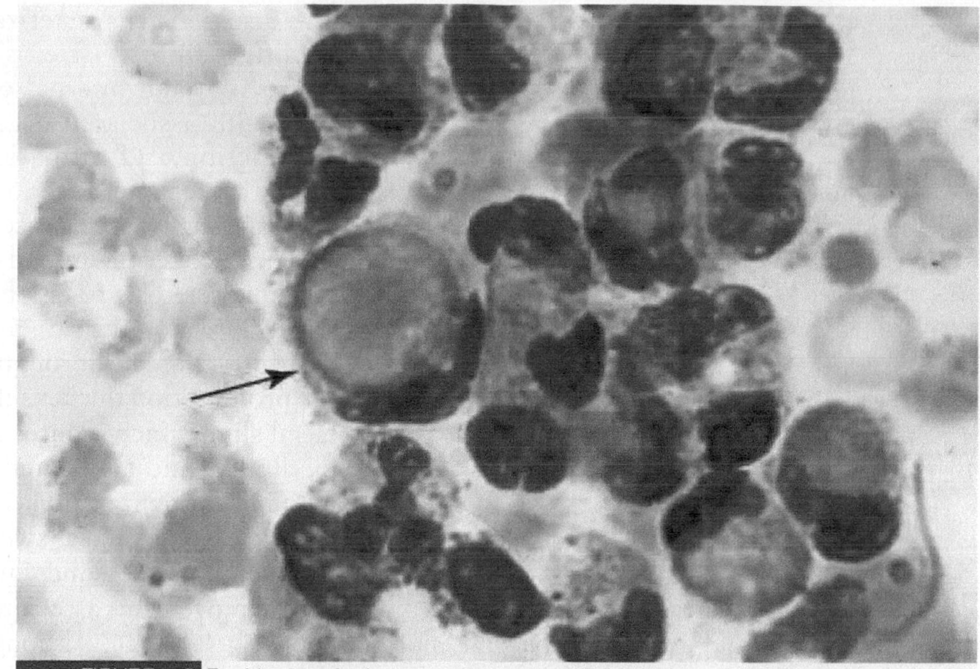

FIGURE 9 Positive test for lupus erythematosus. Spherical mass derived from damaged nucleus (*arrow*) engulfed by neutrophil (original magnification × 1,000).

activated, which generates an inflammatory reaction where the immune complexes are deposited. A characteristic feature of lupus erythematosus is the presence of antinucleoprotein antibodies in the patient's blood, which can be demonstrated by various methods. The original technique consisted of incubating the patient's blood serum with intact white blood cells. The antinucleoprotein antibodies damage many of the leukocytes, causing swelling and loss of structural detail in the cell nuclei. The damaged nuclei are converted into large, homogeneous, spherical "blobs" of blue-staining nuclear debris that becomes surrounded and phagocytized by polymorphonuclear leukocytes. The phagocytized spherical mass fills the cytoplasm of the cell and displaces the nucleus to the edge of the cell, resulting in the characteristic appearance called an LE cell. This classic method of demonstrating antinucleoprotein antibodies was described in 1948 by Hargraves and two associates from the Mayo Clinic in Minnesota and now is primarily of historical interest. The test has been superseded by newer, more sensitive techniques, but the method does clearly illustrate the damaging effect of nucleoprotein antibodies on intact cell nuclei (FIGURE 9).

The pathogenesis of lupus is not well understood but appears to be initiated by some event, possibly a viral infection or other antigenic stimulation in a genetically predisposed individual that damages normal MHC antigens so that they are no longer recognized as self-antigens by the immune system. Helper T lymphocytes and B lymphocytes directed against the abnormal self-antigens are activated. The helper T lymphocytes stimulate the B lymphocytes to proliferate. Then the B lymphocytes form the various autoantibodies and generate the antigen–autoantibody complexes that are responsible for the organ damage characteristic of this disease.

SCLERODERMA (SYSTEMIC SCLEROSIS)

Another connective tissue disease with widespread systemic manifestations has some lupuslike features and other manifestations that resemble rheumatoid arthritis.

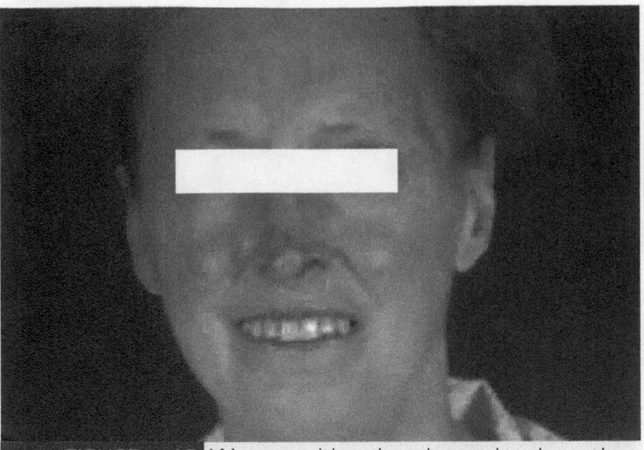

FIGURE 10 Woman with scleroderma in whom the appearance of the skin around the mouth and chin reflects loss of normal skin flexibility.

The disease is characterized by diffuse fibrosis (sclerosis) in the skin and internal organs with associated organ dysfunction and formation of characteristic autoantibodies. Usually, the disease is called scleroderma instead of systemic sclerosis to emphasize its effect on the skin and deeper tissues. The fibrous tissue proliferation thickens the facial skin, which reduces its flexibility, and also extends into the subcutaneous fat and skin appendages (sweat glands, sebaceous glands, and hair follicles). As the thickened skin becomes less mobile, facial movements associated with normal speech and expression become more difficult (FIGURE 10). Although the skin changes may be a source of concern, usually they are not life threatening. Unfortunately, the organ damage caused by the fibrosis can be devastating. The kidneys, esophagus, heart, and lungs are the most frequently and severely affected. Pulmonary fibrosis leads to serious respiratory complications and is the most frequent cause of death in severely affected persons.

QUESTIONS FOR REVIEW

1. What is meant by the following terms: *acquired immunity*, *cell-mediated immunity*, *humoral immunity*, and *hypersensitivity*?
2. What is the role of the lymphocyte in acquired immunity? What is the role of the macrophage?
3. How does the physician manipulate the body's immune reaction to allow kidney transplantation?
4. What is meant by the following terms: *B lymphocyte*, *T lymphocyte*, and *lymphokine*?
5. What are immunoglobulins? What is their basic structure? How do they function?
6. What is meant by the following terms: *light chains*, *macroglobulin*, and *allergy*?
7. What is an autoantibody? What are some of the postulated mechanisms that result in autoantibody formation? What is the effect of autoantibody directed against the patient's own blood cells?
8. What is a connective tissue disease? What are its manifestations? What is an LE cell?
9. What are antigen–antibody complexes? How do they cause tissue injury?
10. How can the immune response be suppressed? Why is this sometimes necessary?

SUPPLEMENTARY READINGS

Dalakas, M. C. 2004. Intravenous immunoglobulin in autoimmune neuromuscular diseases. *Journal of the American Medical Association* 19:2367–75.

- Injections of immunoglobulins are a safe, effective treatment for many autoimmune neuromuscular diseases, although the optimal doses and frequency of administration are still being investigated. The immunoglobulins act by interfering with virtually all of the processes that generate the cytotoxic cells, cytokines, and autoantibodies responsible for autoimmune damage to the target organ or tissue, such as interference with T cell functions, suppression of cytokines, suppression of autoantibody production by B cells, and interference with its ability to bind to its target.

Delves, P. J., and Roitt, I. M. 2000. The immune system. *New England Journal of Medicine* 343:37–49, and 343:108–17.

- A review of current knowledge on this complex system.

Gabrielli, A., Avvedimento, E. V., and Krieg, T. 2009. Scleroderma. *New England Journal of Medicine* 360:1989–2003.

- Scleroderma is a serious autoimmune disease characterized by skin and organ fibrosis preceded by vasculitis, pulmonary hypertension, sometimes associated with lupuslike and rheumatoid arthritislike manifestations, usually associated with autoantibodies directed against various tissue components. The kidneys, esophagus, heart, and lungs are the most frequently and severely affected. Pulmonary involvement is the most frequent cause of death.

Klein, J., and Sato, A. 2000. The HLA system. *New England Journal of Medicine* 343:702–9, and 343:782–6.

- A review of current knowledge about our system of self-antigens, how they function, and the abnormalities of genes linked to the HLA complex. The roles of the HLA system in cancer and transplantation are considered.

OUTLINE SUMMARY

The Body's Defense Mechanisms

Immunity

CHARACTERISTICS OF IMMUNE RESPONSE

Depends on lymphocytes and antigen-processing cells.
Specific populations of lymphocytes perform specific functions.
Cells of immune system communicate and produce their effects by secreting cytokines.

TYPES OF IMMUNITY

AUTOIMMUNITY

DEVELOPMENT OF THE LYMPHATIC SYSTEM

Immature lymphocytes develop immune competence in thymus (T lymphocytes) or bone marrow (B lymphocytes).
Lymphocytes are programmed to develop receptors for the antigens that they will eventually recognize.
T lymphocytes are classified into major groups based on CD antigens on cell membranes.
NK cells lack T or B receptors and can destroy infected or abnormal cells without prior antigenic contact.

RESPONSE OF LYMPHOCYTES TO FOREIGN ANTIGENS

B lymphocytes can respond to intact antigen and proliferate with T cell help.
T lymphocytes require macrophage-processed antigen in order to respond.
Antigens are presented to responding cells complexed with MHC proteins.

TYPES OF RESPONDING T CELLS

Helper T cells: promote immune response.
Cytotoxic T cells: attack and destroy infected cells, cancer cells, transplants.
Delayed hypersensitivity cells: attract and activate macrophages, cytotoxic T cells, NK cells.
Memory cells: set aside to respond rapidly if the same antigen is encountered again.
Response of effector T cell is determined by type of MHC protein displayed with processed antigen.

GENETIC CONTROL OF ABILITY TO GENERATE IMMUNE RESPONSE

THE FUNCTION OF COMPLEMENT

Antibodies (Immunoglobulins)

STRUCTURE

Composed of two light and two heavy chains.

Constant part of molecule determines class of antibody.

Variable part of molecule determines specificity.

Five types of immunoglobulins.

- *IgM: forms large complex pentamer.*
- *IgG: principal antibody formed against majority of infectious agents.*
- *IgA: produced by cells in respiratory and gastrointestinal tracts. Combines with antigens to prevent absorption.*
- *IgD: on surface of lymphocytes.*
- *IgE: increased in allergic persons. Attaches to mast cells and basophils.*

Hypersensitivity Reactions: Immune System–Related Tissue Injury

Cell-tissue injury resulting from immune response.

Classified on pathogenesis of injury.

TYPE I. IMMEDIATE HYPERSENSITIVITY

Localized response: allergy.

- *Tendency to form IgE antibodies to antigens that do not sensitize most individuals.*
- *IgE attaches to mast cells and basophils.*
- *Subsequent contact with allergen leads to antigen–antibody interaction with release of mediators and allergic manifestations.*
- *Antihistamines block some effects.*
- *Desensitization induces formation of IgA and IgG, which combine with allergen before it can interact with IgE.*

Systemic response: anaphylaxis.

Generalized mediator release from mast cells and basophils may be life threatening.

Prompt treatment essential.

TYPE II. CYTOTOXIC HYPERSENSITIVITY

Antibody attaches to cell or tissue antigen.

Complement activated and cell-tissue damage follows.

TYPE III. IMMUNE COMPLEX DISEASE

Circulating antigen–antibody complexes deposited in tissues.

Complement activated and cell-tissue injury follows.

TYPE IV. DELAYED HYPERSENSITIVITY

Sensitized T lymphocytes secrete cytokines that attract lymphocytes, macrophages, and other inflammatory cells, which produce tissue injury.

Mantoux test based on delayed hypersensitivity response to proteins from tubercle bacillus as indication of previous infection.

Suppression of the Immune Response

UNWANTED EFFECTS OF IMMUNE RESPONSE

Autoimmune disease.

Rejection of transplanted organs.

Rh hemolytic disease in newborn infants (discussed in prenatal development and diseases associated with pregnancy).

METHODS FOR SUPPRESSING THE IMMUNE RESPONSE

Radiation: destroys lymphocytes.

Cytotoxic drugs: suppress growth of lymphocytes.

Adrenal corticosteroids: suppress inflammatory reaction, impair phagocytosis, and inhibit protein synthesis.

Antibodies: prevent body from reacting to corresponding antigen.

TISSUE GRAFTS AND IMMUNITY

Graft contains foreign antigens.

Lymphocytes recognize foreign antigen and attempt to eliminate (rejection).

Immune response must be suppressed to prevent rejection of transplant.

Autoimmune Diseases

PATHOGENESIS

Antibodies formed to altered antigens and react with normal antigens.

Antibodies formed to foreign antigens and cross-react with normal tissue antigens.

T lymphocytes fail to control immune response.

TREATMENT

Corticosteroids.

Cytotoxic drugs.

CONNECTIVE TISSUE (COLLAGEN) DISEASES

Clinical features:

- *Autoimmune disease characterized by necrosis and degeneration of fibrous connective tissue.*
- *Clinical features depend on organs affected.*

LUPUS ERYTHEMATOSUS

A connective tissue disease of young women.

Associated with formation of autoantibodies and immune complexes.

SCLERODERMA (SYSTEMIC SCLEROSIS)

Autoimmune disease characterized by progressive fibrosis of skin and internal organs with associated organ damage.

http://health.jbpub.com/humandisease/9e

Human Disease Online is a great source for supplementary human disease information for both students and instructors. Visit this website to find a variety of useful tools for learning, thinking, and teaching.

Abnormalities of Blood Coagulation

LEARNING OBJECTIVES

1. Describe the functions of blood vessels and platelets in controlling bleeding.
2. Explain the three phases of coagulation, and list the coagulation factors involved.
3. Describe the laboratory tests used to evaluate hemostasis.
4. List the most common clinically significant disturbances of hemostasis and describe their clinical manifestations.

Hemostasis

If a person cuts his or her finger with a knife, the cut bleeds, but the bleeding soon stops and healing ensues. The body has a complex mechanism for causing blood to clot when and where it is necessary, while keeping the blood fluid within the capillaries and larger blood vessels.

FACTORS CONCERNED WITH HEMOSTASIS

The proper functioning of the hemostatic mechanism depends on the proper integrated functioning of the five major factors that affect hemostasis:

1. Integrity of the small blood vessels
2. Adequate numbers of structurally and functionally normal platelets
3. Normal amounts of coagulation factors (proteins present in small quantities in the blood plasma)
4. Normal amounts of coagulation inhibitors
5. Adequate amounts of calcium ions in the blood

Blood Vessels and Platelets

The small blood vessels and blood platelets function together to prevent bleeding. The small blood vessels are the body's first line of defense. If a blood vessel is injured, it automatically contracts (reflex vasoconstriction), narrowing its caliber and facilitating closure of the vessel by a blood clot. Injury to the vessel also leads to disruption of the endothelium, exposing the underlying connective tissue. Platelets accumulate and adhere to the site of injury, where they perform three important functions:

1. They plug the defect in the vessel wall.
2. They liberate chemical compounds (vasoconstrictors) that cause the vessel to contract and compounds that cause platelets to aggregate.
3. They release substances (phospholipids) that initiate the process of blood coagulation.

Platelets, which play an essential role in blood coagulation, are very small fragments of the cytoplasm from large precursor cells in the bone marrow called megakaryocytes. Platelets have an average survival in the circulation of about 10 days, and when they wear out, they are removed by macrophages in the spleen.

Platelets contain contractile proteins and various enzyme systems that produce products essential for normal platelet functions. When platelets come in contract with a roughened or damaged endothelial surface, they undergo a dramatic change. They swell and become sticky. Long processes (pseudopods) extend from their cytoplasm, and they release various products that cause further platelet swelling and platelet aggregation to form a platelet plug. Activation of platelets also starts the blood coagulation process, as illustrated in FIGURE 1.

Platelets play a very important part in preventing bleeding from capillaries. Small breaks in the walls of capillaries occur frequently, but the defects are promptly sealed by platelets, and bleeding does not occur. However, if the quantity of platelets in the blood is seriously reduced, as occurs in some diseases, the "platelet sealing mechanism" is impaired. As a result, the affected individual develops multiple small pinpoint areas of bleeding (called **petechiae** or petechial hemorrhages) in the skin and deeper tissues resulting from leakage of blood through minute defects in the capillary endothelium.

Petechia (pe-tē′kēy-uh) *A small pinpoint hemorrhage caused by decreased platelets, abnormal platelet function, or capillary defect.*

Plasma Coagulation Factors

The blood plasma contains several different proteins called coagulation factors, which are designated by both name and roman numerals. When these factors are activated, they interact to produce a blood clot. The process of blood coagulation is a chain reaction in which each component of the chain is formed from an inactive precursor in the blood, and each activated component in turn activates the next member of the chain. The process has been compared with what happens when the first in a long chain of dominoes is knocked over. Tipping the first domino represents the initiation of the clotting mechanism, and the fall of the last domino represents the formation of a firm blood clot.

The process of blood coagulation is a highly complex and bewildering sequence of interactions involving plasma and tissue components, platelets, and calcium. At the risk of oversimplifying its complexities, however, it is convenient to divide it into three phases for descriptive purposes (Figure 1).

Phase 1 leads to the formation of **thromboplastin**, which may be produced by either of two different mechanisms. One mechanism depends on the interaction of platelets and plasma coagulation factors. If the wall of a blood vessel is injured, platelets accumulate at the site and release a phospholipid that interacts with plasma components to form thromboplastin. This is called the intrinsic system because the thromboplastin is produced from substances present in the bloodstream. Tissues also have thromboplastic activity, and thromboplastin is also liberated from injured tissues. This is called the extrinsic system because the thromboplastin is not derived from the blood but primarily from tissue outside of the vascular compartment.

Thromboplastin (throm-bō-plas′tin) *A component formed during blood coagulation from interaction of platelets and plasma components* (intrinsic system) *or liberated from injured tissues* (extrinsic system).

Actually, the intrinsic and extrinsic pathways are not completely independent. Usually both pathways are activated at the same time when tissues are injured, and both pathways interact to initiate the blood clotting process.

The conversion of prothrombin into thrombin takes place in phase 2. The thromboplastin formed in either the intrinsic or the extrinsic system interacts with additional plasma factors and platelet phospholipid to form a complex (called prothrombin

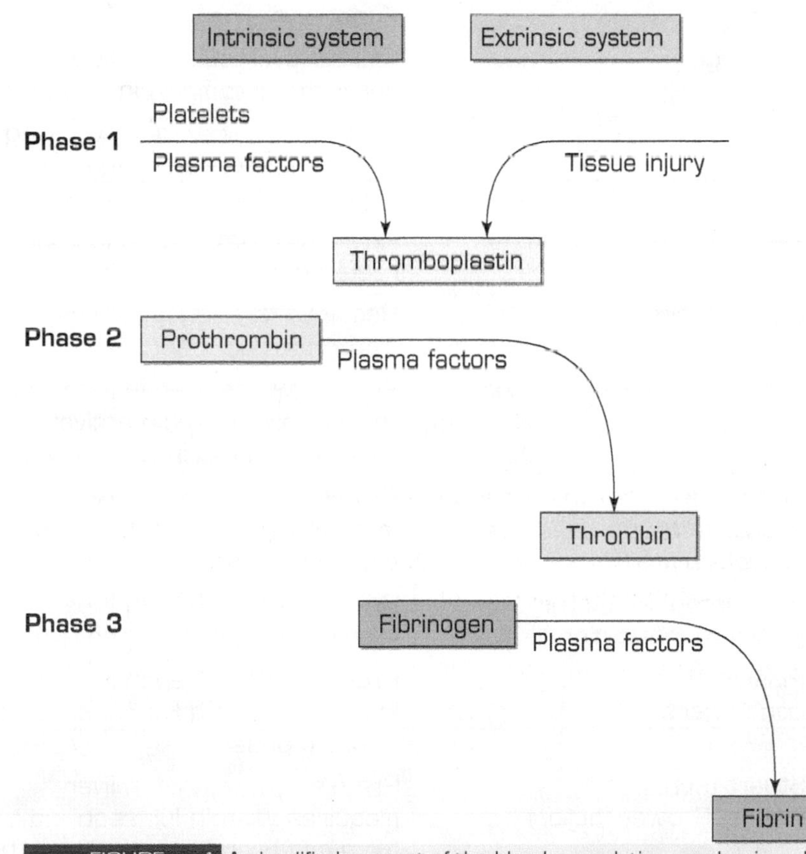

FIGURE 1 A simplified concept of the blood coagulation mechanism. In the intrinsic system, plasma factors (XII, XI, and IX) are activated, and they interact with factor VIII and platelets to yield intrinsic thromboplastin. In the extrinsic system, tissue injury yields extrinsic thromboplastin that reacts with a plasma factor (VII). Then the thromboplastin formed by either the intrinsic or extrinsic system interacts with additional components (factors V, X, and platelet phospholipid) to form the complex (prothrombin activator) that converts prothrombin into thrombin in the second phase. Thrombin converts fibrinogen into fibrin in the third phase.

Thrombin
A coagulation factor formed by activation of prothrombin in the process of blood coagulation.

Fibrinogen
(fī-brin′ō-jen)
A precursor in plasma converted into fibrin by thrombin during blood coagulation.

Fibrin
The meshwork of protein threads that form during the clotting of the blood.

Fibrin monomer
(mă′nō-mer)
A derivative of fibrinogen that polymerizes to form the fibrin clot during blood coagulation.

activator) that converts the prothrombin into thrombin. Prothrombin is a protein manufactured in the liver. It is split into several fragments by thromboplastin. One of these is the active component **thrombin,** an enzyme capable of digesting protein. The formation of thrombin from prothrombin requires other plasma coagulation factors (called accessory factors) that function by speeding the rate of the conversion.

Phase 3 leads to the conversion of **fibrinogen** into **fibrin** by thrombin. Fibrinogen is a high molecular weight protein produced by the liver. Thrombin splits off a part of the fibrinogen molecule, forming a smaller molecule called **fibrin monomer.** The fibrin monomer molecules then become joined end to end (polymerized) to form long strands of fibrin, and the fibrin strands also become linked together side to side. Another plasma factor (fibrin stabilizing factor) acts by strengthening the bonds between the fibrin molecules and increasing the strength of the fibrin clot. The blood clot is the end stage in the clotting process. It consists of an interlacing meshwork of fibrin threads containing entrapped plasma, red cells, white cells, and platelets.

TABLE 1 summarizes the coagulation factors and their role in the clotting process.

TABLE 1

Coagulation factors

Factor number	Name	Functions
I	Fibrinogen	Protein synthesized in liver; converted into fibrin in phase 3
II	Prothrombin	Protein synthesized in liver (requires vitamin K); converted into thrombin in phase 2
III	Tissue thromboplastin	Released from damaged tissue; required in extrinsic phase 1
IV	Calcium ions	Required throughout entire clotting sequence
V	Proaccelerin (labile factor)	Protein synthesized in liver; required to form prothrombin activator in both intrinsic and extrinsic phase 1
VII	Serum prothrombin conversion accelerator (stable factor, proconvertin)	Protein synthesized in liver (requires vitamin K); functions in extrinsic phase 1
VIII	Antihemophilic factor (antihemophilic globulin)	Protein synthesized in liver; required for intrinsic phase 1
IX	Plasma thromboplastin component	Protein synthesized in liver (requires vitamin K); required for intrinsic phase 1
X	Stuart factor (Stuart-Prower factor)	Protein synthesized in liver (requires vitamin K); required to form prothrombin activator in both intrinsic and extrinsic phase 1
XI	Plasma thromboplastin antecedent	Protein synthesized in liver; required for intrinsic phase 1
XII	Hageman factor	Protein required for intrinsic phase 1
XIII	Fibrin-stabilizing factor	Protein required to stabilize the fibrin strands in phase 3

Coagulation Inhibitors and Fibrinolysins

Coagulation factors are counterbalanced by various coagulation inhibitors that restrict the clotting process to a limited area. One coagulation inhibitor called protein C and another called protein S function together to inactivate two coagulation factors (V and VIII). Another important member of this group is antithrombin, which inhibits not only thrombin but also several other activated coagulation factors generated in the clotting process.

An equally important control system is one that dissolves fibrin after it has formed. A precursor compound in blood plasma called plasminogen (profibrinolysin) is activated to form plasmin (fibrinolysin), which dissolves fibrin in blood clots. The fibrinolytic system is activated at the same time that the coagulation process is initiated, and thrombin produced in the coagulation process also activates this system. Another important plasminogen activator is a substance called tissue plasminogen activator, which is released from endothelial cells in the region where the clot is forming. As described in the discussion on cardiovascular system, tissue plasminogen activator or another plasminogen activator called streptokinase, produced by streptococci, is administered intravenously to dissolve blood clots in the coronary arteries of patients who have had a recent heart attack. Prompt administration of one of these plasminogen activators within a few hours after onset of symptoms dissolves the clot and restores flow through the artery, which minimizes heart muscle damage resulting from the blockage.

Calcium and Blood Coagulation

Adequate amounts of calcium ions (Ca^{2+}) are required in all phases of blood coagulation, and blood will not clot in the absence of calcium. However, there are no diseases in which a disturbance of blood coagulation results from an abnormally low level of blood calcium because calcium levels sufficiently low to affect blood coagulation would be incompatible with life.

Clinical Disturbances of Blood Coagulation

Disturbances of blood coagulation may be classified as one of four major categories:

1. Abnormalities of small blood vessels
2. Abnormalities of platelet function
3. Deficiency of one or more of the plasma coagulation factors
4. Liberation of thromboplastic material into the circulation

ABNORMALITIES OF SMALL BLOOD VESSELS

Some rare diseases characterized by abnormal bleeding have been found to result from abnormal function of the small blood vessels. Normally, small blood vessels contract after injury, helping to seal the defect by a blood clot. Sometimes this function is defective, leading to excessive bleeding. In a few other rare diseases, the small blood vessels are abnormally formed and cannot function properly.

ABNORMALITIES OF PLATELET NUMBERS OR FUNCTION

A decrease in platelets is called **thrombocytopenia** (*thrombus* = clot + *cyte* = cell + *penia* = deficiency). This decrease may be a result of injury or disease of the bone

Thrombocytopenia (throm′bō-sī-tō-pē′ny-yuh) *A deficiency of platelets.*

marrow, which damages the megakaryocytes in the marrow, the precursor cells of the platelets. In other cases, thrombocytopenia occurs because the bone marrow has been infiltrated by leukemic cells or by cancer cells that have spread to the skeletal system and the megakaryocytes have been crowded out by the abnormal cells. Thrombocytopenia may also occur if antiplatelet autoantibodies destroy the platelets in the peripheral blood (as seen in some autoimmune diseases). Sometimes platelets are normal in quantity but abnormal in function, and so they are ineffective in initiating the clotting process.

Bleeding associated with defective or inadequate platelets is generally manifested by small petechial hemorrhages rather than by large areas of hemorrhage (FIGURE 2A).

DEFICIENCY OF PLASMA COAGULATION FACTORS

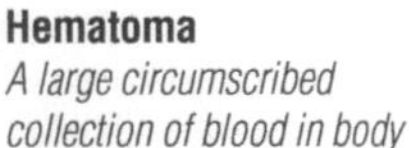
Hematoma
A large circumscribed collection of blood in body tissues.

Deficiencies of plasma coagulation factors often lead to large areas of hemorrhage called **hematomas** (*heme* = blood + *oma* = swelling) (FIGURE 2B). Deficiencies of factors concerned with the first phase of coagulation are usually hereditary and are relatively rare. Only three hereditary bleeding diseases occur with any frequency. Hemophilia, an X-linked hereditary disease affecting males, is the most common and best known. Clinically, the disease is characterized by episodes of hemorrhage in joints and internal organs after minor injury. There are two forms of hemophilia. Both have the same clinical manifestations and X-linked method of transmission. The most common type, which is called hemophilia A or classic hemophilia, is characterized by a decrease in coagulation factor VIII, which is also called antihemophilic factor. Its method of inheritance was considered in the discussion on congenital and hereditary diseases. The less common form of hemophilia is called hemophilia B or Christmas disease. It is caused by a deficiency of coagulation factor IX, which is also called Christmas factor (named after an affected patient, not the holiday). Both factors VIII and IX, which are produced in the liver, are required in the first phase of coagulation.

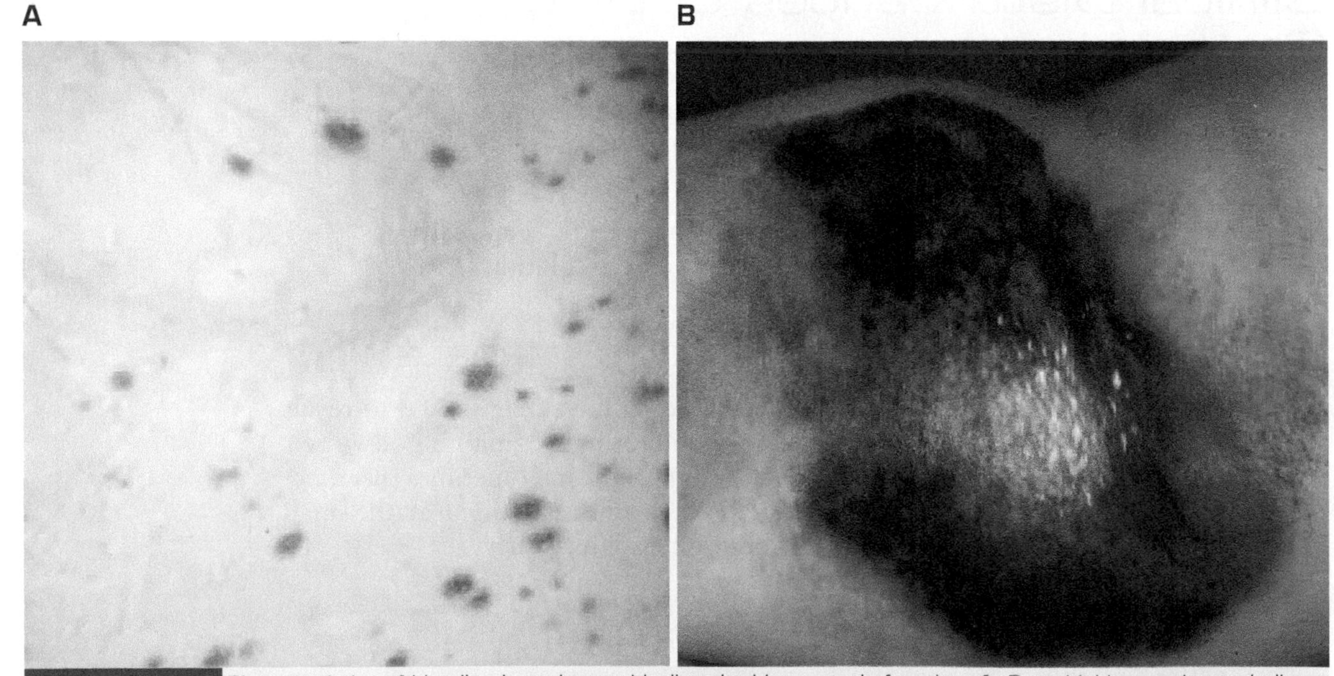

FIGURE 2 Characteristics of bleeding in patients with disturbed hemostatic function. **A**, Petechial hemorrhages indicative of thrombocytopenia or defective platelet function. **B**, A large hemorrhage (hematoma) associated with a deficiency of plasma coagulation factors.

A third hereditary bleeding disease is called von Willebrand disease and is usually transmitted as a Mendelian dominant trait. This disease also is characterized by excessive bleeding after a minor injury, but usually the bleeding is not in the joints, as is so characteristic of hemophilia. The manifestations of von Willebrand disease result from a deficiency of a large protein molecule that is produced primarily by the endothelial cells lining blood vessels. This factor is required in order for platelets to adhere to the vessel wall at the site of injury. The protein is also released into the bloodstream, where it forms a complex in the circulation with factor VIII, and it is needed in order to maintain a normal level of factor VIII in the blood.

Von Willebrand's factor functions by adhering to the vessel wall where the endothelium is disrupted, forming a latticelike framework that allows platelets and coagulation factors to adhere, interact, and form a blood clot.

The level of factor VIII is low in patients with von Willebrand disease, as it is in hemophilia A, but for a different reason. Patients with von Willebrand disease can synthesize factor VIII, but an adequate level of von Willebrand's factor is required to form a complex with factor VIII and maintain a normal amount of factor VIII in the circulation. The factor VIII deficiency in von Willebrand disease occurs because the affected persons lack adequate amounts of circulating von Willebrand's factor with which the factor VIII can combine.

Because von Willebrand's factor is also required in order for platelets to adhere at the site of vascular injury, some platelet functions also are disturbed in persons with this disease, which can be identified by special laboratory tests.

Patients with hemophilia A, hemophilia B, and von Willebrand disease who have bleeding episodes can be treated by administration of factor concentrates prepared from human blood plasma. A factor VIII concentrate prepared by recombinant DNA technology also has become available and can be used to treat patients with classic hemophilia.

Disturbances affecting the second phase of blood coagulation result from a deficiency of prothrombin or various accessory coagulation factors that are required for the conversion of prothrombin into thrombin. These factors are produced in the liver, and vitamin K is required for the synthesis of most of these factors (called vitamin K–dependent factors). Vitamin K is synthesized by intestinal bacteria and also can be obtained from foods, especially green leafy vegetables. It is a fat-soluble vitamin, and bile is required for its absorption.

A disturbance of blood coagulation caused by a deficiency of prothrombin or related factors suggests four possibilities:

1. Administration of anticoagulant drugs
2. Inadequate synthesis of vitamin K
3. Inadequate absorption of vitamin K
4. Severe liver disease

Anticoagulant drugs such as warfarin and similar compounds are sometimes used to treat patients who have shown an increased tendency to develop blood clots in their leg veins, such as patients having a total hip or total knee replacement procedure or other surgical procedures that increase their risk of forming leg vein clots. The drug is also given to patients with some types of heart disease in which blood clots tend to form within the cardiac chambers and to patients with some types of artificial heart valves to prevent clot formation within the artificial valve, which would disrupt the function of the valve. The amount of warfarin or related anticoagulant given to the patient must be monitored closely to reduce blood coagulability sufficiently to prevent unwanted blood clots forming in the heart chambers, leg veins, or other locations without reducing the coagulation factors to such an extent that spontaneous bleeding occurs. Anticoagulant drugs act by inhibiting the synthesis of biochemically active vitamin K–dependent factors. Inadequate synthesis of vitamin K also occurs if the intestinal bacteria have been eradicated by prolonged antibiotic therapy, as sometimes occurs in seriously ill, hospitalized patients. Another cause of inadequate uptake of vitamin K is blockage of the common bile duct by a gallstone or tumor, preventing bile from entering the intestine to promote absorption of the vitamin. Patients with severe liver diseases have deficiencies of prothrombin and accessory factors because the liver is so badly damaged that it can no longer synthesize adequate amounts of coagulation factors.

Intramuscular administration of vitamin K corrects coagulation disturbances resulting from Coumadin anticoagulants, inadequate synthesis of vitamin K, or insufficient absorption of the vitamin. The coagulation disturbance associated with severe liver disease does not respond because the diseased liver is no longer capable of synthesizing sufficient coagulation factors to provide efficient hemostasis.

Another vitamin K–deficient group is newborn infants who lack the intestinal bacteria to make the vitamin and are not yet eating foods that contain the vitamin. They are at risk for serious bleeding called *hemorrhagic disease of the newborn.* In order to prevent this condition, all newborn infants routinely receive a vitamin K injection to prevent spontaneous bleeding caused by lack of the vitamin.

A number of other anticoagulant drugs are available that interfere with some other phase of the coagulation mechanism, which may have advantages over warfarin in specific clinical situations, such as an antithrombin drug that impedes the second phase of blood coagulation. Some newer anticoagulant drugs act by interfering with factor X in the first phase of blood coagulation. The anticoagulant can be given as a standard daily dose without requiring laboratory tests, which simplifies the patient's treatment.

LIBERATION OF THROMBOPLASTIC MATERIAL INTO THE CIRCULATION

In a number of diseases associated with shock, overwhelming bacterial infection, or extensive necrosis of tissue, products of tissue necrosis and other substances with thromboplastic activity are liberated into the circulation, leading to widespread intravascular coagulation of the blood (FIGURE 3). In the process of clotting, platelets and the various plasma coagulation factors are utilized, and the levels of these components in the blood drop precipitously.

In order to defend itself against widespread intravascular clotting, the body activates the fibrinolysin system; this dissolves clots and prevents potentially lethal obstruction of the circulatory system by massive intravascular coagulation. The breakdown products produced during degradation of the fibrin act as additional inhibitors of the clotting process.

The net effect of these various events is a bleeding disturbance, sometimes in a patient already seriously ill because of an underlying disease that caused the blood-clotting mechanism to be activated. This abnormal bleeding state is called **disseminated intravascular coagulation syndrome** or **consumption coagulopathy**. The latter term alludes to consumption of the clotting factors as a result of the pathogenic coagulation process. FIGURE 4 summarizes the pathogenesis of this bleeding syndrome.

Disseminated intravascular coagulation syndrome
A disturbance of blood coagulation as a result of activation of the coagulation mechanism and simultaneous clot lysis.

Consumption coagulopathy
See disseminated intravascular coagulation syndrome.

RELATIVE FREQUENCY OF THE VARIOUS COAGULATION DISTURBANCES

In one group of 350 hospitalized patients with bleeding problems that I studied, most of the disorders were caused by inadequate numbers of platelets or abnormal platelet function. Next in frequency were coagulation disturbances caused by

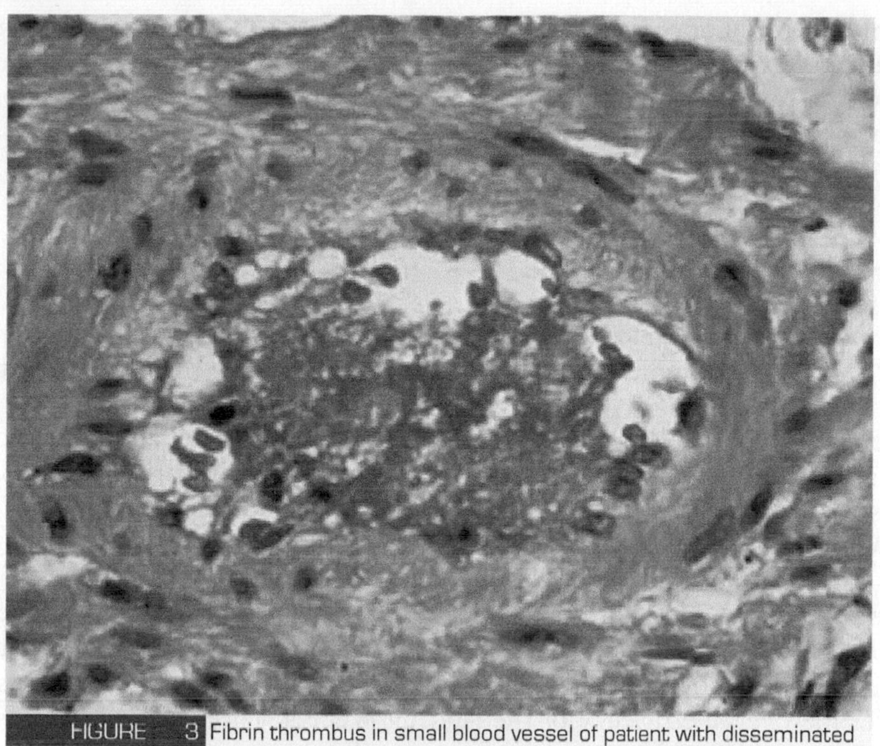

FIGURE 3 Fibrin thrombus in small blood vessel of patient with disseminated intravascular coagulation syndrome (original magnification × 400).

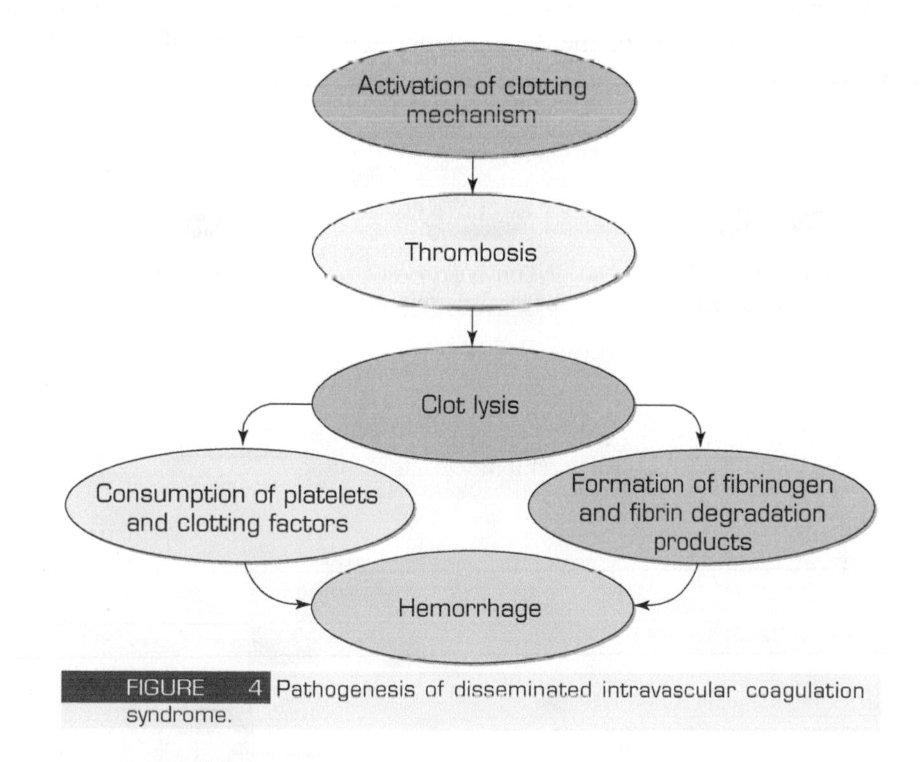

FIGURE 4 Pathogenesis of disseminated intravascular coagulation syndrome.

deficient formation of coagulation factors in patients with liver disease. In acutely ill patients, the majority of acquired coagulation disturbances are the result of disseminated intravascular coagulation, with depletion of both platelets and plasma coagulation factors.

Laboratory Tests to Evaluate Hemostasis

Several laboratory tests can evaluate the overall efficiency of the coagulation process, detect the presence of inhibitors of coagulation, and estimate the number and function of the platelets (FIGURE 5).

The number of platelets in the blood can be estimated by examining the blood smear, and more precise data can be obtained by a numerical platelet count. Special tests also are available to evaluate platelet function. The function of the capillaries in the hemostatic process is evaluated by the bleeding time, which reflects the time it takes for a small, standardized skin incision to stop bleeding.

A few relatively simple tests can be used to evaluate the various proteins concerned with blood coagulation (coagulation factors). The time it takes for blood to clot in a test tube under standard conditions is a crude and relatively insensitive test that measures the overall efficiency of the clotting process. Three other tests are more often used to evaluate the coagulation system. The tests, which are performed on plasma obtained from blood collected in tubes containing an anticoagulant, are the partial thromboplastin time, the prothrombin time, and the thrombin time. Each test measures a different phase of the coagulation process. When the tests are used together, one can assess separately each of the three phases of blood coagulation and can identify the location of the coagulation factor deficiency if any of the tests yield an abnormal result.

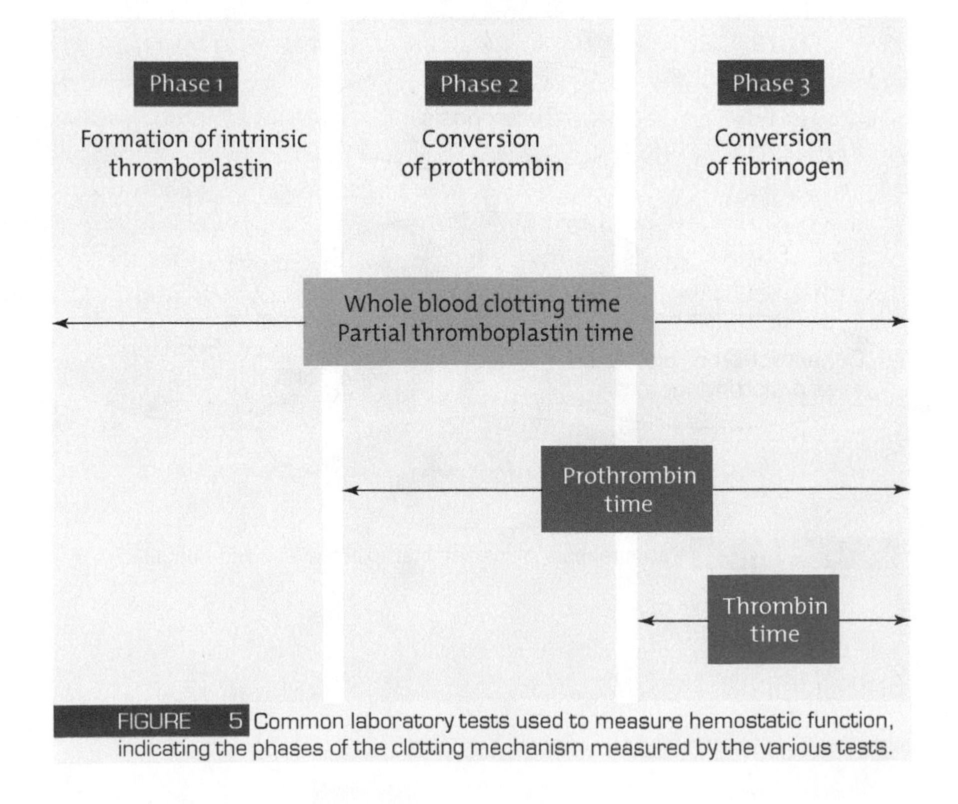

FIGURE 5 Common laboratory tests used to measure hemostatic function, indicating the phases of the clotting mechanism measured by the various tests.

The **partial thromboplastin time (PTT) test** measures the time it takes for blood plasma to clot after a lipid substance is added to the plasma along with calcium to start the clotting process. The lipid added is similar to the lipid material released from platelets to initiate the first phase of blood coagulation, which in turn is followed by activation of the second and third phases of the coagulation process. If a plasma factor in any of the three coagulation phases is deficient, the coagulation process is slowed, and the partial thromboplastin time is prolonged.

Partial thromboplastin time (PTT) test (throm-bō-plas′tin) *A test that measures the overall efficiency of the blood coagulation process.*

The **prothrombin time test** measures the time it takes for blood plasma to clot after adding a commercially available preparation of thromboplastin made from rabbit brain along with calcium to start the coagulation. The thromboplastin added to start the reaction is essentially the same material as the thromboplastin produced by the interaction of platelets and plasma coagulation factors in the first phase of blood coagulation. A normal prothrombin time test indicates that the second and third phases of blood coagulation are normal. If the prothrombin time is prolonged, an abnormality in either the second or third stages of coagulation is indicated. The abnormality cannot be in the first phase of blood coagulation because the first phase is concerned with the formation of intrinsic thromboplastin, and thromboplastin has already been supplied as the test reagent. The first phase has been bypassed, and the test is only measuring the coagulation factors involved in the second and third phases. The prothrombin time test is commonly used to monitor the effect of Coumadin anticoagulants administered to patients in order to reduce the coagulability of the blood. When using the test to monitor the amount of Coumadin to give to a patient who is taking Coumadin to reduce the coagulability of the blood, it is essential that any clinical laboratory performing the test obtains the same result. If the results of a test varied depending on the laboratory performing the test, the physician prescribing the Coumadin would have great difficulty determining how much to give. The physician might give too much, which could cause bleeding, or not enough, which would be undesirable by increasing the coagulability of the patient's blood. The problem was solved by standardizing the thromboplastin against an international standard to achieve uniformity, and the prothrombin time result is reported by comparing the patient's result with normal controls obtained using a standardized thromboplastin.

Prothrombin time test *A test that measures the phase of the coagulation mechanism after the formation of thromboplastin.*

The **thrombin time test** bypasses the first two phases of blood coagulation. One determines the clotting time of plasma after the addition of thrombin, which is normally generated in the second phase of the clotting process. Therefore, the test primarily measures the level of fibrinogen, which may be deficient in some conditions. The level of fibrinogen can also be measured directly by other tests, and one can also test for fibrinogen and fibrin degradation products, which are increased if fibrinolysis is excessive.

Thrombin time test *A laboratory test measurement that determines the concentration of fibrinogen in the blood by determining the clotting time of the blood plasma after addition of thrombin.*

In the event that abnormalities are detected in any phase of coagulation, it is necessary to determine whether they have occurred because a coagulation factor is deficient or because an inhibitor is impairing the action of the factor. If necessary, one can also determine the concentrations of the various factors.

Case Studies

The following cases illustrate the spectrum of coagulation abnormalities encountered in clinical medicine. The cases also illustrate how laboratory tests can help to determine the nature of the abnormality and suggest a proper course of treatment.

CASE 1

FACTOR VIII DEFICIENCY A 10-month-old child was admitted to the hospital through the emergency room because he was bleeding profusely from a cut under the lip that he received when falling. The history revealed easy bruising since birth but no episodes of bleeding into the joints, and the child was considered by the parents to be in good health.

Physical examination revealed ecchymoses over the left chest and a small bruise on the abdomen. Small bruises were noted on both lower extremities. Laboratory studies revealed moderate anemia and normal platelets. Coagulation studies revealed a normal plasma prothrombin time, but the partial thromboplastin time was significantly prolonged.

The bleeding was controlled by applying pressure for about 10 minutes. The next day, the child had a tarry stool, apparently caused by swallowed blood. After this, the stools became normal in color, and no further bleeding was noted.

In this case, the abnormal partial thromboplastin time indicated an abnormality of blood coagulation, but the normal prothrombin time indicated that the abnormality was not in the second or third stages of coagulation. Therefore, the defect must have been in the first phase, which suggests either hemophilia or von Willebrand disease as diagnostic possibilities. Further tests showed a very low level of factor VIII (antihemophilic factor), and additional diagnostic tests established the diagnosis of von Willebrand disease.

CASE 2

VITAMIN K DEFICIENCY A 55-year-old woman was admitted to the hospital with a severe staphylococcal pneumonia that was complicated by an accumulation of pus in the left pleural cavity. She received intensive antibiotic therapy. She was unable to take food or fluid orally because of severe nausea and vomiting and was maintained almost entirely on intravenous fluids. It was difficult to maintain a satisfactory fluid balance and nutrition. After several weeks in the hospital, she developed bleeding from her urinary tract and rectal bleeding.

Coagulation studies revealed a prolonged partial thromboplastin time, and prolonged plasma prothrombin time (27 seconds, control 13 seconds). The patient was given a vitamin K preparation. Both the partial thromboplastin time and the prothrombin time returned to normal, and she had no further bleeding.

In this case, the coagulation data indicate an acquired depression of vitamin K–dependent coagulation factors primarily caused by deficient synthesis of vitamin K by intestinal bacteria, which were eliminated by the intensive antibiotic treatment. The excellent response to vitamin K confirmed the diagnosis.

CASE 3

CHRONIC LIVER DISEASE A 57-year-old man was admitted to the hospital because of bleeding from his urinary tract. Blood coagulation studies revealed a prolonged partial thromboplastin time and prothrombin time. The plasma prothrombin time was 18 seconds (control 13 seconds). Other studies revealed that his liver function was very abnormal. The prothrombin time did not return to normal after administration of a vitamin K preparation. A needle biopsy of the liver revealed a type of chronic liver and biliary system disease called *cirrhosis*.

Here the abnormality was localized to the second stage of blood coagulation. Failure to respond to vitamin K suggested chronic liver disease rather than vitamin K deficiency or a decrease in coagulation factors caused by anticoagulant therapy. The needle biopsy confirmed the presence of chronic liver disease.

CASE 4

DISSEMINATED INTRAVASCULAR COAGULATION SYNDROME AS A RESULT OF RETAINED DEAD FETUS A 36-year-old pregnant woman was admitted to the hospital at 38 weeks' gestation. She had not felt fetal movement for the previous month, and no fetal heart tones were detected by her physician. Coagulation studies revealed prolonged partial thromboplastin time and prothrombin time. Fibrinogen was markedly reduced. The patient's blood contained high levels of fibrinogen and fibrin degradation products. Labor was induced, and delivery was accomplished with very little loss of blood. The next day, the fibrinogen returned to normal, and all coagulation studies were within normal limits.

In this case, all of the coagulation factors were decreased because they had been used up in the coagulation process induced by release of thromboplastic material into the maternal circulation from the retained dead fetus. The high levels of fibrinogen and fibrin degradation products were the result of activation of the fibrinolytic system—the body's defense against a potentially lethal intravascular coagulation process.

QUESTIONS FOR REVIEW

1. How does blood clot?
2. What are some of the common disturbances of blood coagulation?
3. What is thrombocytopenia? What type of bleeding is produced when platelets are markedly reduced? What types of diseases are associated with thrombocytopenia?
4. What types of diseases produce abnormalities in the first phase of blood coagulation?
5. What is the consequence of liberation of thromboplastic material into the circulation?
6. What laboratory tests are used to evaluate the coagulation of blood?
7. A patient with a bleeding tendency has a prolonged partial thromboplastin time with a normal prothrombin time. In what phase of the clotting process is the disturbance located? Name one possible disease that could produce these findings.
8. What are the effects of Coumadin anticoagulants on the clotting mechanism? How do they work? What laboratory test can be used to monitor the effect of the anticoagulant?

SUPPLEMENTARY READINGS

Ansell, J. E., Kurnar, R., and Deykin, D. 1977. The spectrum of vitamin K deficiency. *Journal of the American Medical Association* 238:40–2.

► A common problem, especially in postoperative patients and those with cancer or renal failure. Treatment with parenteral vitamin K confirms the diagnosis and stops bleeding.

Crowley, L. V. 1968. Diagnosis of blood clotting disorders in a community hospital. *The Journal—Lancet* 88:295–302.

► Thrombocytopenia, chronic liver disease, and disseminated intravascular coagulation were the common problems when this article was written in 1968, and more recent data reveal comparable distribution of coagulation problems in community hospital patients.

Hylek, E. M. 2010. Therapeutic potential of oral factor Xa inhibitors. *New England Journal of Medicine* 363:2559–61.

► Two factor Xa inhibitors, which do not require laboratory test monitoring, have proven very useful as prophylaxis against venous thromboembolism in patients undergoing total hip replacement and is much safer than warfarin; Xa inhibitors may also be useful to prevent atrial thrombi in patients with atrial fibrillation.

Kumar, V., Abbas, A. K., Fausto, N., et al. 2010. *Robbins and Contran pathologic basis of disease.* 8th ed. Philadelphia: Elsevier Saunders.

► Good section on coagulation.

Lassen, M. R., Gallus, A., Raskob, G. E., et al. 2010. Apixaban versus enoxaparin for thromboprophylaxis after hip replacement. *New England Journal of Medicine* 363:2487–98.

► Among patients undergoing hip replacement, treatment with apixaban (a factor X antagonist) compared with enoxaparin (a low molecular weight heparin) was associated with lower rates of venous thrombosis without increased bleeding.

OUTLINE SUMMARY

Hemostasis

FACTORS CONCERNED WITH HEMOSTASIS

Blood vessels and platelets

Reflex contraction of blood vessels after injury.

Platelets adhere to site of injury: plug vessel, liberate vasoconstrictors, release phospholipids to initiate clotting.

Small breaks in capillaries are sealed by platelets as they occur.

Plasma Coagulation Factors

Phase 1: generation of prothrombin activator:

Intrinsic system: components derived from blood.

Extrinsic system: tissue injury yields tissue thromboplastin.

Phase 2: formation of thrombin.

Phase 3: formation of fibrin.

Coagulation Inhibitors

Calcium

Required for all phases of coagulation.

No clinical disturbances of coagulation caused by low calcium.

Clinical Disturbances of Blood Coagulation

ABNORMALITIES OF SMALL BLOOD VESSELS

Abnormal function of small blood vessels.

Abnormal structure of small blood vessels.

ABNORMALITIES OF PLATELET NUMBERS OR FUNCTION

Thrombocytopenia:

As a result of bone marrow infiltration.

As a result of autoantibodies.

Defective platelet function.

DEFICIENCY OF PLASMA COAGULATION FACTORS

First phase:

Usually congenital.

Hemophilia is best-known defect.

Second phase:

Administration of anticoagulant drugs.

Inadequate synthesis of vitamin K.

Inadequate absorption of vitamin K.

Severe liver disease.

Liberation of thromboplastic material into circulation:

Activation of coagulation mechanism by products of tissue injury.

Intravascular coagulation.

Activation of fibrinolysin.

Consumption of coagulation factors and platelets.

Products of fibrin breakdown have anticoagulant activity.

FREQUENCY OF COAGULATION DISTURBANCES

Frequently a result of inadequate platelets or defective platelet function.

Chronic liver disease.

Disseminated intravascular coagulation syndrome.

Laboratory Tests to Evaluate Hemostasis

PLATELETS

Platelet count.

Examination of blood smear for platelet numbers.

OVERALL EVALUATION OF COAGULATION MECHANISM

Clotting time of whole blood.

Partial thromboplastin time.

SECOND AND THIRD STAGES

Evaluation by prothrombin time.

Test bypasses first stage of blood coagulation.

THIRD STAGE

Thrombin time.

Determine fibrinogen and fibrin degradation products.

http://health.jbpub.com/humandisease/9e

Human Disease Online is a great source for supplementary human disease information for both students and instructors. Visit this website to find a variety of useful tools for learning, thinking, and teaching.

Circulatory Disturbances

LEARNING OBJECTIVES

1. Describe the causes and effects of venous thrombosis.
2. Explain the pathogenesis of pulmonary embolism. Describe the clinical manifestations and compare the techniques of diagnosis.
3. Describe the causes and effects of arterial thrombosis.
4. List the four factors regulating the circulation of fluid between capillaries and interstitial tissue. Explain the major clinical disturbances leading to edema.
5. Describe the pathogenesis of the hypercoagulable state sometimes seen in patients with carcinoma.

Intravascular Blood Clots

Normally, blood does not clot within the vascular system. Under unusual circumstances, however, intravascular clotting may occur because of one or more of the following factors:

1. Slowing or stasis of the blood flow
2. Damage to the walls of the blood vessel
3. An increase in the coagulability of the blood

An intravascular clot is called a thrombus; the condition is termed **thrombosis.** Intravascular thrombi may form within veins or arteries and occasionally within the heart itself. A clot in the vascular system may become detached and may be carried in the circulation. Such a clot is termed an embolus (*embolus* = plug or stopper); the condition is termed **embolism.** Depending on where the blood clot was formed initially, the embolus may be carried into either the pulmonary circulation or the systemic arterial circulation. Eventually, it is arrested in an artery of smaller caliber than the diameter of the clot. When the embolus plugs the vessel, it blocks the blood flow to the tissue beyond (distal to) the obstruction, and the damaged tissue may undergo necrosis if the collateral blood supply is inadequate. The area of tissue breakdown is called an **infarct** or infarction.

Thrombosis
A blood clot formed within the vascular system.

Embolism
(em′bō-lizm)
A condition in which a plug composed of a detached clot, mass of bacteria, or other foreign material (embolus) occludes a blood vessel.

Infarct (in′färkt)
Necrosis of tissue caused by interruption of its blood supply.

Venous Thrombosis and Pulmonary Embolism

Formation of blood clots within leg veins is primarily a result of slowing or stasis of the blood in the veins. This is likely to occur during periods of prolonged bed rest or after a cramped position has been maintained for a long period of time. Under these circumstances, the "milking action" of the leg musculature, which normally promotes venous return, is impaired, leading to stasis of the blood. Varicose veins or any condition preventing normal emptying of veins predisposes an individual to thrombosis by causing venous stasis.

Postoperative thrombosis in leg veins is a common problem. The surgical patient is susceptible to venous thrombosis because of the combined effects of venous stasis resulting from inactivity and increased blood coagulability resulting from an increased concentration of coagulation factors. (Blood coagulation factors usually increase as a result of tissue injury or necrosis from any cause.)

A venous thrombosis may partially block venous return in the leg, making the leg swell. However, the major complication of venous thrombosis is related to detachment of the clot from the wall of the vein. The thrombus often is not firmly attached to the vein wall. It may break loose, forming an embolus that is carried rapidly up the inferior vena cava into the right side of the heart. From there, it is ejected into the pulmonary artery, where it may become lodged in either the main pulmonary artery or one of its branches. The clinical manifestations of a pulmonary embolism depend on the size of the embolus and where it lodges in the pulmonary artery.

LARGE PULMONARY EMBOLI

A large embolus that completely blocks the main pulmonary artery or its two major branches obstructs the flow of blood through the lungs (FIGURE 1). The right side of the heart becomes overdistended with blood because blood cannot be expelled into the lungs. The pulmonary artery leading to (proximal to) the obstructing embolus also becomes overdistended with blood, and the pressure in the pulmonary artery rises. Because less blood flows through the lungs into the left side of the heart, the left ventricle is unable to pump an adequate volume of blood to the brain and other vital organs. The systemic blood pressure falls, and the patient may go into shock. Blood still flows into the lungs from the bronchial arteries, which arise from the descending aorta and interconnect with the pulmonary arteries by means of collateral channels. This flow normally prevents infarction of the lung (FIGURE 2).

Clinically, the patient becomes very short of breath, and the skin and mucous membranes assume a bluish coloration (cyanosis) because of inadequate oxygenation

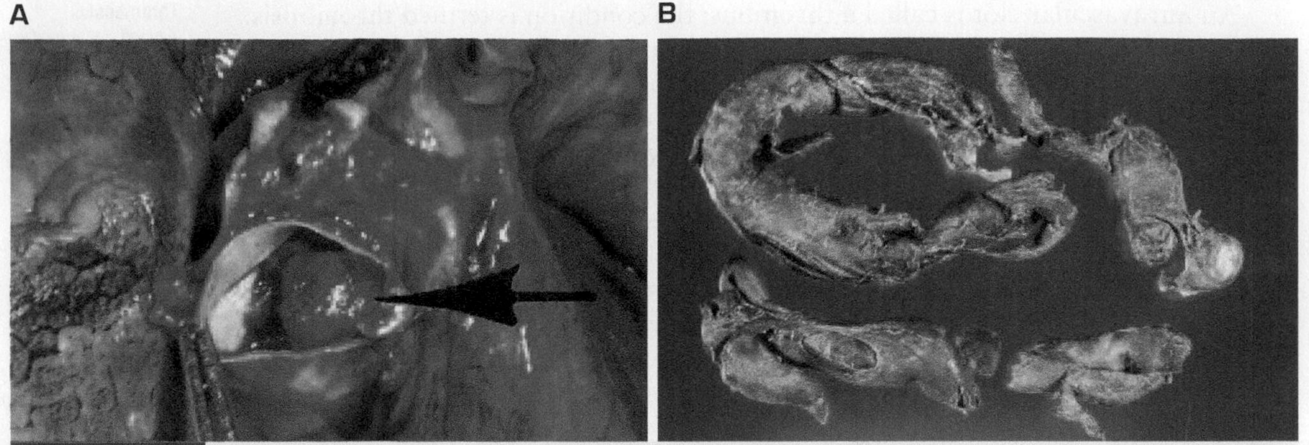

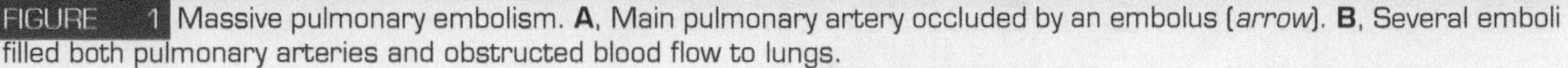
FIGURE 1 Massive pulmonary embolism. **A**, Main pulmonary artery occluded by an embolus (*arrow*). **B**, Several emboli filled both pulmonary arteries and obstructed blood flow to lungs.

of the blood. If the massive embolism is not immediately fatal, some blood may be able to flow around the embolus and circulate through the lungs, because the caliber of the pulmonary artery is increased by overdistention, and the high arterial pressure forces blood around the site of obstruction. In favorable circumstances, the embolus is eventually dissolved by the body's normal clot-dissolving mechanisms, and blood flow through the pulmonary artery is restored. In unfavorable cases, however, thrombus material builds up on the surface of the obstructing embolus and enlarges it. The sluggishly flowing blood in the branches of the pulmonary artery distal to the obstructing embolus may also become thrombosed. These events further impair pulmonary blood flow and may ultimately cause death several days after the initial embolization.

SMALL PULMONARY EMBOLI

If emboli are small, they may pass through the main pulmonary arteries and become impacted in the peripheral branches, usually in the arteries supplying the lower lobes of the lungs. Smaller emboli impede the flow of blood through the lungs and raise pulmonary artery pressure, but they have a less devastating effect than large emboli.

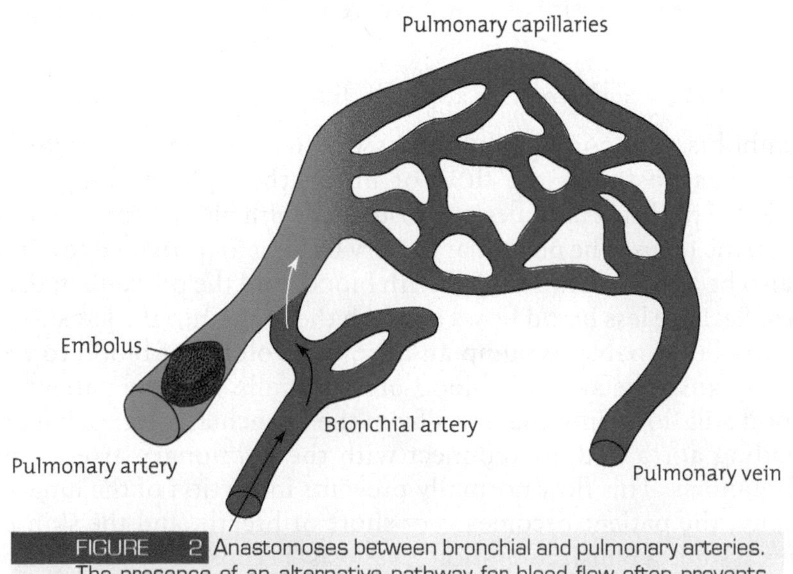

FIGURE 2 Anastomoses between bronchial and pulmonary arteries. The presence of an alternative pathway for blood flow often prevents infarction of the lung when the pulmonary artery is blocked by an embolus.

Frequently, the segment of lung supplied by the obstructed pulmonary artery undergoes necrosis, resulting in a pulmonary infarct. The alveolar septa break down, and blood flows from the ruptured capillaries into the pulmonary alveoli, which become distended with blood. The typical infarct is a wedge-shaped hemorrhagic area that extends to the pleural surface (FIGURE 3). Infarction does not always follow a pulmonary embolism because anastomoses between the bronchial artery and pulmonary artery distal to the obstruction provide an alternative pathway for blood flow. If the pulmonary venous pressure is elevated, however, as occurs in heart failure or when the lungs are poorly expanded, an adequate collateral circulation often does not develop and the lung becomes infarcted.

The clinical manifestations of smaller pulmonary emboli are quite variable and are frequently minimal if the lung does not become infarcted. Common symptoms of pulmonary infarction are difficulty in breathing (dyspnea), pleuritic chest pain, cough, and expectoration of bloody sputum. The chest pain occurs because the pleura overlying the infarct become inflamed and rubs against the overlying parietal pleura as the

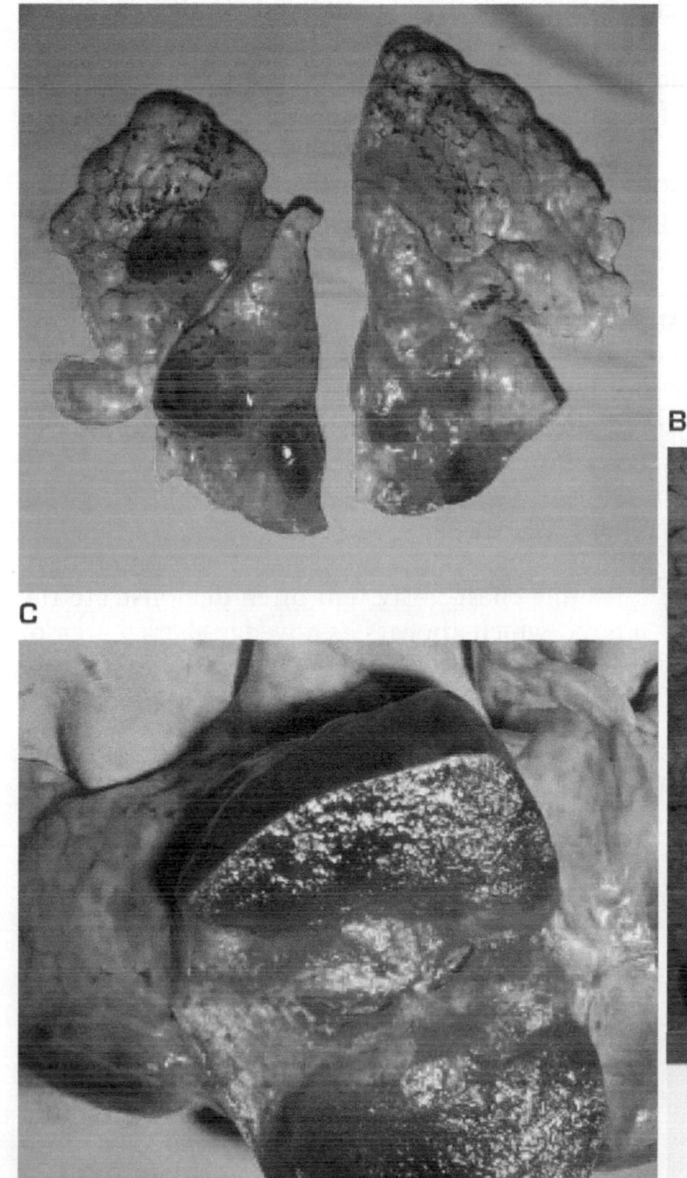

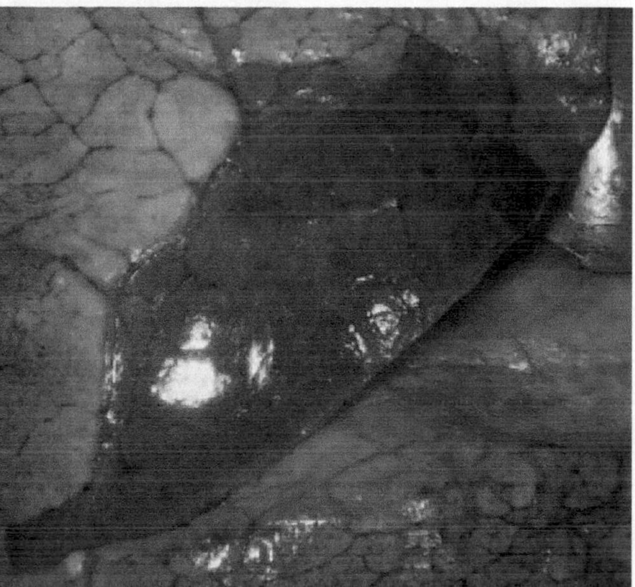

FIGURE 3 **A**, Multiple hemorrhagic pulmonary infarcts in both lungs. **B**, Closer view of infarct illustrating typical wedge-shaped hemorrhagic area that extends to pleural surface. **C**, Cut surface of pulmonary infarct, illustrating the hemorrhage in the infarcted lung segment and the sharp demarcation between infarct and adjacent normal lung tissue.

lung expands and contracts during respiration. The cough is caused by irritation of the bronchi in the injured area. The bloody sputum appears because blood escapes from the infarcted segment of lung into the bronchi and is subsequently coughed up.

SEPTIC PULMONARY EMBOLI

Sometimes, thrombi form in pelvic veins as a result of a bacterial infection in adjacent pelvic organs, as may occur after a uterine infection, and the bacteria may spread to infect the venous thrombi as well. If an infected thrombus breaks loose and causes a pulmonary infarct, the bacteria transported to the lung in the embolus invade the infarcted tissue, which breaks down to form a lung abscess. An infected embolus is called a septic embolus. If a patient sustains a pulmonary infarct owing to a septic embolus, the usual manifestations of pulmonary infarction are overshadowed by those of the systemic infection and the pulmonary abscess.

DIAGNOSIS OF PULMONARY EMBOLISM

A diagnosis of pulmonary embolism requires a high index of suspicion. Unexplained dyspnea, cough, or pleuritic chest pain in a predisposed patient may be the only manifestations of a pulmonary embolism. These symptoms should alert the physician to undertake further diagnostic studies. Sometimes, a blood test is helpful to confirm the physician's clinical impression of a possible pulmonary embolism. The test (called the *d-dimer test*) measures a by-product formed when fibrin within a blood clot is being broken down (fibrinolysis) by the body's normal clot-dissolving process, which would be activated in response to an intravascular thrombus or embolus. If the d-dimer concentration is not elevated, the possibility of a pulmonary embolism is less likely. On the other hand, an elevated d-dimer concentration would support the physician's clinical evaluation, and further studies are required. Some of the more useful tests are required. Some of the more useful studies are chest x-ray, radioisotope lung scans, and pulmonary angiography using either a standard radiologic method or a computed tomography (CT) procedure.

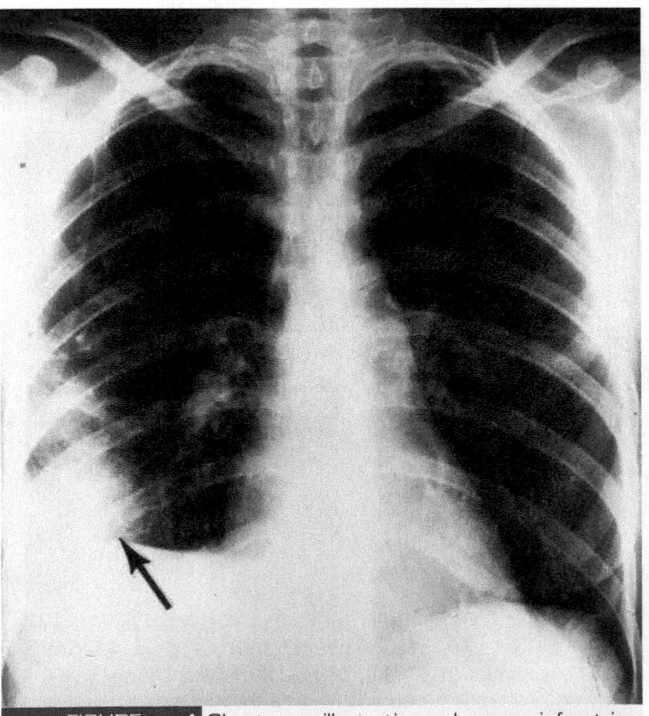

FIGURE 4 Chest x-ray illustrating pulmonary infarct in lower part of right lung (*left side* of photograph), which appears as an area of increased density (*arrow*). The opposite lung appears normal.

Chest X-Ray

If the embolus has caused pulmonary infarction, a routine chest x-ray will often demonstrate the infarct, which appears as a wedge-shaped area of increased density in the lung (FIGURE 4). Because emboli cannot be visualized on x-ray films, the lung will appear normal if it is not infarcted.

Radioisotope Lung Scan

To perform a radioisotope lung scan, one first injects a peripheral vein with a solution of specially prepared albumin labeled with a radioisotope. The injected material flows through the lung and is filtered out in the pulmonary capillaries. The radioactivity in the lungs, which is related to pulmonary blood flow, is then recorded by special instruments. If pulmonary blood flow is normal, the isotope is uniformly distributed throughout both lungs, and a uniform pattern of radioactivity appears on the lung scan. When blood flow to a part of the lung is blocked by an embolism, however, the

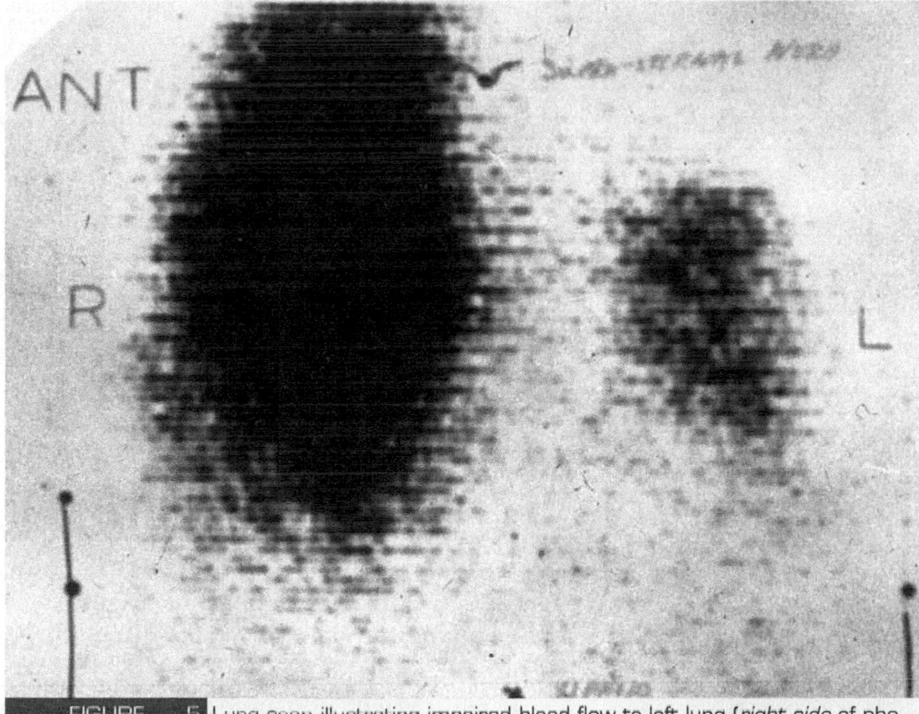

FIGURE 5 Lung scan illustrating impaired blood flow to left lung (*right side* of photograph), representing decreased radioactivity. Radioactivity of the opposite lung is normal (*uniform dark appearance*), indicating normal pulmonary blood flow.

isotope does not flow into the portion of lung supplied by the blocked artery, and no radioactivity is detected in the affected part of the lung. The isotope study does not actually demonstrate the embolus; it indicates only that a part of the lung has a reduced blood supply. Nevertheless, the isotope study does detect the abnormal pulmonary blood flow caused by the embolus (FIGURE 5). Consequently, the lung scan will be abnormal even when the lung is not infarcted, and the routine chest x-ray appears normal.

Pulmonary Angiography

The definitive diagnostic method to identify a pulmonary embolism is a pulmonary angiogram, which directly visualizes the pulmonary artery and its branches. A catheter is inserted into a vein in the arm and advanced up the vein through the superior vena cava, into the right side of the heart, and out the pulmonary artery. A radiopaque material is then injected into the artery through the catheter, and the flow of the material through the pulmonary arteries is visualized by means of serial x-ray films. If the pulmonary artery or one of its branches is completely obstructed by an embolus, no contrast material flows into the blocked vessel (FIGURE 6). If the embolus does not completely obstruct the artery, some contrast medium flows around the embolus, which appears as a filling defect in the column of contrast material within the partially occluded vessel. New advanced CT equipment can provide similar information and does not require insertion of a catheter into the pulmonary artery, although an intravenous injection of radiopaque contrast material is required. The equipment can monitor the flow of contrast material through the pulmonary artery and its branches and can detect an obstruction of blood flow within the pulmonary circulation, indicating a pulmonary embolus.

TREATMENT OF PULMONARY EMBOLISM

Treatment of patients with pulmonary embolism includes general supportive care and administration of anticoagulants. Heparin, which has an immediate effect, is

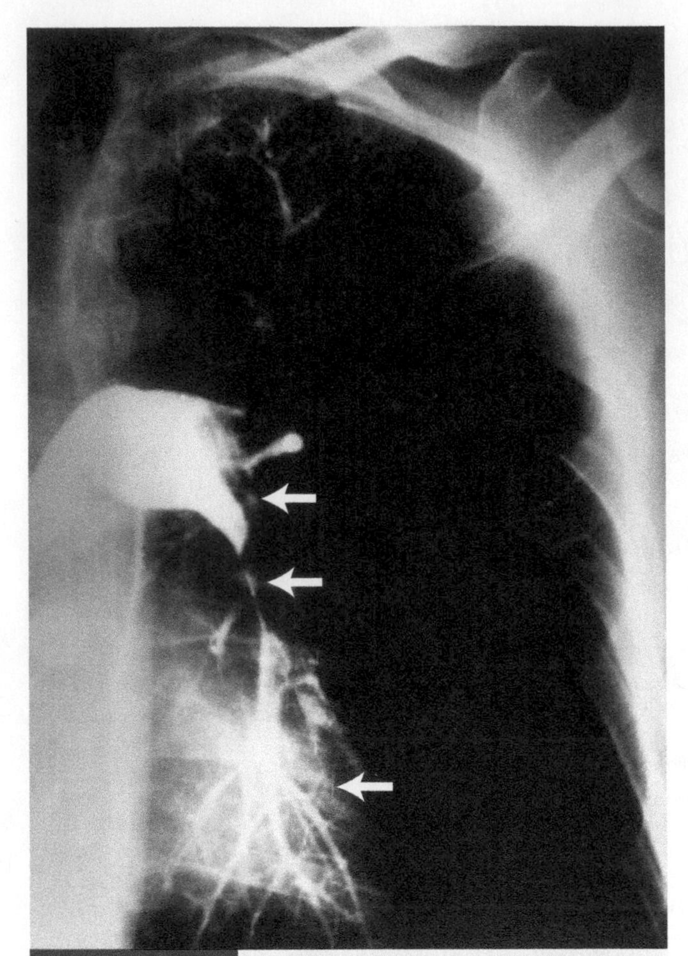

FIGURE 6 An angiogram used to identify pulmonary embolism illustrated by view of the left lung and pulmonary artery. A catheter has been inserted into the pulmonary artery and radiopaque contrast material injected. Flow of contrast material is almost completely blocked (*upper arrow*) by a large pulmonary embolus obstructing the left main pulmonary artery. Only a thin trickle of contrast material flows around the embolus (*middle arrow*) to fill the pulmonary artery branches supplying part of the lower lobe (*lower arrow*).

generally used initially, followed by administration of coumadin-type anticoagulants, which act by depressing hepatic synthesis of coagulation factors. The purpose of anticoagulant therapy is twofold: (1) to prevent recurrent pulmonary emboli by preventing the formation of more thrombi in leg and pelvic veins and (2) to prevent thrombus formation in branches of the pulmonary artery distal to the embolism. If adequate therapy is given, further thromboembolism is prevented, and the embolus will slowly dissolve. Rarely, if the patient has sustained a massive embolus and is in critical condition because blood flow through a main pulmonary artery is blocked, it is necessary to remove the embolus surgically or dissolve the embolus rapidly by administering clot-dissolving (thrombolytic) drugs. These are the same drugs that are given to a heart attack patient in order to dissolve a thrombus blocking a coronary artery (discussion on the cardiovascular system).

If the patient continues to have pulmonary emboli despite adequate anticoagulant therapy, it may be necessary to perform surgery on the inferior vena cava to interrupt the passage of clots from the peripheral veins to the lungs. Generally, the operative procedure consists of either complete or partial interruption of the vena cava below the level of the renal veins. Complete interruption is accomplished by surgical ligation of the vein. Partial interruption has been performed by various methods in such a way as to allow normal blood flow and yet trap emboli.

The following case illustrates the clinical features of a large pulmonary embolism treated successfully by anticoagulant therapy.

A 26-year-old woman consulted her physician because of cough and marked shortness of breath. Physical examination revealed that she was in severe respiratory distress with a dry, hacking cough. Her lips and fingernails were slightly cyanotic, indicating poor oxygenation of the blood. Chest x-ray revealed prominent pulmonary arteries but no evidence of pulmonary consolidation suggesting an infarct. The oxygen saturation of the arterial blood was reduced, which was compatible with a pulmonary embolus. An angiographic study revealed that the left main pulmonary artery was occluded by a pulmonary embolus. The patient received anticoagulant therapy and supplementary oxygen. Her condition gradually improved. Past medical history was significant in that the patient was taking a relatively high-estrogen contraceptive pill for control of a menstrual irregularity. The pill apparently predisposed her to thrombosis of a leg vein, which was followed by a pulmonary embolus.

Arterial Thrombosis

Blood flow in arteries is rapid, and intravascular pressure is high; so stasis of blood is not a factor in arterial thrombosis. The main cause of arterial thrombosis is injury to the wall of the vessel, usually secondary to arteriosclerosis. The arteriosclerotic deposits cause ulceration and roughening of the lining of the artery, and thrombi form on the roughened area. The effects of arterial thrombus formation depend on the location and size of the artery that has become obstructed. Blockage of a coronary artery frequently causes infarction of the heart muscle and consequent "heart attack." If a major artery supplying the leg is occluded, the extremity undergoes necrosis, usually called **gangrene** (FIGURE 7). (This differs from gas gangrene, which is caused by a species of ***Clostridium***.) Occlusion of an artery to the brain leads to infarction of a portion of the brain, commonly called a "stroke."

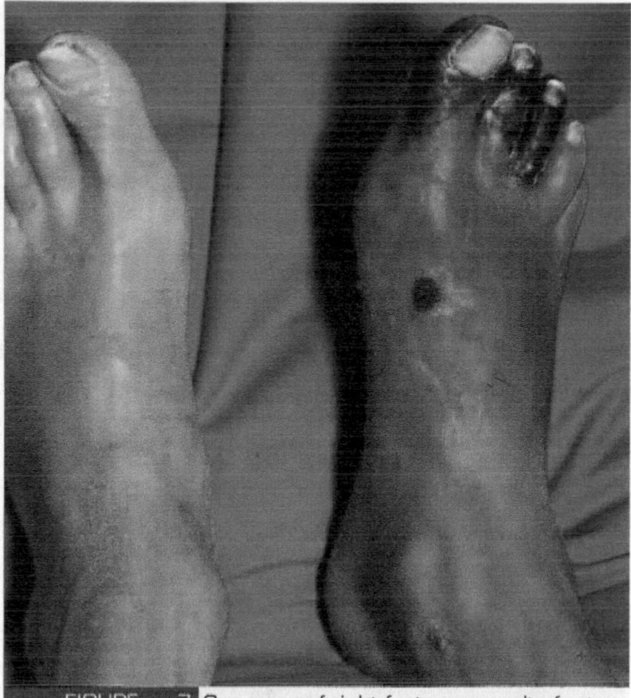

FIGURE 7 Gangrene of right foot as a result of arterial obstruction.

Intracardiac Thrombosis

Occasionally, blood clots may form within the heart itself. Thrombi may form within the atrial appendages when heart function is abnormal, as in heart failure, or when the atria are not contracting normally. Thrombi may also form on the surfaces of heart valves that have been damaged as a result of disease. Occasionally, thrombi may form on the internal lining of the ventricle adjacent to an area where the heart muscle is infarcted. Intracardiac thrombi may become dislodged and may be carried into the systemic circulation, resulting in infarction of the spleen, kidneys, brain, or other organs. The symptoms produced depend on the size and location of the infarction.

Gangrene
(gang-grēn′)
Term has two different meanings. Refers to (1) infection caused by gas-forming anaerobic bacteria (gas gangrene) *or (2) necrosis of an extremity caused by interruption of its blood supply* (ischemic gangrene).

Clostridium
(klä-strid′ē-yum)
Anaerobic gram-positive spore-forming rod-shaped bacterium.

Thrombosis Caused by Increased Blood Coagulability

In some conditions, the concentration of various blood coagulation factors is elevated, increasing the coagulability of the blood and predisposing the individual to intravascular clotting. After injury or operation, products of tissue necrosis with thromboplastic activity stimulate the synthesis of many clotting factors. This increases the likelihood of postoperative thrombosis in leg veins.

The estrogen in contraceptive pills has been found to stimulate synthesis of coagulation factors, raising their concentration and predisposing the women who use the pills to both venous and arterial thrombosis. This observation has led to concern about the safety of "the pill" when used for long periods of time.

Hereditary gene mutations affecting the synthesis of coagulation factors may also increase blood coagulability and the risk of venous thrombosis. One is a relatively common mutation, present in about 5% of the population, that codes for synthesis of coagulation factor V. This is one of the factors involved in the conversion of prothrombin to thrombin in the second phase of blood coagulation. Normal factor

V is inactivated by a coagulation inhibitor called protein C, which terminates its activity. The abnormal factor, called factor V Leiden (after a city in the Netherlands), is more resistant to inactivation, which prolongs the activity of the mutant factor, thereby increasing the coagulability of the blood and the risk of venous thrombosis. The other significant mutation, found in 2% of the population, affects a gene regulating synthesis of prothrombin. The mutation leads to a higher than normal level of prothrombin and is also associated with an increased risk of venous thrombosis.

THROMBOSIS IN PATIENTS WITH CANCER

Many patients with advanced cancer have elevated platelets and increased concentrations of coagulation factors in their blood, and they are predisposed to both venous and arterial thromboses. This tendency results from the release of thromboplastic materials into the circulation from deposits of tumor. The same basic mechanism induces hemorrhage in patients with a disseminated intravascular coagulation syndrome (discussed on abnormalities of blood coagulation). The variations in clinical manifestations result from differences in the rate at which the thromboplastic material enters the circulation. In the acute process, a large quantity of thromboplastic material is rapidly released into the circulation. Platelets and coagulation factors are consumed faster than they can be replenished, and bleeding results. In patients with widespread cancer, the thromboplastic material is liberated slowly but continuously from the tumor. The blood coagulation mechanism is activated, and clot lysis occurs. Production of coagulation factors and platelets increases in response to an increased demand, but the body overcompensates. Production exceeds destruction, which leads to a hypercoagulable state. FIGURE 8 compares these two processes.

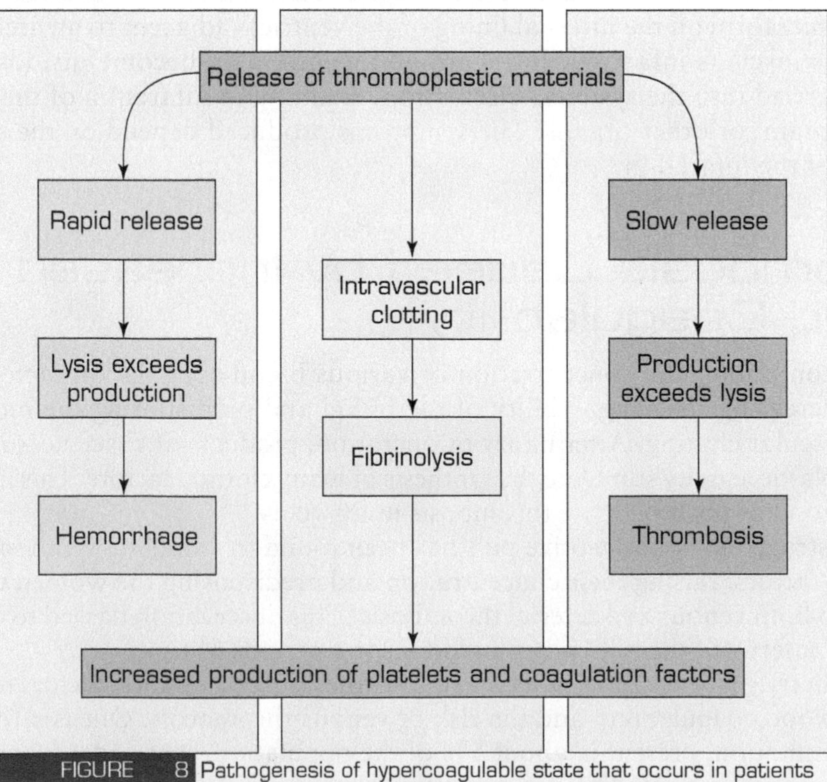

FIGURE 8 Pathogenesis of hypercoagulable state that occurs in patients with cancer, contrasted with the pathogenesis of disseminated intravascular coagulation syndrome. Different clinical manifestations reflect differing rates of fibrinolysis and compensatory regeneration of hemostatic components.

Embolism as a Result of Foreign Material

Most emboli are caused by blood clots, but other materials occasionally gain access to the circulation. Fat, air, and foreign particles within the vascular system may sometimes cause serious difficulties.

FAT EMBOLISM

After a severe bone fracture, fatty bone marrow and surrounding adipose tissue may be disrupted. The emulsified fat globules may be sucked into the veins and carried into the lungs, leading to widespread obstruction of the pulmonary capillaries. Some of the fat may be carried through the pulmonary capillaries and may reach the systemic circulation, eventually blocking small blood vessels in the brain and other organs.

AMNIONIC FLUID EMBOLISM

This condition is an uncommon but devastating complication of pregnancy that usually occurs during labor when the pressure of uterine contractions forces a large volume of amnionic fluid through a tear in fetal membranes into a torn uterine vein at the site of a cervical or uterine laceration. The amnionic fluid, which contains desquamated fetal epithelial cells and hair, fatty material (vernix), debris from the fetal respiratory and gastrointestinal tract, and thromboplastic material, is carried in the maternal venous circulation to the lungs, where it plugs the pulmonary capillaries. Manifestations are severe dyspnea, shock, and often an acute disseminated intravascular coagulation syndrome induced by the thromboplastic material in the amnionic fluid (Figure 8).

AIR EMBOLISM

Sometimes, a large amount of air is sucked into the venous circulation after a chest wound with injury to the lung. Air may also be accidentally injected into the circulation in attempts at abortion by persons without medical training. The air is carried to the heart and accumulates in the right heart chambers, preventing filling of the heart by returning venous blood. As a result, the heart is unable to pump blood, and the individual dies rapidly of circulatory failure.

EMBOLISM OF PARTICULATE FOREIGN MATERIAL

Various types of particulate material may be injected into veins by drug abusers, who crush and dissolve tablets intended for oral use and inject the material intravenously. The material is usually trapped within the small pulmonary blood vessels, producing symptoms of severe respiratory distress caused by obstruction of the pulmonary capillaries by the foreign material.

Edema

The term **edema** refers to accumulation of fluid in the interstitial tissues. Edema is most conspicuous in the skin and subcutaneous tissues of the dependent parts of the body and is usually noted first in the legs and ankles. When the edematous tissue is compressed by indenting the tissue with the fingertips, the fluid is pushed aside, leaving a pit or indentation that gradually refills with fluid. This characteristic is responsible for the common term pitting edema. Fluid may also accumulate in the pleural cavity (**hydrothorax**) or in the peritoneal cavity (**ascites**).

Edema may result from any condition in which the circulation of extracellular fluid between the capillaries and the interstitial tissues becomes disturbed.

Edema
(e-dē′muh)
Accumulation of an excess of fluid in the interstitial tissues.

Hydrothorax
(hī-drō-thor′ax)
Accumulation of fluid in the pleural cavity.

Ascites
(a-si′tēz)
Accumulation of fluid in the abdominal cavity.

FACTORS REGULATING FLUID FLOW BETWEEN CAPILLARIES AND INTERSTITIAL TISSUE

The flow of fluid through the interstitial space depends on four factors:

1. The capillary hydrostatic pressure, which tends to filter fluid from the blood through the capillary endothelium.
2. The permeability of the capillaries, which determines the ease with which the fluid can pass through the capillary endothelium.
3. The osmotic pressure exerted by the proteins in the blood plasma (called colloid osmotic pressure), which tends to attract fluid from the interstitial space back into the vascular compartment. Osmotic pressure, which was considered in cells and tissues: their structure and function in health and disease discussion, may be defined as the property causing fluid to migrate in the direction of a higher concentration of molecules. The osmotic pressure of the plasma depends primarily on the concentration of the plasma proteins. Because the capillaries are impermeable to protein, the protein tends to draw water from the interstitial fluid into the capillaries and to hold it there.
4. The presence of open lymphatic channels, which collect some of the fluid forced out of the capillaries by the hydrostatic pressure of the blood and return the fluid to the circulation.

FIGURE 9 illustrates the mechanism by which fluid flow is regulated through interstitial tissues.

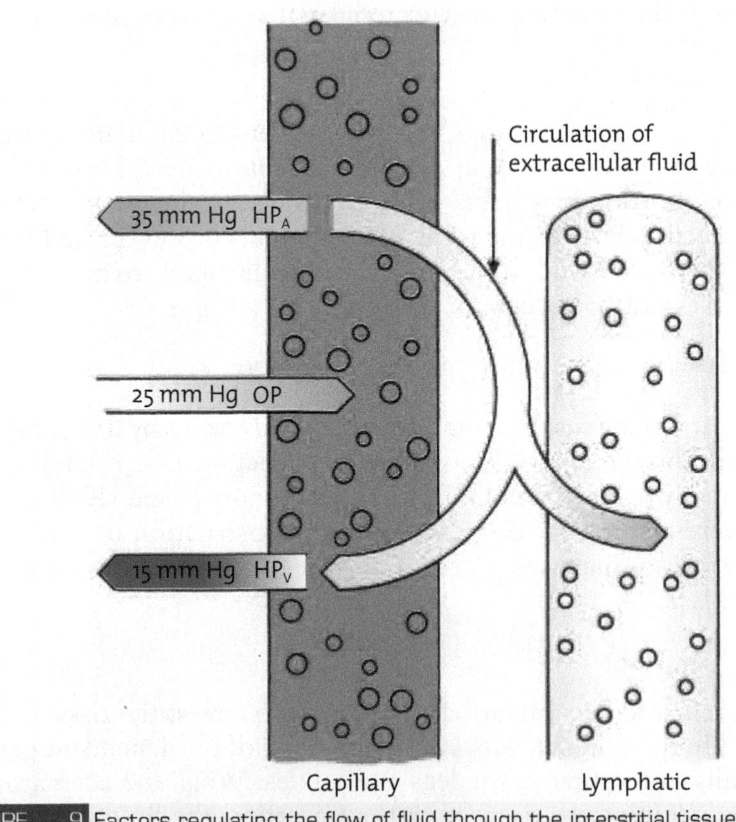

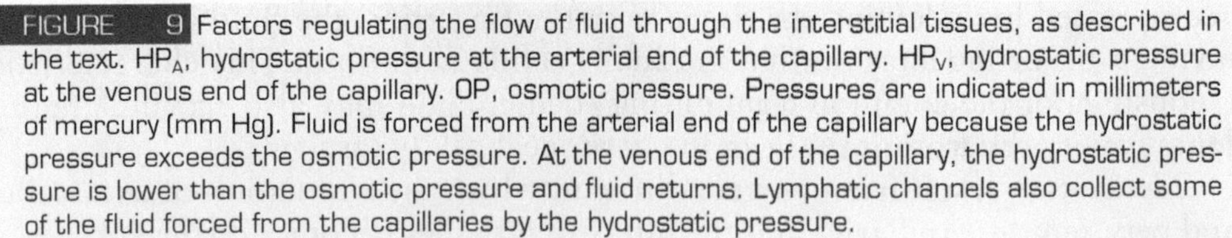
FIGURE 9 Factors regulating the flow of fluid through the interstitial tissues, as described in the text. HP_A, hydrostatic pressure at the arterial end of the capillary. HP_V, hydrostatic pressure at the venous end of the capillary. OP, osmotic pressure. Pressures are indicated in millimeters of mercury (mm Hg). Fluid is forced from the arterial end of the capillary because the hydrostatic pressure exceeds the osmotic pressure. At the venous end of the capillary, the hydrostatic pressure is lower than the osmotic pressure and fluid returns. Lymphatic channels also collect some of the fluid forced from the capillaries by the hydrostatic pressure.

Flow of Fluid Into and Out of Capillaries

The pressure of the blood at the arterial end of the capillary is higher than the colloid osmotic pressure, which causes fluid to be filtered through the endothelium of the capillaries into the interstitial space. The capillary endothelium acts as a semipermeable membrane and limits the rate at which fluid is filtered from the blood. At the venous end of the capillary, the hydrostatic pressure is lower than the colloid osmotic pressure, and fluid tends to diffuse back into the capillaries. In this way, the fluid containing dissolved nutrients is carried from the blood into the interstitial tissues to nourish the cells, and waste products are returned to the circulation for excretion.

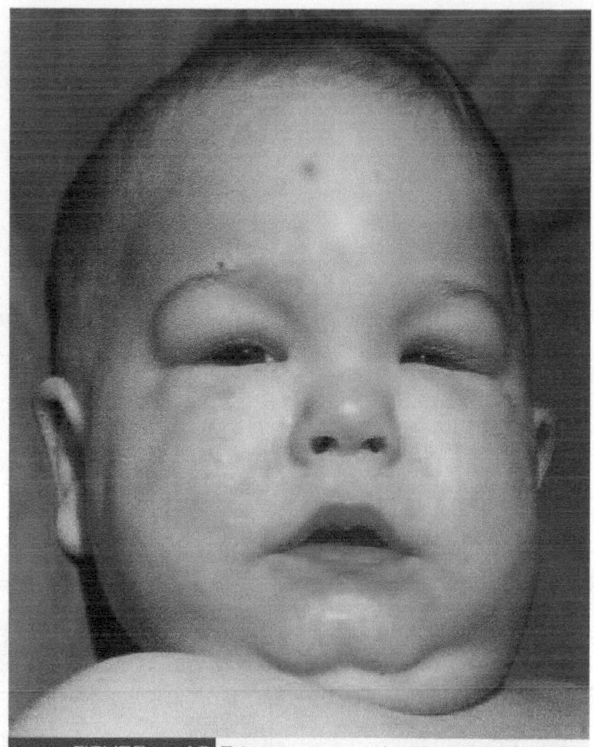

FIGURE 10 Edema as a result of increased capillary permeability. Note the swelling of the eyelids and face.

PATHOGENESIS AND CLASSIFICATION OF EDEMA

Increased Capillary Permeability

Normally, the endothelium of the capillaries limits the amount of fluid filtered from the blood. If the capillaries are excessively permeable, filtration of fluid into the interstitial space is greater than normal. Increased capillary permeability is responsible for the swelling of the tissues associated with an acute inflammation such as a boil or a severe sunburn. Some systemic diseases also cause a generalized increase in capillary permeability, which leads to widespread edema of the subcutaneous tissues (FIGURE 10).

Low Plasma Proteins

If the concentration of plasma proteins is decreased, the colloid osmotic pressure is reduced correspondingly. Consequently, less fluid is attracted back into the capillaries, and the fluid accumulates in the tissues. A low concentration of plasma proteins may result from excessive loss of plasma proteins in the urine, as occurs in patients with some types of kidney disease or from inadequate synthesis of plasma proteins as a result of malnutrition or starvation (FIGURE 11). Hypoproteinemia caused by inadequate protein intake may be encountered in patients with chronic debilitating diseases who are unable to eat an adequate amount of food and in patients with intestinal diseases in whom assimilation of food is impaired.

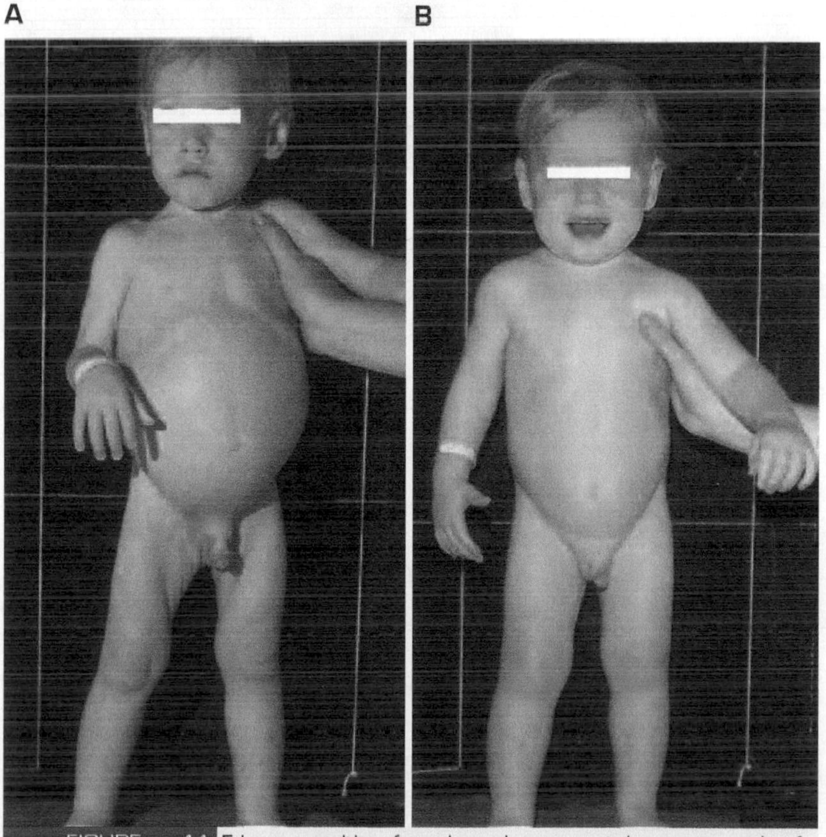

FIGURE 11 Edema resulting from low plasma proteins as a result of malnutrition. **A**, Child prior to treatment, illustrating emaciation, abdominal distention caused by accumulation of fluid in the peritoneal cavity, and edema of legs. **B**, Same child after treatment by a nutritious high-protein diet.

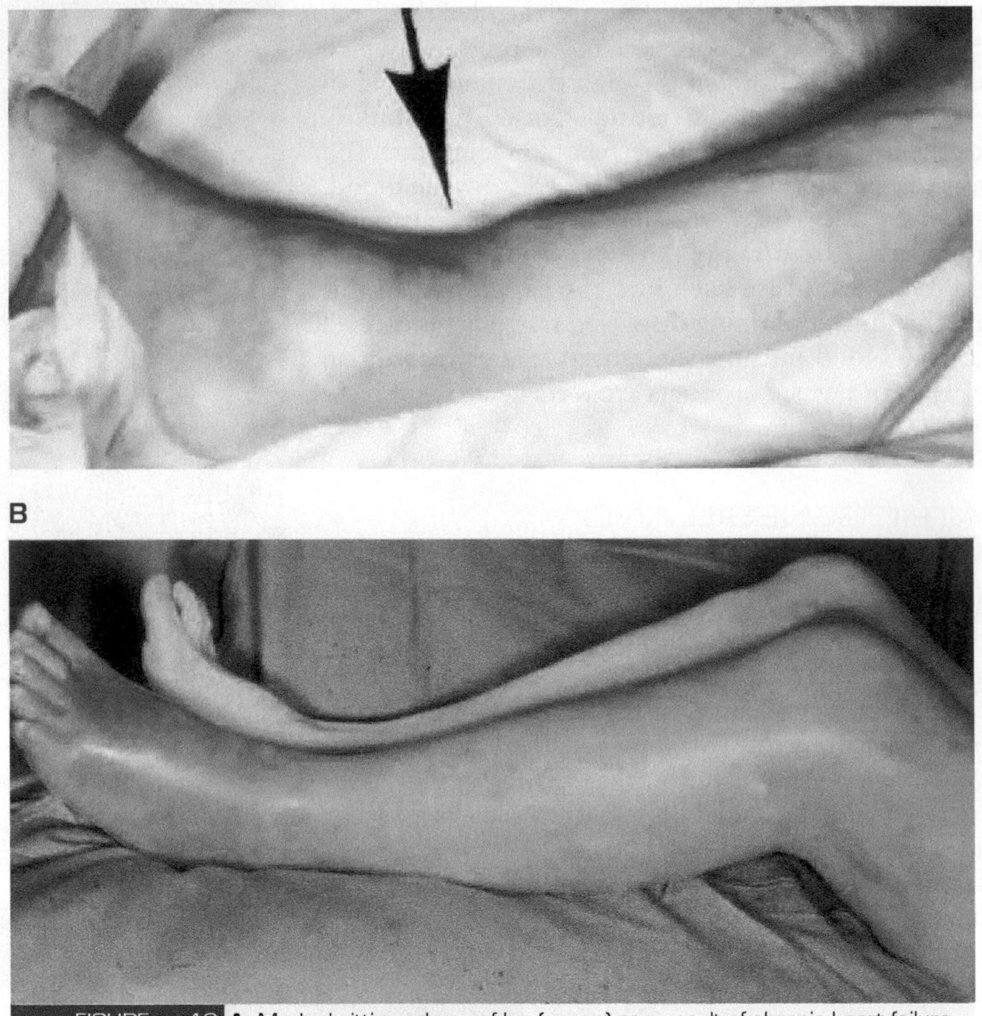

FIGURE 12 **A**, Marked pitting edema of leg (*arrow*) as a result of chronic heart failure. **B**, Localized edema of left leg caused by venous obstruction. Right leg appears normal.

Increased Hydrostatic Pressure

Increased pressure in the veins draining the capillaries is reflected as a higher than normal pressure at the venous end of the capillaries. As a result, more fluid is filtered from the capillaries, causing it to accumulate in the tissues. A localized increase in venous pressure may be encountered if the veins draining a part of the body become compressed, twisted, or obstructed by a blood clot that fills the lumen. More commonly, the increased venous pressure is a manifestation of heart failure, and the pressure is elevated in all the systemic veins (FIGURE 12).

Lymphatic Obstruction

Sometimes, lymphatic channels draining a part of the body become obstructed because of disease. The obstruction blocks a pathway by which fluid is returned from the interstitial space into the circulation and leads to edema in the region that is normally drained by the obstructed lymphatic vessels (FIGURE 13).

Shock
A general term for any condition leading to such a marked fall of blood pressure that body tissues do not receive an adequate amount of oxygen, most often caused by acute blood loss or severe infection (sepsis).

Shock

Shock is a general term to describe any condition in which the blood pressure is too low to provide adequate blood flow to the body cells and organs, and is a serious,

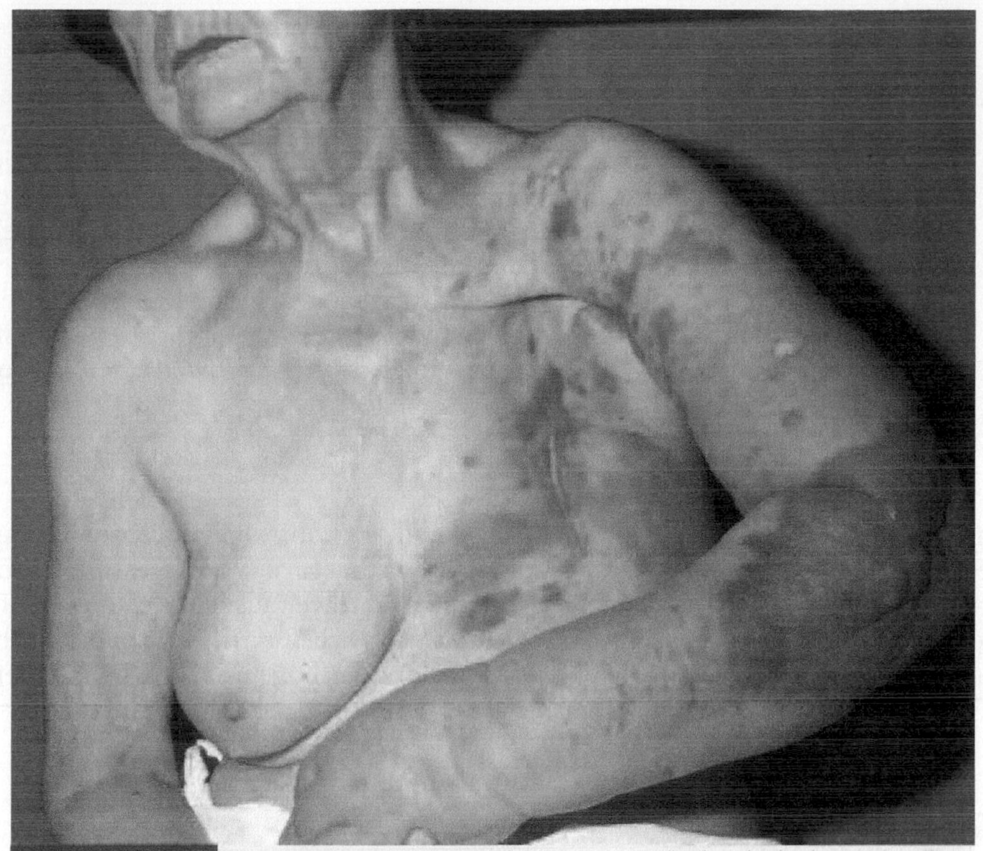

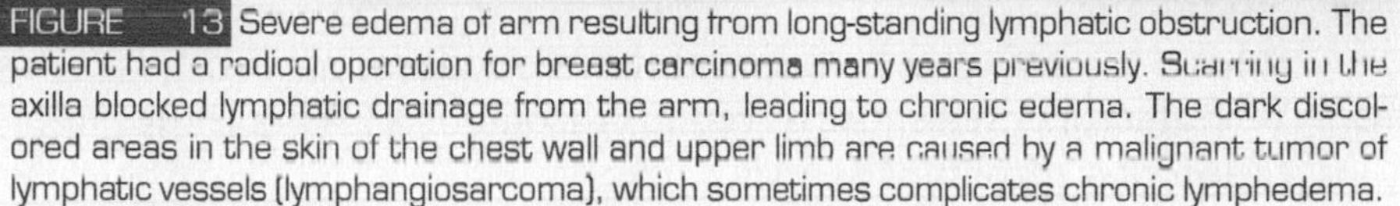
FIGURE 13 Severe edema of arm resulting from long-standing lymphatic obstruction. The patient had a radical operation for breast carcinoma many years previously. Scarring in the axilla blocked lymphatic drainage from the arm, leading to chronic edema. The dark discolored areas in the skin of the chest wall and upper limb are caused by a malignant tumor of lymphatic vessels (lymphangiosarcoma), which sometimes complicates chronic lymphedema.

potentially life-threatening condition. Shock results from a disproportion between the volume of blood in the circulatory system and the capacity of the vascular system that carries the blood. Blood pressure falls if the volume of blood filling the circulatory system falls or if marked dilation of blood vessels expands the capacity of the vascular system to such an extent that the existing blood volume is insufficient to fill the vessels adequately.

CLASSIFICATION

Often shock is classified in four categories based on its cause (pathogenesis).

1. Hypovolemic shock is caused by low blood volume, leading to a corresponding drop in blood pressure. Most cases result from a large hemorrhage that significantly reduces the circulating blood volume, but any excessive depletion of body fluids such as fluid losses from a severe burn, from severe diarrhea, or from excessive fluid loss in urine resulting from diuretics can also reduce blood volume as fluid shifts from the vascular compartment into the depleted extravascular body fluids.
2. Cardiogenic shock is caused by inadequate or impaired cardiac pumping function, which reduces cardiac output. Cardiogenic shock usually is a complication of a myocardial infarction, but the pumping function of the heart can also be impaired if the heart is compressed by accumulation of

blood or fluid within the pericardial sac, which prevents filling of the heart in diastole, or by other conditions that cause acute heart failure.

3. Septic shock results from excessive dilation of the body's blood vessels, in which the volume of circulating blood is insufficient to fill adequately the greatly expanded capacity of the blood vessels. Marked vasodilation results from the severe infection in which microbial toxins and mediators of inflammation that are released at the site of infection dilate the vessels.
4. Anaphylactic shock (described in the discussion on immunity, hypersensitivity, allergy, and autoimmune diseases) also results from excessive vasodilation caused by the widespread release of mediators of inflammation from mast cells and basophils, which is often followed by circulatory collapse.

PROGNOSIS AND TREATMENT

The outcome of shock depends on its cause and how quickly it is recognized and treated. Treatment consists of administering drugs that raise blood pressure by constricting blood vessels, restoring blood volume by intravenous fluids or blood if the shock is caused by a severe hemorrhage, and treating the underlying condition that leads to the shock. Unfortunately, septic shock or cardiogenic shock in an elderly patient with other medical problems has a very poor prognosis.

QUESTIONS FOR REVIEW

1. What is the difference between a thrombus and an embolus? What is an infarct?
2. What factors predispose to venous thrombosis? What is the major complication of a thrombus in a leg vein?
3. What factors predispose to arterial thrombosis?
4. What are the causes and effects of intracardiac thrombi?
5. What conditions predispose to thrombosis by increasing the coagulability of the blood?
6. What factors regulate the flow of fluid between capillaries and interstitial tissue? What are the major causes of edema?
7. What coagulation disturbances may be encountered in patients with tumors?
8. What is the difference between a pulmonary embolus and a pulmonary infarct? What are the clinical manifestations of a pulmonary infarct?

SUPPLEMENTARY READINGS

Alperin, J. B. 1987. Coagulopathy caused by vitamin K deficiency in critically ill, hospitalized patients. *Journal of the American Medical Association* 258:1916–9.

- Vitamin K deficiency in hospitalized patients is common and can be misdiagnosed as disseminated intravascular coagulation syndrome. It can be prevented by prophylactic vitamin K in seriously ill patients receiving antibiotics.

Blom, J. W., Doggen, C. J., Osanto, S., et al. 2005. Malignancies, prothrombotic mutations, and the risk of venous thrombosis. *Journal of the American Medical Association* 293:715–22.

- Patients with cancer have a sevenfold greater risk of venous thrombosis than a comparable control group of patients, especially in the first few months after diagnosis and in the presence of distant metastases. Two hereditary gene mutations increase the risk even more by greatly increasing the coagulability of the blood. One is a relatively common mutation of a gene coding for the synthesis of coagulation factor V called *factor V Leiden*. Normal factor V is inactivated by a coagulation inhibitor called *protein C* during coagulation of the blood, but factor V Leiden is less efficiently inhibited. Mutation of another gene that regulates prothrombin synthesis leads to a higher than normal concentration of prothrombin in the blood.

Goldhaber, S. Z. 2005. Multislice computed tomography for pulmonary embolism—a technological marvel. *New England Journal of Medicine* 352:1812–4.

- CT scanning of the chest has revolutionized the diagnostic approach to pulmonary embolism and has largely replaced radioisotope lung scans to evaluate suspected pulmonary emboli.

Hull, R. D. 2006. Diagnosing pulmonary embolism with improved certainty and simplicity. *Journal of the American Medical Association* 295:213–5.

- Ultrasound has supplanted venography for diagnosing a deep vein thrombosis. Spiral CT provides information about a possible pulmonary embolus. D-dimer is a degradation product of fibrin, which is elevated if there is a leg vein thrombus, and rapid tests are available. Judicious application of these methods improves diagnostic accuracy and allows the clinician to detect a pulmonary embolus or exclude the possibility with more assurance than was available previously.

Litin, S. C., and Gastineau, D. A. 1995. Current concepts in anticoagulant therapy. *Mayo Clinic Proceedings* 70:266–72.

- Discusses various anticoagulation strategies for treating venous thromboembolic disease and methods for monitoring anticoagulant therapy.

Miller, G. H., and Feied, C. F. 1995. Suspected pulmonary embolism. The difficulties of diagnostic evaluation. *Postgraduate Medicine* 97:51–8.

- Discusses the use of various diagnostic procedures in the diagnosis of pulmonary embolism.

OUTLINE SUMMARY

Intravascular Blood Clots

Thrombosis and Embolism

PATHOGENESIS

Slowing or stasis of blood flow.
Damage to wall of blood vessel.
Increased coagulability of blood.

TERMINOLOGY

Thrombosis: intravascular clot.
Embolus: detached clot carried in circulation.
Infarct: tissue necrosis caused by interruption of blood supply.

Venous Thrombosis

PREDISPOSING FACTORS

Stasis of blood in veins.
Varicose veins.
Increased blood coagulability.

Pulmonary Embolism

LARGE PULMONARY EMBOLI

Obstructs main pulmonary artery or major branches.
Obstructs blood flow to lungs.
Causes severe dyspnea and cyanosis.
May cause shock and sudden death.
Usually lung is not infarcted because adequate collateral blood flow is provided by bronchial arteries.

SMALL PULMONARY EMBOLI

Become impacted in peripheral branches of pulmonary artery.
Collateral circulation may be inadequate, and lung infarct develops.
Causes chest pain, cough, and bloody sputum secondary to infarct.

DIAGNOSIS

Chest x-ray: detects infarct, not embolus.
Lung scan: detects impaired lung perfusion secondary to embolus.
Pulmonary angiography: detects blocked pulmonary artery.

TREATMENT

Anticoagulants.

Operation on inferior vena cava to prevent passage of clots if anticoagulants ineffective.

SEPTIC PULMONARY EMBOLI

Thrombi form in pelvic veins after pelvic infection.

Bacteria invade thrombi.

Infected thrombus is transported to lungs and causes pulmonary infarct.

Bacteria in clot invade infarct, which becomes infected and forms lung abscess.

Arterial Thrombosis

PATHOGENESIS

Roughening of arterial wall caused by arteriosclerosis.

Thrombus forms on roughened surface.

CLINICAL MANIFESTATIONS DEPEND ON VESSEL AFFECTED

Heart attack.

Stroke.

Gangrene of extremity.

Intracardiac Thrombosis

LOCATION

Atrial appendage: in heart failure.

Heart valves: secondary to valve injury.

Left ventricle: secondary to infarct of heart muscle.

Thrombosis Caused by Increased Blood Coagulability

PREDISPOSING FACTORS

Postoperative increase in coagulation factors.

Estrogens in contraceptive pills.

Malignant tumors: induce hypercoagulable state.

Embolism as a Result of Foreign Material

SOURCES

Fat embolism: after fracture.

Amnionic fluid embolism during labor.

Air embolism: after chest injury.

Particulate material: associated with illicit drug use.

Edema

FACTORS REGULATING FLOW OF FLUID BETWEEN CAPILLARIES AND INTERSTITIAL TISSUE

Hydrostatic pressure.

Capillary permeability.

Osmotic pressure.

Open lymphatic channel.

PATHOGENESIS AND CLASSIFICATION

Increased capillary permeability.

Low plasma proteins:

Excess protein loss: kidney disease.

Inadequate synthesis: malnutrition.

Increased hydrostatic pressure:

Heart failure.

Localized venous obstruction.

Lymphatic obstruction.

Shock

BLOOD PRESSURE TOO LOW TO SUPPLY BODY

Classified by pathogenesis.

Hypovolemic shock: low blood volume.

Cardiogenic shock: impaired cardiac pumping function.

Septic shock: excessive vasodilation.

Anaphylactic shock: excessive vasodilation.

PROGNOSIS DEPENDS ON EARLY RECOGNITION AND RAPID APPROPRIATE TREATMENT

http://health.jbpub.com/humandisease/9e

Human Disease Online is a great source for supplementary human disease information for both students and instructors. Visit this website to find a variety of useful tools for learning, thinking, and teaching.

The Cardiovascular System

LEARNING OBJECTIVES

1. Explain the basic anatomy and physiology of the heart as they relate to the common types of heart disease.
2. Describe the common causes of congenital heart disease and valvular heart disease. Explain the effects of these diseases. Describe the methods of treating congenital and acquired valvular heart disease.
3. Describe the pathogenesis of coronary heart disease. List the four most important risk factors. Describe the clinical manifestations of coronary heart disease. Explain the methods of treatment and their rationales.
4. List the major complications of myocardial infarction and describe their clinical manifestations.
5. Explain the general principles applied to the diagnosis and treatment of coronary heart disease and myocardial infarction.
6. Explain the current concepts regarding the effect of diet on coronary heart disease. Describe how cholesterol is transported by lipoproteins. Distinguish between "good" and "bad" cholesterol.
7. Describe the adverse effects of hypertension on the cardiovascular system and the kidneys.
8. Differentiate between pathogenesis of acute and chronic heart failure. Describe the pathogenesis of each, and list the principles of treatment.
9. Differentiate between the pathogenesis and clinical manifestations of arteriosclerotic and dissecting aneurysms of the aorta. Explain the principles of treatment.
10. List the common diseases affecting veins, their clinical manifestations, and methods of treatment.

Cardiac Structure and Function

The heart is a muscular pump that propels blood through the lungs and to the peripheral tissues. Heart disease is caused by a disturbance in the function of the cardiac pump. A working knowledge of the normal structure and function of the heart is essential to an understanding of the various types of heart disease.

STRUCTURE OF THE HEART AND ITS CHAMBERS

The heart is a cone-shaped muscular pump that weighs about 350 g, enclosed within a fibrous sac called the pericardial sac located in the mediastinum. The pericardium is lined by a layer of mesothelial cells that is continuous with a similar layer of mesothelial cells covering the external surface of the heart.

The heart is composed of three layers: (1) the epicardium consisting of a layer of mesothelial cells overlying a small amount of loose fibrous and adipose tissue; (2) the myocardium, a thick layer of muscle that forms the bulk of the heart; and (3) the endocardium, a thin layer of endothelial cells that lines the chambers and covers the surfaces of the heart valves. The heart is divided into four chambers by partitions. The two upper chambers are separated by the interatrial septum into the right and left atria, which receive venous blood returning to the heart. The two lower chambers are separated by the interventricular septum into the right and left ventricles. The right ventricle pumps blood through the pulmonary artery to the lungs, where it is oxygenated and returned to the left atrium, and the left ventricle pumps oxygen-rich blood throughout the body, which is then collected into veins and returned to the right atrium. Although the right and left cardiac chambers work together, no direct communications normally exist between the chambers on the right and left sides of the heart, and it is convenient clinically to consider each half as an independent structure. The "right heart" circulates blood into the pulmonary artery and through the lungs (the pulmonary circulation), and the "left heart" pumps blood into the aorta for distribution to the various organs and tissues in the body (the systemic circulation) (FIGURE 1).

The atrial and ventricular muscle is arranged in bundles that encircle the heart and attach to a layer of dense fibrous tissue called the fibrous framework of the heart located between the atria and ventricles, which also extends into the upper part of the interventricular septum and surrounds the openings of the cardiac valves. The fibrous framework separates the atrial muscle fibers from those in the ventricles so that the atrial and ventricular muscles can function independently. Contraction of cardiac muscle reduces the size of the atria or ventricles, raising the pressure of the blood within the compressed chambers, which squeezes blood out of the chambers. The fibrous framework also provides a firm support to which the heart valves can attach, and contains a small opening to allow the atrioventricular bundle (bundle of His), which is part of the impulse conducting system, to carry impulses to the ventricles.

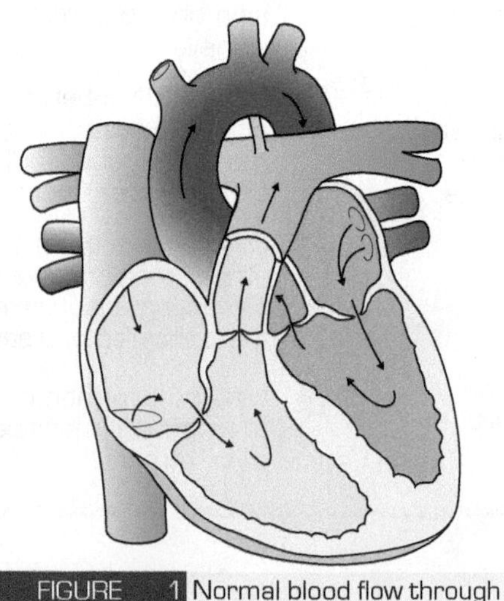

FIGURE 1 Normal blood flow through the right and left cardiac chambers: the pulmonary and systemic circulations.

CARDIAC VALVES

The flow of blood into and out of the cardiac chambers is controlled by a system of valves that normally permits flow in only one direction. The **atrioventricular** (**AV**) **valves** are flaplike valves surrounding the orifices between atria and ventricles. The free margins of the valves are connected to the papillary muscles of the ventricular walls by narrow, stringlike bands of fibrous tissue called the *chordae tendineae* (FIGURE 2A). These bands prevent the valves from prolapsing into the atria during ventricular systole. The **semilunar valves** surrounding the orifices of the aorta and pulmonary artery are positioned so that the free margins of the valves face upward. This structural arrangement defines cuplike pockets between the free margins of the valves and the roots of the blood vessels to which the valves are attached (FIGURE 2B).

Atrioventricular (AV) valve
(a′trē-o-ven-trik′ū-lar)
The flaplike heart valve located between the atrium and ventricle.

Semilunar valve
The cup-shaped valve located between the ventricles and the aorta or pulmonary artery.

A

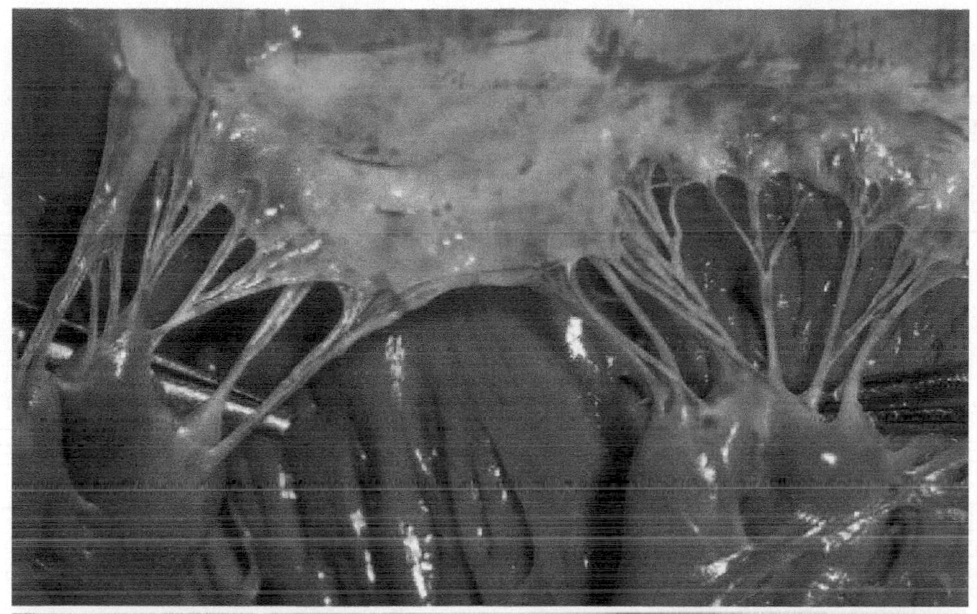

B

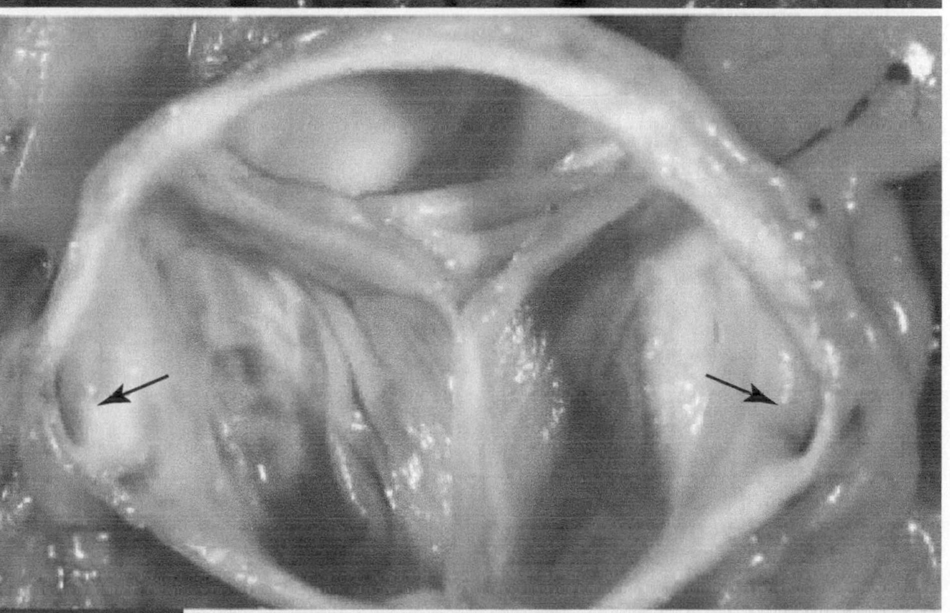

FIGURE 2 **A**, Normal mitral valve, illustrating thin chordae extending from valve leaflets to papillary muscles. **B**, Aortic valve viewed from above, illustrating a cup-shaped configuration of valve leaflets. Note the openings of coronary arteries (*arrows*) arising from base of aorta adjacent to aortic valve leaflets.

When the heart relaxes in diastole, the chordae produce tension on the valves and pull the atrioventricular valves apart. When the ventricles contract, the chordae are no longer under tension, and the force of the blood flow pushes the valves together so that no blood flows from the ventricles into the atria. During ventricular contraction, the semilunar valves are forced apart by the jets of blood leaving the ventricles. When ventricular contraction ceases, the weight of the column of ejected blood forces the valves back into position, preventing reflux of blood into the ventricles during diastole. The atrioventricular and semilunar valves function reciprocally. Ventricular contraction relaxes tension on the chordae, causing the atrioventricular valves to close at the same time that the jets of blood open the semilunar valves. Closure of the semilunar valves in diastole is also associated with opening of the atrioventricular valves. FIGURE 3 illustrates the reciprocal action of the two sets of valves, which is responsible for the unidirectional flow required for normal cardiac function.

BLOOD SUPPLY TO THE HEART

The Left and Right Coronary Arteries

The heart is supplied by two large coronary arteries that arise from the aortic sinuses at the root of the aorta (FIGURE 4). The left coronary artery is a short vessel that soon divides into two major branches. The left anterior descending artery descends

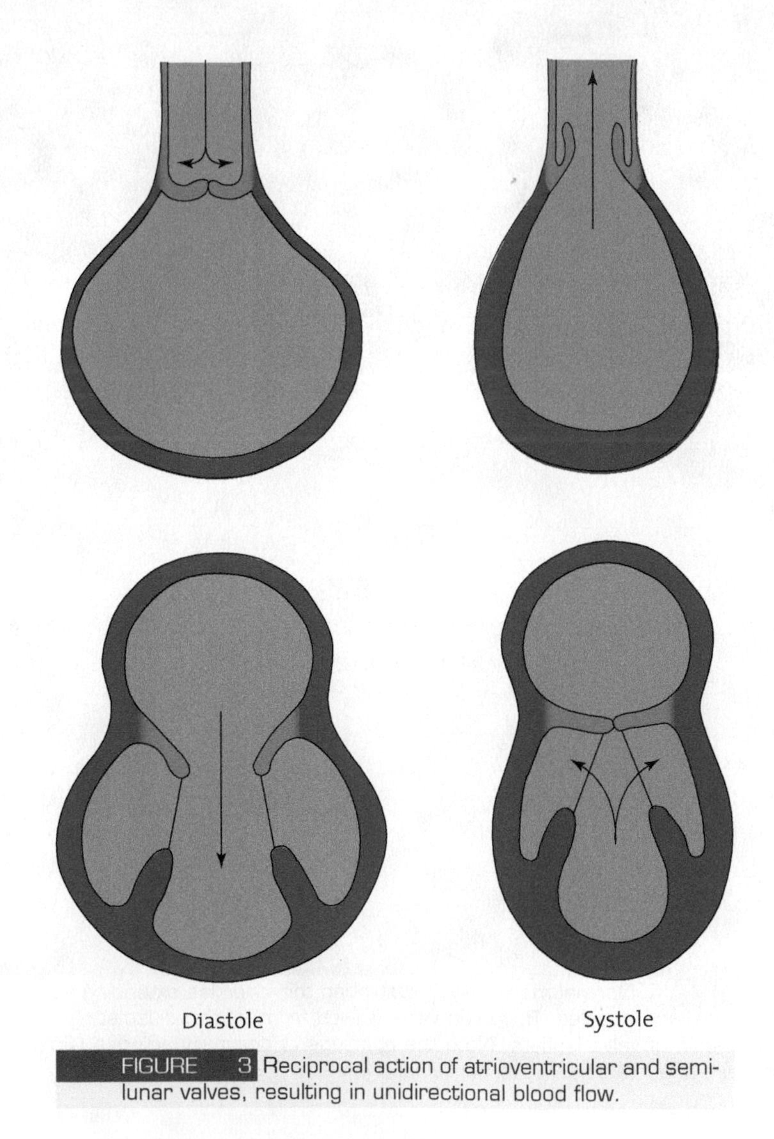

FIGURE 3 Reciprocal action of atrioventricular and semilunar valves, resulting in unidirectional blood flow.

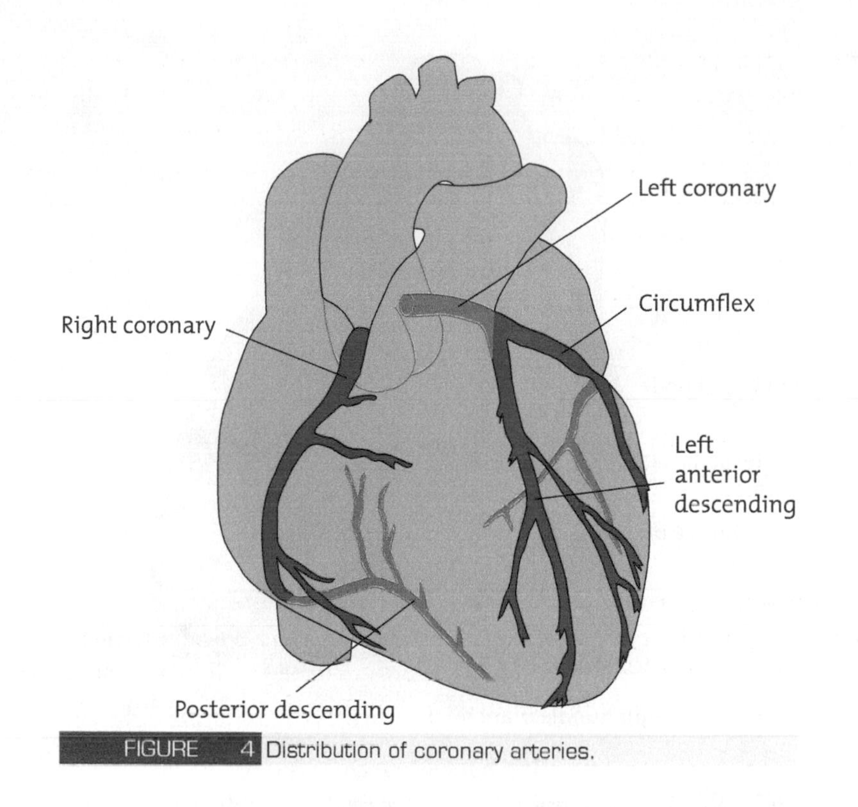

FIGURE 4 Distribution of coronary arteries.

to supply the front of the heart and the anterior part of the interventricular septum. The circumflex artery swings to the left (*circum* = around + *flex* = bend) to supply the left side of the heart. The right coronary artery swings to the right, supplying the right side of the heart, and then descends to supply the back of the heart and the posterior part of the interventricular septum. Each coronary artery gives off many branches that supply the heart muscle. The terminal branches of the coronary arteries frequently communicate with each other by means of connections called **anastomoses.** Because of these connections, obstruction of one of the arteries does not necessarily completely interrupt the blood flow to the tissues supplied by the blocked vessel. There may be enough blood flow through anastomoses with other arteries to supply the heart muscle. This is called a **collateral circulation.**

Anastomosis
(ä-nas-ta-mō′sis)
A communication between two blood vessels or other tubular structures. Also refers to a surgical connection of two hollow tubular structures, such as the divided ends of the intestine or a blood vessel (surgical anastomosis).

Collateral circulation
An accessory circulation capable of delivering blood to a tissue when the main circulation is blocked, as by a thrombus or embolus.

CONDUCTION SYSTEM OF THE HEART

The impulses that cause the heart to beat are initiated and propagated by groups of specialized muscle cells that depolarize spontaneously, which is called the conduction system of the heart (FIGURE 5). Impulses normally are generated in the sinoatrial (SA) node, which is located in the right atrium near the opening of the superior vena cava. Small bundles of fibers called internodal tracts connect the SA node to the atrioventricular (AV) node, which is located posteriorly in the lower part of the atrial septum. The atrioventricular bundle (bundle of His) is the continuation of the AV node, which transmits the impulse to the ventricles by passing through a small opening in the fibrous framework of the heart, the fibrous tissue that separates the atrial muscle from the ventricular muscle. After entering the ventricles, the AV bundle divides into right and left bundle branches in the upper part of the interventricular septum, then descends in the septum and extends into the ventricles, where they terminate as Purkinje fibers that activate the heart muscle. The depolarization rate is also influenced by the autonomic nervous system. Sympathetic nervous system impulses increase the rate, and parasympathetic impulses slow it. The normal rhythm established by the cardiac conduction system is often called a normal sinus rhythm

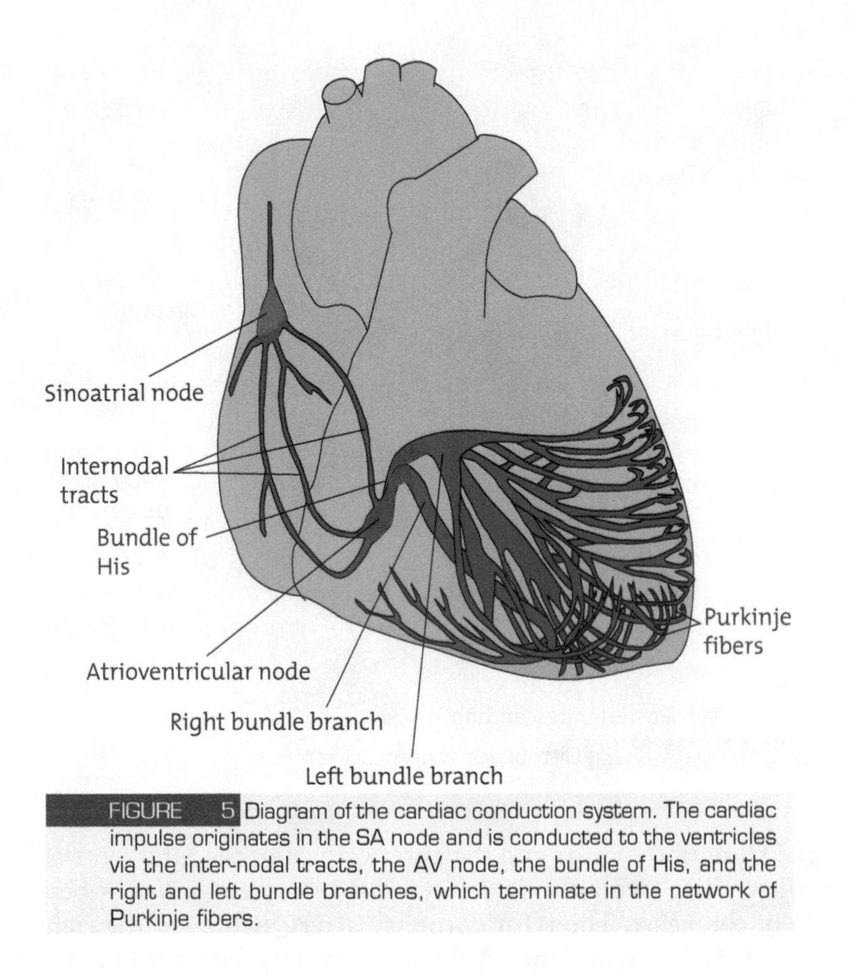

FIGURE 5 Diagram of the cardiac conduction system. The cardiac impulse originates in the SA node and is conducted to the ventricles via the inter-nodal tracts, the AV node, the bundle of His, and the right and left bundle branches, which terminate in the network of Purkinje fibers.

to emphasize that the normal cardiac rhythm is controlled by the sinoatrial node (which is often called simply the sinus node).

Although any part of the conduction system can depolarize spontaneously and generate an impulse, the SA node normally functions as the cardiac pacemaker because it depolarizes about 60 to 70 times per minute, which in turn depolarizes the other parts of the conduction system that depolarize at a slower rate. However, if impulse transmission from the SA node is interrupted by damage to the conduction system, the AV node, which discharges at about 50 times per minute, can take over, and if this system fails, then the bundle or bundle branches can initiate impulses but at a still slower rate of about 30 to 40 times per minute.

THE CARDIAC CYCLE

The sequence of events that occurs during a single contraction and relaxation of the cardiac chambers is called a cardiac cycle. During diastole, both the atria and ventricles are relaxed, the chambers are dilated, and the pressure of the blood within the chambers is very low. In a normal person at rest, each ventricle in diastole contains about 120 ml of blood, and much of the blood that fills the ventricles flows passively into the ventricles through the open atrioventricular valves. Atrial systole expels an additional 30 ml of blood into the ventricles. If the heart rate is normal, the additional blood pumped into the ventricles by atrial contractions is not essential for reasonably normal cardiac function because most of the blood flows into the ventricles during diastole. Atrial systole delivers a relatively small additional amount. However, the additional blood pumped into the ventricles during atrial systole becomes progressively more important as the heart rate increases, which shortens the length of diastole and reduces the volume of blood flowing passively into the ventricles. Atrial systole makes a much greater contribution to ventricular filling when the heart beats rapidly.

The ventricles contract following completion of atrial systole, ejecting blood into the aorta at high pressure and into the pulmonary artery at much lower pressure. Both ventricles contract at the same time, and each ventricle ejects the same volume of blood. Only about 70 ml is ejected from each ventricle during a systolic contraction, which is called the stroke volume, and is about 60% of the blood contained within the ventricles. The percentage of the ventricular volume ejected during systole is called the ejection fraction, and this measurement is often used when evaluating patients with heart failure.

Cardiac output is the output of blood from a single ventricle in 1 minute, and is the product of the stroke volume (about 70 ml) multiplied by the heart rate (about 72 beats per minute), which equals about 5,000 ml per minute. This is approximately the total blood volume of the average adult. During vigorous activity, the normal heart of a healthy young person can double its stroke volume and greatly increase its heart rate, which can increase cardiac output from 4 to 7 times over resting cardiac output.

BLOOD VESSELS

The heart pumps blood into a system of conduction, distribution, and collection tubes that differ in both their structure and function. It is convenient to consider them as four separate groups:

1. Large elastic arteries conduct the blood to various locations throughout the body. They distend as blood is ejected from the heart during systole and recoil during diastole to maintain flow between contractions.
2. Arterioles are smaller vessels with muscular walls that function like a nozzle on a garden hose to regulate flow from the large arteries into the capillaries. They lower the pressure and dampen the amplitude of the pulsations.
3. Capillaries are thin endothelium-lined channels that deliver nutrients to cells and remove waste products.
4. Veins return blood to the heart under low pressure and usually travel with the arteries.

A separate system of channels carrying fluid called lymph is part of the lymphatic system. Its functions and relation to the circulatory system are considered in the discussion on circulatory disturbances.

BLOOD PRESSURE

The flow of blood in the arteries is a result of the force of ventricular contraction. The pressure within the arteries varies rhythmically with the beating of the heart. The highest pressure is reached during ventricular contraction as blood is ejected into the aorta and its branches (systolic pressure). The pressure is lowest when the ventricles are relaxed (diastolic pressure), and the recoil of the stretched arteries provides the force to propel the blood between contractions. The peripheral arterioles regulate the rate of blood flow into the capillaries by varying the degree of arteriolar constriction. In many respects, the effect is analogous to the resistance to outflow of water from a garden hose, which can be varied by tightening or loosening the nozzle on the hose. Because of the resistance offered by the arterioles, the blood pressure during cardiac diastole does not fall to zero but declines slowly as blood leaves the large arteries through the arterioles into the capillaries.

The elasticity of the large arteries also influences the systolic pressure. Some of the pressure rise caused by the blood ejected from the ventricle is absorbed by the stretch of the arteries so that the systolic pressure does not rise as high as would occur if the arteries were more rigid and unable to stretch normally. In summary, the systolic blood pressure is a measure of the force of ventricular contraction as blood is ejected into the large arteries. The diastolic pressure is a measure of the rate of "run off" of blood into the capillaries, which is governed by the peripheral resistance caused by the small arterioles throughout the body. The mean (average) pressure of blood in the large arteries is approximately midway between systolic and diastolic pressure.

The Electrocardiogram

The electrocardiogram (ECG) is a measure of the electrical activity of the heart as measured on the surface of the body by means of electrodes attached to the legs, arms, and chest. Voltage differences are recorded as a series of upward (positive) and downward (negative) deflections that form a characteristic pattern of deflections named in order: P, Q, R, S, and T (FIGURE 6). The P wave reflects the initial wave of depolarization associated with atrial systole. The Q, R, and S waves, called collectively as the QRS complex, reflect the depolarization of the ventricles, which is followed by ventricular systole. The T wave represents repolarization of the ventricles during diastole. The time interval from the beginning of the P wave to the beginning of the QRS complex, which is called the PR interval, reflects the time required for the depolarization wave to pass through the AV bundle from the atria to the ventricles.

Usually, the positive and negative deflections are recorded on calibrated graph paper, each horizontal line representing a standard voltage difference and each vertical line representing a standard time interval. However, the ECG tracing also can be displayed on a fluorescent screen, as when continuously monitoring a patient in a coronary care unit.

The ECG is a valuable diagnostic aid that can identify characteristic disturbances in the heart rate or rhythm and abnormalities in the conduction of impulses through the heart. The ECG can also identify heart muscle injury, as occurs following a heart attack, and can also determine the extent of the damage to the heart muscle.

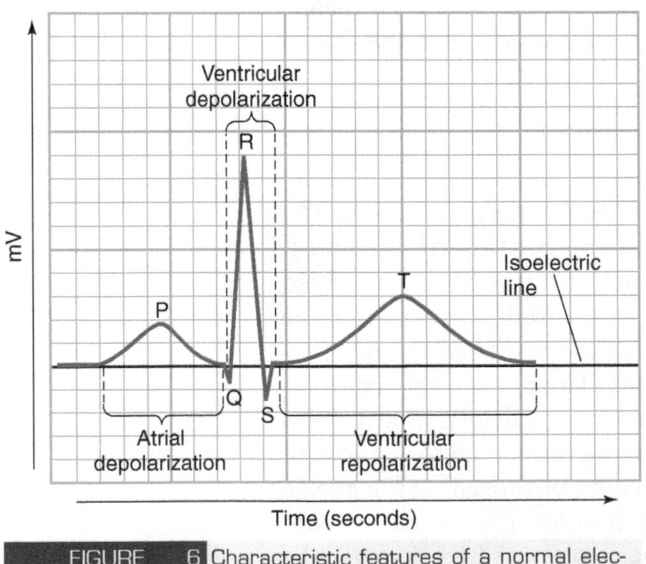

FIGURE 6 Characteristic features of a normal electrocardiogram.

CARDIAC ARRHYTHMIAS

The orderly depolarization and repolarization of the conduction system that directs the contraction and relaxation of the atria and ventricles do not always function perfectly, which leads to disturbances in the heart rate or rhythm, called cardiac arrhythmias.

Atrial Fibrillation

One of the more common abnormal cardiac rhythms is a condition called atrial fibrillation (AF), in which the atria fail to contract normally. The condition often occurs in older persons, especially those with cardiovascular disease or chronic pulmonary disease, but may also occur in persons whose thyroid glands produce an excess of thyroid hormone (hyperthyroidism) and in a few other conditions. Occasionally, AF occurs in apparently normal healthy persons for no apparent reason.

AF starts as an abnormal focus of electrical activity in the atrium, which abruptly evolves into multiple areas of depolarization throughout the atria that stimulate atrial muscle fibers continuously in a haphazard disorganized manner at a very rapid rate of up to 400 impulses per minute. The intense disorderly stimulation of multiple groups of atrial muscle fibers causes the atrial muscle to quiver ineffectively instead of contracting normally. The abnormal electrical impulses are also relayed to the AV node, which is overwhelmed and unable to respond to such a large number of stimuli. Only a relatively small number of impulses are able to travel through the AV node and AV bundle (bundle of His) to reach the ventricles, which beat irregularly at about 140 to 160 times per minute (FIGURE 7A). At such a fast ventricular contraction rate, the duration of diastole is very short. The duration of diastole also varies from beat to beat because the rate at which impulses can be delivered to the ventricles from the quivering atria is not uniform. As a result, the time available for ventricular filling in diastole also varies from beat to beat, which causes the volume of blood filling the ventricles and ejected during each ventricular contraction (stroke volume) to vary. Some of the ventricular contractions occur before the ventricles are adequately filled with blood, and the volume of blood ejected may not always be enough to be detected as a pulse in the radial artery at the wrist. Consequently, the radial pulse detects fewer beats per minute than the number of ventricular contractions per minute heard with a stethoscope placed on the chest. This discrepancy is called a pulse deficit. The diagnosis of atrial fibrillation is made by examination of the ECG, which reveals a lack of P waves and indicates that the atria are not contracting normally, associated with some variability in the QRS complexes related to the variable ventricular stroke volumes, as manifested by the pulse deficit (Figure 7A).

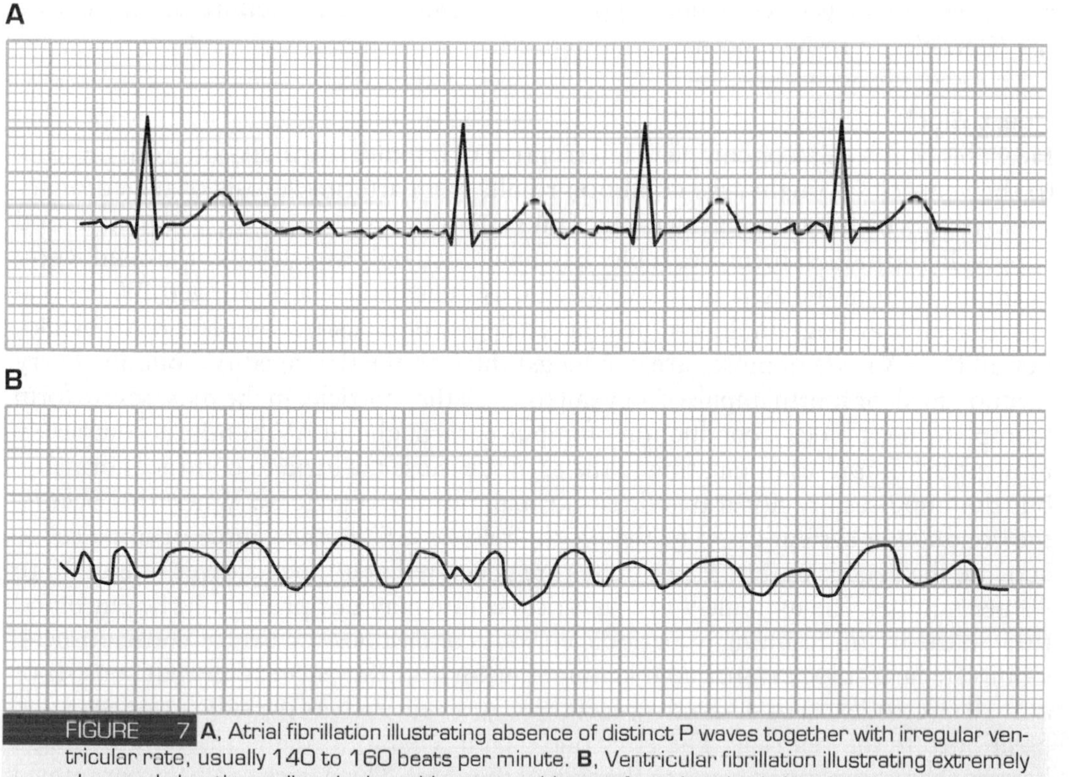

FIGURE 7 **A**, Atrial fibrillation illustrating absence of distinct P waves together with irregular ventricular rate, usually 140 to 160 beats per minute. **B**, Ventricular fibrillation illustrating extremely abnormal chaotic cardiac rhythm without any evidence of synchronized electrical impulses. (From Garcia, T. B., and Holtz, N. E. 2003. Introduction to 12-Lead ECG. Boston: Jones and Bartlett Publishers.)

Treatment of Atrial Fibrillation

The rapid irregular heart rate shortens the time available for ventricular filling in diastole, and the lack of normal atrial contractions further compromises ventricular filling. The cardiac output falls, which may not be well tolerated by a person with pre-existing cardiovascular disease.

The first treatment step is to improve the cardiac output by slowing the heart rate, which provides more time for passive ventricular filling during diastole. This can be accomplished by giving a medication that impedes the transmission of impulses through the AV node and bundle so that fewer impulses reach the ventricles. A digitalis preparation can be used (digoxin), but other pharmacologic agents are also effective.

When the heart rate has been slowed, the next step is to restore a normal heart rhythm by terminating the fibrillation. This can be accomplished either by an electrical cardioversion, which involves the application of an electrical shock by paddles applied to the patient's chest to terminate the arrhythmia, or by pharmacologic therapy, which uses drugs that terminate the arrhythmia by interfering with some phase in the abnormal impulse formation to "break up" the arrhythmia. Once the normal rhythm is restored, the patient may need to continue taking some medication to maintain the normal rhythm.

Further details on the management of atrial fibrillation and its complications along with two case studies illustrating both acute atrial fibrillation and chronic atrial fibrillation are available at the web site that accompanies this text at http://health.jbpub.com/humandisease/9e.

Ventricular Fibrillation

In contrast to atrial fibrillation, ventricular fibrillation is incompatible with life because the ventricles are unable to contract normally and the circulation ceases (FIGURE 7B). Ventricular fibrillation sometimes occurs following a heart attack. If recognized promptly, it is often possible to stop the fibrillation by delivering an electric shock to the heart by means of electrodes applied to the chest. The procedure usually causes the ventricles to resume normal contractions.

Heart Block

Heart block is a delay or complete interruption of impulse transmission from the atria to the ventricles. Usually, the condition results from arteriosclerosis of the coronary arteries in which parts of the conduction system fail to receive an adequate blood supply. In the mildest form, heart block is manifested only as a delay in the conduction of impulses from the atria to the ventricles, as indicated by a prolonged PR interval in the electrocardiogram. In a more marked degree of block (incomplete heart block), not all the SA node impulses are conducted through the damaged AV bundle. Every second, third, or fourth impulses may fail to reach the ventricle. In the most severe form (complete heart block), conduction of impulses through the AV bundle is completely interrupted. Impulses originating in the SA node cause the atria to contract normally, but the impulses are not transmitted normally to the ventricles. When this occurs, the conduction system distal to the block "takes over" as the source of impulses to activate the ventricles, but the impulses are generated at a much slower rate of 30 to 40 per minute. The extremely low ventricular rate may not provide sufficient blood flow to the brain, resulting in periodic episodes of dizziness or loss of consciousness. Complete heart block is treated by implanting an artificial pacemaker that consists of a small electrode inserted into the heart through a vein such as the subclavian vein and positioned in the ventricle. The electrode is connected to a small device containing a battery that is implanted beneath the skin of the chest. The device can be programmed to generate impulses that stimulate ventricular contractions at a predetermined rate. Many different types of pacemakers are available, each having specific applications.

Heart Disease as a Disturbance of Pump Function

For a pump to function properly, several conditions are required:

1. The pump must be properly constructed so that it is free of mechanical defects.
2. The pump must have a system of valves that is properly synchronized to allow unidirectional flow. If valves do not function properly, the force of the pump stroke is dissipated, and effective pumping is impaired.
3. The pump must have an adequate fuel supply. It will not run properly if the fuel line is dirty or plugged.
4. The pump must be used within its rated capacity. One must not use a pump rated at 3 horsepower to perform a job requiring a 10-horsepower pump. Either the pump will not function at all, or it will wear out very rapidly.
5. The pump motor must function smoothly and efficiently. If the motor functions erratically, the efficiency of the pump is reduced greatly.

The heart is a muscular pump that is subject to the same requirements as any mechanical pump. Each type of heart disease can be roughly compared with one of the derangements that would impair the function of a mechanical pump (TABLE 1).

Congenital heart disease corresponds to faulty pump construction. The term valvular heart disease indicates that heart valves have been damaged by rheumatic fever or other diseases, and so they fail to open and close properly. It is comparable to a malfunction in the unidirectional valve system of a mechanical pump. Coronary heart disease is a result of deposits of fatty material in the arterial walls that narrow their lumens and eventually may completely block the flow of blood through the arteries. This type of heart disease corresponds to failure of a mechanical pump caused by a dirty or plugged fuel line. Hypertensive heart disease results when the heart is forced to pump blood at high pressure against an excessively high resistance in the peripheral arterioles and corresponds to overloading a mechanical pump. Primary myocardial disease corresponds to malfunction of the pump motor.

THE ROLE OF ECHOCARDIOGRAPHY IN DIAGNOSIS OF CARDIOVASCULAR DISEASE

Ultrasound examinations described in the discussion on general concepts of disease: principles of diagnosis have many applications in medicine. An ultrasound examination of the cardiovascular system is usually called an **echocardiogram**. The procedure can identify valve and chamber abnormalities, and the dimensions of a narrowed valve orifice can be calculated from the rate of flow through the valve.

Echocardiogram
(eko′-kar-dē-o-gram′)
A record obtained from an ultrasound examination of the heart and related blood vessels; used to assist in the diagnosis of cardiovascular disease.

TABLE 1

Heart disease compared with mechanical pump dysfunctions

Mechanical abnormality	Comparable heart disease
Faulty pump construction	Congenital heart disease
Faulty unidirectional valves	Valvular heart disease
Dirty or plugged fuel line	Coronary heart disease
Overloaded pump	Hypertensive heart disease
Malfunctioning pump	Primary myocardial disease

Abnormal blood flow patterns between chambers can be detected. On the other hand, if a cardiac valve abnormality is suspected because a faint heart murmur was heard during a routine physical examination and the echocardiogram is normal, the subject can be reassured that there are no cardiovascular problems. Some faint murmurs result from turbulent blood flow within a normal heart, which are called functional murmurs. The subject need not restrict his or her activities based on the information obtained from the echocardiogram. A normal echocardiogram can exclude a valve abnormality, an abnormal communication between adjacent atria or between adjacent ventricles, or an abnormal communication between the major blood vessels leaving the heart.

Congenital Heart Disease

CARDIAC DEVELOPMENT AND PRENATAL BLOOD FLOW

The heart undergoes a complex developmental sequence. It is formed from a tube that undergoes segmental dilatations and constrictions along with considerable growth and change in configuration. Eventually the individual chambers, valves, and large arteries develop, culminating in the final structural characteristics of a normal fully developed heart.

As the heart is developing, the blood flow through the fetal heart differs from its final postdelivery flow pattern. Much of the blood flow in the pulmonary artery is diverted away from the lungs, which are nonfunctional in the fetus, and used instead to supply other fetal tissues. One bypass called the **ductus arteriosus** is a large communication connecting the pulmonary artery with the aorta that shunts much of the blood pumped into the pulmonary artery directly into the aorta. As soon as the infant is born and begins to breathe air, the lungs expand and the ductus arteriosus constricts, which blocks blood flow through the ductus arteriosus. Consequently, pulmonary artery blood can flow only into the newly-expanded lungs, and the non-functional ductus eventually becomes converted into a fibrous cord called the ligamentum arteriosum. The other bypass is an opening in the atrial septum called the **foramen ovale**, which maintains blood flow between the two atria as the atrial septum is developing. Blood flow across the foramen ovale is controlled by a flap of atrial tissue on the left atrial side of the septum that covers (overlaps) the opening in the foramen ovale. In this position, the flap functions as a one-way valve that allows blood to flow from the right atrium into the left atrium but does not allow flow in the opposite direction (FIGURE 8). The right-to-left flow is determined by pressure differences between the two chambers. In the fetus, the blood pressure is higher in the right atrium than in the left atrium because only a relatively small volume of blood flows through the lungs and is returned to the left atrium. Most is directed into the aorta through the ductus arteriosus. After birth, the left atrial pressure rises when the lungs expand and a large volume of blood flows through the lungs and into the left atrium. The higher left atrial pressure presses the flap valve against the left atrial surface of the septum, closing the communication between the atria. Usually, the tissue flap fuses with the atrial septum to form a solid partition between the two atria. Often, the fusion is incomplete but no flow of blood from right to left atria is possible as long as the left atrial pressure exceeds the pressure in the right atrium, which holds the flap against the atrial septum.

A diagram and additional details on the prenatal fetal circulation and the postnatal circulatory adjustments are available at the web site that accompanies this text at http://health.jbpub.com/humandisease/9e.

Ductus arteriosus
A fetal artery connecting the pulmonary artery with the aorta that permits pressure determined blood flow from pulmonary artery into the aorta, bypassing blood flow to the nonfunctional fetal lungs.

Foramen ovale
An opening in the atrial septum covered by a one-way flap valve regulated by pressure differences between the atria, permitting blood flow from right to left atrium but not in the opposite direction, thereby bypassing blood flow from right cardiac chambers to the nonfunctional fetal lungs.

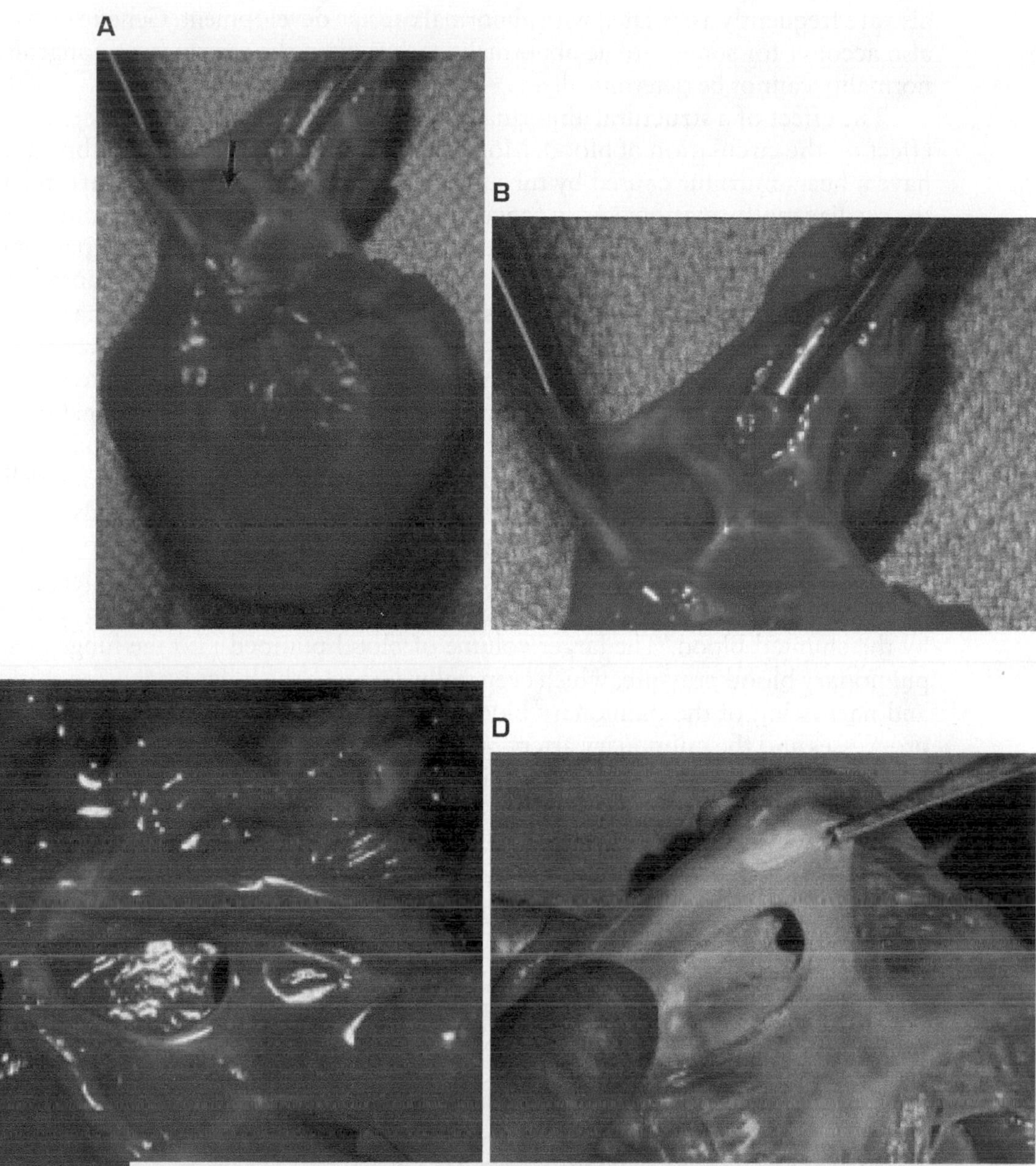

FIGURE 8 Structure and function of the foramen ovale. **A**, Overview of fetal heart with the right atrium opened to show the atrial septum. The foramen ovale appears as a depression in the right atrial surface of the septum (*arrow*). **B**, Closer view of foramen ovale, illustrating flap of atrial septum tissue forming the base of the foramen, which would be displaced toward the left atrium by the higher pressure of blood in the right atrium, allowing blood to flow into the left atrium. **C**, View of septal surface of the fetal right atrium stretched to reveal the free margin of the flap of septal tissue, which would be displaced by the higher right atrial pressure in the fetus, allowing blood to flow into the left atrium. **D**, Similar view of stretched right atrium from adult heart with patent foramen ovale to illustrate how a high right atrial pressure allows blood to flow from right to left atrium but normally would prevent left-to-right blood flow when the flap is in its normal position.

PATHOGENESIS AND MANIFESTATIONS OF CONGENITAL HEART DISEASE

Sometimes the heart fails to develop normally. Partitions between cardiac chambers may be defective. The cardiac valves may be malformed, or the large vessels entering and leaving the heart may not communicate normally with the appropriate atrium or ventricle. Some viral infections, such as German measles or other maternal illnesses during the early phases of fetal development, may cause improper development of the heart as well as other organs. Some drugs or medications taken by the mother may disrupt normal fetal development. Some chromosomal abnormalities, such as Down syndrome, also are frequently associated with abnormal cardiac development. Genetic factors may also account for some cardiac abnormalities, but often the reason for a congenital abnormality cannot be determined.

The effect of a structural abnormality depends on the nature of the defect and its effect on the circulation of blood. Most persons with congenital heart abnormalities have a heart murmur caused by turbulent flow of blood within the heart, related to the cardiac malformation. Many congenital heart abnormalities result from abnormal communications between the systemic and pulmonary circulations that permit blood to be shunted between the adjacent chambers. The amount of blood shunted and the direction of the shunt depend on the size of the opening between the chambers, and the blood pressure difference between the chambers determines the direction of flow.

Most shunts are left-to-right shunts from left cardiac chambers (systemic circulation) into right cardiac chambers (pulmonary circulation). A left-to-right shunt mixes oxygenated blood from the left cardiac chambers with deoxygenated blood in the right chambers, but the admixture does not affect the oxygen content of the blood delivered to the tissues by the left ventricle. The amount of blood shunted depends on the size of the septal defect. A small defect shunts very little blood and has no significant effect on cardiovascular function. However, a large septal defect can shunt a large volume of blood, which puts an additional burden on the right ventricle, which is overfilled by the shunted blood. The larger volume of blood pumped into the lungs raises the pulmonary blood pressure, which eventually damages the lungs by causing thickening and narrowing of the pulmonary blood vessels. As the pulmonary vascular damage progresses and the pulmonary artery pressure continues to rises, the right ventricle has to work even harder to overcome the increasing resistance to blood flow through the lungs. The higher right ventricular pressure also causes the right atrial pressure to rise, reducing the pressure differences between the left and right atria. Consequently, the amount of blood shunted from the left to the right atrium also falls. Little or no blood shunting occurs when left and right atrial pressures equalize, and if right atrial pressure exceeds left atrial pressure, blood shunts between the atria in the opposite direction.

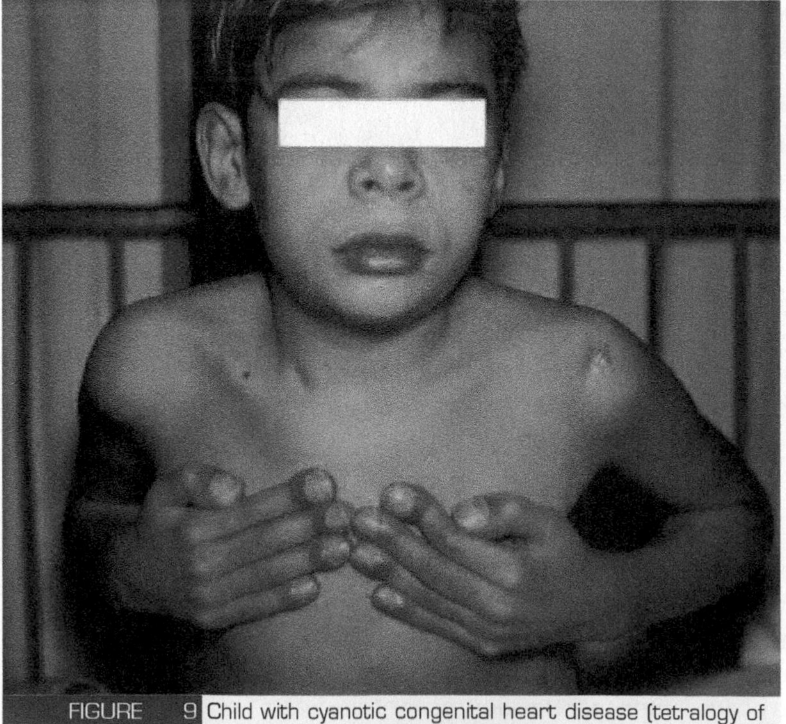

FIGURE 9 Child with cyanotic congenital heart disease (tetralogy of Fallot) illustrating cyanosis of skin and prominent clubbing of fingers caused by deoxygenated blood mixing with oxygenated blood (right-to-left shunt).

In contrast, right-to-left shunts mix poorly oxygenated blood from the right cardiac chambers with normally oxygenated blood contained in the left cardiac chambers, which reduces the oxygen content of the blood pumped by the left ventricle to supply the body. The affected person's activities usually are severely restricted because of the low oxygen content of the arterial blood. The skin and mucous membranes acquire a blue color called cyanosis, which is caused by the low oxygen saturation of arterial blood, and congenital cardiovascular abnormalities associated with cyanosis are grouped together under the general term cyanotic congenital heart disease. Usually the finger tips and toes become swollen (called clubbing). The condition results from overgrowth of connective tissue and blood vessels at the tips of the fingers and toes caused by the low oxygen content of the arterial blood (FIGURE 9). The poorly oxygenated blood also stimulates the bone marrow to increase red cell production (called polycythemia) in an attempt to increase oxygen delivery to the tissues, which unfortunately has some disadvantages. The heart has to work harder to pump the more viscous blood, and the increased blood viscosity also predisposes to formation of blood clots within the circulation.

COMMON CARDIOVASCULAR ABNORMALITIES

The more common and important cardiovascular abnormalities fall into four major groups:

1. Failure of the normal fetal bypass channels to close.
2. Atrial and ventricular septal defects.
3. Abnormalities that obstruct blood flow through the heart, pulmonary artery, or aorta.
4. Abnormal formation of the aorta and pulmonary artery, or abnormal connection of the arteries to the appropriate ventricles.

Patent Ductus Arteriosus

Normally the ductus closes spontaneously soon after birth in full-term infants. A large patent ductus shunts blood from the aorta into the pulmonary artery and causes the same clinical manifestations and complications as an intracardiac left-to-right shunt, and is treated by surgical closure of the ductus.

Patent Foramen Ovale

The foramen ovale normally becomes nonfunctional after birth, caused by the rapid postdelivery changes in atrial pressures. The left atrial pressure rises when pulmonary blood flow increases after the ductus arteriosus closes. The higher left atrial pressure pushes the flap valve of the foramen ovale against the atrial septum, where it usually fuses with the septum.

In newborn infants, the foramen ovale may remain patent and functional if the infant has a congenital cardiac abnormality that is associated with a high right atrial pressure, which forces right-to-left blood flow through the foramen ovale.

In about 25% of adults the flap valve does not fuse completely, but the foramen ovale remains nonfunctional as long as the left atrial pressure remains higher than the right atrial pressure. Some uncommon late neurologic problems have been identified that may be related to a patent foramen ovale, which will be considered in the discussion on the nervous system.

Atrial and Ventricular Septal Defects

Usually, an atrial septal defect results from defective development of the partitions that divide the atria, and the defect is located in the middle of the septum at the site usually occupied by the foramen ovale. Small defects in children often close spontaneously. Larger defects should be closed, which usually can be accomplished using a device inserted into the heart through a peripheral vein. Sometimes an open surgical procedure is required to place a patch over the defect. Ventricular septal defects are also very common (FIGURE 10).

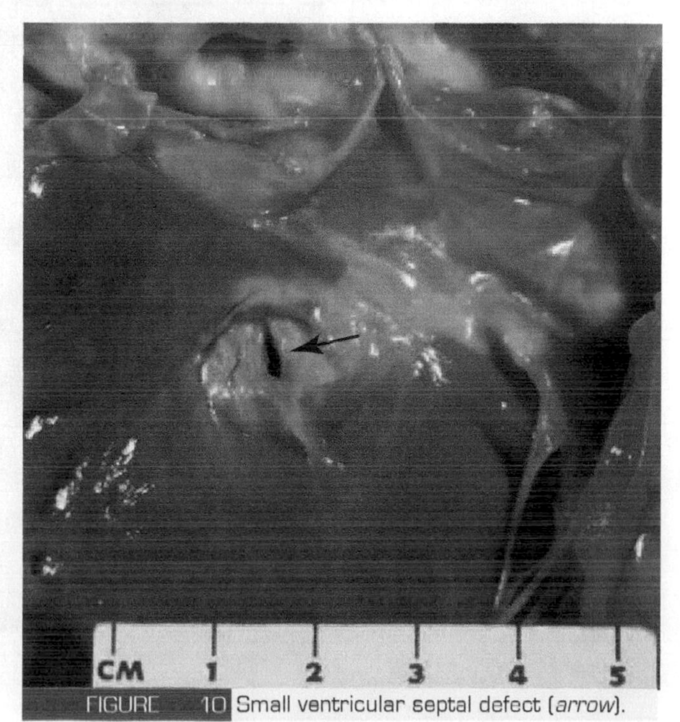

FIGURE 10 Small ventricular septal defect (*arrow*).

Many are less than 3 mm in diameter and often close spontaneously, but larger defects require surgical closure.

Generally, all large septal defects need to be closed because of the harmful effects of a large open left-to-right shunt on the heart and pulmonary blood vessels, as described previously.

Pulmonary or Aortic Valve Stenosis Caused by Semilunar Valve Maldevelopment

Abnormal development of the semilunar valve leaflets narrows the valve opening, which can vary from 2 to 10 ml diameter, and the degree of obstruction depends on the diameter of the orifice (FIGURE 11). Pulmonary stenosis obstructs outflow from the right ventricle, and aortic stenosis impedes outflow from the left ventricle. Treatment consists of dilating the valve opening by inserting a balloon-like device into the narrow valve opening.

Coarctation of the Aorta

Coarctation is a Latin word meaning narrowing, and the term describes a localized narrowing of the proximal aorta that restricts blood flow into the distal aorta. Usually, the constriction is located distal to the origin of the large arteries arising from the arch of the aorta. The blood pressure in the aorta and its branches proximal to the coarctation is much higher than normal because the heart has to pump blood at a much higher pressure in order to deliver blood through the narrowed segment of aorta, but the higher pressure is not adequate to deliver a normal volume of blood through the constriction. The pressure and volume of blood flowing into the aorta distal to the coarctation are both lower than normal, and a collateral circulation develops to bypass the obstruction. Branches of the subclavian arteries proximal to the coarctation communicate with chest arteries distal to the coarctation (intercostal arteries) to deliver blood into the aorta distal to the obstruction. A subject with a coarctation may appear normal except for high blood pressure identified when measuring pressure in the brachial arteries, but lower-than-normal blood pressure in the arteries of the lower extremities. Often, a coarctation is first identified during a

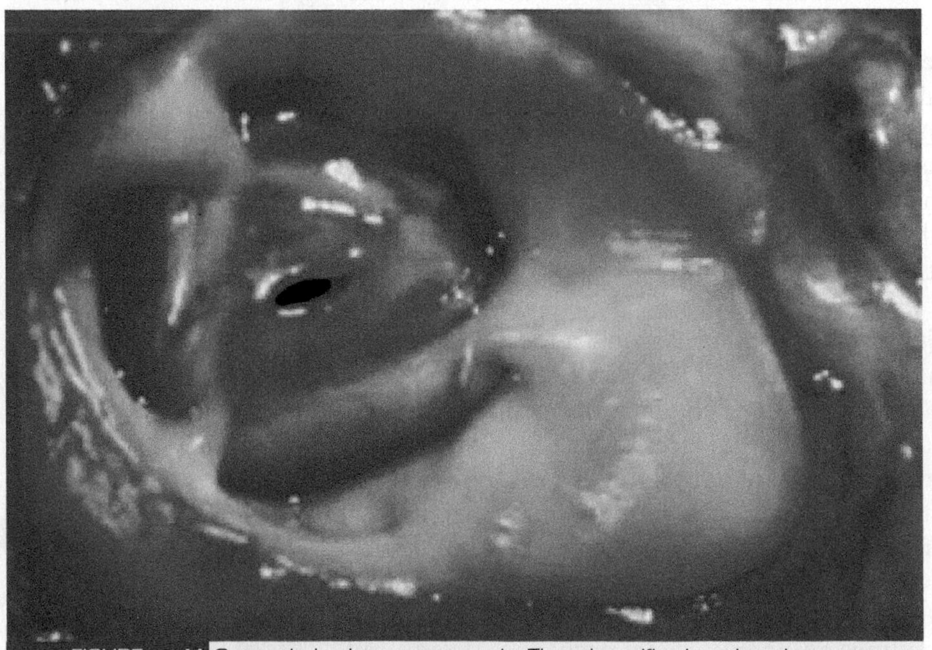

FIGURE 11 Congenital pulmonary stenosis. The valve orifice is reduced to a narrow slit, obstructing outflow from the right ventricle.

medical examination for an unrelated condition in which an unexpected hypertension is detected. Usually, the narrowed segment of aorta is relatively short and can be treated by resecting the constricting segment and reconnecting the aorta so that its caliber is normal throughout its entire length.

The Tetralogy of Fallot and Transposition of the Great Arteries

Both of these conditions result from abnormal division of a single channel called the truncus arteriosus, which extends from the developing ventricles and will be divided by a partition to form the aorta and the pulmonary artery. The partition, called the aorticopulmonary septum, takes a spiral course as it divides the truncus arteriosus, which is why the aorta and the pulmonary artery spiral around each other as they attach to their respective ventricles. The two abnormalities caused by abnormal division of the truncus arteriosus are relatively common, and both cause intermixing of deoxygenated blood with oxygenated blood, which leads to marked cyanosis and related problems, as described in the subject illustrated in Figure 9.

The tetralogy of Fallot results if the aorticopulmonary septum divides the truncus unequally. As a result, the pulmonary artery is smaller than it should be and the aorta is too large; the upper part of the ventricular septum, which is formed in part from the aorticopulmonary septum, does not connect properly to the aorta and the pulmonary artery that extend from the ventricles. The failed connection results in a large ventricular septal defect that is straddled by the enlarged aorta and receives blood ejected from both ventricles. The four abnormalities composing the tetralogy are (1) a ventricular septal defect, (2) pulmonary stenosis, (3) an enlarged aorta that overrides the septal defect, and (4) right ventricular hypertrophy that develops as a consequence of the pulmonary stenosis. In this condition, poorly oxygenated blood in the right ventricle flows through the septal defect to mix with blood from the left ventricle flowing into the aorta, which overrides the septal defect. Treatment consists of enlarging the opening of the narrowed pulmonary artery and closing the septal defect.

Transposition of the great arteries results if the aorticopulmonary septum divides the truncus arteriosus without following its normal spiral course when it divides the truncus into the aorta and pulmonary artery. Consequently, the aorta and pulmonary artery develop parallel to each other. The aorta becomes located to the right of the pulmonary artery instead of behind and to the left of the pulmonary artery, which changes the relationship of the arteries to their "correct" ventricles. The aorta becomes connected to the right ventricle and the pulmonary artery attaches to the left ventricle, which severely disrupts blood flow in both the pulmonary and systemic circulations. The right ventricle pumps blood into the aorta (instead of the pulmonary artery) to be distributed to the body, and the blood is returned by the superior and inferior vena cava to the right atrium. Consequently, the body is supplied by poorly oxygenated blood that is continuously circulated in the systemic circulation. In contrast, the left ventricle pumps oxygenated blood into the pulmonary artery (instead of the aorta), which returns in the pulmonary veins to the left atrium. The flow of oxygenated blood remains confined to the pulmonary circuit, where it serves no useful purpose. After birth, the condition is not compatible with life unless there is a communication that permits some intermixing of blood between the pulmonary and systemic circulations such as a patent foramen ovale, atrial septal defect, or ventricular septal defect (FIGURE 12). Generally, such communications do not provide enough oxygenated blood to supply the infant's needs.

The current treatment of this condition is called the arterial switch operation, which involves cutting across the bases of the aorta and pulmonary artery above their attachments to the ventricles. Then the aorta is connected to the left ventricle, and the pulmonary artery is attached to the right ventricle. It is also necessary to reposition the coronary

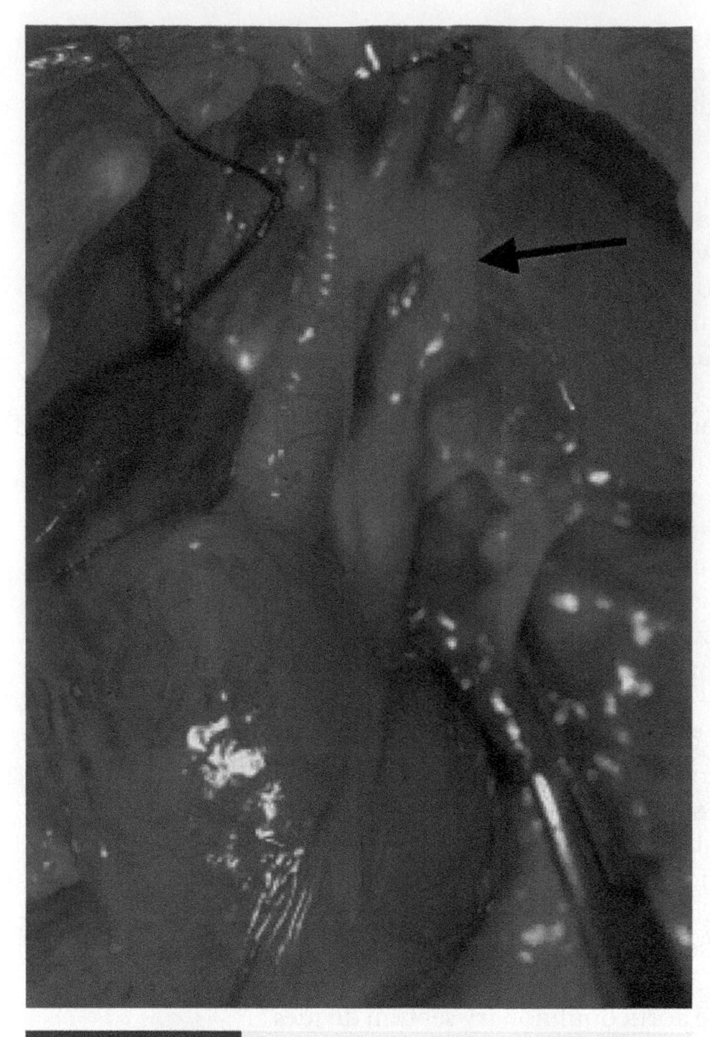

FIGURE 12 Transposition of the great arteries showing the parallel course of the aorta and pulmonary artery. Aorta is located to the right of the pulmonary artery (*left* of photograph) and is connected to the right ventricle, and the pulmonary artery is attached to the left ventricle. Some intermixing of blood between the aortic and pulmonary circulations is achieved by the large patent ductus arteriosus (*arrow*), and also by the foramen ovale, which is not demonstrated in the photograph.

arteries so that they are connected properly to the artery supplying blood to the left ventricle.

TABLE 2 summarizes the principal features of the congenital cardiovascular malformations described in this section, which are also illustrated in FIGURE 13.

PREVENTION OF CONGENITAL HEART DISEASE

The only way to prevent congenital heart disease is to attempt to protect the developing fetus from intrauterine injury during the early phases of pregnancy when it is extremely vulnerable. The factors that may cause intrauterine fetal injury are discussed in the discussion on congenital and hereditary diseases.

Valvular Heart Disease

Rheumatic fever is much less frequent now than formerly. As a result, rheumatic valvular heart disease has also declined, and other conditions that cause valve malfunction have assumed greater importance. These include various degenerative conditions of the aortic valve and an abnormality of the mitral valve that causes it to prolapse into the atrium during ventricular systole.

RHEUMATIC FEVER AND RHEUMATIC HEART DISEASE

Rheumatic fever
A disease caused by hypersensitivity to antigens of the beta streptococcus, characterized by fever, joint pains, and inflammation of heart valves and muscle.

Rheumatic fever is a complication of infection by the group A beta hemolytic streptococcus, the organism responsible for streptococcal sore throat and scarlet fever. This disease, encountered most commonly in children, is a febrile illness associated with inflammation of connective tissue throughout the body, especially in the heart and joints. Clinically, the affected individual has an acute arthritis affecting multiple joints (which is why the disease is called "rheumatic" fever) and evidence of inflammation of the heart.

Rheumatic fever is not a bacterial infection but a type of hypersensitivity reaction induced by various antigens present in the streptococcus. This reaction develops several weeks after the initial streptococcal infection. It is uncertain exactly how the streptococcus induces the development of rheumatic fever. Apparently, some persons form antibody against antigens present in the streptococcus, and the antistreptococcal antibody cross-reacts with similar antigens in the individual's own tissues. The antigen–antibody reaction injures connective tissue and is responsible for the febrile illness. Fortunately, rheumatic fever develops in only a small proportion of persons with group A beta streptococcal infections.

TABLE 2

Features of common congenital cardiovascular abnormalities

Abnormality	Physiologic disturbance	Complications	Treatment
Patent ductus arteriosus	Aorta to pulmonary artery shunt	Pulmonary hypertension	Ligate or excise ductus
Patent foramen ovale	Right-to-left atrial shunt	Usually nonfunctional as long as left atrial pressure exceeds right atrial pressure	Usually no treatment required
Atrial, ventricular, and combined septal defects	Left-to-right shunt	Pulmonary hypertension damages lungs. Right ventricular hypertrophy.	Close defect
Pulmonary stenosis	Obstructed outflow from right ventricle	Right ventricular hypertrophy	Dilate narrowed valve opening
Aortic stenosis	Obstructed outflow from left ventricle	Left ventricular hypertrophy	Dilate narrowed valve opening
Aortic coarctation	Obstructed flow into aorta distal to coarctation	Hypertension in arteries supplying head and upper limbs	Excise coarctation and reconnect aorta
Tetralogy of Fallot	Right-to-left shunt. Ventricular septal defect straddled by enlarged aorta. Pulmonary stenosis. Right ventricular hypertrophy.	Cyanosis. Polycythemia. Clubbing of fingers and toes.	Enlarge pulmonary artery opening. Close septal defect.
Transposition of great arteries	Aorta attached to right ventricle and pulmonary artery attached to left ventricle	Only communication between systemic and pulmonary circulations is through ductus arteriosus and foramen ovale	Reattach aorta and pulmonary artery to proper ventricles. Reposition coronary arteries.

Some patients with acute rheumatic fever die as a result of severe inflammation of the heart and consequent acute heart failure. In most instances, however, the fever and signs of inflammation eventually subside. Healing is often associated with some degree of scarring. In the joints and in many other tissues, scarring causes no difficulties, but scarring of heart valves may produce various deformities that impair function.

Unfortunately, rheumatic fever is likely to recur when the patient develops another streptococcal infection because any subsequent contact with the streptococcus reestablishes the sequence of hypersensitivity and connective tissue damage.

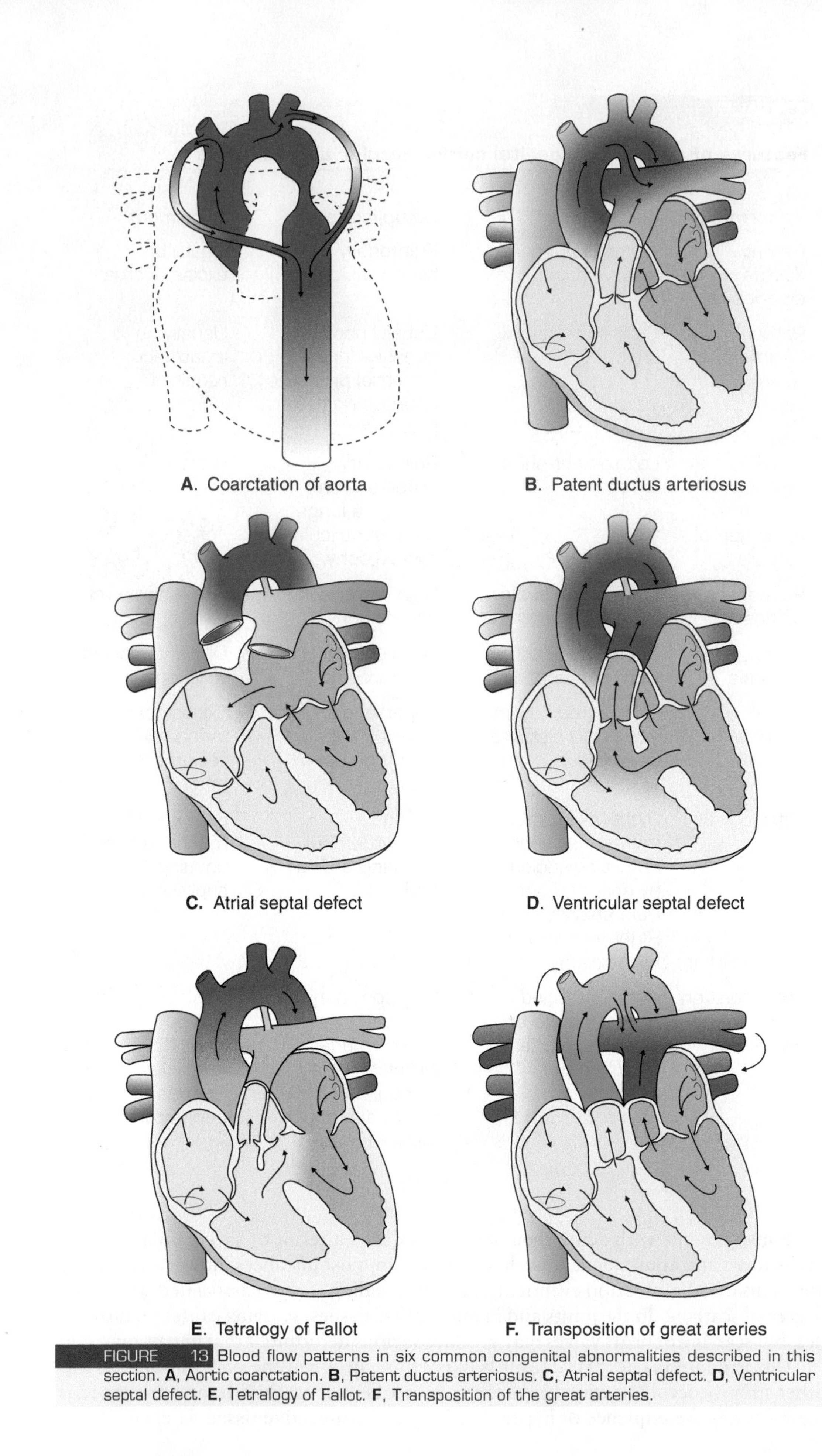

FIGURE 13 Blood flow patterns in six common congenital abnormalities described in this section. **A**, Aortic coarctation. **B**, Patent ductus arteriosus. **C**, Atrial septal defect. **D**, Ventricular septal defect. **E**, Tetralogy of Fallot. **F**, Transposition of the great arteries.

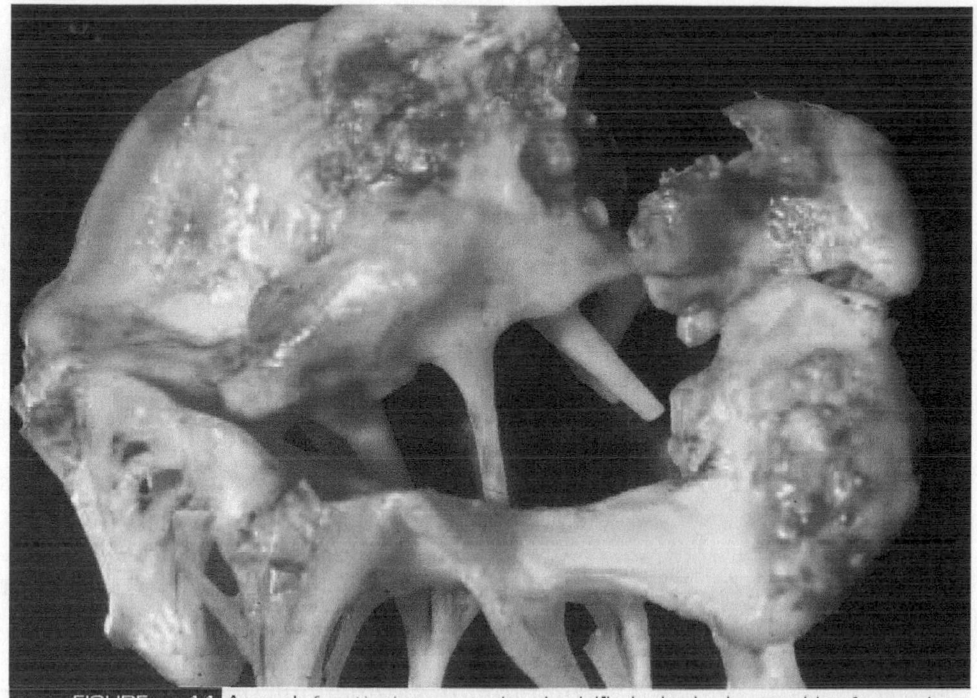

FIGURE 14 A poorly functioning scarred and calcified mitral valve resulting from valve damage caused by prior rheumatic fever. The valve was excised and replaced by an artificial heart valve.

Rheumatic heart disease, a complication of rheumatic fever, is caused by scarring of the heart valves subsequent to the healing of a rheumatic inflammation. This complication is relatively common and primarily affects the valves of the left side of the heart, the mitral and aortic valves (FIGURE 14). If the valve does not close properly, blood refluxes back through it (called regurgitation). Frequently, the damaged valve also does not open properly, and the valve orifice is narrowed. This is called a valve stenosis. Valve lesions impair cardiac function. When valvular stenosis is present, the heart must exert more effort than normal to force blood through the narrowed orifice. In regurgitation, a portion of the ventricular output is not expelled normally and leaks through the incompetent valve. This is a serious disadvantage because the heart must repump the volume of regurgitated blood to deliver the same amount of blood to the peripheral tissues.

An individual with a mild rheumatic valvular deformity that does not seriously interfere with cardiac function may experience little or no disability. However, a severe valve deformity may place a serious strain on the heart, eventually causing heart failure many years after the initial attack of rheumatic fever. When a person is seriously disabled by a rheumatic valvular deformity, it is possible to excise the abnormal, scarred heart valve surgically and replace it with an artificial valve.

Prevention of Rheumatic Heart Disease

Rheumatic heart disease can be largely prevented by treating beta streptococcal infection promptly, thereby forestalling the hypersensitivity state that causes rheumatic fever. Because a person who has once had rheumatic fever is susceptible to recurrent attacks after beta streptococcal infections, many physicians recommend that persons who have had rheumatic fever receive prophylactic penicillin therapy throughout childhood and young adulthood. Penicillin treatment prevents streptococcal infections and reduces the risk of recurrent rheumatic fever and further heart valve damage.

NONRHEUMATIC AORTIC STENOSIS

In about 2% of all people, the aortic valve has two rather than the usual three cusps. This abnormality is called a congenital bicuspid aortic valve. The valve functions satisfactorily for a time but is subjected to unusual stress during opening and closing because of its bicuspid configuration. As a result, the valve gradually becomes thickened and may eventually become calcified after many years, leading to marked rigidity of the valve when a person reaches middle age (FIGURE 15). This condition is called aortic stenosis secondary to bicuspid aortic valve.

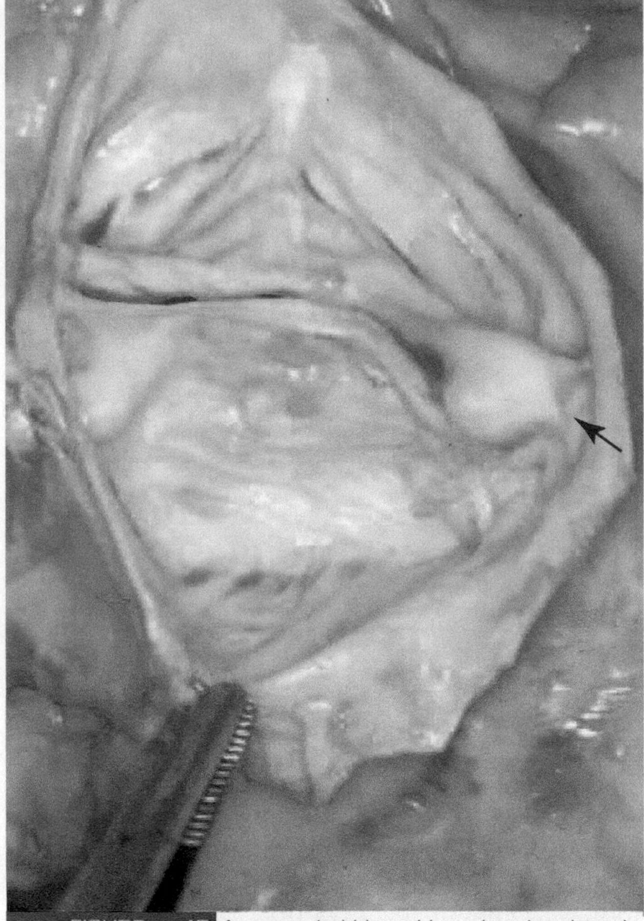

FIGURE 15 A congenital bicuspid aortic valve viewed from above. Beginning scarring is seen at the right margin of the valve (*arrow*).

Fibrosis and calcification of the valve leaflets of a normal three cusp aortic valve may also occur in older persons, and sometimes the valve becomes so rigid that it is unable to open properly. This entity is called calcific aortic stenosis (FIGURE 16).

Mild degrees of aortic stenosis may not greatly compromise cardiac function, but severe aortic stenosis places a great strain on the left ventricle, which must expel blood through the greatly narrowed and rigid valve orifice. This leads to marked left ventricular hypertrophy and eventual heart failure. Treatment of severe aortic stenosis consists of surgically replacing the stenotic valve with an artificial heart valve.

Aortic stenosis usually is considered to be caused by degenerative changes in valve leaflet connective tissue, a consequence of the stresses placed on the

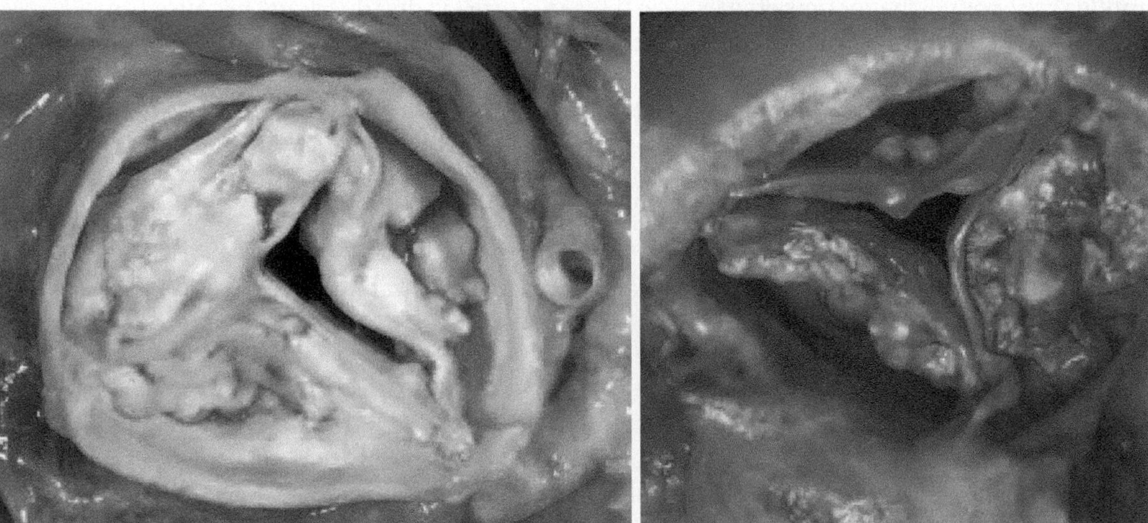

FIGURE 16 An aortic valve viewed from above, illustrating marked thickening and nodularity of valve leaflets. **A**, Partial fusion of valve cusps (*left side* of photograph). A normal coronary artery is seen in a cross section at right of aortic valve. **B**, Severe calcific aortic stenosis. Extensive calcium deposits within cusps severely limit valve mobility.

valve resulting from the repeated opening and closing of the valve leaflets over many years, followed by calcification that restricts valve mobility. More recent studies, however, have demonstrated deposits of lipids and accumulation of macrophages in the valve leaflets similar to the changes found in coronary atherosclerosis. On the basis of these studies, it now appears that the same risk factors that predispose to coronary artery disease, such as high cholesterol, diabetes, and hypertension, also may contribute to the valve changes leading to aortic stenosis. Control of these risk factors may retard or perhaps even prevent the fibrosis and calcification of the valve leaflets that impair valve function.

As our population ages, aortic stenosis is becoming one of the most common types of valvular heart disease. Case 1 describes a common clinical presentation of aortic stenosis and also illustrates the management of a patient with this condition.

MITRAL VALVE PROLAPSE

Mitral valve prolapse is a common condition, and only a very small percentage of persons ever develops any problems related to the prolapse. In this condition, one or both mitral leaflets are enlarged and redundant and prolapse into the left atrium during ventricular systole. Sometimes, the prolapsing free margins of the valve leaflets do

CASE 1

During a routine physical examination, a 73-year-old man was found to have a systolic murmur. He was in good health and had not had any serious illnesses in the past, and there was no history of previous rheumatic fever.

Physical examination was completely normal except for the heart murmur. Temperature, pulse, and blood pressure were all within normal limits. Routine laboratory tests and an electrocardiogram were all normal.

An echocardiogram was performed in order to determine the cause of the murmur and revealed that he had mild aortic stenosis. The aortic valve was calcified, and there was a mild to moderate restriction of the aortic valve opening. The aortic valve did not appear to be bicuspid, although this possibility could not be excluded completely. The aortic valve opening was calculated to be 1.2 sq. cm., in contrast to a normal valve opening which should be 3 to 4 sq. cm. when fully open. The mean pressure gradient across the aortic valve was 17 mm Hg, indicating that the pressure within the left ventricle during systole was higher than that in the aorta because outflow of blood from the left ventricle was impeded by the valve stenosis. Normally, there should be no pressure difference between the pressure in the aorta and the pressure within the ventricular chamber. However, there was as yet no significant hypertrophy of the left ventricle.

The patient was told that he had a mild degree of aortic stenosis that was likely to progress over time and that he probably would eventually require a valve replacement. He did not need to restrict his activities, but he was advised to take prophylactic antibiotics before any dental procedures or surgical procedures that could cause transient entry of bacteria into his circulation in order to reduce his risk of endocarditis. He was also advised to take one 81-mg aspirin tablet daily (a "baby aspirin" tablet) both to reduce his risk of coronary heart disease and also to prevent platelets from adhering to the roughened surface of the stenotic aortic valve. He was also advised to have the echocardiogram repeated in 2 years to evaluate possible progression of the stenosis.

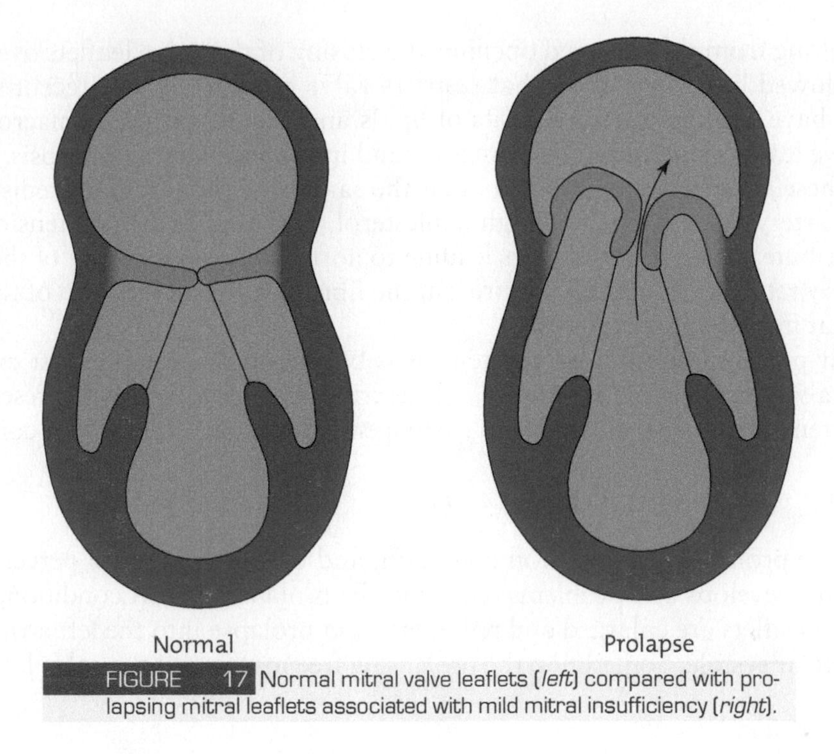

FIGURE 17 Normal mitral valve leaflets (*left*) compared with prolapsing mitral leaflets associated with mild mitral insufficiency (*right*).

not fit together tightly, which allows some blood to leak across the closed mitral valve into the atrium, which is called mitral regurgitation. The extent of the prolapse is quite variable, and the amount of blood that leaks into the left atrium through the prolapsing valve depends on how tightly the free margins of the prolapsing valve leaflets come together during ventricular systole (FIGURE 17).

The mitral valve leaflets, like other cardiac valve leaflets, are attached to a ring of dense connective tissue called the mitral annulus, which circumscribes the valve opening. The annulus is part of the fibrous framework of the heart to which the valves and cardiac muscle bundles are attached. Normally, the valve leaflets close at the level of the mitral annulus or just below the annulus. The closure position is determined by the length of the valve leaflets, the chordae to which the leaflets are attached, and the length of the papillary muscles.

When one listens to the heart sounds with a stethoscope, one first hears a click sound during systole when the leaflets come together, which is often followed by a faint systolic murmur caused by reflux of blood between the closed valve leaflets into the left atrium.

In some cases, the prolapse appears to be caused by degenerative changes in the connective tissue of the valve leaflets, which permits the affected valve leaflets to gradually stretch as a result of the degeneration of the valve connective tissue. Eventually, one or both leaflets may become enlarged and redundant. When this occurs, the stretched prolapsing mitral valve, held at its margin by the chordae, somewhat resembles an open parachute (FIGURE 18), and a significant amount of blood may reflux into the left atrium. The prolapsing valve may also produce excessive strain on the chordae and papillary muscles, which may provoke bouts of ventricular arrhythmia. Sometimes, the excessive stress causes one of the chordae to rupture.

SEROTONIN-RELATED HEART VALVE DAMAGE

Some uncommon types of heart valve damage seem to be related to high concentrations of serotonin in the blood. Serotonin (5-hydroxytryptamine) is a biologic compound produced by many cells throughout the body and has many different

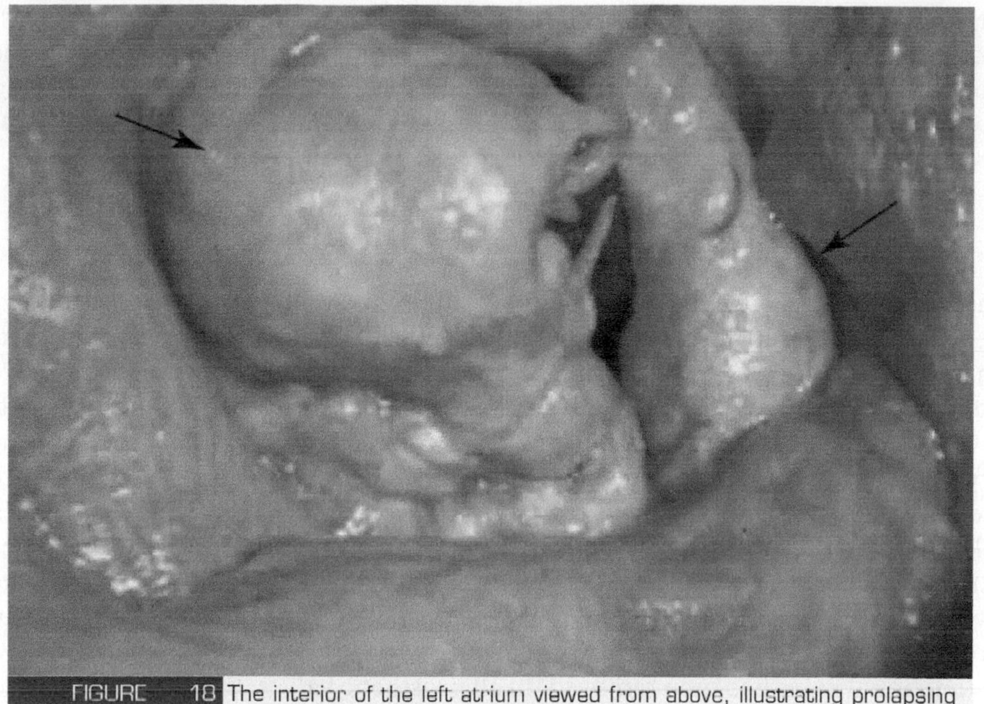

FIGURE 18 The interior of the left atrium viewed from above, illustrating prolapsing mitral valve leaflets ballooning into the left atrium (*arrows*). Prolapse was complicated by a rupture of mitral valve chorda tendinea.

functions. Serotonin produces different effects on body tissues and organs because there are several different types of serotonin receptors, and the biologic effects of serotonin in a specific tissue are governed by the characteristics of the receptor to which the serotonin attaches. (Usually, the receptor is designated by the chemical name of serotonin [5-hydroxytryptamine], abbreviated 5-HT, with the type of receptor indicated by a subscript, such as 5-HT_{2B}). Serotonin is produced by specialized cells (called neuroendocrine cells), which are scattered among the secretory and absorptive cells within the epithelium of the gastrointestinal tract, where the serotonin regulates some gastrointestinal functions. Similar neuroendocrine cells are also present in the epithelium of other organs. Platelets contain large amounts of serotonin, which constricts blood vessels to decrease bleeding when it is released along with histamine as platelets aggregate during blood coagulation. Serotonin is also released from nerve endings within the nervous system, where it is involved in the transmission of nerve impulses.

Sometimes, tumors arise from the neuroendocrine cells of the gastrointestinal tract or other organs and produce large amounts of serotonin. Patients with serotonin-producing tumors of this type often develop marked thickening of their heart valves caused by proliferation of connective tissue within the valves, which distorts the valves and impairs their functions. The heart valve damage occurs because the receptor to which the serotonin attaches (designated 5-HT_{2B}) stimulates the valve connective tissue cells (fibroblasts) to proliferate and form an excess of connective tissue fibers, which leads to fibrous thickening of the valves.

Some drugs and chemicals other than serotonin have a chemical structure that enables them to attach to heart valve serotonin receptors (5-HT_{2B}) and cause the same type of valve injury as serotonin. These drugs are called 5-HT_{2B} receptor agonists (*ago* = to act or do something) because they mimic the effects of serotonin. Some of these drugs are derived from ergot, which constricts blood vessels, and are used to treat persons with migraine headaches; other ergot-derived drugs are used to treat persons with a neurologic disease called Parkinson disease (described in the discussion on the nervous system). Two appetite suppressant drugs used together about 10 years ago to treat overweight and obese patients caused heart valve damage because one of the drugs stimulated proliferation of connective tissue in the heart valves by attaching to serotonin receptors (5-HT_{2B}) on the heart valves.

PROSTHETIC (ARTIFICIAL) HEART VALVES

A heart valve that has been so badly damaged by disease that it no longer can function adequately can be replaced by an artificial valve, which is usually called a prosthetic heart valve (*prosthesis* = replacement). There are two major types, mechanical valves and tissue valves. Each type has advantages and disadvantages, and no prosthetic valve can function as well as a normal heart valve. Mechanical valves, which are very durable, are composed of metal components. The valves are classified into three categories according to how they function: (1) a caged-ball valve, (2) tilting circular disk valve, or (3) a two leaflet (bi-leaflet) valve. The valves come in various sizes and the appropriate size is selected for the replacement. The periphery of all valves have a rim of synthetic flexible material for attachment of sutures to hold the valve in proper position when anchoring the valve within the heart after the patient's own dysfunctional valve has been removed. In all prosthetic valves, the opening and closing of the valve is governed by blood pressure differences on opposite sides of the valve, as in a normal heart valve.

Caged-ball valve
An artificial heart valve consisting of a small ball in a metal cage in which the position of the ball in the cage determines the blood flow through the valve.

Tilting disk valve
An artificial heart valve in which the flow through the valve is determined by the position of a flat circular disk within the valve.

Two leaflet valve
An artificial heart valve in which the flow through the valve is determined by two flat "half moon" leaflets that pivot to open and close the valve.

In the **caged-ball valve** (FIGURE 19A), the ball is shown against the valve opening (orifice) at the base of the valve, which closes the valve. When used to replace an aortic valve, the column of blood ejected from the aorta during ventricular systole pushes the ball away from the valve opening at the base of the cage. When the blood pressure within the ventricle falls lower than the intra-aortic pressure during diastole, the ball returns to the base of the cage to close the valve opening, thereby preventing reflux of ejected blood from the aorta into the left ventricle. A lateral x-ray of a patient with a caged-ball prosthesis is illustrated in FIGURE 19B. The metal parts of the prosthesis are demonstrated but the ball is not radio-opaque.

In a **tilting disk valve** (FIGURE 19C), the circular disk is held within the valve by two struts that extend from the metal valve ring on opposite sides of the disk, which allows the disk to open or close the valve in response to blood pressure difference on opposite sides of the valve. When used to replace a mitral valve, the disk moves (tilts) away from the valve opening during diastole, allowing blood to flow from the left atrium into the left ventricle. During ventricular systole, the rising ventricular pressure pushes the disk against the valve opening to prevent reflux of blood into the left atrium.

In a **two leaflet valve**, the single circular disk of a tilting disk valve is replaced by two "half leaflets" that pivot on a hinge to open or close the valve, which perform essentially the same function as the tilting disk (FIGURE 19D). Despite the durability of mechanical valves, they have one disadvantage; blood clots can form on the metal parts of the prosthesis unless the patient takes an anticoagulant continuously to prevent formation of thrombi, which would disrupt the function of the prosthesis and could also lead to embolism of pieces of blood clot from the prosthesis, blocking major systemic arteries. Tissue valves, which more closely resemble normal valves, are composed of specially treated animal tissues, such as "pig valves." The patient does not have to take anticoagulants, since thrombi do not form on tissue valves, but they are not as durable as mechanical valves and tend to wear out in 10 to 15 years. Consequently, their use is usually limited to older individuals, such as elderly persons with severe calcific aortic stenosis.

Obviously, a prosthetic valve is not the same as a normal valve, and a person with a valve prosthesis has an increased risk of developing infective endocarditis, as

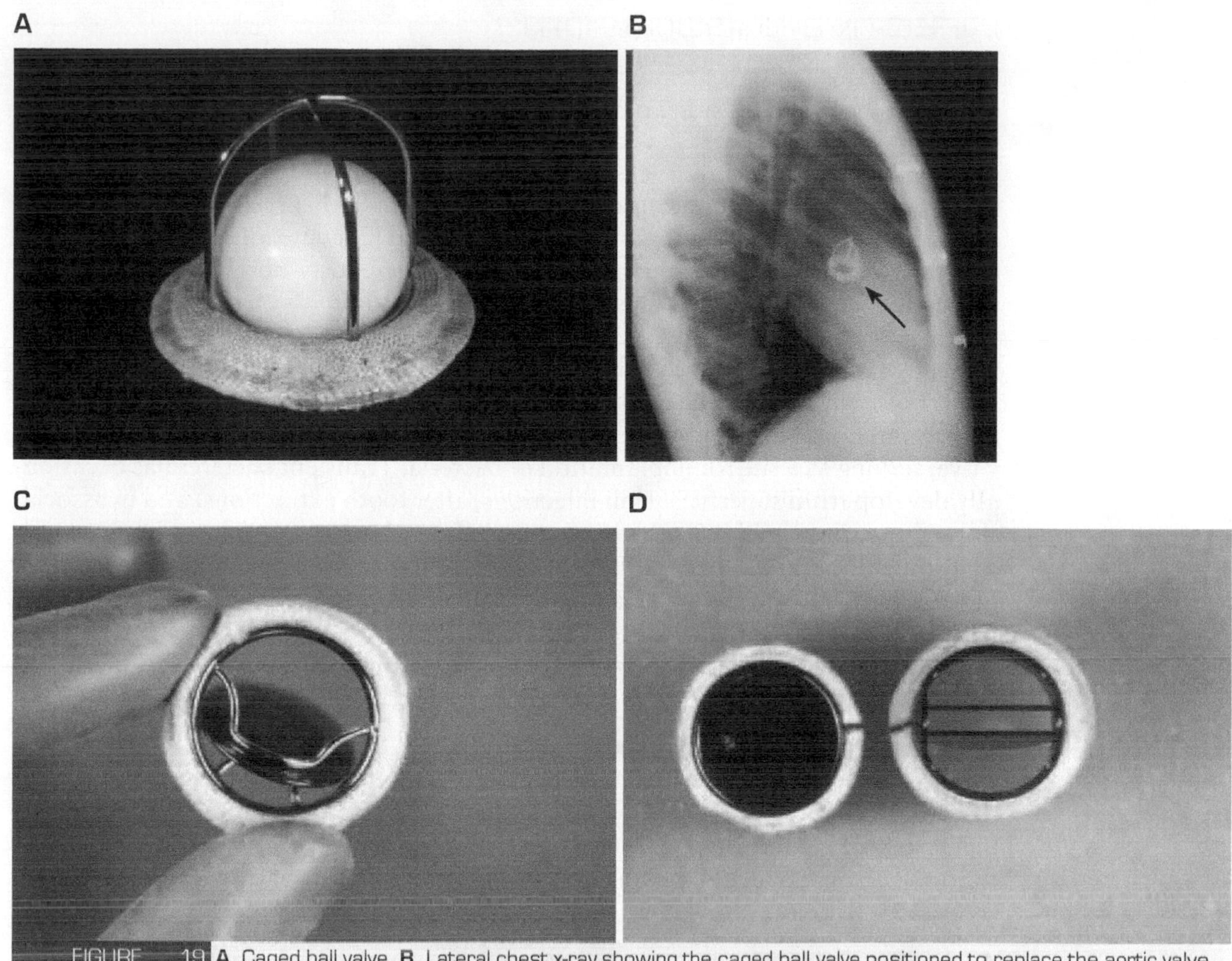

FIGURE 19 A, Caged ball valve. B, Lateral chest x-ray showing the caged ball valve positioned to replace the aortic valve. The base of the valve is positioned in the aortic valve opening with the cage extending into the base of the aorta (*arrow*). The ball is not radio-opaque and is not seen in the x-ray film. C, Tilting disk valve viewed from superior surface with the disc in open-valve position to allow flow from atrium to ventricle during diastole, as when replacing a mitral valve. D, Two views of two leaflet valves viewed from undersurface with leaflets closed (*left*) and opened (*right*).

described in the following section. Infection of a prosthetic heart valve is a very serious complication. If this unfortunate complication occurs, the infection is often at the site where the valve is attached to the myocardial tissues surrounding the valve opening.

Methods of Valve Replacement

The standard method for replacing a poorly functioning heart valve, such as a narrowed calcified aortic stenosis in an elderly patient, as illustrated by the valve in Figure 16, requires an extensive surgical procedure. The sternum must be divided and separated to reach the heart, followed by a cardiopulmonary bypass procedure assisted by a heart lung machine to divert blood from the heart while the calcified valve is removed and usually replaced by a tissue valve, such as a pig valve. Many elderly patients with other health problems in addition to aortic stenosis may be too ill for such an extensive procedure. Consequently, other less invasive procedures to replace heart valves are being developed, such as passing the replacement valve retrograde into the heart through the femoral artery, or directly into the left ventricle through a small chest incision. Advances in valve design and development of newer ways to place the valves in the heart should improve the safety of valve replacement.

INFECTIVE ENDOCARDITIS

Infective endocarditis is an infection of a heart valve, usually caused by bacteria but occasionally caused by other pathogens. In most cases, the infection is in the valves in the left side of the heart. It is customary to classify infective endocarditis into two groups: (1) subacute infective endocarditis, which is caused by organisms of low virulence, may be a complication of any type of valvular heart disease and is associated with relatively mild symptoms of infection; and (2) acute infective endocarditis, caused by highly virulent organisms that infect previously normal heart valves, is associated with symptoms of a severe systemic infection.

Subacute Infective Endocarditis

An abnormal or damaged valve is susceptible to infection because small deposits of agglutinated platelets and fibrin may accumulate on the roughened surface of the valve, serving as a site for implantation of bacteria. Transient bacteremias occasionally develop from superficial skin infections, after tooth extractions, and in association with various minor infections. In normal persons, transient bacteremia causes no problems because the organisms are normally destroyed by the body's defenses. However, an individual with a damaged valve runs the risk that bacteria may become implanted on the valve and incite an inflammation (FIGURE 20). Frequently, thrombi form at the site of the valve infection, and bits of thrombus may be dislodged and carried as emboli to other parts of the body, producing infarcts in various organs.

Antibiotic Prophylaxis to Prevent Endocarditis

Infective (bacterial) endocarditis is relatively uncommon, but it is a very serious disease. Persons with damaged heart valves or other cardiac abnormalities are at increased risk. Some surgical procedures and many dental procedures, such as cleaning and removal of dental plaque, tooth extractions, and root canal treatment, may

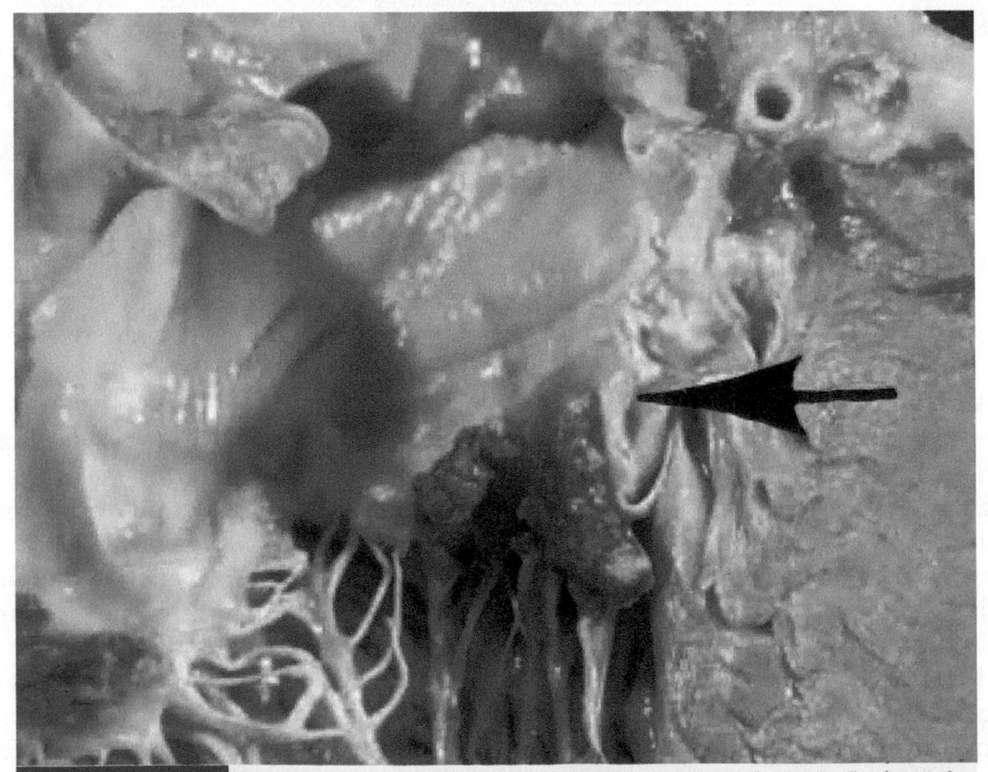

FIGURE 20 Bacterial endocarditis illustrating vegetations on mitral valve leaflet (*arrow*). Normal coronary artery is seen in cross section (*upper right*).

cause a shower of bacteria to be discharged into the bloodstream, which was considered a potential risk to patients with damaged or abnormal heart valves. Therefore, prophylactic antibiotics were given to susceptible persons about to undergo dental procedures because small deposits of agglutinated platelets and fibrin may have accumulated on the roughened surface of the valve, on which bacteria may implant. The American Heart Association provides guidelines regarding who should receive antibiotic prophylaxis, the types of surgical procedures requiring antibiotic prophylaxis, the recommended antibiotics to use, and the recommended dosage and duration of antibiotic treatment.

Recently, these guidelines were modified by a committee of physicians because the low risk of bacterial endocarditis in most persons with heart murmurs did not justify routine use of prophylactic antibiotics in all persons with heart murmurs. Now, prophylactic antibiotics are only recommended for dental patients who are at high risk of endocarditis. This latter group includes:

1. Persons with heart valve damage who have been treated previously for endocarditis
2. Persons in whom a diseased valve has been replaced by an artificial heart valve
3. Most persons who have had surgically treated congenital heart disease

Although the current recommendations are less restrictive, the committee concedes that possibly a very small number of cases of infective endocarditis could be prevented by a more liberal use of prophylactic antibiotics prior to dental procedures. Ultimately, the dental patient who has a heart murmur but is not at high risk of endocarditis must make the final decision about the use of prophylactic antibiotics, guided by the advice of the physician or dentist who is involved in the patient's care.

Acute Infective Endocarditis

Acute infective endocarditis results when highly pathogenic organisms spread into the bloodstream from an infection elsewhere in the body and infect a previously normal heart valve. Virulent staphylococci are a common cause of acute endocarditis and may cause considerable destruction of the affected valve (FIGURE 21).

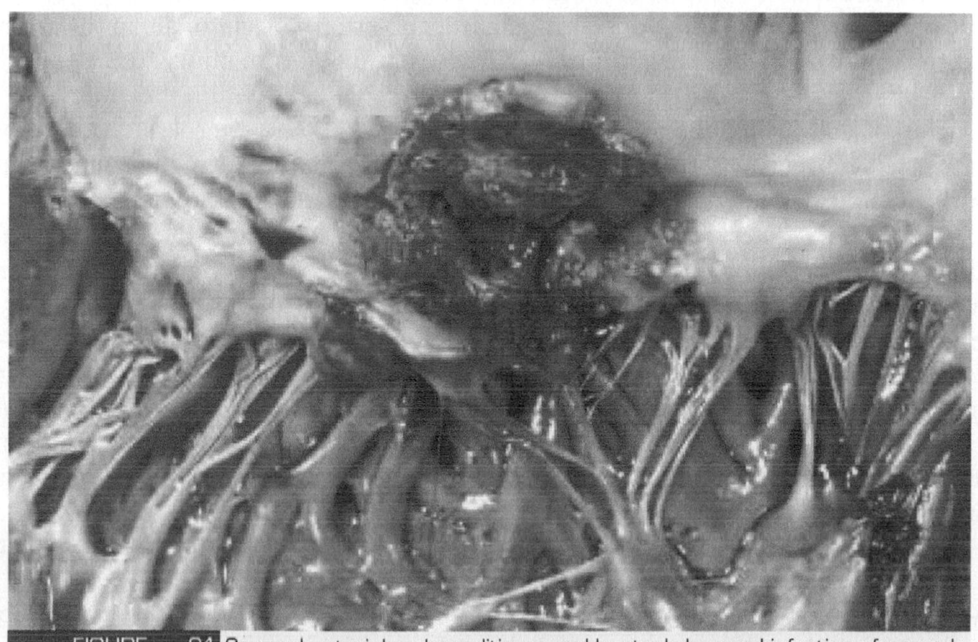

FIGURE 21 Severe bacterial endocarditis caused by staphylococcal infection of normal mitral valve. Infection has caused extensive destruction and perforation of valve leaflet.

CASE 2

A thirty-two-year-old hospital employee was admitted to the hospital because of chills and fever of about 2 weeks' duration. She was an intravenous cocaine user. Physical examination revealed numerous needle marks on the extremities and neck. Laboratory studies revealed increased numbers of polymorphonuclear leukocytes in the blood, suggesting an infection, and blood culture revealed *Staphylococcus aureus*. Special cardiac studies (echocardiograms) demonstrated a large vegetation on the tricuspid valve, and chest x-ray revealed multiple densities throughout both lungs, suggesting pulmonary infarcts secondary to emboli from the infected tricuspid valve. She eventually required surgical removal of the tricuspid valve and entered a drug treatment program.

Another group at high risk are intravenous drug abusers; in this group, the infection is usually in the tricuspid valve rather than the valves on the left side of the heart. Infection results from using unsterile materials to dissolve and inject the drug. In addition to bacterial contamination, undissolved particles and other debris contaminate the injected material. Intravenous injection carries the contaminated solution directly to the right side of the heart, where the particles and debris abrade the surface of the tricuspid valve. Platelets adhere to the site of injury and form thrombi, providing a favorable site for the injected microorganisms to implant and start an infection. Often, large bacteria-laden vegetations form on the valve. Pieces often break loose and are swept into the pulmonary arteries where they lodge in the lungs, causing multiple infected pulmonary infarcts and lung abscesses. Case 2 illustrates some of the clinical features of an acute endocarditis in a drug abuser.

Coronary Heart Disease

Coronary heart disease results from arteriosclerosis of the large coronary arteries. The arteries narrow owing to accumulation of fatty materials within the vessel walls. The lipid deposits, consisting of neutral fat and cholesterol, accumulate in the arteries by diffusion from the bloodstream. The initial event may be an injury to the endothelium of the vessel, which is followed by proliferation of cells within the inner layer of the arterial wall (called the intima) and accumulation of cholesterol and other lipids within their cytoplasm (FIGURE 22). Some of the cells accumulate so much cholesterol that it precipitates as crystals within the cytoplasm, disrupting the cells and causing cell necrosis. Cholesterol crystals, debris, and enzymes escape from the disrupted cells, inducing secondary fibrosis, calcification, and other degenerative changes in the arterial wall. The end result is an irregular mass of yellow, mushy debris that encroaches on the lumen of the artery and extends more deeply into the muscular and elastic tissue of the arterial wall. Often, the smooth internal lining of the vessel becomes ulcerated over the surface of the fatty deposits, leaving a roughened surface that predisposes to thrombus formation. The plaquelike deposit of material is called an atheromatous plaque or **atheroma** (*athere* = mush); the term for this type of arteriosclerosis is **atherosclerosis** (FIGURE 23).

Atheroma
(ah-ther-ō'muh)
A mass of lipids and debris that accumulates in the intima lining of an artery and narrows its lumen.

Atherosclerosis
A thickening of the lining (intima) *of blood vessels caused by accumulation of lipids, with secondary scarring and calcification.*

The initial stage in the development of atherosclerosis is reversible, and the newly formed plaques are called unstable plaques. The later stages, characterized by crystallization of cholesterol and secondary degenerative changes, are irreversible. The plaques, which become surrounded by fibrous tissue, are called stable plaques, and the vessel becomes permanently narrowed (FIGURE 24).

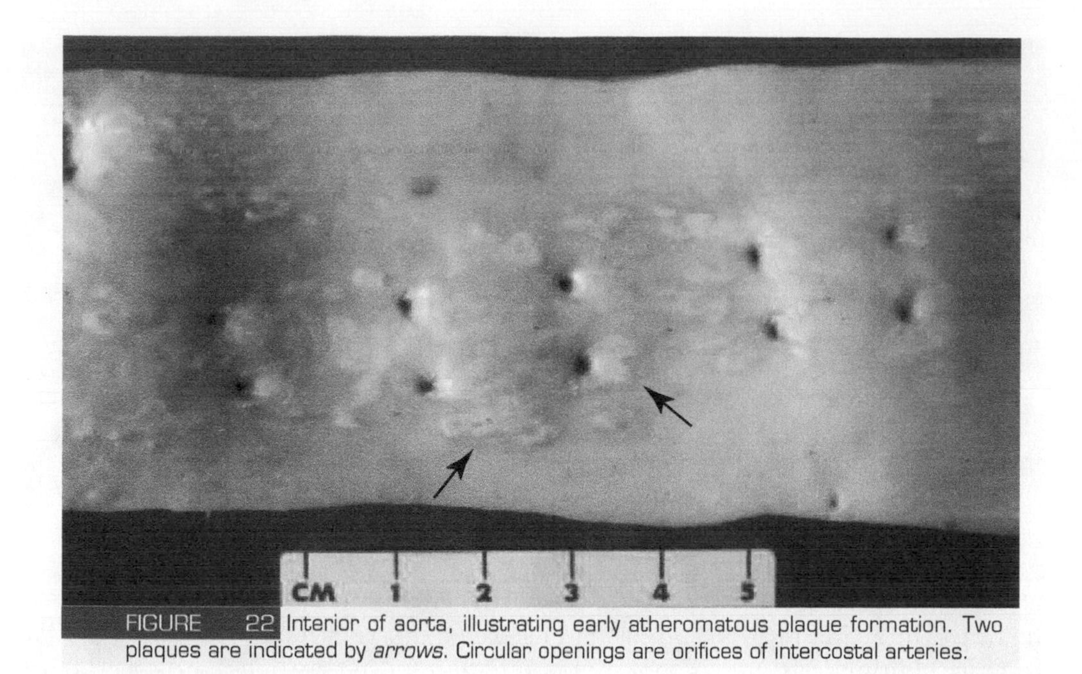

FIGURE 22 Interior of aorta, illustrating early atheromatous plaque formation. Two plaques are indicated by *arrows*. Circular openings are orifices of intercostal arteries.

RISK FACTORS

A number of factors are known to increase the risk of developing coronary heart disease and its associated complications. The four most important of these are (1) elevated blood lipids, (2) high blood pressure, (3) cigarette smoking, and (4) diabetes. If one risk factor is present, the likelihood of coronary heart disease and heart attacks is twice that in an individual lacking risk factors. If two risk factors are present, the risk increases fourfold, and if three factors are present, the risk of heart attack is seven times that for an individual with none.

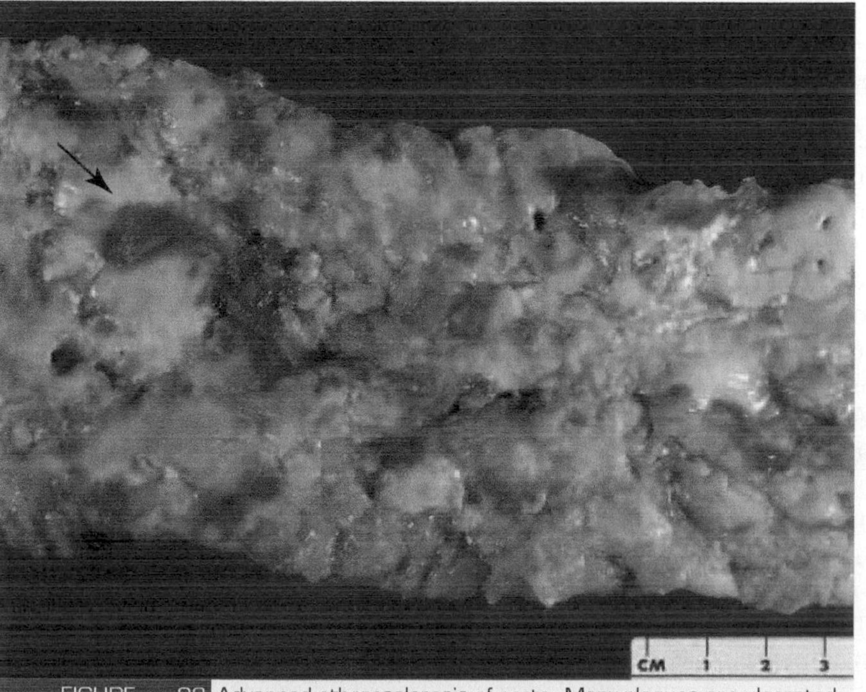

FIGURE 23 Advanced atherosclerosis of aorta. Many plaques are ulcerated and are covered by thrombus material (*arrow*).

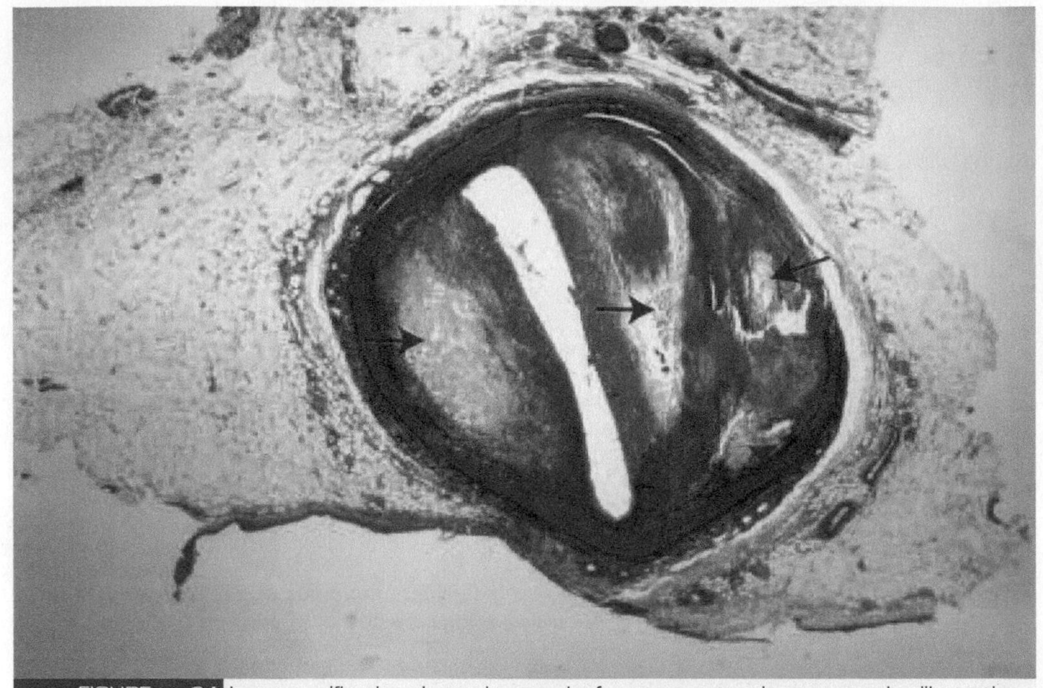

FIGURE 24 Low-magnification photomicrograph of coronary artery in cross section illustrating several stable atheromatous plaques (*arrows*) surrounded by dense fibrous tissue. Atheromatous deposits reduce lumen of artery to a narrow slit (original magnification × 40).

Other factors also may increase risk but play a less important role. Obesity increases the risk, but probably because an obese person usually has high blood lipids and elevated blood pressure. The personality of the individual may also play a role. One investigator has classified individuals on the basis of personality traits into two large groups. The type A person is aggressive, hard driving, and competitive and is thought to have a greater risk of coronary heart disease than the type B person, who is less aggressive and more easygoing.

MANIFESTATIONS

If atherosclerotic plaques narrow the coronary arteries by 50% or more, the arteries may still be able to supply enough blood to the heart muscle if the individual is not very active and no excessive demands are placed on the heart (FIGURE 24). However, blood supply may become inadequate if the subject exerts himself or herself and the heart requires more blood to satisfy the increased demands. Myocardial ischemia is the term commonly used to describe a reduced blood supply to the heart muscle caused by narrowing or obstruction of the coronary arteries, and the term **ischemic heart disease** is frequently used interchangeably with coronary heart disease. Although the flow rate through a tube falls as the tube narrows, the decrease is related not directly to the tube diameter but to the fourth power of the diameter. Consequently, a moderate decrease in the caliber of a coronary artery causes a disproportionately large reduction in its flow rate (FIGURE 25).

Ischemic heart disease (iss-kē′mik) *Used synonymously with coronary heart disease. Designates heart disease as a result of inadequate blood flow through the coronary arteries.*

The clinical manifestations of coronary heart disease are quite variable. Although many individuals are free of symptoms, some experience bouts of oppressive chest pain that may radiate into the neck or arms. The pain, which is caused by myocardial ischemia, is called angina pectoris, which means literally "pain of the chest." The usual type of angina is a midsternal pressure discomfort that occurs on exertion and subsides when the person rests or takes a nitroglycerine tablet, which dilates the coronary arteries and increases blood flow to the heart muscle. This kind of angina is often called stable angina to distinguish it from unstable angina, which is a manifestation of more severe and progressive narrowing of the coronary arteries. Unstable angina is characterized by episodes of pain that occur more frequently, last longer, and are less completely relieved by nitroglycerine.

A few patients exhibit another type of angina that characteristically occurs at rest rather than on exertion and is caused by a coronary artery spasm. This type of angina is usually called Prinzmetal's angina, named after the physician who first described it. Although angina is a common manifestation of coronary artery disease, it is not invariably present even though the coronary arteries are severely narrowed.

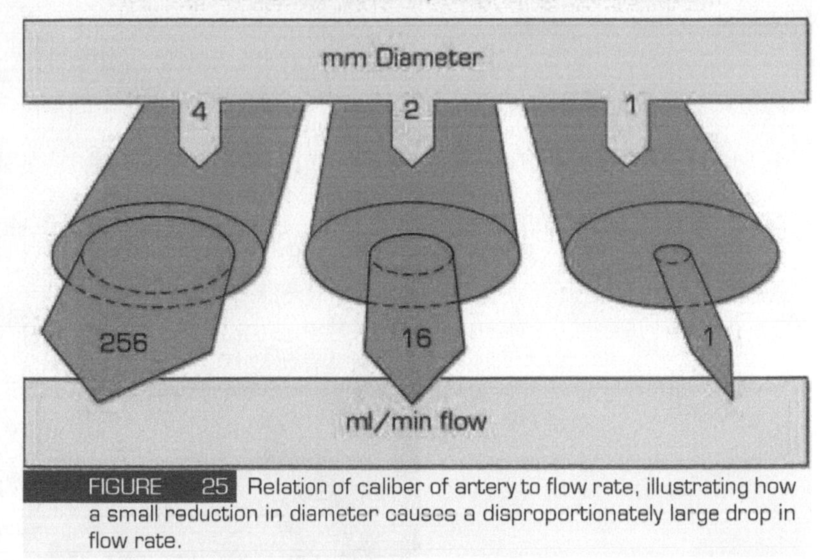

FIGURE 25 Relation of caliber of artery to flow rate, illustrating how a small reduction in diameter causes a disproportionately large drop in flow rate.

DIAGNOSIS OF CORONARY ARTERY DISEASE

Physicians can now evaluate the extent of coronary artery disease as well as the exact sites where the main coronary arteries are obstructed. This is accomplished by passing a catheter into the aorta and injecting a radiopaque dye directly into the orifices of the coronary arteries. The filling of the coronary arteries can be observed, along with the location and degree of arterial obstruction (FIGURE 26). This procedure is called a coronary angiogram (discussion on general concepts of disease: principles of diagnosis).

CORONARY DISEASE MANIFESTATIONS WITH APPARENTLY NORMAL CORONARY ARTERIES

Sometimes patients have symptoms of coronary artery disease, but coronary arteriograms reveal apparently normal coronary arteries or only evidence of small arteriosclerotic plaques that do not narrow the coronary arteries significantly. There are three possible reasons for the discrepancies between clinical manifestations and the apparently normal coronary angiograms.

1. There is arteriosclerosis of the coronary arteries, but the angiogram cannot detect it.

   For example, a coronary artery may be involved diffusely and uniformly by arteriosclerosis rather than forming discrete plaques that lead to localized narrowing of the artery, and the artery may appear to have a small lumen without evidence of disease. In other cases, isolated plaques may expand outward rather than extending into the lumen of the vessel and may escape detection.
2. The coronary arteries are normal, but marked sympathetic nervous system vasoconstrictor impulses may reduce myocardial blood flow by causing coronary artery spasm.

   This is the cause of the type of angina pectoris called Prinzmetal's angina, described previously. Other examples include stress-induced coronary artery

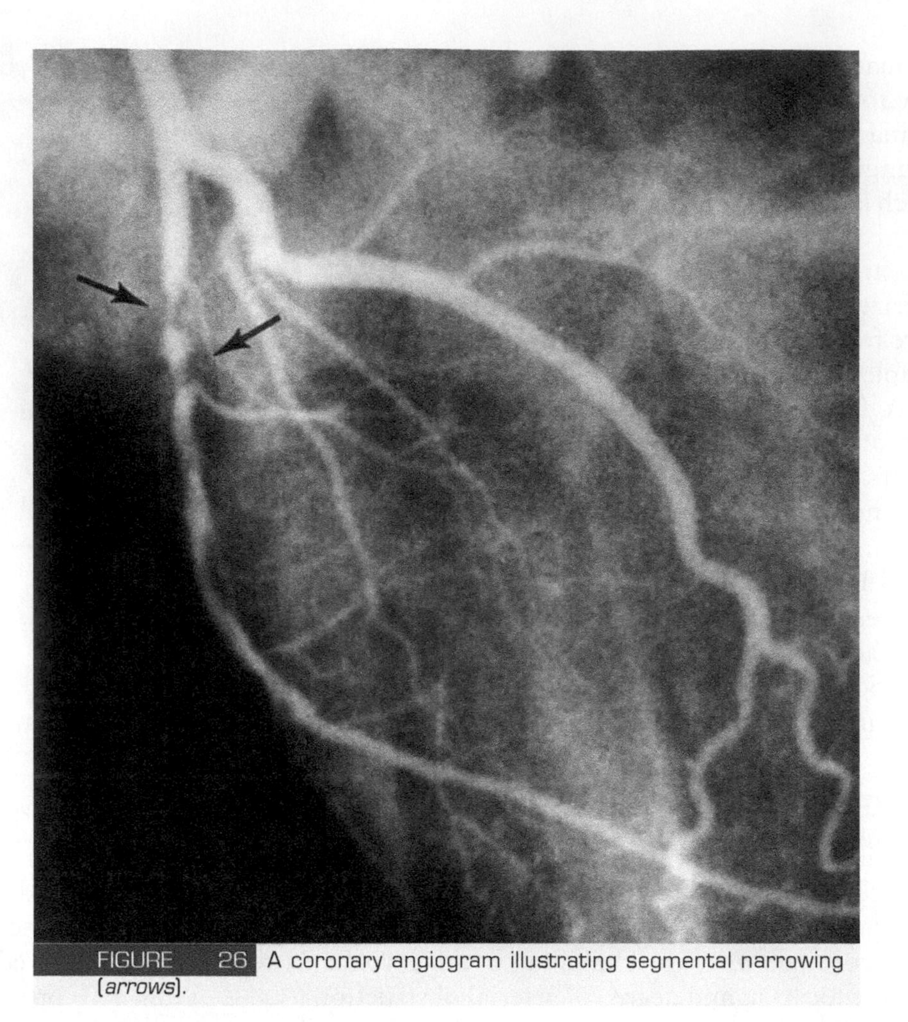

FIGURE 26 A coronary angiogram illustrating segmental narrowing (*arrows*).

vasoconstriction, which may actually lead to myocardial damage, as documented in a recent study of 19 women without coronary artery disease. In these women, severe emotional stress caused coronary artery vasospasm and myocardial injury as demonstrated by abnormal electrocardiograms, elevated cardiac enzymes, and impaired left ventricular function.

3. The coronary arteries are normal, but the function of the coronary arterioles is not.

   Normal coronary arterioles regulate blood flow to the heart muscle in response to myocardial oxygen requirements. When the arterioles are completely dilated, they can increase myocardial blood flow up to five times over basal levels when heart muscle needs more blood during exercise or exertion. In some persons, however, studies have demonstrated that the coronary arterioles are unable to dilate sufficiently to provide adequate blood to the heart muscle during exertion, which leads to symptoms of myocardial ischemia.

TREATMENT OF CORONARY ARTERY DISEASE

Medical Treatment

Medical treatment of coronary heart disease consists of administering drugs that reduce myocardial oxygen consumption and improve coronary circulation (antianginal drugs). If the patient exhibits cardiac irregularities, drugs that reduce myocardial irritability also are prescribed (antiarrhythmial drugs). Factors that potentiate coronary artery disease also are controlled or eliminated as follows whenever possible (FIGURE 27):

1. Cessation of smoking, which has an adverse effect on the coronary circulation
2. Control of hypertension, which increases myocardial work and accelerates development of atherosclerosis
3. An "anti-coronary diet," which lowers levels of cholesterol and fat in the blood
4. Weight reduction
5. A program of graduated exercises, which seems to improve myocardial performance

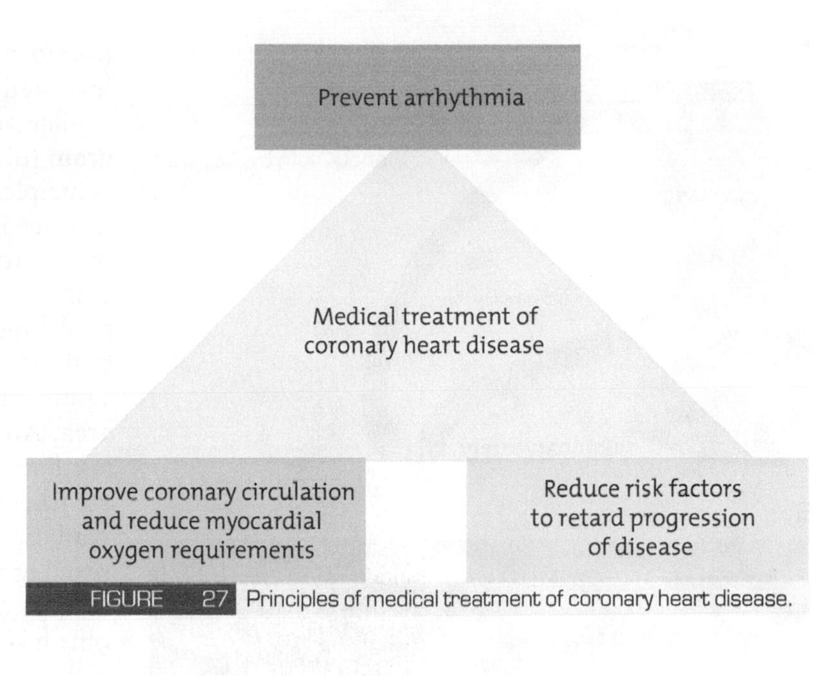

FIGURE 27 Principles of medical treatment of coronary heart disease.

Surgical Treatment

Several surgical approaches, called myocardial revascularization procedures, have been devised to improve blood supply to the heart muscle. Surgery is often recommended for patients who do not respond satisfactorily to medical treatment. The usual surgical method is to bypass the obstructions in the coronary arteries by means of segments of saphenous vein obtained from the patient's legs. The proximal ends of the grafts are sutured to small openings made in the aorta above the normal openings of the coronary arteries, and the distal ends are sutured into the coronary arteries beyond the areas of narrowing (FIGURE 28). Myocardial revascularization operations are generally reserved for patients with severe sclerosis of all three major coronary arteries, and usually grafts are used to bypass all three arteries. The operation alleviates or greatly improves symptoms of angina and may also improve survival in some groups of patients. Unfortunately, the high arterial pressure carried by the vein grafts sometimes causes the grafts to undergo progressive intimal thickening, which may lead to complete occlusion of the grafts. Many of the grafts eventually also develop the same type of atherosclerosis that occurred in the coronary arteries.

The internal thoracic arteries, which are more often called by their older name of internal mammary arteries, also can be used to bypass obstructed coronary arteries. The internal mammary arteries are paired arteries that arise from the aorta and descend along the undersurface of the thoracic cavity just lateral to the sternum. They can be dissected from their normal location and connected to the coronary arteries, thereby delivering blood directly from the aorta to the coronary arteries beyond the narrowed or blocked areas. Because the arteries are able to carry blood under much higher pressure than veins, artery grafts are less likely to become narrowed or obstructed. In some patients, both vein grafts and internal mammary arteries are used to restore adequate blood flow to the myocardium.

Coronary Angioplasty

Many patients with less extensive coronary artery disease can be treated successfully by dilating narrowed areas in the coronary arteries instead of bypassing them, thereby avoiding major surgery. The procedure is called coronary angioplasty (*angio* = vessel + *plasty* = molding) and is illustrated in FIGURE 29. By means of a technique similar to that used to perform a coronary arteriogram (discussion on general concepts of disease: principles of diagnosis), a guiding catheter is introduced through the skin and into a large artery in the arm or leg, threaded under fluoroscopic control into the narrowed coronary artery, and positioned at the site of narrowing. Then the balloon catheter is threaded through the guide catheter until the balloon lies within the narrowed area. After the balloon is properly positioned, it is inflated briefly under very high pressure, which smashes the plaque and pushes it into the arterial wall, enlarging the lumen of the artery and improving blood flow to the myocardium. At first, the procedure was used to treat patients who had only a single narrowed artery, but it is now used to treat patients who have multiple obstructing plaques in their coronary arteries and can also be used to dilate saphenous vein grafts that have become narrowed or obstructed.

Successful dilatation of a narrowed coronary artery restores normal blood flow through the artery. Unfortunately, in about 35% of successfully treated patients, the stenosis recurs within 6 months after balloon angioplasty and may require redilatation. In an attempt to solve the problem of restenosis, most physicians now perform balloon angioplasty using a **stent**, which is a short, expandable metal mesh tube that is placed over the balloon catheter with the metal mesh collapsed. The stent expands as the balloon is inflated to enlarge the lumen of the artery and functions as a rigid support to help keep the vessel open (FIGURE 29). This procedure is usually supplemented by administration of drugs that prevent accumulation of platelets at the site where the stent was placed. The arterial wall responds to the metal stent by proliferation of connective tissue and smooth muscle cells that grow through the meshes in the stent and cover its inner surface, followed by gradual ingrowth of endothelial cells to provide a smooth interior lining for the stent. Consequently, platelets are less likely to adhere at the site of the stent placement and cause thrombosis of the stented vessel.

Although use of stents has been helpful, restenosis of the dilated artery still occurs in about 25% of patients, resulting from ingrowth of tissue extending from the inner layers of the stented artery into the lumen of the vessel between the meshes of the stent. In an attempt to avoid this problem, stents have been

A

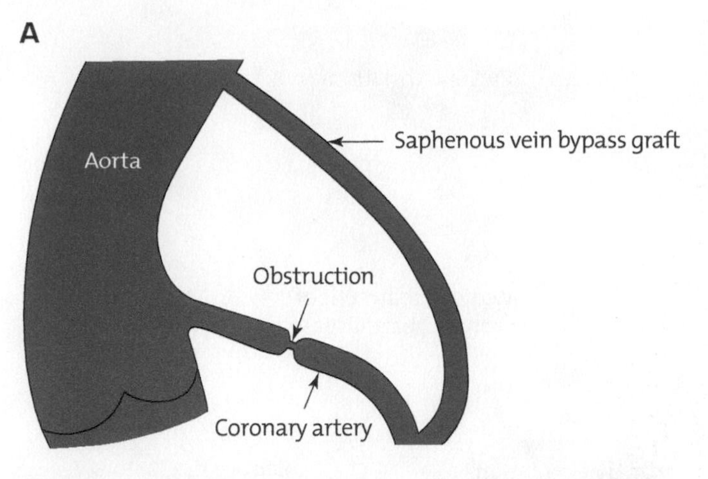

B

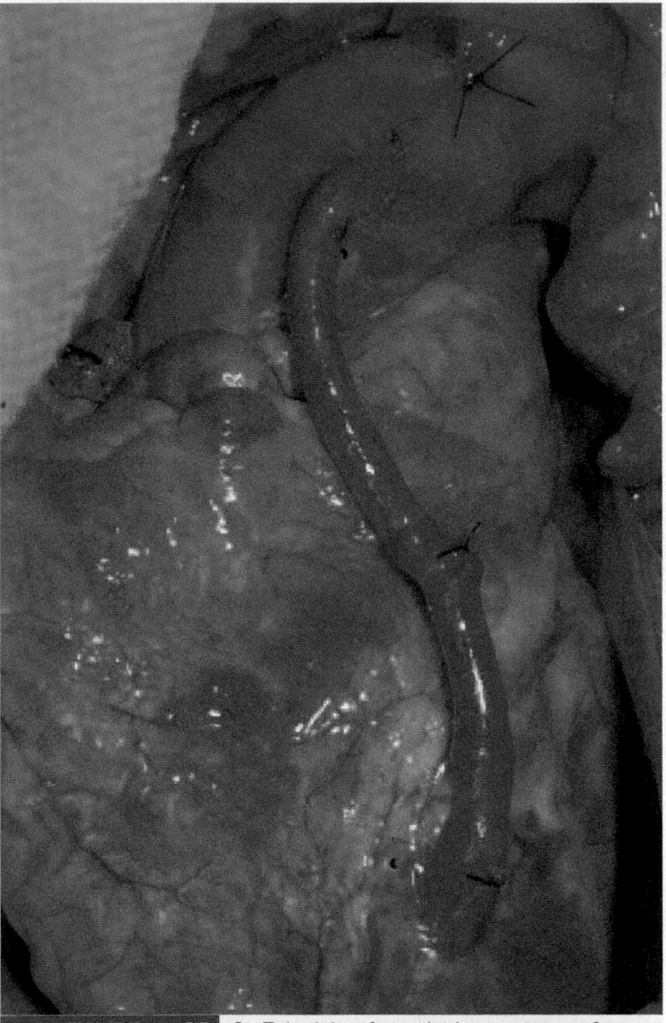

FIGURE 28 **A**, Principle of surgical treatment of coronary heart disease by means of saphenous vein grafts that bypass obstructions in coronary arteries. **B**, Vein graft extending from aorta above the origin of the coronary arteries to the anterior interventricular (descending) coronary artery distal to the site of arterial narrowing.

Stent
An expandable metal hollow tubular device placed within the lumen of a structure such as a blood vessel, often used to expand the lumen of the vessel, where it functions as a support to prevent narrowing of the dilated vessel.

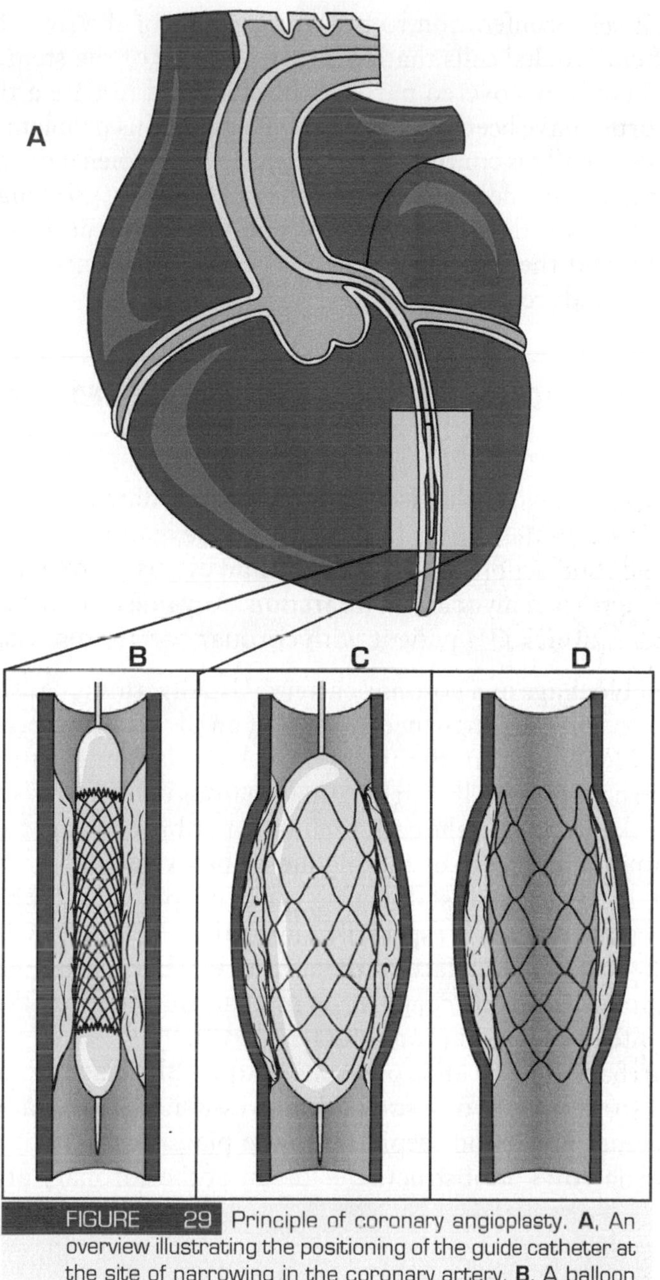

FIGURE 29 Principle of coronary angioplasty. **A**, An overview illustrating the positioning of the guide catheter at the site of narrowing in the coronary artery. **B**, A balloon catheter covered by unexpanded stent advanced through guide catheter and positioned within narrowed segment of artery. **C**, Balloon inflated, relieving arterial obstruction by smashing plaque and simultaneously expanding the stent. **D**, Balloon catheter withdrawn, leaving an expanded stent that forms a rigid support to maintain the caliber of the dilated artery.

produced that are coated with drugs that suppress the cell proliferation responsible for narrowing the stented artery.

After a drug-releasing stent has been inserted in an artery, the patient is treated with antiplatelet drugs for several months to prevent formation of a thrombus within the lumen of the stented artery, as is also done when using bare metal stents. Drug-releasing stents are less prone to stenosis, but are slightly more likely to become thrombosed than are bare metal stents, which usually occurs after the antiplatelet drugs have been discontinued. Apparently, the chemicals in the drug-releasing stent that inhibit cell proliferation to prevent stenosis of the stent also impede the proliferation of endothelial cells that cover the interior of the stent. Consequently, platelets can adhere to uncovered parts of the stent and initiate a thrombosis after the antiplatelet drugs have been discontinued. To avoid this problem, treatment with antiplatelet drugs usually is continued for at least a year when a drug-releasing stent is used, in order to allow adequate time for the more slowly growing drug-inhibited endothelial cells to cover the interior of the stent. Currently, both types of stents are used successfully, and the type used depends on the preference of the cardiologist performing the procedure.

Severe Myocardial Ischemia and Its Complications: A "Heart Attack"

Severe and prolonged myocardial ischemia may precipitate an acute episode called a "heart attack" (see FIGURE 30). This event may be manifested as either cessation of normal cardiac contractions, called a **cardiac arrest**, or an actual necrosis of heart muscle, which is termed a **myocardial infarction**. Any one of four basic mechanisms may trigger a heart attack in a patient with coronary artery disease.

Cardiac arrest
Complete cessation of cardiac activity.

Myocardial infarction
(mī-o-kar′dī-ul in-färk′ shun)
Necrosis of heart muscle as a result of interruption of its blood supply. May affect full thickness of muscle wall (transmural infarct) *or only part of the wall* (subendocardial infarct).

1. Sudden blockage of a coronary artery. Usually, this is cause by a blood clot that forms on the roughened surface of an ulcerated atheromatous plaque. This is called a coronary thrombosis. A less common cause of blockage is an obstruction of the lumen by atheromatous debris. This sometimes occurs if a break develops in the endothelium and fibrous tissue covering a plaque, allowing the contents of the plaque to be extruded and block the lumen (FIGURE 31A). An unstable atheromatous plaque (lacking a fibrous cap covering the plaque) is especially vulnerable to rupture, which disrupts the endothelium-lined surface of the artery. Platelets accumulate, followed by activation of the blood coagulation mechanism and formation of a thrombus at the site of plaque rupture (FIGURE 31B).
2. Hemorrhage into an atheromatous plaque. Bleeding into a plaque usually results from rupture of a small blood vessel in the arterial wall adjacent to the plaque. The blood seeping into the plaque causes it to enlarge, which further narrows or obstructs the lumen of the coronary artery.

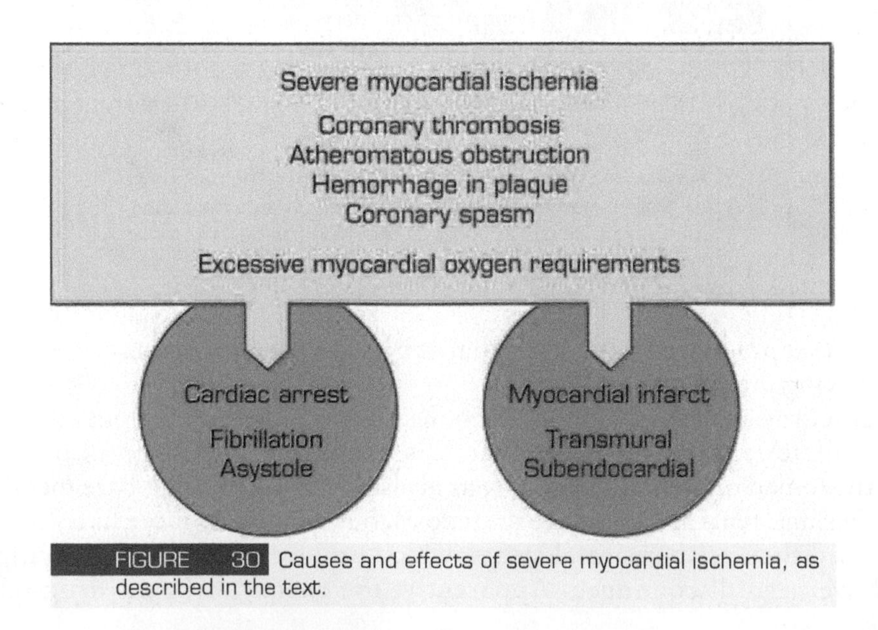

FIGURE 30 Causes and effects of severe myocardial ischemia, as described in the text.

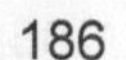

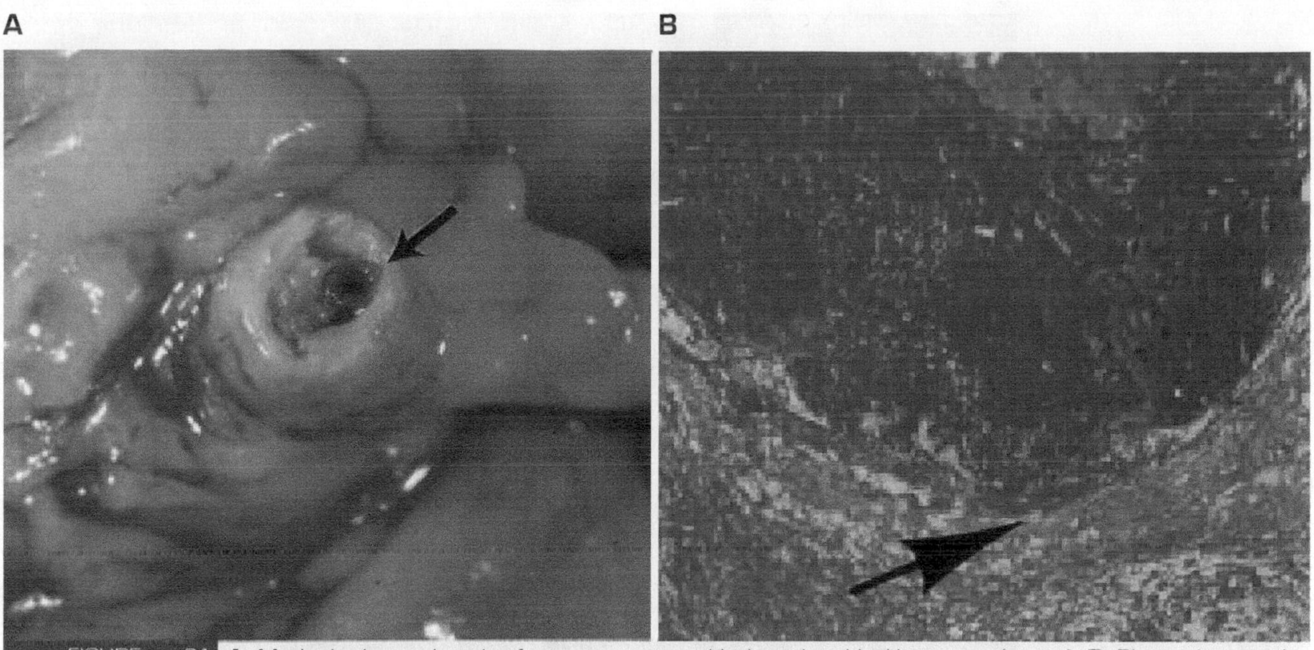

FIGURE 31 **A**, Marked atherosclerosis of coronary artery with thrombus blocking artery (*arrow*). **B**, Photomicrograph illustrating thrombosis of coronary artery at the site of a ruptured unstable atheromatous plaque. Note absence of fibrous tissue (*arrow*) covering the inner surface of the plaque.

3. Arterial spasm. A spasm of coronary arteries has been shown to occur adjacent to atheromatous plaques. This may be the mechanism that precipitates arterial obstruction in some patients with heart attacks.
4. Sudden greatly increased myocardial oxygen requirements. Vigorous activity such as running, snow shoveling, or tennis abruptly increases cardiac output, which in turn raises myocardial oxygen consumption. However, the sclerotic coronary arteries are incapable of delivering an adequate blood supply to the heart muscle, and severe myocardial ischemia develops.

Cardiac Arrest

Myocardial ischemia increases myocardial irritability, which may lead to disturbances of cardiac rhythm called cardiac **arrhythmias**. A cardiac arrest occurs when an arrhythmia induced by prolonged or severe myocardial ischemia disrupts the pumping of the ventricles. The most devastating arrhythmia is an uncoordinated quivering of the ventricles that is called ventricular fibrillation. It is the most common cause of cardiac arrest and sudden death in patients with coronary heart disease. Ventricular fibrillation is rapidly fatal because the normal pumping action of the ventricles ceases. If the condition is recognized promptly, it is often possible to stop the fibrillation by delivering an electric shock to the heart by means of electrodes applied to the chest. This procedure frequently causes the ventricles to resume normal contractions, but in many cases, ventricular fibrillation occurs without warning, and the patient dies before medical attention can be obtained. A less common cause of cardiac arrest is complete cessation of cardiac contractions, which is called asystole (*a* = without + *systole*).

Arrhythmia
(a-rith'mi-uh)
An irregularity of the heartbeat.

Myocardial Infarction

A myocardial infarct is a necrosis of heart muscle resulting from severe ischemia (FIGURE 32). It occurs when blood flow through one of the coronary arteries is insufficient to sustain the heart muscle and when collateral blood flow into the

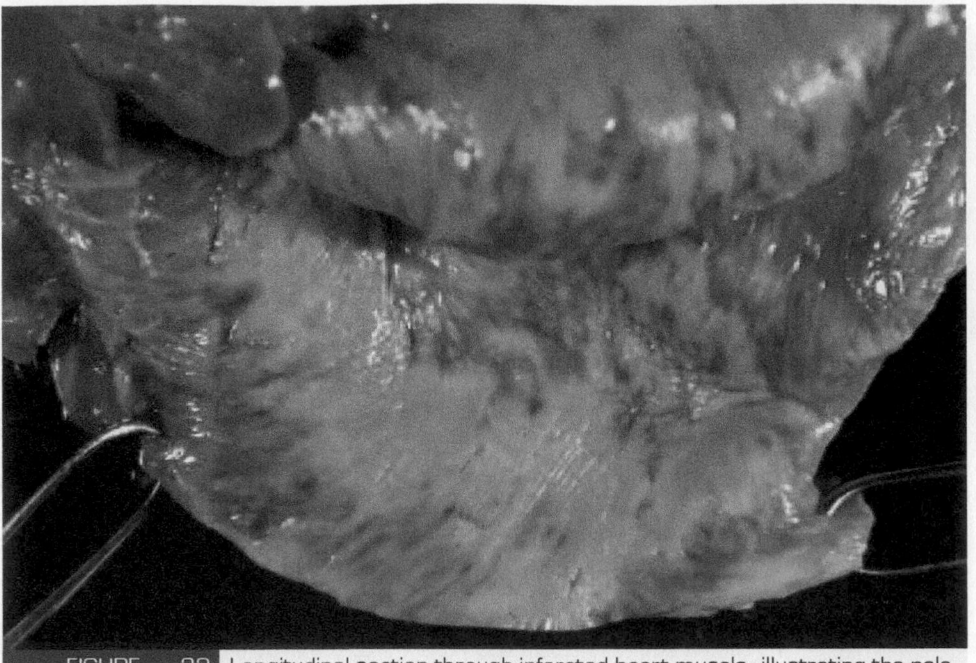

FIGURE 32 Longitudinal section through infarcted heart muscle, illustrating the pale zone of necrotic muscle that has been infiltrated by inflammatory cells.

ischemic muscle from other coronary arteries is inadequate. The infarction is usually associated with severe chest pain and often with shock and collapse.

The manifestations of a myocardial infarct results from partial to complete obstruction of a coronary artery, and prognosis is related to the amount of muscle damage, which often can be minimized by prompt treatment to restore blood flow to the damaged heart muscle.

An infarct may involve the full thickness of the muscular wall or only part of the wall. A full-thickness infarct extending from endocardium to epicardium is called a transmural infarct (*trans* = across + *muris* = wall) and is usually the result of thrombosis of a major coronary artery. If only a part of the wall undergoes necrosis, the term subendocardial infarct is used.

LOCATION OF MYOCARDIAL INFARCTS

Myocardial infarcts involve the muscle of the left ventricle and septum almost exclusively. Only rarely are the walls of the atria or right ventricle involved. This is because the left ventricle is much more vulnerable to interruption of its blood supply than are other parts of the heart. The left ventricular wall is much thicker than the walls of the other chambers, and it works much harder because it must pump blood at high pressure into the systemic circulation. Consequently, it requires a very rich blood supply. In contrast, the other chambers have much thinner walls, pump blood under much lower pressures, need a less abundant blood supply, and can usually "get by" by means of collateral blood flow if a major coronary artery is blocked.

The size and location of myocardial infarcts are determined by both the location of the obstructions in the coronary arteries and the amount of collateral blood flow. Generally, an obstruction of the left anterior descending artery leads to an infarct of the anterior wall and often of the adjacent anterior part of the interventricular septum as well. If the circumflex artery is blocked, it is usually the lateral wall that is damaged. Occlusion of the right coronary artery generally causes an infarction of the back wall of the left ventricle and adjacent posterior part of the interventricular septum. A block of the main left coronary artery, which fortunately is quite uncommon, causes an extensive infarction of both the anterior and the lateral walls of the left ventricle and is frequently fatal.

MAJOR COMPLICATIONS OF MYOCARDIAL INFARCTS

Patients who sustain a myocardial infarct are subject to a number of complications. The most important are

1. Disturbances of cardiac rhythm (arrhythmias)
2. Heart failure
3. Intracardiac thrombi
4. Cardiac rupture.

Complications are not inevitable, and prompt restoration of blood flow through the blocked artery can reduce the damage sustained by the heart muscle and improve the patient's prognosis.

Arrhythmias

Heart block
Delay or complete interruption of impulse transmission from the atria to the ventricles.

Disturbances of cardiac rhythm are common subsequent to a myocardial infarct. The arrhythmias result from the extreme irritability of the ischemic heart muscle adjacent to the infarct and can frequently be controlled by drugs that reduce myocardial irritability. The most serious arrhythmia is ventricular fibrillation, which leads to cessation of the circulation. Another type of disturbance of cardiac rhythm occurs if the conduction system of the heart is damaged by the infarct. Conduction of impulses from the atria to the ventricles may be disturbed, which is called a **heart block**. The conduction disturbance may subside spontaneously as the infarct heals, but sometimes it is necessary to insert various types of electrodes directly into the heart in order to stimulate the ventricles to contract properly. A device of this type is called a cardiac pacemaker.

Heart Failure

The ventricle may be so badly damaged that it is unable to maintain normal cardiac function, and the heart fails (Figure 32). Heart failure may develop abruptly (acute heart failure) or more slowly (chronic heart failure), as described in a subsequent section, and may be difficult to treat.

Intracardial Thrombi

If the infarct extends to involve the endocardium, thrombi may form on the interior of the ventricular wall and cover the damaged endocardial surface. This is called a mural thrombus (FIGURE 33). Bits of the thrombus may break loose and be carried as emboli into the systemic circulation, causing infarctions in the brain, kidneys, spleen, or other organs. Some physicians attempt to forestall this

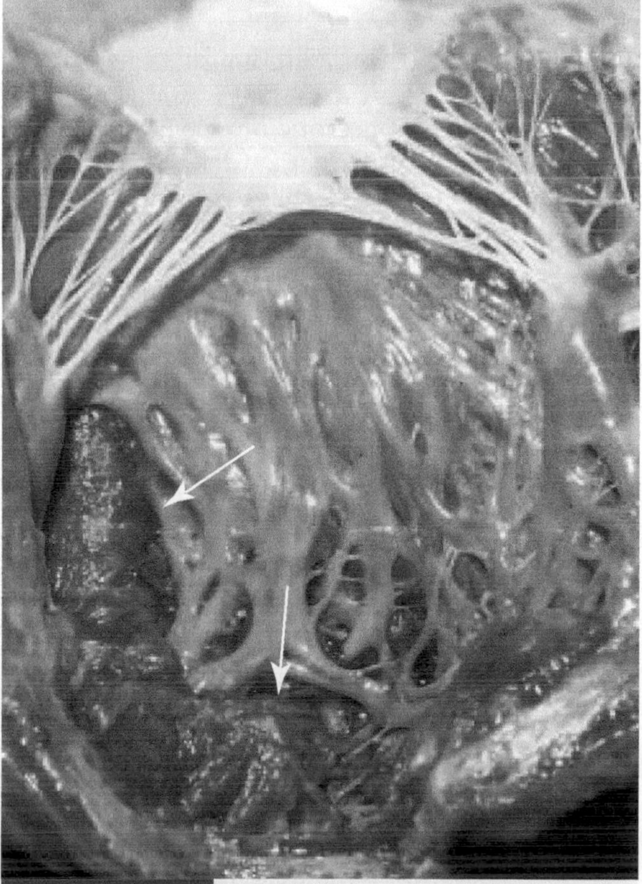

FIGURE 33 Interior of left ventricle, illustrating mural thrombus (*arrows*) adherent to endocardium adjacent to myocardial infarct. Normal mitral valve leaflets and chordae are seen on *top* of photograph.

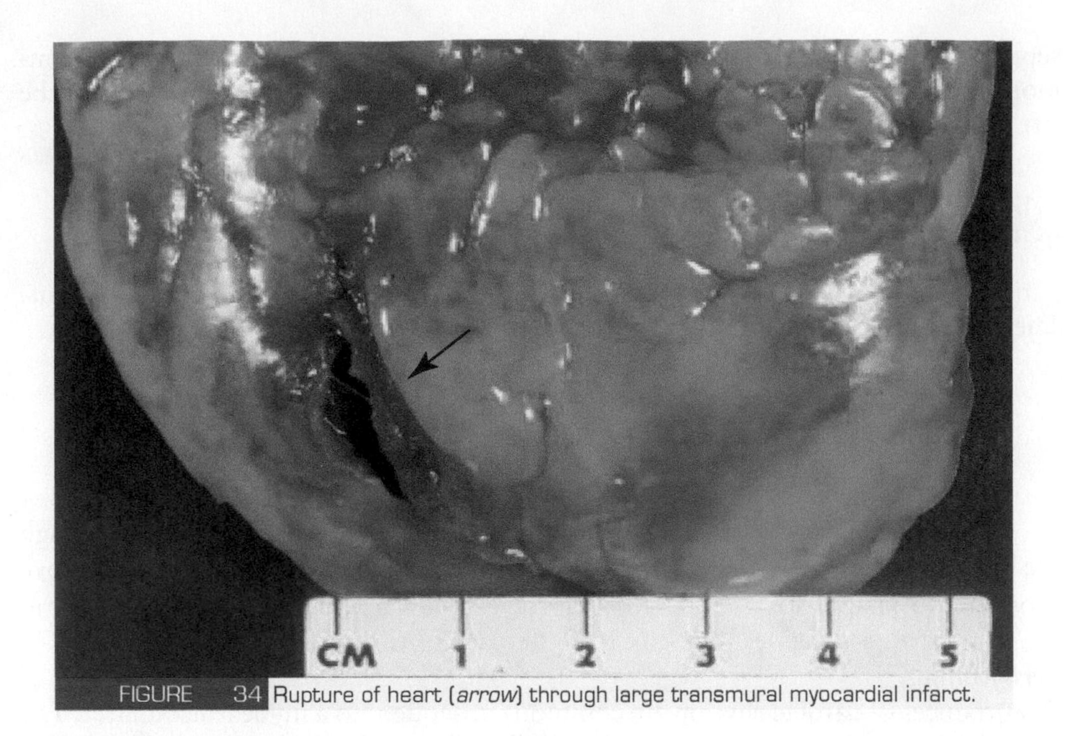

FIGURE 34 Rupture of heart (*arrow*) through large transmural myocardial infarct.

complication by administering anticoagulants when a patient has sustained a severe infarction.

Cardiac Rupture

If a patient sustains a transmural infarct, a perforation may occur through the necrotic muscle (FIGURE 34). This permits blood to leak through the rupture into the pericardial sac, and as the blood accumulates, it compresses the heart so the ventricles cannot fill in diastole. Eventually, the circulation ceases because the heart is no longer able to pump blood.

SURVIVAL AFTER MYOCARDIAL INFARCTION

The survival rate of patients who have had a myocardial infarct depends on many factors, the more important being (1) the size of the infarct, which is related to how rapidly the blood flow to the damaged muscle can be restored, (2) the patient's age, (3) the development of complications, and (4) the presence of other diseases that would adversely affect the patient's survival. Mortality rates vary from about 6% in patients who have had small infarcts and who do not develop heart failure to more than 50% in patients with large infarcts who develop severe heart failure. Major causes of death after myocardial infarction are fatal arrhythmia, heart failure, and cardiac rupture. Coronary care units staffed by specially trained personnel have reduced the mortality from cardiac arrhythmias, which are prone to occur in the first several days after myocardial infarction, but these facilities have not had any significant effect on the rates of death from heart failure or cardiac rupture.

If we consider all hospitalized patients as a group, about 95% survive and are able to leave the hospital. The data on survival, however, relate only to patients with myocardial infarction who are admitted to the hospital. They do not include patients with severe heart attacks who die suddenly or within a few hours. This is a significant number of patients because it is estimated that one-third of all deaths from heart attacks occur outside the hospital. On the other hand, the survival data also do not include patients with small infarcts that may not be detected clinically.

Many small myocardial infarcts cause relatively mild symptoms and heal without complications. The patients may ascribe the chest discomfort associated with the infarction to indigestion or other causes and never seek medical attention. Some studies indicate that as many as 25% of all patients with myocardial infarcts have very few symptoms and do not consult a physician.

DIAGNOSIS OF MYOCARDIAL INFARCTION

Diagnosis of myocardial infarction rests on evaluation and interpretation of the medical history, physical examination, and laboratory data. The clinical history may at times be inconclusive because severe angina may be quite similar to the pain of a myocardial infarction. Conversely, many patients who develop subendocardial myocardial infarcts may have minimal symptoms. Physical examination will usually not be abnormal unless the subject exhibits evidence of shock, heart failure, or a heart murmur as a result of papillary muscle dysfunction. Consequently, the physician must rely on specialized diagnostic studies to demonstrate infarction of heart muscle. The most helpful diagnostic aids are the electrocardiogram and determination of blood levels of various enzymes that leak from damaged heart muscle.

The Electrocardiogram

The **electrocardiogram** (ECG or EKG), which measures the transmission of electrical impulses associated with cardiac contraction, reveals rather characteristic abnormalities when heart muscle becomes infarcted. By means of the electrocardiogram, the physician can often determine the location and approximate size of the infarct. The process of healing can be followed by means of serial cardiograms. The electrocardiogram can also detect arrhythmias and various disturbances in the transmission of impulses through the cardiac conduction system.

Electrocardiogram (ē lek-trō-kär′dē-ō-gram) *A technique for measuring the serial changes in the electrical activity of the heart during the various phases of the cardiac cycle. (Often called ECG or EKG.)*

Blood Tests to Identify Cardiac Muscle Necrosis

Heart muscle is rich in proteins and enzymes that regulate the metabolic activities of cardiac muscle cells. When heart muscle is damaged, some of these components leak from the injured cells into the bloodstream, where they can be detected by laboratory tests on the blood of the affected patient. The most important proteins used as diagnostic tests of muscle necrosis are called troponin T and troponin I, which are not detectable in the blood of normal persons. Cardiac muscle damage causes the proteins to leak from the damaged cardiac muscle fibers.

Elevated troponin blood levels appear within 3 hours after muscle necrosis, with the highest levels attained within 24 hours, and the elevations persist as long as for 10 to 14 days. In general, the larger the infarct, the higher the troponin elevation and the longer it takes for the levels to return to normal. The pattern of rapid troponin rise and subsequent fall over the succeeding days is characteristic of myocardial necrosis. Troponin tests are so sensitive that even very small areas of muscle necrosis are sufficient to produce a positive test. Consequently, the troponin tests have become the preferred blood tests for evaluating patients with a suspected myocardial infarct because the tests can detect a very small area of heart muscle damage as well as a large myocardial infarct.

Another diagnostic test for heart muscle damage is measurement of the creatine phosphokinase (CK) enzyme present in heart muscle called CK-MB. The test is less sensitive than troponin tests but usually becomes positive when a large amount of heart muscle has been damaged. Consequently, the CK-MB has been used to assess the severity of the heart muscle damage. The original World Health Organization definition of a major myocardial infarction requires an elevated CK-MB test as well as an elevated troponin test result. Using both tests together was considered to help the clinician assess the extent of muscle damage because a small infarct which raises the sensitive troponin test may not elevate the less sensitive CK-MB test. Although the CK-MB is still used by some clinicians along with the troponin test, many cardiologists use only the troponin test as the preferred biochemical test of muscle necrosis. The test result is used in conjunction with the clinical features and the electrocardiogram to assess the patient's condition. Then this information is used to determine the most effective way to restore blood flow to the injured heart muscle.

THE ACUTE CORONARY SYNDROME CLASSIFICATION OF CORONARY ARTERY DISEASE: A GUIDE TO PROGNOSIS AND TREATMENT

This classification system assigns all patients with suspected inadequate blood flow to the heart muscle (myocardial ischemia) into three categories of progressively increasing severity based on the clinical manifestations, enzyme tests, and ECG findings under the general heading of *acute coronary syndromes*, often shortened to ACS. The term *myocardial infarction* is applied to any degree of heart muscle necrosis, which can vary from minor myocardial injury to extensive heart muscle damage resulting from complete obstruction of a large coronary artery. The categories, which also serves as a guide to prognosis and treatment, include (1) unstable angina without evidence of muscle necrosis, (2) non-ST segment elevation myocardial infarction, and (3) ST segment myocardial infarction.

Acute coronary syndromes
A classification of patients with coronary artery disease complaining of chest pain into one of three separate groups (unstable angina, non-ST elevation myocardial infarction, and ST elevation myocardial infarction) based on ECG and cardiac enzyme tests, used to assess prognosis and guide treatment.

The physician usually can assess the amount of heart muscle damage by correlating the changes in the ECG (FIGURE 35) and cardiac enzyme test results with the patient's clinical condition, which can be used to classify patients with chest pain into one of three groups called **acute coronary syndromes**. The information helps to guide proper treatment, and also provides an indication of the patient's prognosis (TABLE 3).

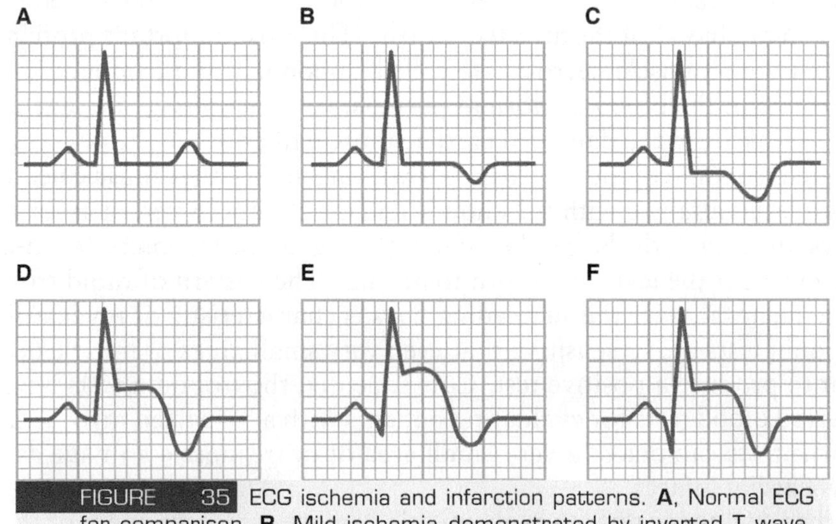

FIGURE 35 ECG ischemia and infarction patterns. **A**, Normal ECG for comparison. **B**, Mild ischemia demonstrated by inverted T wave. **C**, Moderate ischemia demonstrated by slight ST-segment depression and inverted T wave. **D** and **E**, ST-segment elevation myocardial infarction. **F**, ST-segment myocardial infarction with prominent Q wave indicating more severe myocardial damage. (Slightly modified from Garcia, T. B., and Holtz, N. E., 2003. *Introduction to 12-Lead ECG*. Boston: Jones and Bartlett Publishers.)

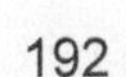

TABLE 3

Acute coronary syndrome (ACS) classification of coronary heart disease

Condition	ECG	Enzymes	Evaluation and treatment
Unstable angina	ST depression during angina returns to normal when angina subsides	Not elevated	Treat angina. May progress to minor myocardial damage. Consider adding anti-platelet and anticoagulant drugs. Minimize cardiovascular risk factors.
Non ST-segment elevation myocardial infarction	ST-segment depression	Troponin elevated. Creatine kinase not elevated, if test is performed.	Minor myocardial damage caused by atheromatous debris from ruptured coronary plaque blocking distal branches of artery, or artery partially blocked by thrombus. Treat with anticoagulant and antiplatelet drugs to keep artery open. Consider angioplasty (percutaneous coronary intervention) if anticoagulant-antiplatelet treatment is not successful.
ST-segment elevation myocardial infarction	ST-segment elevation	Troponin elevated. Creatine kinase also elevated if test is performed.	Artery completely blocked. Identify site of block by arteriogram and open blocked coronary artery preferably by angioplasty (percutaneous coronary intervention) as quickly as possible to salvage as much cardiac muscle as possible. If facilities not available for angioplasty, attempt to dissolve clot by thrombolytic drugs.

ST Segment Elevation Myocardial Infarction

Complete obstruction of a major coronary artery by a thrombus leads to a large transmural infarction. The extensive myocardial injury causes a characteristic elevation of the ST segment in the ECG, and is also associated with marked elevation of cardiac muscle enzymes that leak from the damaged muscle and can be detected in the bloodstream by laboratory tests. This type of myocardial infarct usually is named after its characteristic ECG pattern as a ST-segment elevation myocardial infarction, which sometimes is called by its acronym, STEMI.

A ST elevation myocardial infarction is a medical emergency and should be treated by an angioplasty or thrombolytic drugs to unblock the artery as soon as possible. The faster the blood flow can be restored through the blocked artery, the less severe the heart muscle damage and the better the prognosis.

Non-ST Segment Elevation Myocardial Infarction

Incomplete obstruction of a coronary artery causes less damage. The blood clot may not completely block the artery, or the atheromatous debris contained within a ruptured plaque may be extruded into the lumen and carried distally (downstream) to plug small arterioles and capillaries in the distribution of the ruptured plaque instead of completely occluding the artery. Some blood still flows to the damaged myocardium, which leads to a more favorable prognosis than a large transmural infarct. The ECG may show minor abnormalities but does not reveal the ST-segment elevation of a large infarct, and the rise of cardiac enzymes is less pronounced. The very sensitive troponin test result is elevated, but the less sensitive CK test result is normal.

Unstable Angina Without Evidence of Muscle Necrosis

Sometimes a patient with a history of stable angina begins to experience more severe chest pain, and it may be difficult clinically to determine whether the patient has unstable angina or is having a myocardial infarction. The ECG and enzyme tests will help make the distinction. The ECG may show minor abnormalities but does not show the ST-elevation pattern of a large infarct, and cardiac enzyme tests indicating muscle necrosis are not elevated. These features favor the diagnosis of unstable angina without evidence of muscle necrosis. The patient requires treatment with anti-angina drugs, but also anticoagulant and antiplatelet drugs, to prevent aggregation of platelets that may initiate a coronary thrombosis.

Restoring Blood Flow Through a Thrombosed Coronary Artery

Two different methods can be used to re-establish blood flow through a thrombosed coronary artery. Each has advantages and limitations. One method is thrombolytic (clot dissolving) treatment, which attempts to dissolve the clot, and the second is a procedure called percutaneous coronary intervention (often abbreviated PCI), which is another name for an angioplasty procedure that is used to open the artery and place a short expandable metal mesh tube called a stent at the site of the occlusion to hold the artery open. The angioplasty procedure is more effective than thrombolytic therapy, but requires a medical center staffed by personnel experienced with PCI procedures.

Thrombolytic Treatment

Thrombolytic therapy offers the advantage of ready availability. Any physician can perform the procedure in a hospital or emergency room setting, which is an advantage when there are no personnel available who are skilled in performing angioplasty procedures, and the additional time required to transfer the patient to a coronary care facility would delay attempting to open the artery and would lead to further myocardial necrosis. The disadvantages are that a significant number of patients are not suitable for thrombolytic therapy. The procedure is less effective than percutaneous coronary intervention, and in some patients may be complicated by a serious hemorrhage.

The thrombolytic method attempts to dissolve the clot by administering a thrombolytic (*thrombus* = clot + *lysis* = dissolving) drug intravenously. In many patients, good results are obtained and mortality is reduced if the drug can be given within 1 hour after the patient experiences the first symptoms of a heart attack.

The benefit of thrombolytic therapy decreases progressively as the time interval between coronary thrombosis and clot lysis lengthens. After about 6 hours, administration of a thrombolytic drug is of no benefit because by this time the heart muscle has progressed from ischemia to complete infarction, and it can no longer be salvaged by restoring blood flow through the occluded vessel.

Various thrombolytic drugs are available for intravenous administration. These include streptokinase and a more slowly acting streptokinase preparation and several preparations of tissue plasminogen activator. All act by converting plasminogen into plasmin, which is the fibrinolytic agent that dissolves the clot. (The coagulation and fibrinolytic mechanisms are described in the discussion on abnormalities of blood coagulation.) Each agent has advantages and disadvantages, and each is quite effective. Tissue plasminogen activator (TPA), which is produced commercially by recombinant DNA technology, is the same material that is normally produced by the endothelial cells of blood vessels to dissolve clots. It binds to the fibrin within the clot in the coronary artery, where it converts plasminogen into plasmin within the clot and dissolves the clot. Several types of TPA preparations are available.

Aspirin and heparin are often used along with thrombolytic agents. Aspirin reduces the tendency of platelets to aggregate and initiate the coagulation process at the site where the clot was dissolved. Heparin reduces the coagulability of the blood and decreases the likelihood that the clot will reform.

Although thrombolytic therapy improves survival and salvages myocardium, it also tampers with the body's coagulation mechanisms, and treatment may be complicated by serious bleeding episodes, including brain hemorrhage (hemorrhagic stroke) that can severely disable the patient or may even be fatal. Consequently, patients who are at greater than normal risk of hemorrhagic complications are not suitable candidates for thrombolytic therapy. In this group are (1) patients who have had a stroke or have any other disease affecting the cerebral blood vessels because they are at greater risk of a hemorrhagic stroke; (2) patients with severe hypertension, which increases the risk of a cerebral hemorrhage; (3) patients who have had a recent operation because the site of the operation may not be completely healed and may bleed if the clotting mechanism is disturbed; and (4) patients with any type of bleeding disorder or with any condition (such as a gastric or duodenal ulcer) in which thrombolytic therapy may precipitate bleeding.

Percutaneous Coronary Intervention (PCI)

The term percutaneous coronary intervention, often abbreviated as PCI, is used frequently to describe a coronary angioplasty (*angio* = vessel + *plasty* = molding), which is used to open a blocked coronary artery, and is the preferred method of treatment if the procedures can be performed by an experienced physician within 12 hours after onset of symptoms and within 90 minutes after the patient reaches the hospital or coronary care unit where PCI is to be performed. The procedure is quite similar to the angioplasty procedure used to dilate stenotic coronary arteries described previously and illustrated in FIGURE 29. The first step required to perform a PCI requires a coronary angiogram to identify the location of the blocked artery. A guiding catheter is introduced through the skin and into a large artery in the arm or leg, and threaded under fluoroscopic control to the openings of the coronary arteries at the base of the aorta. Next, a guidewire is inserted through the thrombus and atheromatous material that is obstructing blood flow through the artery. Then a balloon catheter covered by a collapsed expandable metal mesh tube called a stent is directed over the guide wire, passing through the clot and atheromatous debris obstructing blood flow through the artery. The balloon is inflated, which opens the artery and expands the stent to keep the artery open. Aspirin, heparin, and drugs that block platelet function are also given to prevent thrombus formation at the site of the reopened artery. Generally, blood flow through the artery can be restored in about 90% of the patients, as compared with dissolving the clot with thrombolytic drugs, which has only a 50 to 60% success rate. Unfortunately, although good flow is restored through the blocked artery, the PCI procedure may dislodge small bits of thrombus and atherosclerotic plaque debris from the arterial wall when the artery is opened, which is carried downstream to block small arterioles and capillaries. Consequently, blood flow to the heart muscle is reduced somewhat even though the flow through the artery has been restored. Coronary care units in many hospitals can evaluate a suspected myocardial infarction patient and proceed with a PCI if necessary in as little as 1 hour. Unfortunately, success of the PCI procedure depends on how long the artery has been obstructed before the patient reaches the coronary care unit, not on the elapsed time between the diagnosis and the treatment of a blocked coronary artery in the coronary care unit. Many patients delay seeking treatment for several hours after onset of symptoms, which reduces the chance of a successful outcome in patients with an ST elevation myocardial infarction caused by a completely blocked coronary artery.

The advantage of directly opening the blocked artery is the higher success rate when compared with thrombolytic therapy even though opening the artery does not always guarantee that the blood supply to the damaged heart muscle will be restored completely. The disadvantage is the need to reach a cardiac care facility staffed by highly trained personnel within a very short period of time. These facilities are readily available in large metropolitan communities but may not be easy to access in small communities or rural areas, and transferring the patient to a metropolitan coronary care unit consumes valuable time, which delays restoring blood flow through the blocked artery.

Nevertheless, transferring patients for PCI may still be advantageous, as demonstrated by a study involving 1,100 Canadian patients who were treated initially at a facility where PCI was not available. The patients were divided into two groups. The half underwent immediate transfer to a medical facility for angiography and PCI if needed. The other group received standard medical treatment for an acute myocardial infarction. The PCI patients did better than those receiving medical treatment. There were 11% deaths and infarct-related complications (coronary events) within the first 30 days after the infarction in the PCI group, which compared favorably with the 17% death and complication rate in the medical treatment group.

SUBSEQUENT TREATMENT AND PROGNOSIS OF MYOCARDIAL INFARCTION

After as much myocardium as possible has been salvaged by restoring flow through the occluded artery, further treatment of myocardial infarction consists of bed rest initially, gradually progressing to limited activity and then to full activity. Sometimes, the injured heart is quite irritable and prone to abnormal rhythms. Therefore, various drugs are often given to decrease the irritability of the heart muscle. Development of heart block may require insertion of a cardiac pacemaker. The patient who has sustained a myocardial infarction may develop intracardiac thrombi if the endocardium is injured or may develop thrombi in leg veins as a result of reduced activity. Therefore, some physicians also administer anticoagulant drugs to reduce the coagulability of the blood and thereby decrease the likelihood of thromboses and emboli. If the patient shows evidence of heart failure, various drugs are administered to sustain the failing heart.

Patients recovering from a myocardial infarct are at increased risk of sudden death from a fatal arrhythmia or another infarct, and the risk is greatest within the first 6 months after the infarct. The overall mortality rate within the first 30 days after a major myocardial infarction ranges from about 10% to as high as 25%, depending on the size of the infarct, the patient's condition, and any complications associated with the infarct. Many physicians treat postinfarct patients for at least 2 years with drugs that reduce myocardial irritability (called beta-blockers) because this seems to reduce the incidence of these postinfarct complications and improves survival. Ingesting a small amount of aspirin daily also is beneficial. As mentioned earlier, aspirin inhibits platelet function, making them less likely to adhere to roughened atheromatous plaques and initiate a thrombosis in the coronary artery. Some physicians also recommend insertion of a cardioverter-defibrillator in post-infarct patients considered at high risk of a cardiac arrest or fatal arrhythmia. The device continually monitors the patient's heart rhythm. If ventricular fibrillation or other life-threatening arrhythmia is detected, the device automatically administers an electric shock to terminate the arrhythmia.

Case Studies

The following three cases illustrate some of the clinical features and complications of myocardial infarctions.

CASE 3

A 74-year-old man was admitted to the emergency room because of severe oppressive chest pain of about 5 hours' duration. For the previous 2 weeks, he had also experienced episodes of less severe chest pain when he walked rapidly, but the pain soon subsided when he rested.

Physical examination revealed an older man in no acute distress. Heart sounds were normal. Lungs were clear. Blood pressure was 190/110 (normal about 120/80). Electrocardiogram showed the pattern of acute ST elevation myocardial infarction involving the anterior wall of the left ventricle.

Laboratory studies revealed elevated cardiac enzymes troponin and CK-MB.

Soon after admission, his blood pressure fell precipitously as a result of the severe myocardial damage, and the cardiac monitor recorded ventricular fibrillation. Resuscitative measures were unsuccessful.

An autopsy revealed severe arteriosclerosis of all coronary arteries. The left anterior descending coronary artery was occluded by a thrombus, and there was a large transmural anterolateral myocardial infarction. A myocardial perforation at the apex had permitted blood to fill the pericardial sac.

CASE 4

A 57-year-old man was admitted to the hospital from his place of employment. While at work he complained of a sweaty feeling and then lost consciousness. When he regained consciousness, he noted a constant, oppressive, substernal pain. In the preceding month, he had experienced similar episodes of substernal pain that would last for several minutes and disappear spontaneously. The pain was associated with a feeling of numbness in the arms. The patient had sustained a myocardial infarction 2 years earlier.

Physical examination and blood pressure were normal. An electrocardiogram showed changes of acute myocardial infarction involving the anterior wall and interventricular septum.

Soon after admission, his blood pressure dropped precipitously and the cardiac monitor recorded ventricular fibrillation. Resuscitation was unsuccessful.

The autopsy revealed old scarring in the posterior wall and the posterior portion of the interventricular septum in the distribution of the right coronary artery. There was a recent area of infarction in the anterior and lateral wall and in the anterior portion of the interventricular septum in the distribution of the anterior descending left coronary artery. The coronary arteries showed a variable degree of arteriosclerosis. The main left and circumflex arteries showed from 35 to 50% narrowing. The anterior descending left artery was 85 to 90% narrowed but was not occluded. The right coronary artery was occluded by old thrombus material that extended within the vessel for a distance of 7 to 8 cm. Lungs exhibited marked pulmonary edema.

CASE 5

A 52-year-old man experienced an episode of severe precordial pain associated with nausea and vomiting. He attributed this to indigestion and did not consult a physician. He remained at home on restricted activity but felt quite weak and experienced periodic episodes of sweating and chest pain. Eventually, he was able to be up and about around the house and felt somewhat better. While eating supper 2 weeks later, he experienced a sudden onset of weakness in the right arm and difficulty with speech. When he attempted to get up from the table, his right leg did not support him and he fell to the floor.

On admission to the hospital, he exhibited a paralysis of the right side of the body. His blood pressure was elevated (210/110). The remainder of the physical examination was normal.

The electrocardiogram showed the pattern of a recent anterior-wall myocardial infarction. Serum cardiac enzyme studies on admission, at 24 hours, and at 48 hours were all within normal limits because the myocardial infarct had occurred 2 weeks earlier. The elevated levels of enzyme activity had returned to normal by the time the patient entered the hospital.

The patient's disorder was treated as a recent myocardial infarction. A mural thrombus had apparently formed in the left ventricle at the site of the infarct. A piece of the clot had broken loose and had been carried as an embolus to the brain, where it had obstructed a cerebral artery and caused the paralysis. He made a satisfactory recovery but was left with some residual weakness and speech difficulty.

Additional Factors Influencing Cardiovascular Disease Risk

TAKING ASPIRIN TO REDUCE THE RISK OF CARDIOVASCULAR DISEASE

Aspirin is now widely used in clinical medicine to reduce the risk of heart attacks and strokes. Aspirin works by interfering with platelet function (discussion on abnormalities of blood coagulation). Aspirin permanently inactivates (acetylates) a platelet enzyme needed to produce a chemical compound called thromboxane A_2 that is released by platelets when they adhere to a roughened surface, which causes platelets to clump together and start the clotting process. Blocking platelet function by taking aspirin reduces the likelihood that platelets will adhere to the roughened surface of an atherosclerotic plaque in a coronary or cerebral artery and cause a blood clot to plug the artery.

Aspirin is rapidly absorbed from the stomach and small intestine. Peak levels are obtained in the blood within about 20 minutes after aspirin is ingested, and some inhibition of platelet function can be detected within an hour after the drug is taken. Although not all patients respond uniformly to the beneficial antiplatelet effects of aspirin, the platelets of most persons are extremely sensitive to aspirin. As little as 30 mg per day (less than one-half a baby aspirin) inactivates thromboxane A_2 production, which persists for the entire 10-day life span of the platelets. Because about 10% of the circulating platelets are replaced every 24 hours, after about 10 days almost no functionally normal platelets are present in the circulation.

Although taking aspirin to inactivate platelet function reduces the risk of cardiovascular disease as well as strokes caused by blood clots in cerebral blood vessels, aspirin use to reduce the risk of heart attacks slightly increases the risk of bleeding in the brain if the person does have a stroke.

COCAINE-INDUCED ARRHYTHMIAS AND MYOCARDIAL INFARCTS

Cocaine has very powerful effects on the cardiovascular system, and as the recreational use of cocaine has increased in recent years, so has the number of cocaine-related cardiac deaths.

The drug prolongs and intensifies the effects of sympathetic nerve impulses that regulate the heart and blood vessels. As a result, the heart beats faster and more forcefully, thereby increasing myocardial oxygen requirements. The heart muscle becomes more irritable, which predisposes to arrhythmias, and the peripheral arterioles constrict, which raises the blood pressure. Cocaine also constricts the coronary arteries and may induce coronary artery spasm, which leads to severe myocardial ischemia and may be followed by a myocardial infarction. Cocaine-related fatal arrhythmias and myocardial infarcts may occur in persons with normal coronary arteries, and cocaine users who already have some degree of coronary atherosclerosis are at even greater risk.

BLOOD LIPIDS AND CORONARY ARTERY DISEASE

The level of lipids in the blood has been shown to be an important factor in the pathogenesis of coronary atherosclerosis. The lipids of clinical importance are neutral fat (triglyceride) and cholesterol.

Neutral Fat

Chemically, a fat (triglyceride) is composed of three molecules of fatty acid combined with glycerol. A fatty acid consists of a long chain of carbon atoms joined together by shared (covalent) bonds. The end carbon in each fatty acid chain forms the carboxyl group (COOH), which is the acid group of organic molecules. Glycerol is a three-carbon alcohol containing a hydroxyl group (OH) attached to each carbon molecule. The carboxyl groups of the fatty acids are linked to the hydroxyl groups of glycerol, with loss of a molecule of water, in a linkage called an ester (FIGURE 36A).

A carbon atom has a valence of four, meaning that there are four sites on the carbon atom at which it can combine with other atoms. In the carbon chain of a fatty acid, each carbon atom in the chain is joined to the two adjacent carbon atoms by either a single or double covalent bond, and the remaining bonds are connected to hydrogen atoms.

A fat may be classified as saturated or unsaturated. In a saturated fat, each carbon atom in the chain is joined to the two adjacent carbon atoms, each by a single covalent bond, and the other two bonding sites are occupied by hydrogen atoms (FIGURE 36B). The three fatty acids attached to glycerol form long straight symmetrical molecules "packed" closely together and parallel to one another. This configuration gives rise to a compact, relatively dense fat molecule, which is why saturated fats have a high melting point and are solid at room temperature. Most animal fats such as butter, lard, and beef products are saturated fats.

Most vegetable oils and fats found in fish and poultry are unsaturated. In an unsaturated fat at least one of the three fatty acids in the molecule has a double bond between two adjacent carbon atoms in the carbon chain instead of a single bond, and the two carbon atoms flanking the double bond have only a single attached hydrogen atom instead of two, as in a saturated fat. If the fatty acid molecules contain more than one double bond, the term polyunsaturated fat is used. In almost all naturally occurring unsaturated fats, the hydrogen atoms attached to the carbons flanking the double bond are located on the same side of the carbon chain, which is called a cis configuration (FIGURE 36C).This arrangement "unbalances" the symmetry of the carbon chain and causes the chain to bend sharply at the double bond, which requires the bent chain to occupy more space in the triglyceride molecule (FIGURE 36E). Consequently, the fatty acids in the triglyceride molecule are less closely packed together and occupy more space than the molecules in a saturated fat, which is why unsaturated fats have a lower melting point and are liquid rather than solid at room temperature.

Trans Fats

A trans fat is unsaturated fat in which the hydrogen atoms attached to the carbons flanking the double bond in a fatty acid molecule are located on opposite sides of the carbon chain (FIGURE 36D), which is called a trans configuration (*trans* = across) and causes the carbon chain to maintain a more straight-line configuration, similar to that of a saturated fat instead of bending sharply at the double bond, which causes the fatty acid to adopt a straight-line configuration similar to that of a saturated fat (FIGURE 36F). Almost all trans fats are produced artificially by partial hydrogenation of vegetable oils at high temperature and pressure using a catalyst to facilitate the reaction. Partial hydrogenation adds hydrogen atoms to some of the double bonds that are converted to single bonds, but also changes many of the bonds from cis to trans configuration without hydrogenating the bonds, and may also change the location of some of the double bonds. The cis-to-trans change at the double bonds converts the bent fatty acid chains to straight chains, which causes the fatty acid molecules to resemble those in a saturated fat, and also changes a vegetable oil to a semisolid fat.

We know now that trans fats are "bad fats" because of their harmful effects on blood lipids. They are much more atherogenic (predisposing to atherosclerosis) than saturated fats and should be avoided as much as possible in our diets.

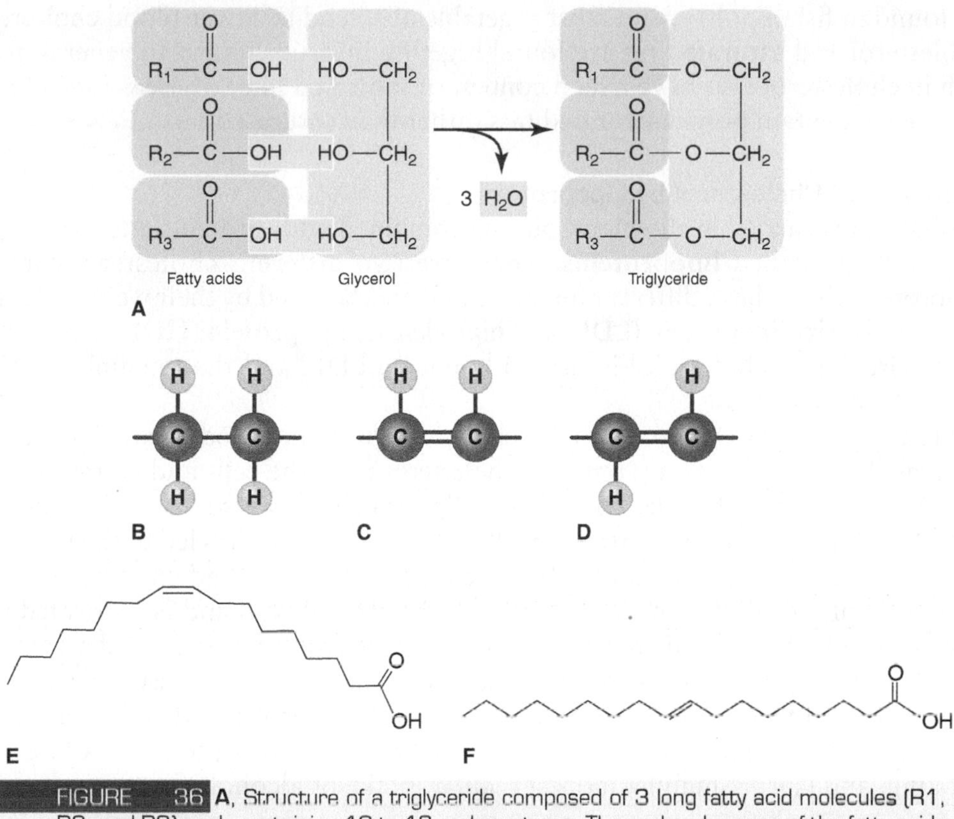

FIGURE 36 **A**, Structure of a triglyceride composed of 3 long fatty acid molecules (R1, R2, and R3) each containing 16 to 18 carbon atoms. The carboxyl groups of the fatty acids are joined to glycerol with loss of water molecules to form the triglyceride. **B**, Single bonds join carbon atoms in the triglyceride molecules of a saturated fat. **C**, Double bond in an unsaturated fat in which the hydrogen atoms are on the same side of the chain (cis configuration). **D**, Double bond in an unsaturated fat in which the hydrogen atoms are on opposite sides of the chain (trans configuration). **E**, Representation of the bent fatty acid chain at the site of a cis position double bond. **F**, Representation of the straight fatty acid chain structure caused by the trans position double bond, which is similar to the chains in a saturated fat.

High levels of neutral fat (along with cholesterol) in the blood promote atherosclerosis. Carbohydrate is converted readily into fat in the body, and much of the blood triglyceride is derived not from ingested fat but from ingested carbohydrate. In clinical medicine, most examples of high blood triglycerides can be traced to diets excessively high in carbohydrate. Sugar has been found to be more potent in elevating blood triglycerides than the more complex carbohydrates derived from cereals and other starches.

Cholesterol

Cholesterol is a complex carbon compound containing several ring structures and is classified as a sterol. Most cholesterol is present in the body in combination with fatty acids as cholesterol esters. Cholesterol is synthesized in the body and is also present in many foods. Normally, cholesterol is excreted in the bile into the gastrointestinal tract.

Much evidence indicates that a high dietary intake of cholesterol leads to high levels of blood cholesterol and premature atherosclerosis. Americans subsist on a diet relatively high in cholesterol; they also have one of the highest rates of death from coronary heart disease. In contrast, other populations whose diet is much lower in cholesterol have much lower rates of death from coronary heart disease.

The level of blood cholesterol is influenced not only by the amount of cholesterol in the diet, but also by the type of dietary fat. Saturated fats, the type found in meats and dairy products, tend to raise blood cholesterol, whereas unsaturated fats, which are found in fish, poultry, and most vegetable oils, tend to lower blood cholesterol. Cholesterol and saturated fat are found together in many foods. In general, foods high in cholesterol also have a high content of saturated fats, whereas foods low in cholesterol contain polyunsaturated fats rather than saturated fats.

Transport of Cholesterol by Lipoproteins

Lipoproteins
A lipid-protein complex that transports cholesterol and triglycerides in the blood stream to various locations throughout the body.

Low-density lipoprotein (LDL) cholesterol (li-pō-prō′tēn kō-les′ter-all)
The fraction of cholesterol carried by low-density lipoproteins, which is correlated with atherosclerosis.

High-density lipoprotein (HDL) cholesterol (li-pō-prō′tēn kō-les′ter-ol)
The fraction of cholesterol carried by high-density lipoprotein, which is correlated with protection against atherosclerosis.

Cholesterol is carried in the blood plasma combined with proteins and other lipids as complexes called **lipoproteins.** There are two different cholesterol-carrying lipoproteins. They have different functions and are classified by their weight (density) into **low-density lipoprotein** (**LDL**) and **high-density lipoprotein** (**HDL**). About 80% of the circulating cholesterol is carried bound to LDL, and the remaining 20% is transported by HDL.

The function of LDL is to transport cholesterol from the bloodstream into the cells, whereas the HDL apparently removes cholesterol from the cells and carries it to the liver for excretion in the bile. High-density lipoprotein may also "tie up" cholesterol so that it cannot infiltrate the arterial wall (FIGURE 37). This has led to the belief that there is a "bad cholesterol" and a "good cholesterol." The "bad cholesterol" is the fraction bound to LDL, which can infiltrate the arterial wall and is correlated with atherosclerosis. The "good cholesterol" is the cholesterol fraction carried attached to HDL, and elevations of this cholesterol fraction actually protect against coronary heart disease. Several factors are known to raise HDL cholesterol and thereby reduce risk of coronary heart disease. These factors include regular exercise, cessation of cigarette smoking, and (surprisingly) a modest regular intake of alcoholic beverages.

Alteration of Blood Lipids by Change in Diet

Various studies have demonstrated that the levels of both cholesterol and triglycerides in the blood can be lowered by dietary change. These studies have also demonstrated that individuals maintained on a modified diet have a lower incidence of coronary artery disease than a comparable group subsisting on an average American diet.

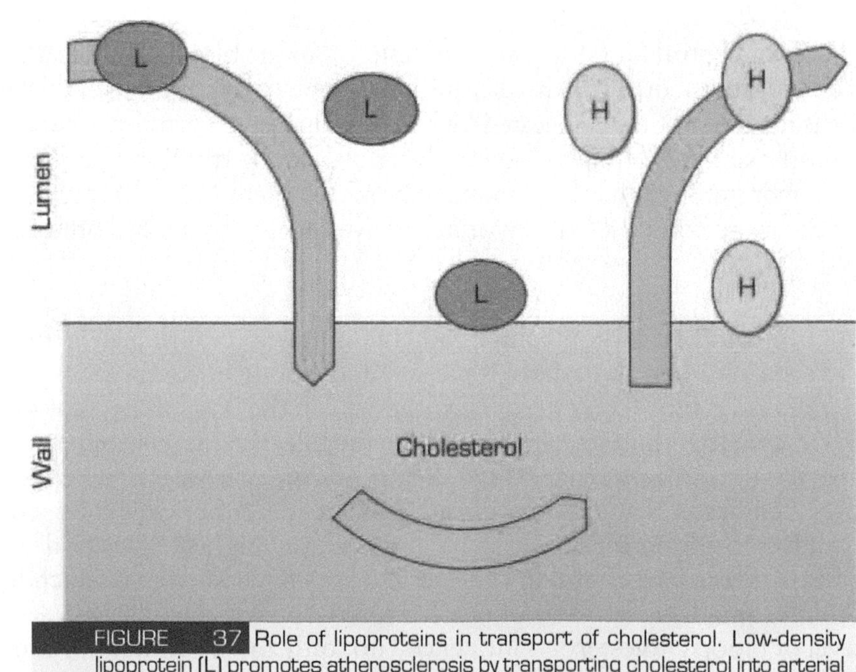

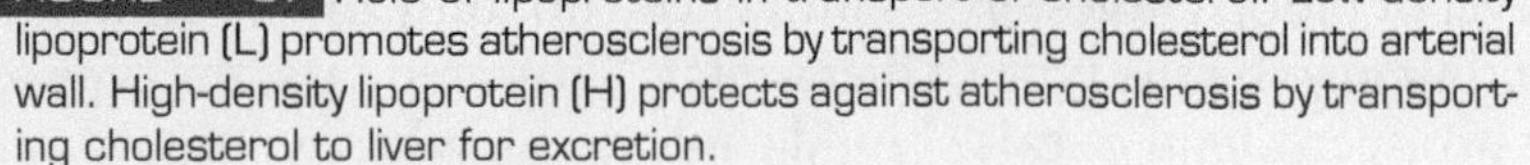
FIGURE 37 Role of lipoproteins in transport of cholesterol. Low-density lipoprotein (L) promotes atherosclerosis by transporting cholesterol into arterial wall. High-density lipoprotein (H) protects against atherosclerosis by transporting cholesterol to liver for excretion.

The diet (often called an "anti-coronary" diet) is modified by decreasing the amount of cholesterol and saturated fat and substituting foods containing polyunsaturated fats. This involves restricting the intake of animal fat and substituting fish and poultry. Carbohydrates are derived primarily from starches and cereals. The consumption of sugar and foods rich in sugar (pies, cakes, candies) is reduced. Alcohol consumption is restricted but not forbidden because of its favorable effect on HDL levels, which seems to protect against coronary heart disease. In addition to raising HDL, modest alcohol intake also helps protect against heart attacks by raising the level of circulating tissue plasminogen activator. This substance, which is one of the body's physiologic clot-dissolving components, is produced by the endothelial cells of blood vessels and diffuses into the circulation. Blood containing a higher concentration of tissue plasminogen activator has increased fibrinolytic activity. Consequently, any small clots that begin to form over atheromatous plaques in coronary arteries would be dissolved by the body's own tissue plasminogen activator before the clots become large enough to occlude the vessel.

Modifying the typical American diet is difficult because it requires breaking old dietary habits. However, some change in diet is desirable because it will significantly reduce the incidence of coronary artery disease. An "anti-coronary" diet is essential for individuals who have high levels of blood lipids because they run a greatly increased risk of death or disability from coronary artery disease.

It should be emphasized that the factors influencing the development of atherosclerosis are complex; an elevated level of blood lipids is only one of many factors concerned with atherogenesis. A number of other conditions, among them obesity, hypertension, cigarette smoking, and genetic factors, also predispose individuals to atherosclerosis.

C-REACTIVE PROTEIN AS A RISK FACTOR FOR CARDIOVASCULAR DISEASE

C-reactive protein (CRP) is one of several proteins produced by the liver and released into the bloodstream in response to tissue injury or inflammation. The protein is one of the body's nonspecific defenses against infection and also provides some protection against the harmful effects of inflammation by neutralizing various products produced by the cells that accumulate at the site of the inflammation. Measurement of CRP has been used for many years to monitor the activity of diseases associated with inflammation such as rheumatic fever and rheumatoid arthritis.

Recently, very sensitive tests have been developed that can detect slight CRP elevations in persons who do not appear to have evidence of an inflammatory or infectious disease. Several studies have demonstrated that an elevated CRP level in an otherwise normal person predicts an increased long-term risk of cardiovascular disease, probably because the elevated CRP is detecting the accumulation of macrophages, lymphocytes, lipids, and products of tissue injury within unstable plaques in coronary arteries. The CRP test has been proposed as an additional screening test to detect persons at risk of coronary artery disease, who then can be offered treatment to reduce their risk factors.

THE METABOLIC SYNDROME AND CARDIOVASCULAR DISEASE

The **metabolic syndrome,** which is also called the syndrome of insulin resistance, is a group of conditions and laboratory abnormalities that leads to development of cardiovascular disease and type 2 diabetes (described in the discussion on the pancreas and diabetes mellitus). The condition is characterized by obesity with concentration of fat around the abdomen (a waist circumference of over 40 in. in men and over

Metabolic syndrome
A group of conditions consisting of obesity, hypertension, elevated blood glucose and blood lipids, which predisposes to cardiovascular disease and diabetes.

35 in. in women, called an "apple shape" body configuration), hypertension, impaired carbohydrate tolerance that may progress to type 2 diabetes, and lipid abnormalities that predispose to coronary artery disease. The condition is estimated to affect about 23% of the adult population in the United States, and about half of those affected also have type 2 diabetes mellitus. Treatment consists of weight loss, a low-calorie and low-cholesterol diet, regular exercise, and appropriate drugs to treat lipid abnormalities and hypertension. Hopefully, treatment will prevent or slow the progression of cardiovascular disease and diabetes in persons with the metabolic syndrome.

HOMOCYSTEINE AND CARDIOVASCULAR DISEASE

Homocysteine is a sulfur-containing amino acid formed enzymatically from methionine, an essential amino acid that is abundant in animal protein. Homocysteine is then metabolized by other biochemical pathways in which vitamin B_6, vitamin B_{12}, and folic acid are required. Blood concentrations of homocysteine are higher in men than in premenopausal women but increase in women after the menopause. Renal function also influences homocysteine blood levels, which are elevated in persons with kidney disease.

Abnormal homocysteine metabolism is characteristic of a rare hereditary disease called *homocystinuria*. The disease results from a gene mutation leading to an enzyme defect that impairs the normal metabolism of homocysteine. Affected persons have an extremely high concentration of homocysteine in their blood and excrete the amino acid in their urine. The affected persons show evidence of marked vascular disease, which has its onset at a very young age. These manifestations include arteriosclerosis of coronary arteries and other major arteries, strokes, and blood clots in arteries and veins.

Because of the relationship of elevated homocysteine and premature vascular disease in persons with homocystinuria, investigators studied the relationship of homocysteine blood levels to cardiovascular disease in large groups of people. Numerous clinical studies have demonstrated that many persons with cardiovascular disease, strokes, and peripheral vascular disease have elevated homocysteine blood levels, and a high homocysteine blood level is a risk factor for arteriosclerosis, comparable to the increased risk associated with hypercholesterolemia, smoking, and hypertension.

In most persons in whom renal function is normal, the elevated homocysteine level seems to be related to a deficiency of vitamin B_6, vitamin B_{12}, or folic acid and can be corrected by vitamin supplements. A significant proportion of the population consumes insufficient amounts of both vitamin B_6 and folic acid.

Since vitamin B and folic acid supplements lower homocysteine blood levels, additional studies were undertaken to determine whether therapy with vitamin B_6, B_{12}, and folic acid would benefit patients with coronary artery disease who had already had a myocardial infarct. A large group of patients with severe cardiovascular disease received homocysteine-lowering vitamin therapy, and their outcomes were compared with a similar group of patients who did not receive vitamins. The homocysteine levels of the vitamin-treated group declined, but vitamin therapy did not reduce their risk of recurrent myocardial infarction or death from cardiovascular disease when compared with the untreated group. Moreover, the risk of a recurrent myocardial infarction was slightly higher in the vitamin-treated group, possibly because folic acid promotes cell proliferation and may have increased the size of some plaques by stimulating proliferation of cells within the plaques. Consequently, supplementary folic acid is no longer recommended for patients who have had a recent myocardial infarct. Supplementary folic acid is probably also inadvisable for patients who have had a stent inserted in one or more of their coronary arteries because cell proliferation in the arterial wall adjacent to the stent may encroach on the lumen of the stented artery and possibly lead to stenosis of the stented artery.

Hypertension and Hypertensive Cardiovascular Disease

PRIMARY HYPERTENSION

The ideal normal blood pressure should be below 120/80. A pressure consistently higher than 140/90 is called hypertension, and the higher the pressure, the greater are its harmful effects. Most cases of hypertension result from excessive vasoconstriction of the small arterioles throughout the body, which raises the diastolic pressure. Because of the high peripheral resistance, the heart needs to pump more forcefully in order to overcome the resistance created by the constricted arterioles and supply adequate blood to the tissues, which leads to a compensatory rise in systolic blood pressure. Therefore, both systolic and diastolic pressure rise when the primary problem is excessive arteriolar vasoconstriction. We do not really understand all of the factors responsible for this condition, which is called primary hypertension or essential hypertension, but we know that severe hypertension exerts injurious effects not only on the heart, but also on the blood vessels and kidneys.

Cardiac Effects

The heart responds to the increased workload resulting from the high peripheral resistance by becoming enlarged. Although the enlarged heart may be able to function effectively for many years, the cardiac pump is being forced to work beyond its "rated capacity." Eventually, the heart can no longer maintain adequate blood flow, and the patient develops symptoms of cardiac failure.

Vascular Effects

Because the blood vessels are not designed to carry blood at such a high pressure, the vessels wear out prematurely. Hypertension accelerates the development of atherosclerosis in the larger arteries. The arterioles also are injured; they thicken and undergo degenerative changes, and their lumens become narrowed. This process is termed **arteriolosclerosis**. Sometimes the walls of the small arterioles become completely necrotic owing to the effects of the sustained high blood pressure. Weakened arterioles may rupture, leading to hemorrhage. The brain is particularly vulnerable, cerebral hemorrhage being a relatively common complication of severe hypertension.

Arteriolosclerosis
(är-tēr-ē-óĺo-skler-ō′-sis)
One type of arteriosclerosis characterized by thickening and degeneration of small arterioles.

Renal Effects

The narrowing of the renal arterioles decreases the blood supply to the kidneys, which, in turn, leads to injury and degenerative changes in the glomeruli and renal tubules. Severe hypertension may cause severe derangement of renal function and eventually leads to renal failure.

SECONDARY HYPERTENSION

In a small proportion of patients, the hypertension results from a known disease or condition such as chronic kidney disease (discussion on the urinary system), endocrine gland dysfunction such as a pituitary or an adrenal tumor, or a hyperactive thyroid gland (discussion on the endocrine glands). The high blood pressure associated with these conditions is called secondary hypertension because the cause of the hypertension is known. In many cases, successful treatment of the underlying condition cures the hypertension.

ISOLATED SYSTOLIC HYPERTENSION

As the name implies, isolated systolic hypertension is characterized by a mild to moderately elevated systolic pressure with a normal or even lower than normal diastolic pressure. This condition occurs primarily in older adults because the aorta and major arteries become less flexible with age. Consequently, when blood is ejected into the aorta during ventricular systole, the more rigid arteries are less able to stretch and absorb some of the force of the ejected blood. As a result, the systolic pressure is higher than it would be if the vessels were more flexible. The diastolic pressure remains normal because there is no excessive arteriolar vasoconstriction. Previously, this condition was considered to be less serious than hypertension in which both pressures were higher than normal, but unfortunately, more recent studies have demonstrated that isolated systolic hypertension causes the same harmful effects on the heart and blood vessels as primary and secondary hypertension.

TREATMENT OF HYPERTENSION

Although the reason for the hypertension cannot be determined in most instances, the blood pressure can be reduced to more normal levels, thereby lowering risk of complications of high blood pressure. This is accomplished by administering various drugs that lower the blood pressure by lessening the vasoconstriction of the peripheral blood vessels. This same approach is used to treat isolated systolic hypertension. Even though the cause of this condition is related to aging and increased rigidity of larger arteries, the same types of drugs used to treat primary and secondary hypertension are also effective.

Primary Myocardial Disease

In a small number of patients, heart disease results not from valvular or coronary disease or hypertension but from primary disease of the heart muscle itself. There are two major types of primary myocardial disease. One type results from inflammation of heart muscle and is called myocarditis. The other type, in which there is no evidence of inflammation, is designated by the noncommittal term cardiomyopathy (*cardio* = heart + *myo* = muscle + *pathy* = disease).

MYOCARDITIS

Myocarditis is characterized by an active inflammation in the heart muscle associated with injury and necrosis of individual muscle fibers. In the United States, most cases are caused by viruses. A few are caused by parasites, such as *Trichinella* (discussion on animal parasites) that lodge in the myocardium and cause an inflammation. Occasionally, other pathogens such as *Histoplasma* are responsible, especially in immunocompromised patients. Some cases are the result of a hypersensitivity reaction such as the myocarditis occurring in acute rheumatic fever.

The onset of myocarditis is usually abrupt and may lead to acute heart failure. Fortunately, in most cases, the inflammation subsides completely and the patient recovers without any permanent heart damage. There is no specific treatment other than treating the underlying condition that caused the myocarditis and decreasing cardiac work by bed rest and limited activity while the inflammation subsides.

CARDIOMYOPATHY

The general term cardiomyopathy encompasses two different conditions: dilated cardiomyopathy and hypertrophic cardiomyopathy. Both conditions are hereditary and transmitted as dominant traits. Often, the responsible gene mutations can be identified by genetic tests. Dilated cardiomyopathy is characterized by enlargement of the heart and dilatation of its chambers. The pumping action of the ventricles is greatly impaired which leads to chronic heart failure.

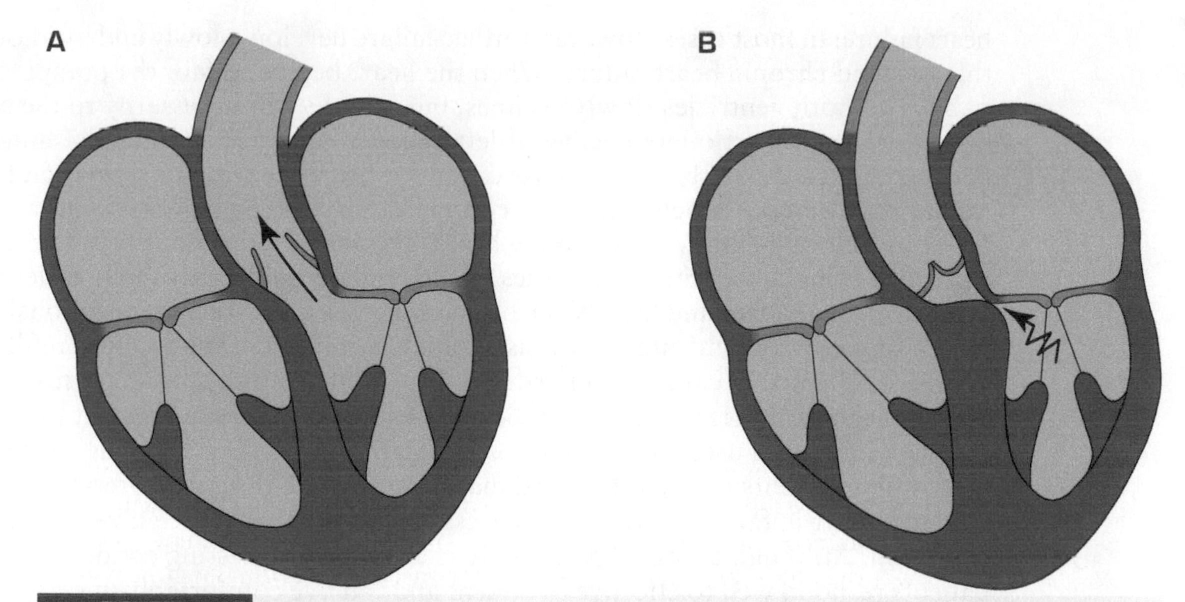

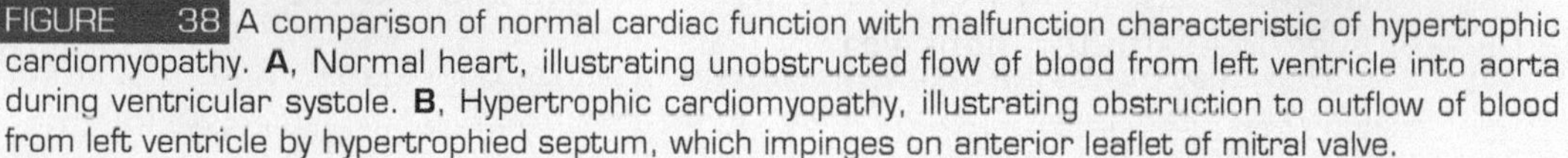
FIGURE 38 A comparison of normal cardiac function with malfunction characteristic of hypertrophic cardiomyopathy. **A**, Normal heart, illustrating unobstructed flow of blood from left ventricle into aorta during ventricular systole. **B**, Hypertrophic cardiomyopathy, illustrating obstruction to outflow of blood from left ventricle by hypertrophied septum, which impinges on anterior leaflet of mitral valve.

Hypertrophic cardiomyopathy is characterized by disarray of muscle fibers that intersect at odd angles with no apparent organized pattern and marked hypertrophy of heart muscle to such an extent that the thick-walled chambers become greatly reduced in size and do not dilate readily in diastole. Frequently, the muscle of the septum is hypertrophied to a greater extent than the rest of the myocardium and hinders outflow of the blood from the ventricle into the aorta. At times, the thick septum may actually impinge on the anterior mitral valve leaflet, intermittently completely blocking the outflow of blood from the left ventricle (FIGURE 38). This type of cardiomyopathy is often called idiopathic hypertrophic subaortic stenosis, usually abbreviated IHSS. The term indicates that the obstruction (stenosis) is located below the aortic valve (subaortic), resulting from myocardial hypertrophy (hypertrophic) of unknown cause (idiopathic).

Patients with IHSS frequently exhibit manifestations related to inadequate cardiac output, such as episodes of excessive fatigue and lightheadedness related to exertion. The characteristic myocardial hypertrophy with greatly thickened septum can be identified by echocardiography (discussion on general concepts of disease: principles of diagnosis). Treatment consists of administering drugs that slow the heart (allowing more time for ventricular filling) and reduce the force of ventricular contraction (which tends to reduce the degree of obstruction caused by the hypertrophied septum). Commonly used drugs are those that block the sympathetic nerve impulses that normally increase heart rate and the force of contraction (beta blockers) and those that decrease myocardial contractility by impeding the flow of calcium into myocardial cells (called calcium channel blocking agents). Persons who do not respond to medical treatment may require surgical resection of part of the thickened septum.

Heart Failure

Heart failure exists whenever the heart is no longer able to pump adequate amounts of blood to the tissues. It may result from any type of heart disease. Rapid failing of the heart, as when a large portion of muscle undergoes infarction, is called acute heart failure. In most cases, however, cardiac failure develops slowly and insidiously; this is called chronic heart failure. When the heart begins to fail, the pumping capability of both ventricles slowly declines, but initially not necessarily to the same extent. A disproportionate decline of left ventricular output causes the lungs to become engorged with blood, which is called left heart failure. The term right heart failure may be used when the right ventricle cannot "keep up" with the volume of venous blood being returned to the heart. The increased venous pressure in the distended veins causes the body tissues to accumulate fluid that usually is detected most easily in the feet and legs. When one compresses the swollen (edematous) skin with a fingertip, the indentation persists for a few minutes until the fluid refills the depression, which is called pitting edema. Because the most prominent feature in chronic heart failure is congestion of the tissues as a result of engorgement by blood, the physician often uses the term congestive heart failure when referring to chronic heart failure and its attendant clinical manifestations. Although the term indicates that the heart is failing, it does not necessarily indicate a severe life-threatening condition. Although chronic heart failure is a slowly progressing condition, many patients respond well to effective treatment and can live comfortably in reasonably good health for many years.

PATHOPHYSIOLOGY AND TREATMENT

Sometimes the terms "forward failure" and "backward failure" are used to describe the mechanisms leading to the development of heart failure. In forward failure, the initial effect of inadequate cardiac output is considered to be insufficient blood flow to the tissues. The inadequate renal blood flow results in retention of salt and water by the kidneys. (This effect is mediated indirectly through the adrenal glands.) Fluid retention, in turn, leads to an increased blood volume, and this is soon followed by a rise in venous pressure. The high venous pressure and high capillary pressure cause excessive transudation of fluid from the capillaries, leading to edema of the tissues. In backward failure, the inadequate output of blood is considered to cause "back up" of blood within the veins draining back to the heart, leading to increased venous pressure, congestion of the viscera, and edema. FIGURE 39 illustrates the interrelation of the various factors concerned in the development of cardiac failure. Probably, both forward failure and backward failure are present to some degree in every patient with heart failure. Treatment consists of diuretic drugs, which promote excretion of excess salt and water by the kidneys, thereby lowering blood volume. In addition, digitalis preparations are sometimes administered. They act to increase the efficiency of ventricular contractions. Other medications called ACE inhibitors are also frequently used. These drugs block an enzyme called angiotensin converting enzyme (abbreviated ACE), which is part of a renal regulatory mechanism called the renin–angiotensin-aldosterone system (discussion on the urinary system) that promotes retention of salt and water by the kidneys and raises blood pressure. Both of these effects are undesirable in heart failure patients, and blocking this mechanism by an ACE inhibitor has been shown to improve survival of patients in congestive heart failure.

COMPARISON OF SYSTOLIC AND DIASTOLIC DYSFUNCTION IN HEART FAILURE

The efficiency of ventricular function in heart failure patients can be measured, which allows the physician to determine whether the heart failure results primarily from inadequate ejection of blood from the ventricles in systole or from inadequate filling

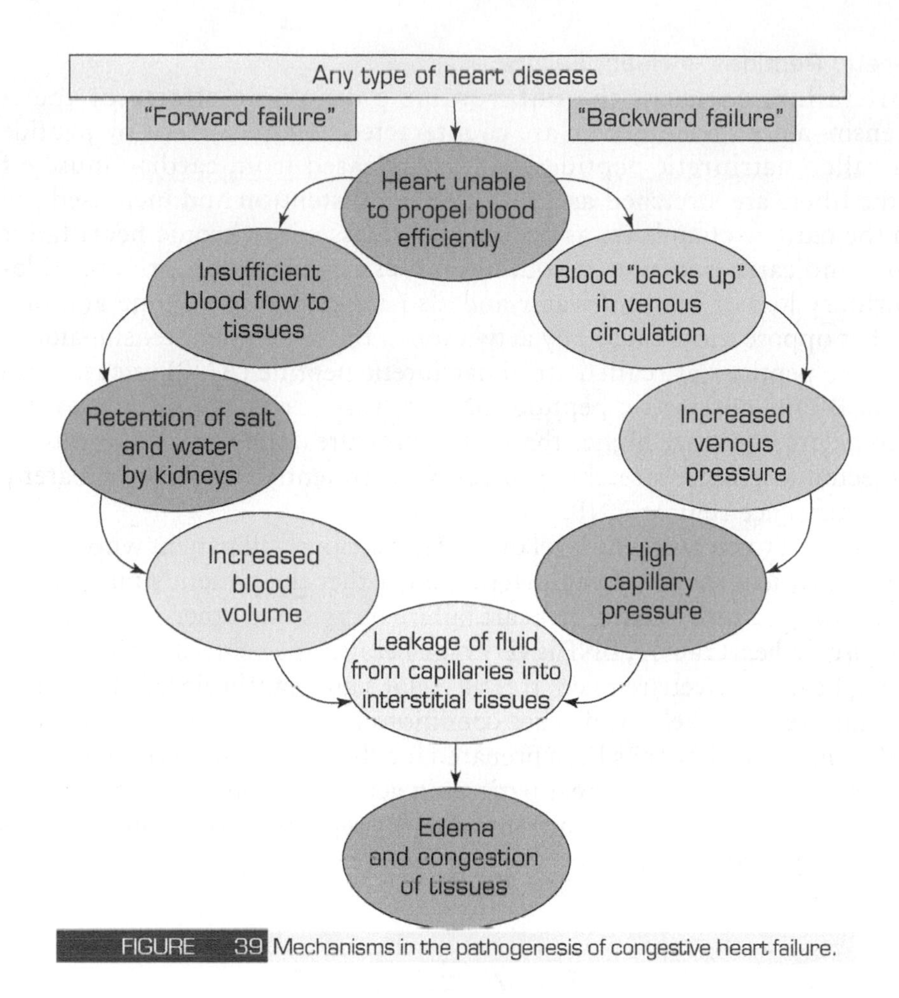

FIGURE 39 Mechanisms in the pathogenesis of congestive heart failure.

of the ventricles in diastole. In most patients with heart failure, the failing ventricles are distended with blood but are unable to expel a normal volume of blood during systole. Consequently, the left ventricular ejection fraction is significantly reduced and may fall from a normal value of about 60% to as low as 20%. This condition is called **systolic heart failure.**

In contrast, the main problem in some heart failure patients is not with the impaired ejection of blood in systole but with inadequate filling of the ventricles during diastole. In this condition, called **diastolic heart failure**, the volume of blood contained in the ventricles during diastole is lower than it should be, and the pressure of the blood within the chambers is elevated. This condition may occur in persons with marked hypertension in whom the thick hypertrophied left ventricular wall cannot relax enough in diastole to allow the left ventricular chamber to expand normally. Consequently, less blood can flow into the ventricle and the pressure of the blood within the ventricle is elevated. Some other less common conditions in which the ventricles are unable to relax normally in diastole may also reduce ventricular filling and raise intraventricular pressure. In all of these conditions, the left ventricle is underfilled in diastole (low end-diastolic volume), and the stroke volume is also low because there is a smaller volume of blood available in the chamber to be ejected. However, the ejection fraction is normal because both end-diastolic volume and stroke volume are reduced proportionately. Nevertheless, the cardiac output is inadequate to supply the body's needs. The clinical manifestations and methods of treatment of both systolic and diastolic heart failure are similar, although diuretics are the preferred treatment for patients with diastolic heart failure.

Systolic heart failure
Heart failure caused by inadequate ejection of blood from the ventricles during systole, in contrast to diastolic heart failure in which filling of the ventricles in diastole is inadequate.

Diastolic heart failure
Heart failure caused by inadequate filling of the ventricles during diastole, in contrast to systolic heart failure in which ejection of blood from the ventricles during systole is inadequate.

Natriuretic Peptides in Heart Failure

In heart failure patients, the unfavorable physiologic effects of the renin–angiotensin–aldosterone system are counteracted to some extent by peptide hormones called natriuretic peptides that are released from cardiac muscle fibers when the fibers are stretched as a result of overdistention and increased pressure within the cardiac chambers, as occurs in patients with chronic heart failure. As the name indicates (*natrium* = sodium + *uresis* = urination), the peptides promote urinary loss of salt and water and also reduce blood volume and pressure, effects that oppose those caused by activation of the renin–angiotensin–aldosterone system. The peptides are called atrial natriuretic peptide (ANP) released from the atria and B-type natriuretic peptide (BNP) released from the ventricles. Because ventricular pressures are higher than atrial pressures, the ventricular muscle cells are subjected to greater stretching forces. Consequently, BNP is of greater physiologic significance than is ANP.

A blood test to measure the level of BNP in a seriously ill patient who is very short of breath may help the physician determine whether the patient's marked dyspnea (shortness of breath) is caused by heart failure or by some other condition, such as lung disease. In heart failure, BNP is very high because the ventricular muscle fibers of the failing heart are overstretched. If BNP is not significantly elevated, the diagnosis of heart failure is unlikely, and other conditions must be considered to explain the patient's symptoms. BNP has been prepared for clinical use by recombinant technology and is sometimes used to treat patients in acute heart failure who are very short of breath. The intravenously administered BNP preparation promotes fluid loss and improves the patient's dyspnea.

Acute Pulmonary Edema

Acute pulmonary edema is a manifestation of acute heart failure and is a very serious life-threatening condition that requires immediate treatment. It is caused by a temporary disproportion in the output of blood from the ventricles. If the output of blood from the left ventricle is temporarily reduced more than the output from the right ventricle, the "right heart" will pump blood into the lungs faster than the "left heart" can deliver the blood to the peripheral tissues. This rapidly engorges the lungs with blood, raises the pulmonary capillary pressure, and produces transudation of fluid into the pulmonary alveoli. The patient becomes extremely short of breath because fluid accumulates within the alveoli, and oxygenation of the blood circulating through the lungs is impaired. The edema fluid becomes mixed with inspired air, forming a frothy mixture that "overflows" into the bronchi and trachea, filling the patient's upper respiratory passages. Treatment consists of supplementary oxygen to get more oxygen to the edematous pulmonary alveoli, intravenous diuretics and other medications to improve cardiac function by reducing the circulating blood volume, morphine to relieve anxiety, and measures directed toward correcting the underlying condition that precipitated the acute heart failure.

Aneurysms

An aneurysm is a dilatation of the wall of an artery or an outpouching of a portion of the wall. Most aneurysms are acquired as a result of arteriosclerosis, which causes weakening of the vessel wall. One type of aneurysm involving the cerebral arteries is the result of a congenital abnormality of the vessel wall and is considered in conjunction with the nervous system (discussion on the nervous system).

ARTERIOSCLEROTIC ANEURYSM

A small artery that undergoes arteriosclerotic change becomes narrowed and may eventually become thrombosed. A large artery such as the aorta has a diameter so large that complete obstruction is uncommon. However, atheromatous deposits tend to damage the wall of the aorta, reducing its elasticity and weakening the wall (FIGURE 40). The aortic wall tends to balloon out under the stress of the high pressure within the vessel. Aortic aneurysms usually develop in the distal part of the abdominal aorta, where the pressure is highest and the atheromatous change is most severe (FIGURES 41 AND 42). Usually, the interior of the aneurysm becomes covered with a layer of thrombus material, and the wall often becomes partially calcified.

As the name implies, arteriosclerosis is the major cause of arteriosclerotic aneurysms, but there appears to be some genetic predisposition as well, as 15 to 20% of patients with an aneurysm also have another affected family member. An aortic aneurysm usually enlarges slowly and does not produce symptoms initially. Because a small aneurysm is difficult to detect by physical examination, current guidelines recommend a routine ultrasound screening examination to identify an asymptomatic aneurysm in any adult older than age 65 who has risk factors that predispose to arteriosclerosis or who has a family history of an aortic aneurysm.

Aortic aneurysms are dangerous because they may rupture, leading to massive and often fatal hemorrhage. The normal cross-section diameter of the abdominal aorta is about 2 cm. An aneurysm exceeding about 5 cm in diameter may rupture

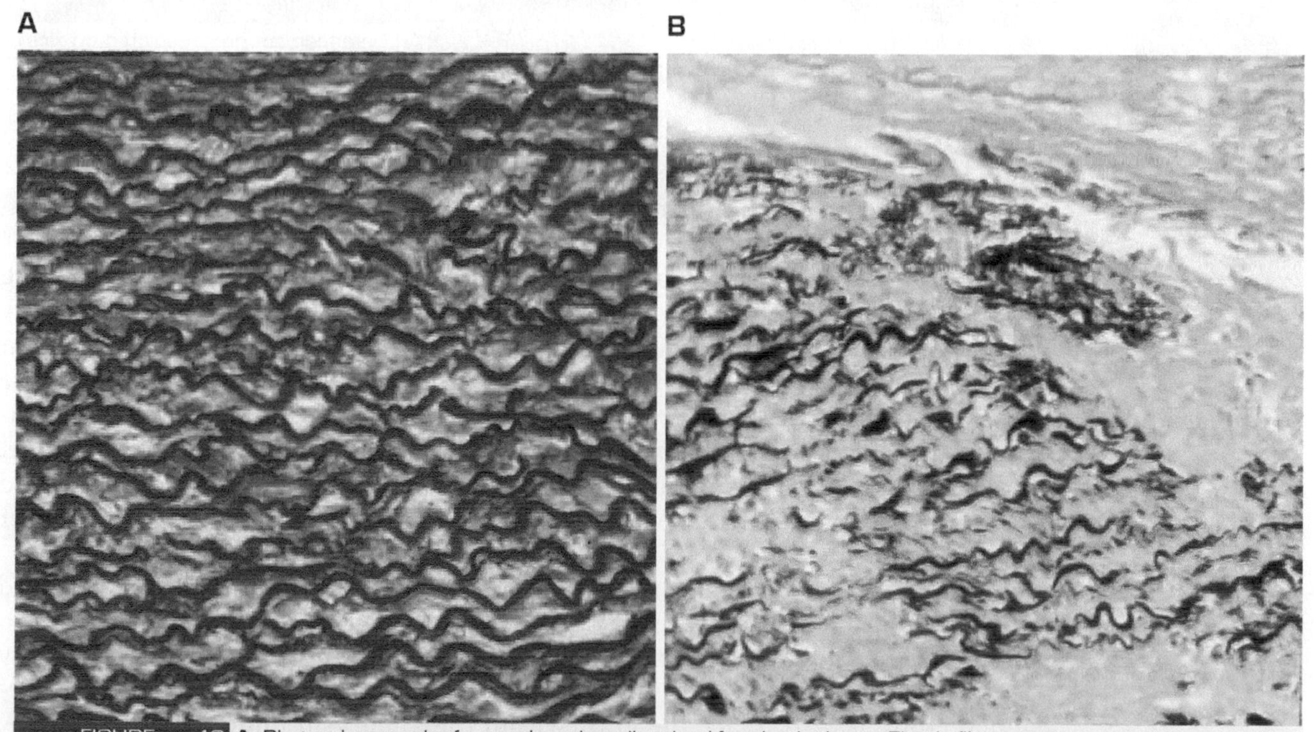

FIGURE 40 **A**, Photomicrograph of normal aortic wall stained for elastic tissue. Elastic fibers appear as dark wavy bands. **B**, Aortic wall from a patient with severe aortic atherosclerosis, illustrating marked fragmentation and destruction of elastic fibers, which weakens wall and predisposes to aneurysm (original magnification × 400).

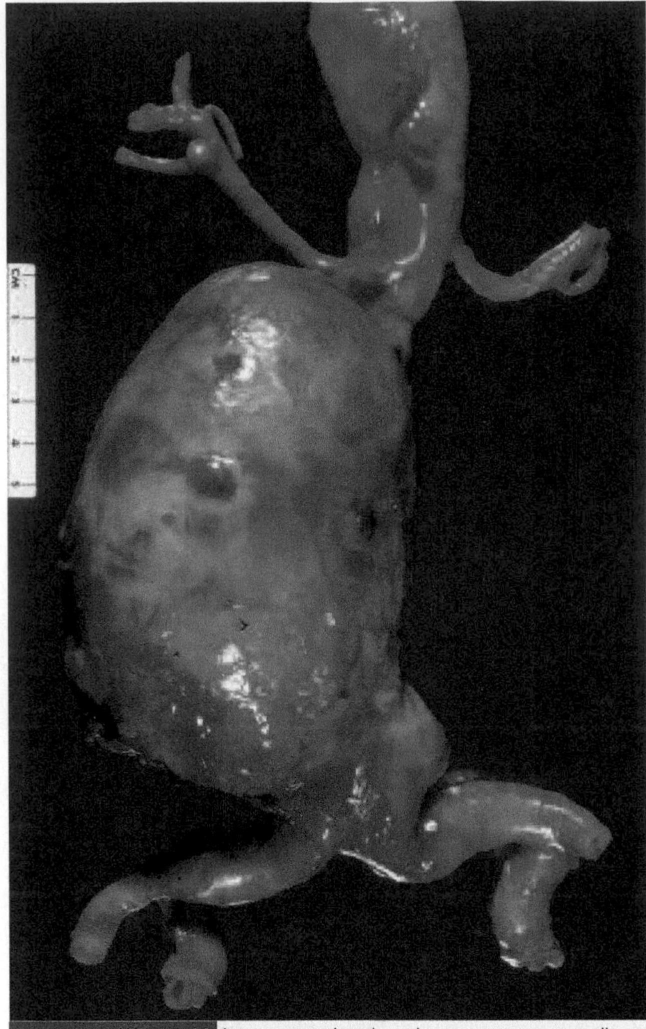

FIGURE 41 Large arteriosclerotic aneurysm extending from renal arteries (*above*) to iliac arteries (*below*).

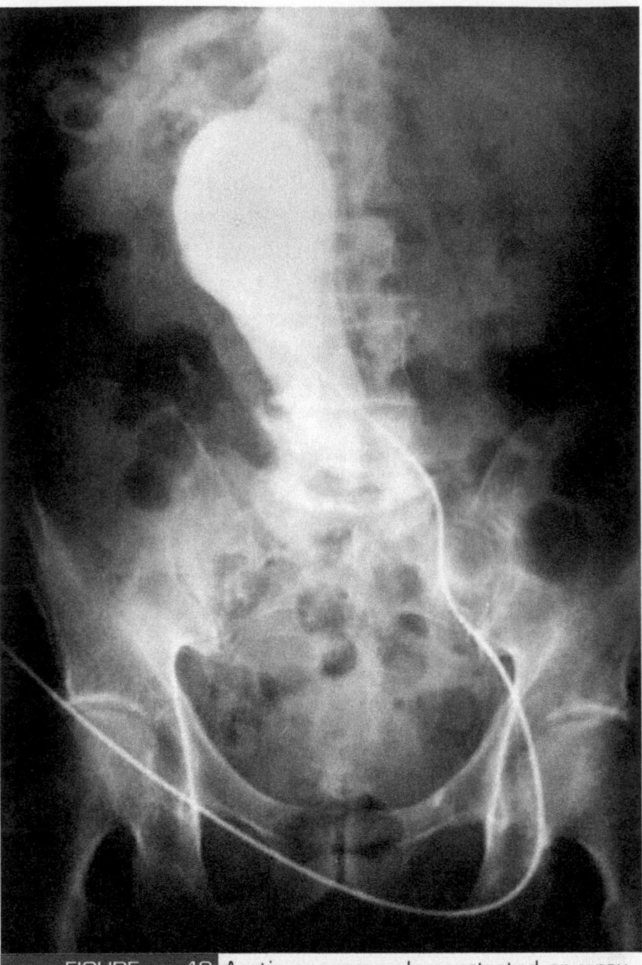

FIGURE 42 Aortic aneurysm demonstrated on x-ray by injection of contrast material into aorta.

Open surgical aneurysm repair
A surgical procedure in which an aortic aneurysm is opened; a graft is placed within the aneurysm sac and sutured to the aorta above and below the aneurysm so that the blood flows through the graft rather than through the aneurysm.

Endovascular aneurysm repair
A nonsurgical treatment of an abdominal aortic aneurysm in which the aneurysm graft is inserted through the femoral arteries, positioned within the aneurysm, and anchored within the aorta above and below the aneurysm.

and should be repaired. In general, the larger the aneurysm, the greater the likelihood of rupture (FIGURE 43).

The standard **open surgical aneurysm repair** procedure consists of opening the aneurysm and sewing a nylon or Dacron graft into the aorta above and below the aneurysmal segment so that the blood flowing through the aorta flows through the graft rather than through the aneurysm (FIGURE 44). It is not necessary to excise the aneurysm that has been bypassed by the graft, and usually the walls of the aneurysm are wrapped around the graft. This procedure is a well-established, reliable, and highly successful method of treatment, but it is a major surgical procedure and poses some risks to older patients who may have coronary artery disease and other medical problems.

In selected patients, an alternative method of treatment is available called **endovascular aneurysm repair** (*endo* = within + *vascular* = blood vessel). Two small incisions are made in the groins to expose the femoral arteries. A specially designed stent graft is inserted through the femoral arteries using a specially designed equipment to place the graft within the aneurysm under x-ray guidance. Then a balloon expands the stent graft, which has hooks or similar attachment devices to fix the graft to the aorta proximally, and to the aorta or iliac arteries distally (FIGURE 45). When properly fixed in position, blood flows through the graft instead of through the aneurysm. Two recently completed large studies comparing endovascular graft repair with standard surgical procedures appear to favor the endovascular graft, which had a lower mortality associated with the graft insertion than the surgical procedure, a shorter hospitalization, and fewer complications. However, the function of the graft after 3 years may not be as good as the open surgical procedure and may require additional treatment.

DISSECTING ANEURYSM OF THE AORTA

The thick middle layer of the aorta is called the media. It is composed of multiple layers of elastic tissue and muscle bonded together by fibrous connective tissue. Degenerative changes sometimes occur in the media, causing the layers to lose their cohesiveness and separate (FIGURE 46). Then the pulsatile force of the blood flowing through the aorta may cause the inner half of the aortic wall to pull away from the outer half in the region where the media has degenerated, and sometimes the inner lining (intima) tears as the media separates. This complication is especially likely to occur in persons with high blood pressure.

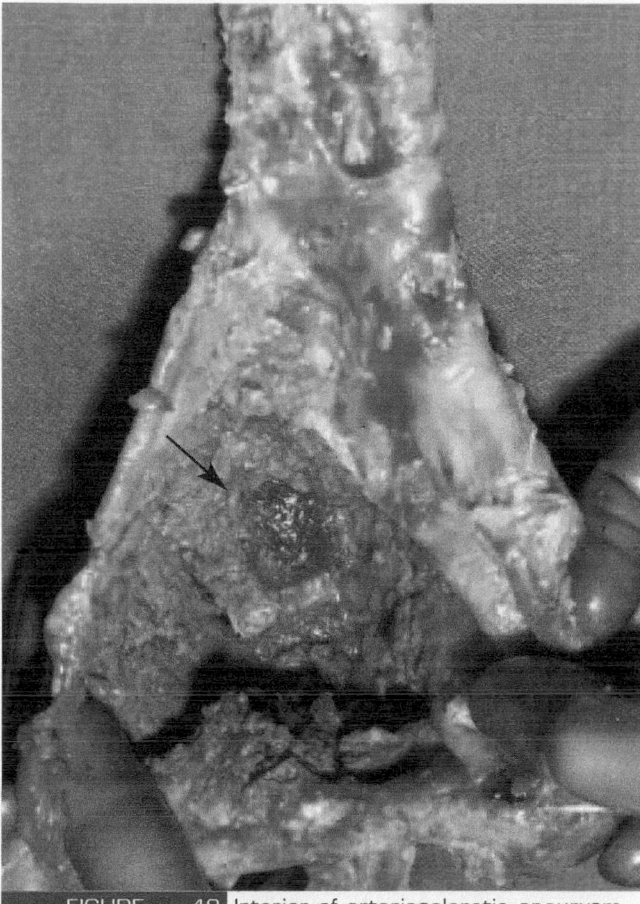

FIGURE 43 Interior of arteriosclerotic aneurysm, illustrating marked degenerative change in wall. Extremely thin area in wall (*arrow*) predisposes to rupture.

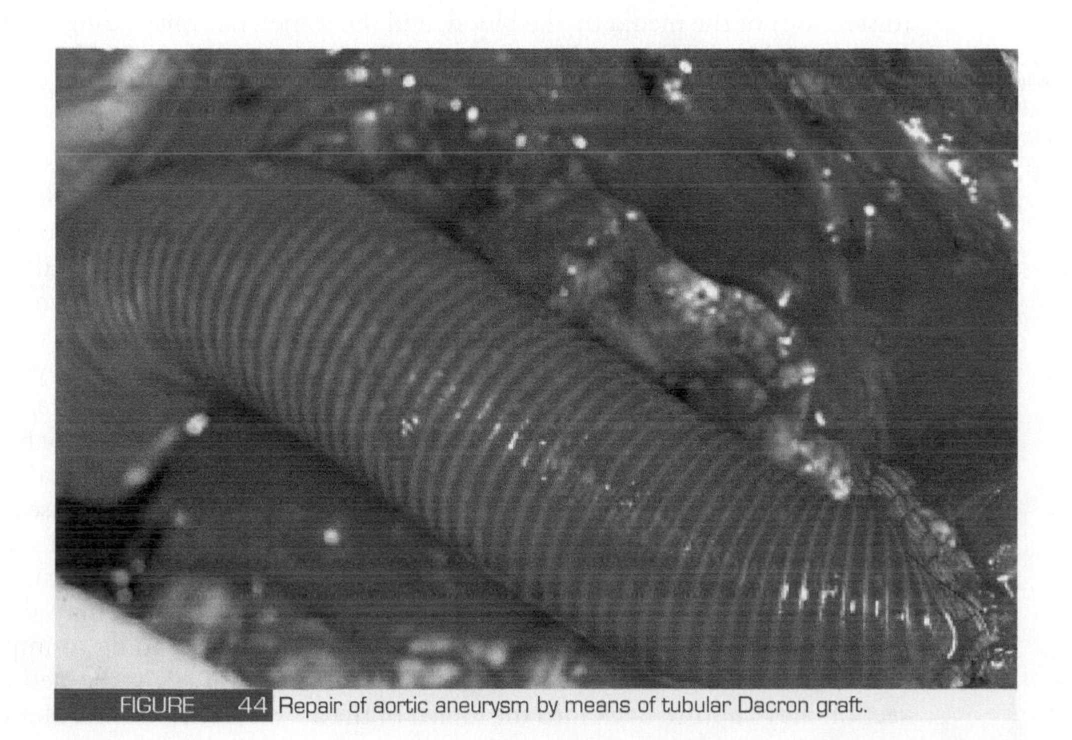

FIGURE 44 Repair of aortic aneurysm by means of tubular Dacron graft.

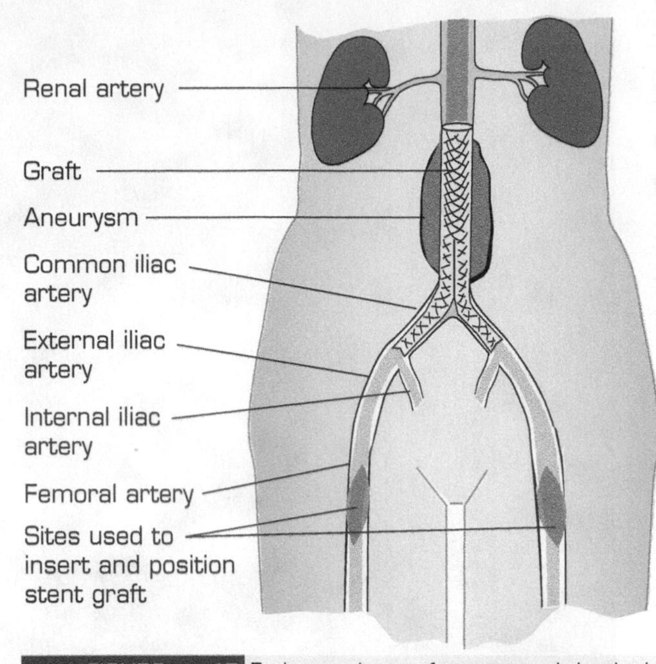

FIGURE 45 Endovascular graft to treat abdominal aortic aneurysm. The graft expands within the aorta, and the stent attachments fix graft to aorta proximally and iliac arteries distally.

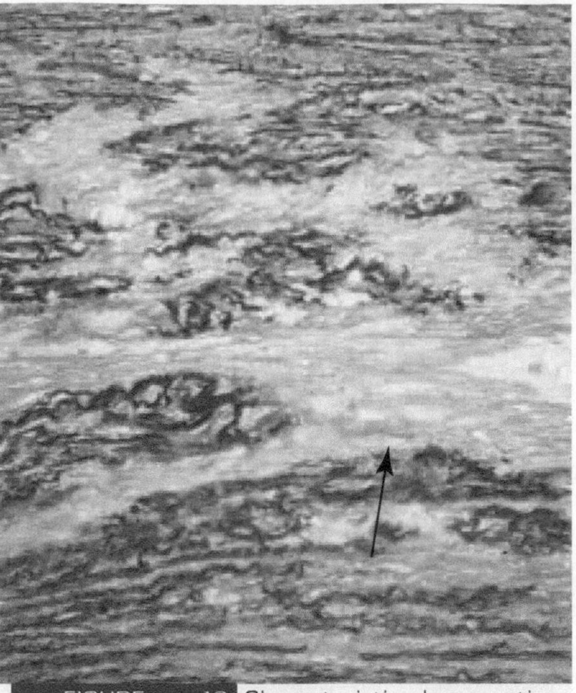

FIGURE 46 Characteristic degenerative changes in the media of the aortic wall (called cystic medial necrosis) illustrated in the center of the photograph (*arrow*), which leads to loss of cohesion between the inner and outer layers of the aortic wall and predisposes to aortic dissection.

Dissecting aneurysm of the aorta
(an'ū r-izm)
A dissection of blood into the wall of the aorta secondary to degeneration of the arterial wall with an associated tear of the lining (intima) *of the artery.*

Aneurysm
(an'ū r-izm)
A dilatation of a structure, such as the aorta, a cerebral artery, or a part of the ventricular wall. See ventricular aneurysm.

After an intimal tear has developed, blood is forced into the aortic wall. The area of medial degeneration forms a cleavage plane that permits the blood to dissect within the media for a variable distance. This event, a **dissecting aneurysm of the aorta,** is associated with severe chest and back pain. The term dissecting refers to the splitting (dissection) of the media by the blood, and the somewhat misleading term **aneurysm** was applied because the affected part of the aorta appears wider than normal. The widening results from the hemorrhage within the aortic wall, but the lumen of the aorta is not dilated.

The intimal tear that starts the dissection is usually either in the ascending aorta just above the aortic valve or in the descending aorta just beyond the origin of the large arteries that arise from the aortic arch (FIGURE 47). If the tear is in the ascending aorta, the blood often dissects proximally as well as distally within the aortic wall, extending into the base of the aorta where the aortic valve attaches and the coronary arteries arise. The dissection may separate the aortic valve from its attachment to the deeper aortic wall so that it no longer functions properly, and severe aortic regurgitation develops. The origins of the coronary arteries may also be compressed by the hemorrhage in the wall, which compromises the blood supply to the heart muscle. A dissection in the ascending aorta is often fatal because the blood frequently ruptures through the outer wall of the aorta at the base of the heart, leading to extensive hemorrhage into the mediastinum or pericardial sac.

If the intimal tear is in the descending aorta, the blood dissects distally and may extend the entire length of the aorta. The blood in the aortic wall may also compress the origins of the large arteries that arise from the aorta, leading to impairment of blood flow to the kidneys, the intestines, or other vital organs. Sometimes the dissection may rupture back into the lumen of the aorta. If this occurs, blood flows not

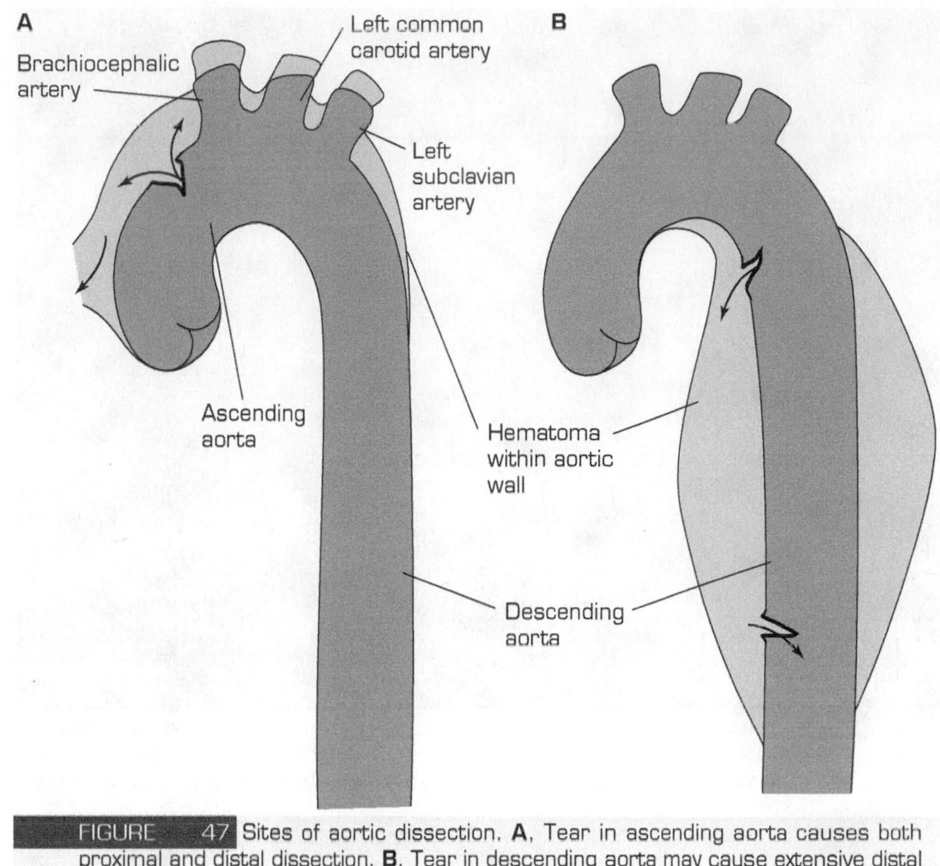

FIGURE 47 Sites of aortic dissection. **A**, Tear in ascending aorta causes both proximal and distal dissection. **B**, Tear in descending aorta may cause extensive distal dissection and may rupture back into lumen of aorta.

only through the lumen of the aorta, but also through the channel in the aortic wall created by the dissection, which communicates with the lumen of the aorta both proximally and distally (FIGURE 48).

Various surgical procedures have been devised to correct this condition.

Diseases of the Veins

The main diseases of veins are (1) venous thrombosis, (2) inflammation of veins, and (3) excessive dilatation and tortuosity of veins.

Venous thromboses occur most commonly in leg veins, but sometimes clots form within veins elsewhere in the body. Inflammation of a vein is called phlebitis (*phleb* = vein + *itis* = inflammation). If there is an associated thrombosis of the affected vein, the term thrombophlebitis is used. Dilated tortuous veins are called varices or varicose veins. (*Varix* is a Latin word meaning dilated vessel; the plural term is varices.) Varicosities occur most often in leg veins but may occur in other veins as well.

VENOUS THROMBOSIS AND THROMBOPHLEBITIS

Thrombus formation in deep leg veins is a frequent problem in postoperative patients and in those confined to bed, and it may be complicated by a pulmonary embolism, as described in the discussion on circulatory disturbances. The risk of leg vein thromboses in susceptible patients can be minimized by encouraging active

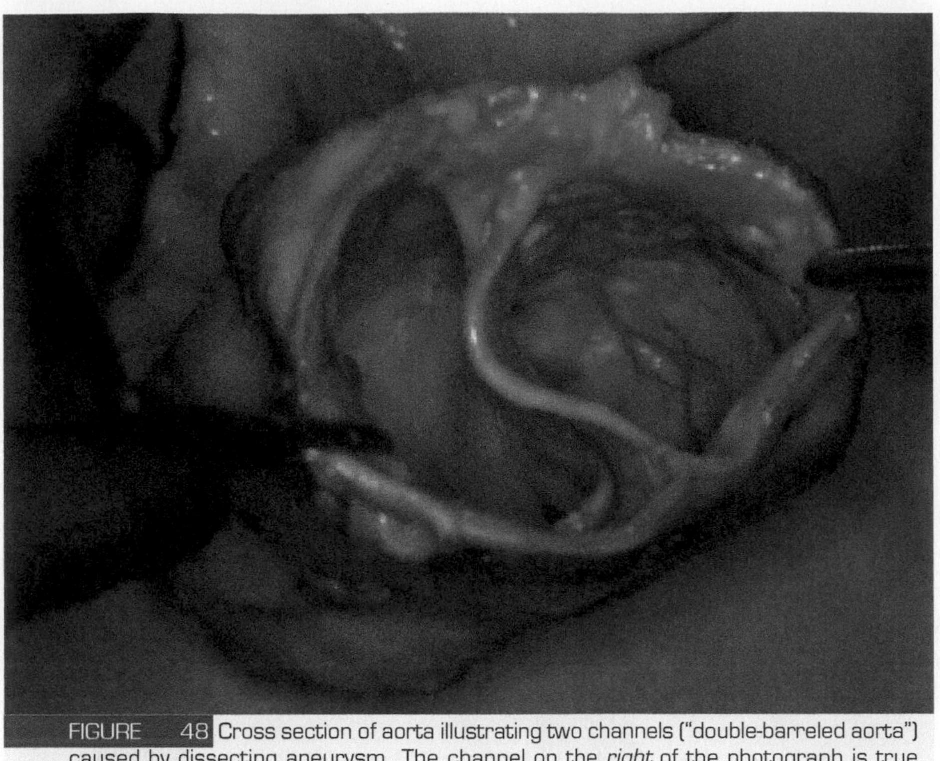

FIGURE 48 Cross section of aorta illustrating two channels ("double-barreled aorta") caused by dissecting aneurysm. The channel on the *right* of the photograph is true lumen of aorta. The channel on the *left* is the channel in the aortic wall created by the dissection.

leg exercises to improve venous blood flow and prevent venous stasis and by early ambulation.

Venous thrombosis and thrombophlebitis are treated by elevation of the leg, heat, and anticoagulant drugs. The anticoagulation stops the progression of the intravascular clotting process while the body's normal protective mechanisms remove the clot. The clot is dissolved by activation of the fibrinolytic mechanism and by ingrowth of connective tissue from the vein wall at the site where the clot adheres to the vein wall. Damage to the vein wall and its valves after thrombophlebitis may disturb venous return and predispose to later development of varicose veins.

VARICOSE VEINS OF THE LOWER EXTREMITIES

Two main groups of veins return blood from the lower limbs: the deep veins and the superficial veins. The deep veins carry most of the venous return. They accompany the major arteries and drain into the iliac veins, which in turn empty into the inferior vena cava. The superficial veins form a network of intercommunicating channels that travel just beneath the skin in the subcutaneous tissue and eventually drain into the deep veins. The largest superficial vein is the great saphenous vein, which extends up the medial surface of the leg from the ankle to the groin and drains into the more deeply placed femoral vein just below the groin. A second large superficial vein called the small saphenous vein ascends the back of the leg and drains into the deep venous system at the back of the knee. Both the superficial and deep veins contain cup-shaped valves, fashioned somewhat like the semilunar valves in the heart, which are interposed along the course of the veins. The arrangement of the valves is such that blood can flow upward in the veins but cannot flow in the reverse direction. The superficial and deep venous systems are also interconnected by short communicating branches that contain valves arranged so that blood normally flows only from superficial to deep veins and not in the reverse direction.

Blood is propelled upward within the deep veins by contraction of the leg and thigh muscles, which intermittently compress the veins and force the blood upward within the veins against gravity. The valves within the veins prevent retrograde flow. In contrast, the superficial veins are relatively unsupported, and venous return is much less efficient. Nevertheless, venous return through the superficial veins is normal provided that the veins do not become excessively dilated and the valves function properly to prevent retrograde flow and venous stasis.

Varicose veins result if the saphenous veins become dilated and their valves become incompetent. As a result, the blood tends to stagnate in the veins instead of flowing back normally to the heart, causing the veins to become elongated and tortuous. The condition tends to run in families, suggesting that the basic cause is a congenital weakness of the vein wall or its valves, which predisposes to the varicosities.

Varicose veins of the saphenous system may also develop if the deeper veins become blocked or if their valves become damaged by previous thrombophlebitis. As a result of damage to the deep veins, more of the venous return is shifted to the unsupported superficial veins, which are unable to cope with the increased flow and become varicose.

Complications of Varicose Veins

Complications result from stasis of blood in the veins, with poor nutrition of the tissues caused by chronic venous engorgement. The skin of the distal leg and ankle becomes thin and atrophic and quite susceptible to infection. Skin ulcers may develop and heal poorly. The dilated veins are easily injured and may rupture, leading to extravasation of blood and chronic discoloration of the skin. Stasis of blood in the veins also predisposes to repeated bouts of thrombophlebitis.

Treatment of Varicose Veins

Varicosities of the saphenous veins are treated by elastic stockings to support the veins and elevation of the legs whenever possible to promote more efficient venous return. Sometimes surgical removal of the varicose veins may be required. This is usually performed in conjunction with ligation of the communicating veins that interconnect the superficial and deep venous systems.

VARICOSE VEINS IN OTHER LOCATIONS

Dilated veins around the rectum are called **hemorrhoids** and are described in the discussion on the gastrointestinal tract in conjunction with disorders of the gastrointestinal tract. Varicose veins of the esophagus often occur in patients with a disease called **cirrhosis of the liver. Esophageal varices** may rupture and cause profuse life-threatening hemorrhage. Their pathogenesis and treatment are considered in the discussion on the liver and the biliary system. Varicose veins of the spermatic cord appear as a mass of vessels in the scrotum above the testicle. The condition is called a **varicocele** (*varix* = vein + *cele* = swelling). The varicosities usually do not cause symptoms but at times may cause mild scrotal discomfort. Rarely, they may impair fertility in some men. Usually no treatment is required.

Hemorrhoids
(hem′or-oyds)
Varicosities of anal and rectal veins.

Cirrhosis of the liver
(si-rō′sis)
A disease characterized by diffuse intrahepatic scarring and liver cell degeneration.

Esophageal varices
(var′i-sēz)
Dilated (varicose) veins of the esophagus, which are often present in patients with cirrhosis of the liver.

Varicocele
(var′-ik-kō-sēl)
Varicose veins within the spermatic cord that drain blood from the testis.

QUESTIONS FOR REVIEW

1. How do the heart valves function to provide unidirectional blood flow? What factors determine the level of the systolic and diastolic blood pressure?
2. What are the major causes of heart disease? What is the difference between rheumatic fever and rheumatic heart disease?
3. What is infective endocarditis? How does it arise? How is it prevented?
4. What is coronary heart disease? What are its manifestations? What is the difference between angina pectoris and myocardial infarction?
5. What is the effect of high blood pressure on the heart and the blood vessels?
6. What is heart failure? What is meant by the following terms: *forward failure, backward failure, acute heart failure, chronic heart failure, systolic heart failure, diastolic heart failure, and acute pulmonary edema*?
7. What is the usual cause of an aortic aneurysm? How is an aneurysm treated?
8. What is the difference between an arteriosclerotic aneurysm of the aorta and a dissecting aneurysm of the aorta?
9. What are the major complications of a large myocardial infarction?
10. What is meant by the following terms: *mitral valve prolapse*, *calcific aortic stenosis*, *atrial fibrillation*, and *ventricular fibrillation*?
11. What factors predispose to thrombus formation in leg veins? What are the major complications of venous thrombi?
12. What are varicose veins? What veins are commonly affected? What are the clinical manifestations?

SUPPLEMENTARY READINGS

Alpert, J. S., Thygesen, K., Antman, E., et al. 2000. Myocardial infarction redefined—a consensus document of The Joint European Society of Cardiology/American College of Cardiology Committee for the redefinition of myocardial infarction. *Journal of the American College of Cardiology* 36:959–69.

- Previously, a myocardial infarction was defined by a combination of two or three characteristics using standard World Health Organization criteria: typical symptoms, typical ECG pattern, and rise of cardiac enzymes. Now the very sensitive and specific cardiac troponin tests performed on patients with chest pain can detect very small foci of myocardial necrosis that are not large enough to cause the MB fraction of creatine kinase (CK-MB) to rise. Using the earlier criteria, these patients would have been considered to have severe unstable angina but now are diagnosed as having a small myocardial infarct.

Al Suwaidi, J., Berger, P. B., and Holmes, D. R., Jr. 2000. Coronary artery stents. *Journal of the American Medical Association* 284:1828–36.

- Intracoronary stents improve clinical outcome and are an essential component of catheter-based treatment of coronary artery disease.

Antman, E. M. 2002. Decision making with cardiac troponin tests. *The New England Journal of Medicine* 346:2079–82.

- Troponin tests are very sensitive and specific and can identify minor myocardial damage that is not sufficient to cause a rise in the cardiac specific fraction of creatine kinase. These observations have led to a reevaluation of the spectrum of coronary artery disease syndromes.

Beckett, N. S., Peters, R., Fletcher, A. E., et al. 2008. Treatment of hypertension in patients 80 years of age or older. *The New England Journal of Medicine* 358:1887–98.

- Reducing elevated blood pressure reduces the risk of strokes and also reduces death rate from cardiovascular disease even in very elderly patients.

Boden, W. E., O'Rourke, R. A., Teo, K. K., et al. 2007. Optimal medical therapy with or without PCI for stable coronary disease. *The New England Journal of Medicine* 356:1503–16.

- Insertion of stents to open narrowed coronary arteries, called percutaneous coronary intervention (PCI), is performed frequently as the initial treatment of patients with stable coronary artery disease along with standard medical therapy. A trial involving 2,287 patients with significant coronary artery disease and angina was undertaken in which the subjects were divided into two groups. PCI did not reduce the risk of death, myocardial infarction, or other cardiovascular events in patients with stable coronary artery disease when added to optimal medical therapy. Addition of elective PCI offers no advantage over medical treatment alone.

Bugiardini, R., and Bairey Merz, C. N. B. 2005. Angina with "normal" coronary arteries: A changing philosophy. *Journal of the American Medical Association* 293:477–84.

- Angina pectoris associated with apparently normal coronary arteries, or with nonobstructive coronary artery disease, is not a benign condition, as this condition occurs in about 10% of women and 6% of men. The various reasons that may explain this paradox are discussed, including the role of emotional stress.

Feldman, T., and Leon, M. B. 2007. Prospects for percutaneous valve therapies. *Circulation* 116:2866–77.

- A comprehensive discussion of percutaneous methods available or under active investigation that can be used to treat patients with valvular heart disease who are not good candidates for a standard surgical method of valve replacement. The percutaneous methodology is a "work in progress," as the valves and their methods of insertion are improved continuously based on clinical experience with the current percutaneous valves and their methods of replacement.

Ford, E. S., Ajani, U. A., Croft, J. B., et al. 2007. Explaining the decrease in U.S. deaths from coronary disease, 1980–2000. *The New England Journal of Medicine* 356:2388–98.

- Although coronary heart disease and its complications is a leading cause of death in the United States, great progress has been made in reducing mortality, which has declined about 50% in the last two decades. About half the mortality reduction resulted from better control of risk factors that promote coronary heart disease, such as lowering blood lipids, better control of hypertension, reduced smoking, and increased physical activity. The other half of the mortality reduction was related to improved methods for diagnosing and treating coronary heart disease and its complications.

Hagan, P. G., Nienaber, C. A., Isselbacher, E. M., et al. 2000. The International Registry of Acute Aortic Dissection (IRAD): New insights into an old disease. *Journal of the American Medical Association* 283:897–903.

- A review of the presentation, management, and outcomes of acute aortic dissection.

Hochman, J. S., and Steg, P. G. 2007. Does preventive PCI work? *The New England Journal of Medicine* 356:1572–74.

- PCI is effective in reducing angina in patients with coronary artery disease, and reduces mortality in patients who have an acute myocardial infarction or high-risk acute coronary syndromes accompanied by myocardial damage. These favorable outcomes have led to more widespread use of PCI to supplement medical therapy in an attempt to improve the long-term prognosis in patients with stable coronary artery disease. PCI offers no additional advantage over standard medical therapy for most patients with stable coronary artery disease.

Judge, D. P. 2009. Use of genetics in the clinical evaluation of cardiomyopathy. *Journal of the American Medical Association* 302:2471–76.

- Inherited forms of cardiomyopathy may be responsible for heart failure that is otherwise unexplained, and often the gene mutations can be identified by genetic tests. Screening of family members who may be at risk for an acquired form of cardiomyopathy may lead to earlier identification of affected family members, which in turn can lead to earlier treatment and a more favorable response to therapy.

Keeley, E. C., and Hillis, L. D. 2007. Primary PCI for myocardial infarction with ST-segment elevation. *The New England Journal of Medicine* 356:47–54.

- Plugging of a coronary artery by a thrombus cuts off the blood supply to the heart muscle in the distribution of the occluded vessel, which is soon followed by necrosis of the ischemic muscle. PCI is the preferred method of treatment. The site of the thrombosis is identified by angiography followed by insertion of a guide wire through the region blocked by the thrombus. Then a balloon catheter covered by a collapsed bare metal or drug-coated stent is directed over the guide wire and positioned at the site of the thrombus. Finally the balloon is inflated, which opens the artery and expands the stent to keep the artery open.

Kloner, R. A., and Rezkalla, S. H. 2003. Cocaine and the heart. *The New England Journal of Medicine* 348:487–88.

- A review of the mechanisms of action of cocaine on the cardiovascular system. The risk of myocardial infarction is highest within the first hour after cocaine use, and there is no clear relationship between the dose of cocaine and the occurrence of an acute myocardial infarction.

Lange, R. A., and Hillis, L. D. 2002. Reperfusion therapy in acute myocardial infarction. *The New England Journal of Medicine* 346:954–55.

- Restoration of blood flow through a blocked coronary artery reduces myocardial damage and improves survival. Thrombolytic therapy is effective but does not always completely dissolve the thrombus. Balloon angioplasty is more effective than thrombolytic therapy. The use of a stent along with antiplatelet drugs helps prevent restenosis of the dilated vessel.

Lederle, F. A. 2005. Endovascular repair of abdominal aortic aneurysm—Round two. *The New England Journal of Medicine* 352:2443–45.

- A review of the costs and benefits of the two procedures. The endovascular repair was associated with a lower postoperative mortality than the open surgical procedure, but the longer term follow-up revealed no survival advantage because there were late complications and deaths related to the endovascular repair. Long-term mortality data were similar for both procedures.

Le May, M. R., So, D. Y., Dionne, R., et al. 2008. A citywide protocol for primary PCI in ST-segment elevation myocardial infarction. *The New England Journal of Medicine* 358:231–40.

- A Canadian metropolitan community developed a protocol in which specially trained paramedics who were able to interpret an ST-elevation myocardial infarction responded to 911 calls. Patients in whom ST-segment myocardial infarction was demonstrated received a chewable aspirin tablet and sublingual nitroglycerine, and were transported directly to a cardiac care center for immediate angiogram and PCI. Overall in-hospital mortality was 4.7% compared with 5.7% mortality for patients not directly transferred to a coronary care center.

Mark, D. B., and Felker, G. M. 2004. B-type natriuretic peptide—A biomarker for all seasons? *The New England Journal of Medicine* 350:718–20.

- BNP is a useful diagnostic tool for evaluating a patient with acute dyspnea in an emergency department. If the BNP level is less than 100 pg per milliliter, the diagnosis of congestive heart failure is very unlikely. If the level is over 500 pg per milliliter, congestive cardiac failure is likely. Intermediate levels are not helpful.

Maron, B. J. 2002. Hypertrophic cardiomyopathy: A systematic review. *Journal of the American Medical Association* 287:1308–20.

- This disease is an important cause of disability, but the prognosis is not ominous and is compatible with normal longevity, which should provide reassurance to patients.

Mukamal, K. J., Conigrave, K. M., Mittleman, M. A., et al. 2003. Roles of drinking pattern and type of alcohol consumed in coronary heart disease in men. *The New England Journal of Medicine* 348:109–18.

- Consumption of alcohol at least three or four times per week reduces the risk of myocardial infarction, and the type of alcohol consumed (beer, red wine, or white wine, etc.) does not have any effect on the favorable result.

Otto, C. M., Kuusisto, J., Reichenbach, D. D., et al. 1994. Characterization of the early lesion of "degenerative" valvular aortic stenosis. *Circulation* 90:844–53.

- Mechanical stresses initiate structural changes in the valve followed by lipid deposition and infiltration of the valve leaflets by macrophages and T lymphocytes, similar to the changes in coronary atherosclerosis.

Pinto, D. S. 2010. A 43-year-old man with angina, elevated troponin, and lateral ST depression: Management of acute coronary syndromes. *Journal of the American Medical Association* 303:54–63.

- All patients with intermediate or high risk non-ST elevation myocardial infarction (NSTEMI) should have coronary angiography, and the cardiologist in consultation with the patient should determine the best way to proceed: (1) to open the coronary artery by angioplasty with stent placement (PCI), (2) to perform a coronary artery bypass graft (CABG), or (3) to continue with medical treatment. In general, patients with diffuse coronary artery disease have better results with CABG than PCI. The various types of antiplatelet and anticoagulant therapy associated with treatment are described and compared.

Roth, B. L. 2007. Drugs and valvular heart disease. *The New England Journal of Medicine* 356:6–9.

- Drugs that activate serotonin receptors in heart valves (agonists of 5-HT_{2B} receptors, a subtype of serotonin receptors) stimulate mitosis and proliferation of valve connective tissue cells and collagen fibers, leading to valve thickening and impaired valve function. More recently, some drugs used to treat Parkinson's disease (pergolide and carbergoline) have been shown to cause heart valve damage by targeting the 5-HT_{2B} serotonin receptors in heart valves.

Sacks, F. M., and Campos, H. 2010. Dietary therapy in hypertension. *The New England Journal of Medicine* 362:2102–12.

- In most cases, primary hypertension is a genetic disorder involving many individual genes which collectively regulate how the body deals with the dietary intake of sodium. Dietary treatment of hypertension includes a sodium intake restricted to 1.5 g per day along with maintaining or achieving a normal weight. A restricted alcohol intake is also recommended. No more than 2 alcoholic drinks per day for men of average size and 1 for women and smaller men. A trial of intensive dietary treatment is warranted for 6 months to achieve a goal of systolic blood pressure of less than 140 mm Hg and diastolic pressure less than 90 mm Hg before considering adding anti-hypertensive drugs.

Schade, R., Andersohn, F., Suissa, S., et al. 2007. Dopamine agonists and the risk of cardiac valve regurgitation. *The New England Journal of Medicine* 356:29–38.

- Ergot-derived dopamine agonists pergolide and cabergoline used to treat Parkinson's disease and restless leg syndrome may increase the risk of cardiac valve regurgitation. The drugs are potent agonists of the serotonin receptor ($5\text{-}HT_{2B}$) expressed on heart valves. Preferential activation of this receptor stimulates mitosis in cardiac valve cells leading to cell and connective fiber proliferation, which may impair valve function. The risk of valve dysfunction is high among subjects who have taken daily doses exceeding 3 mg for a period of 6 or more months. There was no increased risk with the use of other dopamine agonists.

Schermerhorn, M. L., O'Malley, A. J., Jhaveri, A., et al. 2008. Endovascular vs. open repair of abdominal aortic aneurysms in the medicare population. *The New England Journal of Medicine* 358:464–74.

- Endovascular repair compared with open repair is associated with a lower short-term rate of death and complications. Late additional procedures are required more often after endovascular repair, but there are also a comparable number of late procedures and hospitalizations after surgical procedures.

Shah, S. J., and Gheorghiade, M. 2008. Heart failure with preserved ejection fraction: Treat now by treating comorbidities. *Journal of the American Medical Association* 300:431–33.

- Half the patients with heart failure have a normal ejection fraction, and standard treatment for heart failure has had limited success. Most of these patients have other conditions that contribute to the heart failure, primarily coronary artery disease and hypertension.

Svilaas, T., Vlaar, P. J., van der Horst, I. C., et al. 2008. Thrombus aspiration during primary percutaneous coronary intervention. *The New England Journal of Medicine* 358:557–67.

- Primary PCI is effective in opening an infarct-related artery in patients with a ST-elevation myocardial infarction, but embolization of atheromatous debris and thrombus material plugs distal arterioles and reduces myocardial perfusion. Thrombus aspiration can be performed on most patients with ST-segment elevation myocardial infarction, which results in better reperfusion and better clinical outcomes than conventional PCI.

Thompson, R. W. 2002. Detection and management of small aortic aneurysms. *The New England Journal of Medicine* 346:1484–86.

- Routine physical examination cannot detect small aneurysms (between 4.0 to 5.4 cm diameter), but routine ultrasound screening of persons older than the age of 65 would detect almost all small aneurysms. Small aneurysms should be monitored periodically, and surgical repair is advisable if the aneurysm enlarges further or produces symptoms.

Thygesen, K., Alpert, J. S., and White, H. D. 2007. Universal definition of myocardial infarction. *Journal of the American College of Cardiology* 50:2173–95.

- A proposal to designate any degree of heart muscle damage as a myocardial infarction, with a discussion of diagnosis and treatment methods based on the degree of muscle necrosis. The authors believe that a change in the definition of a myocardial infarct will favorably influence the identification, prevention, and treatment of cardiovascular disease throughout the world.

Zanettini, R., Antonini, A., Gatto, G., et al. 2007. Valvular heart disease and the use of dopamine agonists for Parkinson's disease. *The New England Journal of Medicine* 356:39–46.

- Pergolide may cause fibrosis in valve leaflets and in the subvalvular tissues leading to stiffening, retraction, incomplete coaptation, and resulting valve regurgitation. Valve damage has been described following use of this drug to treat Parkinson's disease, and the drug has also been used in low dose to treat hyperprolactinemia. Drugs that mimic the effect of serotonin (serotonin agonist effect) on the serotonin receptor subtype 5-HT_{2B} may damage heart valves by stimulating mitosis of inactive valve connective tissue cells (fibroblasts). Active fibroblast proliferation leads to an excess production of connective tissue (collagen) fibers, which thickens and deforms the heart valves.

Zile, M. R., Baicu, C. F., and Gaasch, W. H. 2004. Diastolic heart failure—Abnormalities in active relaxation and passive stiffness of the left ventricle. *The New England Journal of Medicine* 350:1953–9.

- Patients with heart failure and a normal ejection fraction had higher end diastolic pressures with lower end diastolic volumes than a control group, related to abnormal diastolic function.

OUTLINE SUMMARY

Cardiac Structure and Function

STRUCTURE OF THE HEART AND ITS CHAMBERS

Right heart circulates blood to lung.
Left heart circulates blood to peripheral tissues.

CARDIAC VALVES

AV valves attached to papillary muscles by chordae.
Cup-shaped semilunar valves.

BLOOD SUPPLY TO HEART

Left coronary artery:
Anterior descending: supplies anterior wall.
Circumflex: supplies lateral wall.
Right coronary artery: supplies posterior wall.

CONDUCTION SYSTEM

SA node.
AV node.
AV bundle, branches, and Purkinje fibers.

THE CARDIAC CYCLE

Blood fills ventricles passively during diastole.
Atrial contraction not essential for ventricular filling.
Only about 60% of ventricular blood ejected during systole (ejection fraction).

BLOOD VESSELS

Large elastic arteries stretch during systole and relax in diastole.
Arterioles lower pressure and regulate flow into capillaries.
Capillaries deliver nutrients and carry away waste products.

BLOOD PRESSURE

Systolic pressure: reflects force of ventricular contraction.
Diastolic pressure: measure of peripheral resistance.

THE ELECTROCARDIOGRAM (ECG)

Cardiac arrhythmias: diagnosis and treatment
Atrial and ventricular fibrillation.
Heart block.

Heart Disease as a Disturbance of Pump Function

CONGENITAL HEART DISEASE

Classification
Failure of fetal bypass channels to close normally.
Abnormal communication between cardiac chambers.
Abnormalities that impede blood flow through the cardiovascular system.
Abnormal division of truncus arteriosus:
Left-to-right blood shunts cause pulmonary hypertension and damage lungs.
Right-to-left blood shunts cause cyanosis, polycythemia, and clubbing of digits.
Treatment methods available for many patients.
Prevention: protect fetus from intrauterine injury.

VALVULAR HEART DISEASE

Rheumatic fever and rheumatic heart disease:
Rheumatic fever is a complication of beta-streptococcal infection and causes valvular damage.
Healing leads to valve scarring. Prevented by prompt treatment of beta-streptococcal infection.

Nonrheumatic aortic stenosis:

Bicuspid aortic valve: congenital malformation eventually leads to valve thickening and scarring.

Calcific aortic stenosis: degenerative change in elderly individuals.

MITRAL VALVE PROLAPSE

Valve stretches owing to degeneration of connective tissue and prolapses into left atrium.

Chordae may rupture owing to stress.

Predisposes to arrhythmia.

SEROTONIN-RELATED HEART VALVE DAMAGE

High concentration of blood serotonin damages heart valves.

Valve damage caused by drugs that activate serotonin receptors, causing proliferation of connective tissue in valves.

ANTIBIOTIC PROPHYLAXIS TO PREVENT ENDOCARDITIS

Transient bacteremia often follows dental or surgical procedures.

Bacteria may implant on damaged heart valves and cause endocarditis.

Antibiotic treatment for selected persons.

Prosthetic heart valves.

INFECTIVE ENDOCARDITIS

Subacute: organisms of low virulence implant on damaged valves.

Acute: virulent organisms implant on normal valves and may destroy valve. Intravenous drug abusers at high risk.

Coronary Heart Disease

PATHOGENESIS OF ATHEROSCLEROSIS

Endothelial injury.

Lipids accumulate and precipitate.

Secondary fibrosis and calcification.

MAJOR RISK FACTORS

High blood lipids.

High blood pressure.

Cigarette smoking.

Diabetes.

MANIFESTATIONS

Angina pectoris.

Classification:

Stable angina: pain on exertion, subsides with rest or medication.

Unstable angina: more frequent episodes, last longer, poor response to rest or medications.

Prinzmetal's angina: occurs at rest, caused by coronary artery spasm.

DIAGNOSIS

Angiography: detects extent of disease and localizes sites of obstruction.

CORONARY DISEASE SYMPTOMS WITH NORMAL ANGIOGRAMS

Disease missed by angiography.

Coronary vasospasm.

Failure of arterioles to dilate normally.

TREATMENT

Medical treatment:

Drugs to reduce myocardial oxygen consumption and improve coronary circulation.

Drugs to reduce myocardial irritability.

Reduction of risk factors:

Cessation of smoking.

Control of hypertension.

Anti-coronary diet.

Weight reduction where appropriate.

Graduated exercises.

Surgical treatment: myocardial revascularization.

Coronary angioplasty: balloon catheter smashes atheromatous plaque and dilates artery.

Severe myocardial ischemia and its complications: a "heart attack."

Cardiac arrest: ventricular fibrillation or asystole.

Myocardial Infarction

LOCATION: ALMOST ALWAYS LEFT VENTRICLE

Anterior wall: left anterior descending artery distribution.

Lateral wall: circumflex artery distribution.

Posterior wall: right coronary distribution.

Massive anterior and lateral wall: main left coronary distribution.

MAJOR COMPLICATIONS

Arrhythmias.

Heart failure.

Intracardiac thrombi.

Cardiac rupture: a complication of transmural infarct.

SURVIVAL AFTER MYOCARDIAL INFARCTION

Depends on patient's age, size of infarct, presence of complications.

Average survival: 95% of hospitalized patients.

Survival frequency does not reflect patients who die before entering the hospital or patients with small infarcts who do not consult physician.

DIAGNOSIS

History and physical: often inconclusive.

Electrocardiogram: can detect location and size of infarct.

Enzyme tests: enzymes leak from infarcted muscle.

TREATMENT OF CORONARY THROMBOSIS

Thrombolytic (clot-dissolving) therapy or angioplasty improves survival and salvages myocardium.

Bed rest advancing to graded activity.

Anti-arrhythmia drugs: to reduce myocardial irritability.

Treatment of complications:

Heart block: requires pacemaker.

Heart failure: digitalis and diuretics.

Long-term treatment with antiarrhythmia drugs (beta-blockers) and aspirin improves prognosis.

COCAINE-INDUCED ARRHYTHMIAS/ INFARCTS

Drug intensifies effects of sympathetic nerve impulses.
Rapid heart rate: increases oxygen requirements.
Myocardial irritability: predisposes to arrhythmias.
Constricts blood vessels: raises blood pressure.

Drug may induce coronary artery spasm/severe ischemia/myocardial infarcts.

Fatal arrhythmias/myocardial infarcts may occur in persons with normal coronary arteries. Persons with coronary atherosclerosis are at even greater risk.

Blood Lipids and Coronary Heart Disease

NEUTRAL FAT: TRIGLYCERIDE

Composed of fatty acid combined with glycerol.

Fatty acids may be saturated, unsaturated, or polyunsaturated.

CHOLESTEROL

High levels associated with increased incidence of coronary heart disease.

Transport of cholesterol by lipoprotein.
LDL cholesterol is atherogenic: "bad cholesterol."
HDL cholesterol is protective: "good cholesterol."

ALTERATION OF BLOOD LIPIDS BY CHANGE IN DIET

Decrease cholesterol intake.

Decrease intake of saturated fats.

Derive carbohydrates from complex carbohydrates.

Reduce alcohol intake.

C-REACTIVE PROTEIN AS A CARDIOVASCULAR RISK FACTOR

A protein produced in response to inflammation or infection.

Sensitive CRP tests detect body's response to cells and lipids in unstable coronary artery plaques.

Test proposed as additional screening test to detect persons at risk of coronary artery disease.

The metabolic syndrome and cardiovascular disease:
An obesity-related insulin resistance syndrome.
Predisposes to cardiovascular disease and diabetes.
Effective treatment may reduce risk.

HOMOCYSTEINE AND CARDIOVASCULAR DISEASE

Persons with very high homocysteine blood levels caused by a rare hereditary disease called homocysteinuria have early onset of severe atherosclerosis.

Persons with higher-than-normal homocysteine blood levels are at higher-than-normal risk of cardiovascular disease.

Deficiency of vitamin B_6, B_{12}, or folic acid can raise homocysteine blood concentration, which can be corrected by vitamin supplements, but treatment is harmful to coronary heart disease patients by promoting cell proliferation in coronary artery plaques.

TAKING ASPIRIN TO REDUCE CARDIOVASCULAR DISEASE RISK

Blood clots are initiated by platelets that adhere to roughened areas overlying an atherosclerotic plaque, which initiates an intravascular thrombosis.

Aspirin reduces risk by inactivating a platelet enzyme that is required for platelet aggregation.

Hypertension and Hypertensive Cardiovascular Disease

INCREASED PERIPHERAL RESISTANCE INCREASES WORK OF HEART

Vascular effects:
Vessels wear out prematurely.
Weakened arteries may rupture in brain causing cerebral hemorrhage.

Renal effects: narrowing of arterioles damages kidneys.

CAUSES AND TREATMENT

In most cases cause unknown.

Treatment by drugs that lower blood pressure.

ISOLATED SYSTOLIC HYPERTENSION

Affects older persons.

Rigid aorta unable to stretch to absorb the force of ejected blood.

Systolic pressure rises, but diastolic pressure is normal.

Treatment advisable despite normal diastolic pressure.

Primary Myocardial Disease

MYOCARDITIS

Usually viral; occasionally, other pathogens or hypersensitivity state.

Onset usually abrupt, with eventual complete recovery.

CARDIOMYOPATHY

Dilated cardiomyopathy:
Heart enlarged and dilated.
Cause uncertain, no specific treatment available.

Hypertrophic cardiomyopathy:
Hereditary dominant transmission.
Disorganized muscle fibers and greatly hypertrophied heart.
Thick septum impinging on mitral valve leaflet may block outflow of blood from ventricle (idiopathic hypertrophic subaortic stenosis).
Treated by drugs that slow heart and reduce force of contraction.
Surgical resection of part of septum if medical management fails.

Heart Failure

DEFINITION

Heart no longer able to function efficiently:
Acute heart failure: rapid progression.
Chronic heart failure: slow onset and progression.

Pathogenesis:
Forward failure: inadequate cardiac output leads to salt and water retention by kidneys.
Backward failure: blood backs up in venous circulation.

Systolic and diastolic dysfunction in heart failure.
Failing ventricle cannot eject adequate blood in systole: systolic heart failure.

Ventricle cannot fill adequately in diastole: diastolic heart failure.

Treatment:

Diuretics: promote salt and water excretion.
Digitalis: increases efficiency of cardiac contraction.
ACE inhibitors.
Natriuretic peptide (BNP).

Acute Pulmonary Edema

PATHOGENESIS

Temporary disproportion in output of blood from left and right ventricles.
Blood accumulates in lung.
Extravasation of fluid in alveoli.

Aneurysms

ARTERIOSCLEROTIC ANEURYSM

Arteriosclerosis damages wall, which dilates owing to high intraluminal pressure.
Aneurysm may rupture and cause profuse hemorrhage.
Treatment by replacement with nylon or Dacron graft.
Endovascular repair available for selected cases.

DISSECTING ANEURYSM OF THE AORTA

Splitting of layers of wall.
Blood dissects through intimal tear and may rupture back into lumen or externally.
Can be treated surgically.

Diseases of the Veins

VENOUS THROMBOSIS AND THROMBOPHLEBITIS

Deep veins of lower extremities most commonly affected.
Postoperative and bed patients predisposed.
Predisposing factors, pathogenesis, manifestations, and treatment covered in the discussion on circulatory disturbances.

VARICOSE VEINS OF LOWER EXTREMITIES

Usually a result of congenital weakness of vein wall or valves predisposing to varicosities.
May occur if deeper veins blocked or valves damaged by thrombophlebitis, diverting more blood flow to superficial veins.
Complications:

Stasis ulcers.
Rupture with bleeding.
Thrombophlebitis.

Treatment:

Medical: elastic stockings, elevation of limb.
Surgical: ligation and excision of varicosities.

VARICOSE VEINS IN OTHER LOCATIONS

Hemorrhoids: varicose veins of rectum (see the gastrointestinal tract).
Esophageal varices: in patients with cirrhosis of liver (see the liver and the biliary system).
Varicocele: veins of spermatic cord. Usually asymptomatic, requiring no treatment.

http://health.jbpub.com/humandisease/9e

Human Disease Online is a great source for supplementary human disease information for both students and instructors. Visit this website to find a variety of useful tools for learning, thinking, and teaching.

The Hematopoietic and Lymphatic Systems

LEARNING OBJECTIVES

1. Describe the composition of the blood, and enumerate its functions. Explain the functions of the lymphatic system.
2. Explain the principles by which anemias are classified and treated.
3. List and describe the usual causes of hypochromic microcytic anemia and macrocytic anemia. Explain how these anemias are treated.
4. List the usual causes of anemia as a result of bone marrow damage and anemia caused by accelerated blood destruction. Explain their treatment.
5. Describe the causes and effects of polycythemia and thrombocytopenia.
6. Describe the cause and clinical manifestations of infectious mononucleosis.
7. List the common causes of lymph node enlargement.
8. Explain the role of the spleen in protecting the body against infection. Describe the effects of a splenectomy on the body's defenses, and relate them to the management of the patient who has had a splenectomy.

The Hematopoietic System

Composition and Function of Human Blood

Blood is essential to transporting oxygen and nutrients to the tissues; carbon dioxide and other waste products of cell metabolism to the excretory organs; and leukocytes, hormones, and antibodies to various locations in the body. The volume of blood, which varies with the size of the individual, is about 5 quarts in the average man. Almost half of the blood consists of cellular elements: red cells, white cells (leukocytes), and platelets suspended in a viscous fluid

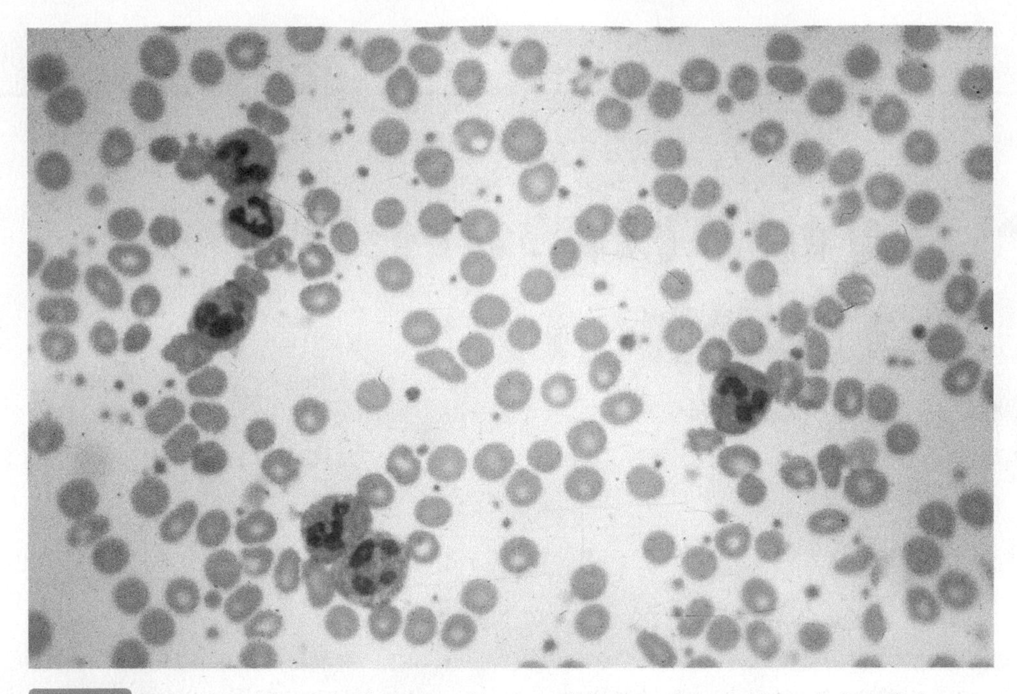

Figure 1 Stained blood film. Red cells appear as biconcave disks. Several neutrophils can be identified near the *center* of the photograph. Small dark structures are platelets (original magnification × 1000).

called blood plasma (Figure 1). All blood cells arise from precursor cells within the bone marrow called stem cells, which undergo further differentiation to form the red cells, white cells, and platelets circulating in the bloodstream. The numbers of circulating red cells, white cells, and platelets are so great that their numbers are expressed as the number per microliter of blood (1 mL = 1000 microliters). This same quantity can also be expressed as the number per cubic millimeter (mm^3) of blood. The terms are equivalent because 1 microliter is the same as 1 cubic millimeter.

Red cells, which are concerned primarily with oxygen transport, are the most numerous cells, averaging about 5 million per microliter of blood. A mature red cell is an extremely flexible biconcave disk measuring about 7 micrometers (microns) in cross-section diameter. Its biconcave configuration is responsible for its characteristic central pallor and more intensely stained periphery, as seen in a stained blood smear. The biconcave configuration also provides the red cell with a large surface area relative to its volume, which facilitates rapid uptake of oxygen as blood flows through the pulmonary capillaries, and a rapid release of oxygen to body cells as blood is delivered to the tissues. The red cell shape also contributes to its extreme flexibility, which allows red cells to squeeze through small blood capillaries less than half the diameter of the red cells. Red cells normally survive for about 4 months in the circulation.

Leukocytes are much less numerous, averaging about 7000 per microliter. The following types of leukocytes are recognized:

1. Neutrophils
2. Eosinophils
3. Basophils
4. Monocytes
5. Lymphocytes

Although lymphocytes are produced chiefly in the lymph nodes and spleen, they are also manufactured in the bone marrow and elsewhere throughout the body where lymphoid tissue is present. Under normal circumstances, production of the other types of white cells is confined to the bone marrow. In contrast with the relatively long survival of red cells, most white cells have a short survival time within the circulation, varying from several hours to several days, and they must be replenished continually. Lymphocytes are an exception. Two populations of lymphocytes are present in the circulation, one surviving about the same length of time as most of the other leukocytes and another surviving for several years.

The proportions of the various leukocytes vary with the age of the individual. The most numerous in the adult are the neutrophils, constituting about 70 percent of the total circulating white cells. Neutrophils are actively phagocytic and predominate in acute inflammatory reactions. Lymphocytes are the next most common type of white cells in adults and are the predominant leukocytes in the blood of children. The lymphocytes in the peripheral blood constitute only a small fraction of the total lymphocytes, most being located in the lymph nodes, spleen, and other lymphoid tissues. Lymphocytes continually recirculate from the bloodstream into lymphoid tissues. Eventually, they leave the lymphoid tissue through the lymphatic channels and the thoracic duct, returning to the circulation and later becoming reestablished for a time in a different site of lymphoid tissue. Lymphocytes take part in cell-mediated and humoral defense reactions.

Small numbers of eosinophils, basophils, and monocytes also are normally present in the blood. **Eosinophils** are related in some manner to allergy. One of their functions appears to be phagocytosis and digestion of antigen–antibody complexes. Eosinophils increase in allergic diseases, in the presence of worm or other animal–parasite infections, and in a few other conditions. **Basophils** are similar to mast cells. Their granules contain histamine and an anticoagulant called heparin. **Monocytes** are actively phagocytic and increase in certain types of chronic infections. A monocyte–lymphocyte interaction is necessary in the initial phase of response to a foreign antigen; it also plays a role in the cell mediated immune reaction.

Blood platelets, which are essential for normal blood coagulation, are much smaller than leukocytes. They represent bits of the cytoplasm of **megakaryocytes**, large precursor cells present in the bone marrow. Platelets have a short survival, comparable to that of most leukocytes.

Normal Hematopoiesis

The bone marrow can be compared to a large manufacturing plant. It replenishes the blood cells that are continually being worn out and removed from the circulation. As with any manufacturing process, adequate quantities of raw materials are required. Moreover, the factory must be able to process these raw materials efficiently into finished products (the blood cells). The major raw materials necessary for hematopoiesis are protein, vitamin B_{12}, folic acid (one of the vitamin B group), and iron. Inadequate supplies of these substances will handicap the production of blood cells.

Development, Maturation, and Survival of Red Cells

Red cells develop from large precursor cells in the bone marrow called **erythroblasts** (*erythro* = red + *blast* = a primitive cell). **Hemoglobin,** the oxygen-carrying protein that is formed by the developing red cells, is composed of four separate pieces called *subunits*, which in turn fit together to form a much larger aggregate called a *tetramer* (*tetra* = four). Each subunit consists of two parts: *heme* and *globin*.

Heme is a complex nitrogen-containing ring structure (called a *porphyrin ring*) containing an iron atom. Globin, which forms the largest part of each hemoglobin subunit, is a short, coiled protein (*polypeptide*) chain. Several types of globin chains, differing in their amino acid composition, are formed at varying times and in differing proportions in the fetus and in the adult. The chains are designated by Greek letters: alpha (α), beta (β), gamma (γ), delta (δ), and epsilon (ε).

The hemoglobin in the red cells of the normal adult is called *hemoglobin A* or *adult hemoglobin*. Two subunits of the tetramer contain alpha chains and two contain beta chains. The hemoglobin can also be designated by the shorthand notation $\alpha_2\beta_2$. (The chain is designated by the Greek letter and the number of subunits by the subscript.)

In the embryo and fetus, hemoglobin containing different globin chains is produced at various times in the course of prenatal development. Beta chain production does not occur until relatively late in prenatal development. Consequently, the predominant hemoglobin in the fetus is a tetramer of alpha and gamma chains that is termed **fetal hemoglobin** (hemoglobin F). Fetal hemoglobin is able to take up and release oxygen more efficiently than adult hemoglobin when the oxygen partial pressure (PO_2) of the blood is low, an ability that is advantageous to the fetus because the PO_2 in fetal blood is lower than the PO_2 of adult blood. Late in pregnancy, fetal production of beta chains replaces gamma chains, and adult hemoglobin (hemoglobin A) begins to replace fetal hemoglobin in the red cells as the fetus prepares for life outside of the uterus.

The hemoglobin of a newborn infant contains both adult and fetal hemoglobin in approximately equal proportions. Normally, no significant fetal hemoglobin synthesis occurs after birth. As new red cells are

eosinophil (ē-ō-sin′o-fil) A cell whose cytoplasm is filled with large, uniform granules that stain intensely red with acid dyes. See also *basophil*.

basophil A cell that contains numerous variable-sized granules that stain intensely purple with basic dyes. See also *eosinophil*.

monocyte (mon′ō-sī-t) A leukocyte having a kidney-shaped nucleus and light blue cytoplasm; a phagocytic cell that forms part of the reticuloendothelial system.

megakaryocyte (mega-car-ry′o-sī-t) A very large bone marrow cell having abundant granular cytoplasm and multilobed nucleus that forms the platelets circulating in the bloodstream.

erythroblast (e-rith′rō-blast) A precursor cell in the bone marrow that gives rise to red blood cells.

hemoglobin An oxygen transport protein within red cells composed of an iron-porphyrin complex (heme) combined with a protein chain (globin).

fetal hemoglobin A type of hemoglobin containing two alpha and two gamma chains, which is able to take up and release oxygen at much lower PO_2 (oxygen partial pressures) than in adult hemoglobin.

reticulocyte (rē-tik′ū-lō-sīt) A young red cell that can be identified by special staining procedures.

erythropoietin (er-ith-rō-poy′e-tin) A humoral substance made by the kidneys that regulates hematopoiesis.

anemia (an-ē′mē-uh) A decrease in hemoglobin or red cells or both.

produced by the infant to replace those containing fetal hemoglobin that have reached the end of their life span, the new "replacement" red cells contain essentially only hemoglobin A. Consequently, the concentration of hemoglobin A rises in the infant's blood as hemoglobin F falls. By about 6 months of age, the hemoglobin is almost entirely hemoglobin A, which functions normally in the circulation.

The developing red cell accumulates increasing amounts of hemoglobin as it matures. When about 80 percent of its total hemoglobin has been synthesized, the nucleus is extruded. The cell is then discharged from the bone marrow into the circulation, where it completes its maturation and hemoglobin synthesis over the succeeding 24 hours. A newly formed red cell, which lacks a nucleus but still retains its mitochondria and other organelles for a short time, is called a **reticulocyte**. The name comes from its special staining characteristics. Certain stains precipitate the organelles within the cell cytoplasm, causing them to appear as a network (reticulum) of dark blue strands and granules. A reticulocyte is slightly larger than a mature red cell, and it also has a faint blue color because it contains less red-staining hemoglobin than a mature cell. These distinguishing features, which differentiate a reticulocyte from a mature red cell, are soon lost as the cell matures within the circulation.

The red cell, which derives its energy from the enzymatic breakdown of glucose, possesses enzyme systems that permit the cell to perform the diverse metabolic functions necessary for survival. Because the cell lacks a nucleus, it cannot synthesize new enzyme molecules to replace those that gradually wear out. As the cell ages, its enzyme systems gradually become depleted until eventually, after about 4 months, the cell is no longer able to function. The worn-out red cell is then removed by the mononuclear phagocyte system (reticuloendothelial system), primarily in the spleen, and its hemoglobin is degraded. The globin chains are broken down, and their component amino acids are used to make other proteins. The iron is extracted and saved to make new hemoglobin. The porphyrin ring, however, cannot be salvaged. It is degraded and is excreted by the liver as bile pigment.

Regulation of Hematopoiesis

Red cell production is regulated by the oxygen content of the arterial blood. Decreased oxygen supply to the tissues stimulates erythropoiesis. However, low oxygen tension does not act directly on the bone marrow. The effect is mediated by the kidneys. Certain specialized cells in the kidneys elaborate a hormonelike erythrocyte-stimulating material called **erythropoietin.**

The factors regulating the production of white blood cells and their delivery into the circulation are not well understood. Products of cell necrosis may cause the number of white blood cells in the peripheral blood to increase. Hormone secretion by the adrenals and some other endocrine glands also influences white cell production.

Anemia

Anemia literally means "without blood." Specifically, the term is used to refer to a decrease in red cells or to subnormal hemoglobin levels. Many classifications of anemia have been proposed, and two different methods of classification are widely used. One system, based on the factor responsible for the anemia, is an etiologic classification. A second system, based on the shape and appearance of the red blood cells (as determined by microscopic examination of a stained blood smear), is a morphologic classification.

Etiologic Classification of Anemia

One simple classification of the anemias is based on the "bone marrow factory" concept (Figure 2). Anemia is classified as being caused by either inadequate production of red cells or an excessive loss of cells. Inadequate production, in turn, may result from an insufficiency of raw materials or from factors that render the factory inoperative and no longer able to deliver enough finished products into the circulation. Examples of the latter would be marrow damage or replacement of marrow by abnormal cells. Excessive loss of red cells may be caused either by external blood loss or by accelerated destruction of the cells (and hence shortened survival) in the circulation. Table 1 presents a classification of the various causes of anemia.

Morphologic Classification of Anemia

An anemia in which the cells are normal in size and appearance is called a normocytic anemia. If the cells are larger than normal, the anemia is called a macrocytic anemia. If the cells are smaller than normal, the anemia is called a microcytic anemia. Many times, microcytic cells also have a reduced hemoglobin content, appearing quite pale when examined under the microscope; here, the term *hypochromic anemia* is used. Often the latter two terms are combined, and the anemia is called a *hypochromic microcytic anemia.* Classification of anemia on the basis of red cell appearance

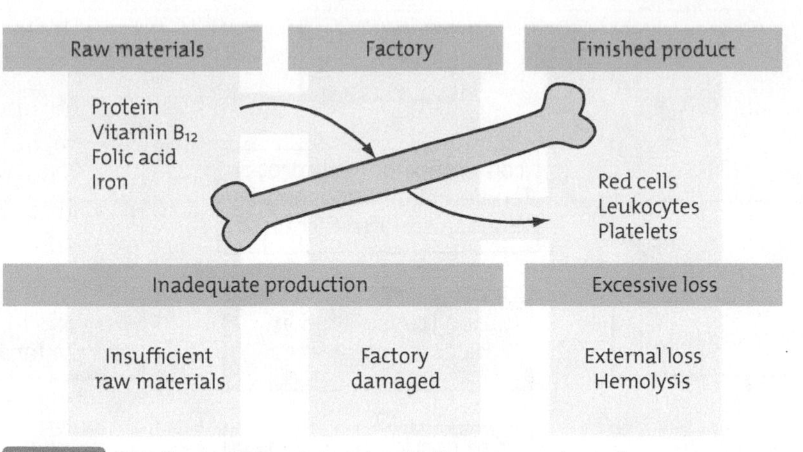

Figure 2 Classification of anemia based on the "bone marrow factory" concept.

Table 1 Etiologic Classification of Anemia

Inadequate Production of Red Cells
Caused by inadequate "raw materials"
Iron deficiency
Vitamin B_{12} deficiency
Folic acid deficiency
Caused by impaired function of bone marrow factory
Anemia of chronic disease
Bone marrow damaged or destroyed (aplastic anemia)
Bone marrow replaced by foreign or abnormal cells (bone marrow replacement anemia)
Excessive Loss of Red Cells
Caused by external blood loss (hemorrhage)
Caused by shortened survival of red cells in the circulation
Defective red cells (hereditary hemolytic anemia)
Abnormal red cell shape
Abnormal hemoglobin within red cells
Defective hemoglobin synthesis within red cells
Deficient red cell enzymes
"Hostile environment"
Anti-red cell antibodies
Mechanical trauma to circulating red cells

is useful because the appearance of the cells provides a clue to the etiology. Iron deficiency anemia is a hypochromic microcytic anemia. Anemia caused by vitamin B_{12} or folic acid deficiency is a macrocytic anemia. Most other types of anemia are normocytic.

Iron Metabolism and Hematopoiesis

The body contains about 4 grams of iron, of which about 75 percent is contained in hemoglobin. Most of the rest is a reserve supply that is stored in the liver, bone marrow, and spleen combined with an iron-binding protein called apoferritin to form an iron–protein complex called ferritin. A small amount of iron also circulates in the blood bound to a protein called transferrin, which is the iron being transported from place to place in the body.

The usual diet of an adult contains from about 10 to 20 mg of iron, but men absorb merely 1 mg per day, and only slightly more iron is absorbed by women and children. Women need more iron to make up for menstrual losses because 1 mL of blood contains about 0.5 mg of iron. Additional iron is also required during pregnancy to supply the needs of the developing fetus. Children require greater amounts of iron in order to synthesize more hemoglobin during periods of growth when the blood volume is increasing. Iron is absorbed with difficulty from the gastrointestinal tract, and iron stores within the body are carefully conserved.

Figure 3 summarizes how iron is handled in the body. Iron is absorbed chiefly in the duodenum, and the amount absorbed depends on the iron content of the duodenal epithelial cells, which in turn is determined by the amount of iron stored as ferritin in the liver, bone marrow, and other iron storage sites. If iron stores are abundant, so also is the iron content of the intestinal epithelial cells, and less dietary iron is absorbed. On the other hand, if body iron stores are depleted, the iron content of the duodenal cells is also reduced, and more iron can be absorbed into the cells for eventual transport to storage sites in order to replenish ferritin stores.

From the duodenal mucosa the iron is transported by transferrin to the bone marrow for hemoglobin synthesis and to the liver and other storage sites where it is available for later use.

As red cells wear out and are destroyed, the iron from the hemoglobin is recycled, transported by transferrin back to the bone marrow, and used to make new hemoglobin. If sufficient recycled iron is not available

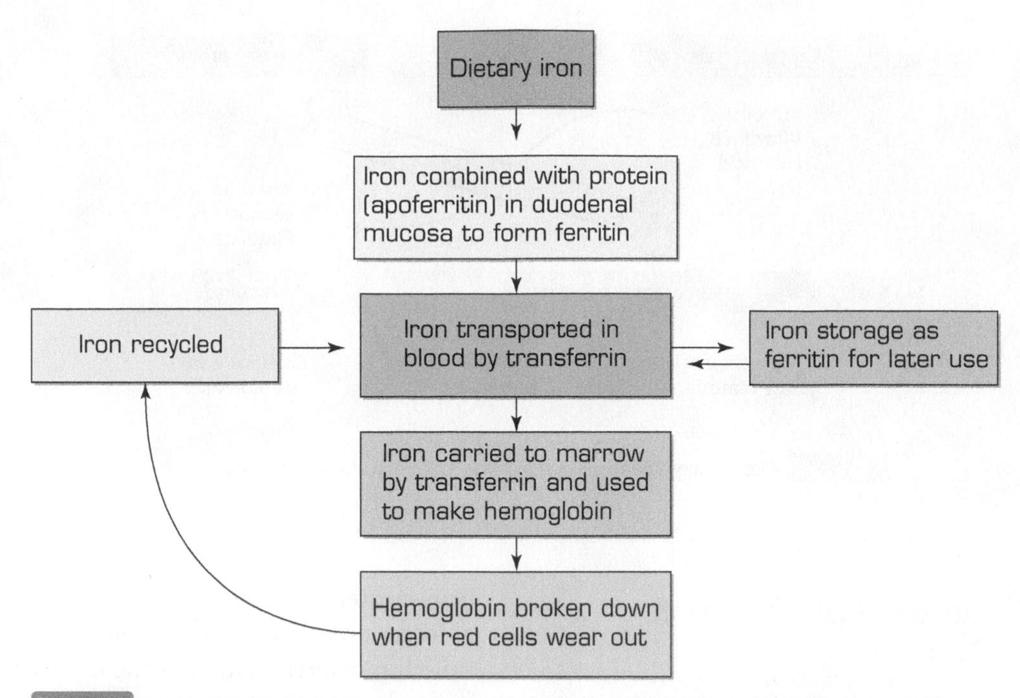

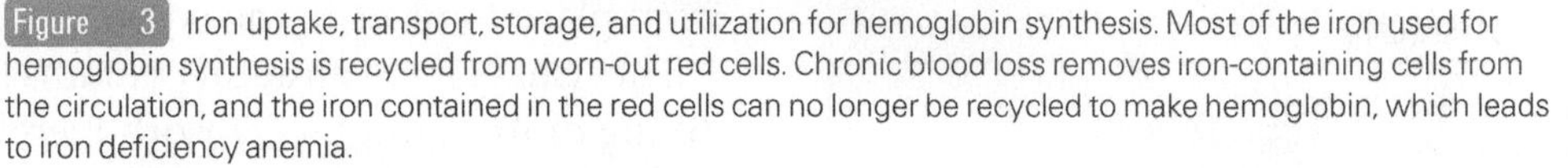
Figure 3 Iron uptake, transport, storage, and utilization for hemoglobin synthesis. Most of the iron used for hemoglobin synthesis is recycled from worn-out red cells. Chronic blood loss removes iron-containing cells from the circulation, and the iron contained in the red cells can no longer be recycled to make hemoglobin, which leads to iron deficiency anemia.

for hemoglobin synthesis, additional iron is mobilized from storage sites.

Iron Deficiency Anemia

Iron deficiency anemia is the most common anemia encountered in clinical practice. Iron forms an essential part of the hemoglobin molecule, and normal synthesis of hemoglobin requires adequate supplies of iron.

When red blood cells, which have a normal life span of about 4 months, become "senile," they are removed from the circulation. The iron from the destroyed cells is transported back to the bone marrow and is reused by the bone marrow to be incorporated into newly formed red cells. Iron deficiency anemia may result from either (1) insufficient intake of iron in the diet, or (2) inadequate reutilization of the iron present in worn-out red cells, which normally is recycled to make new hemoglobin. Chronic blood loss depletes body iron stores because the iron in the hemoglobin is also lost along with the red cell, and is no longer available to be recycled for red cell production.

Iron deficiency caused by inadequate dietary intake may occur in infants during periods of rapid growth. A normal, full-term infant has been provided with a reserve supply of iron that was transferred to the fetus from the mother during the last part of pregnancy. Consequently, the newborn infant generally has an adequate short-term supply of iron available for hematopoiesis during the neonatal period when the production of red cells accelerates to supply the needs of an increasing blood volume. Premature infants, however, may not get their full component of iron stores, and may not have enough reserve to supply their postnatal needs. Even in full-term infants, the reserve supply of iron for hematopoiesis is limited and must be supplemented by iron from the diet. Breast milk contains very little iron, although the amount available is well absorbed. If the diet is not supplemented by cereals, fruits, vegetables, other foods containing iron, or some type of iron supplement, iron stores will become rapidly exhausted, and iron deficiency anemia will develop in the first year of life. For this reason, many physicians gradually add supplementary foods containing additional sources of iron to infants' diets. Occasionally, adolescents subsisting on an inadequate or poorly balanced diet develop iron deficiency anemia.

Most cases of iron deficiency anemia in adults result from a failure to recapture the iron present in red cells for hemoglobin synthesis. This failure is a result of chronic blood loss. The iron contained in red cells that is lost from the circulation by bleeding is no longer available to the body for the production of new red cells. Because each milliliter of blood contains 0.5 mg of iron, a loss of 500 mL of blood represents a loss of 250 mg of iron, which is equivalent to one-fourth of the body's entire iron reserves. Unless dietary intake of iron is extremely liberal, iron stores soon become exhausted, and iron deficiency anemia develops.

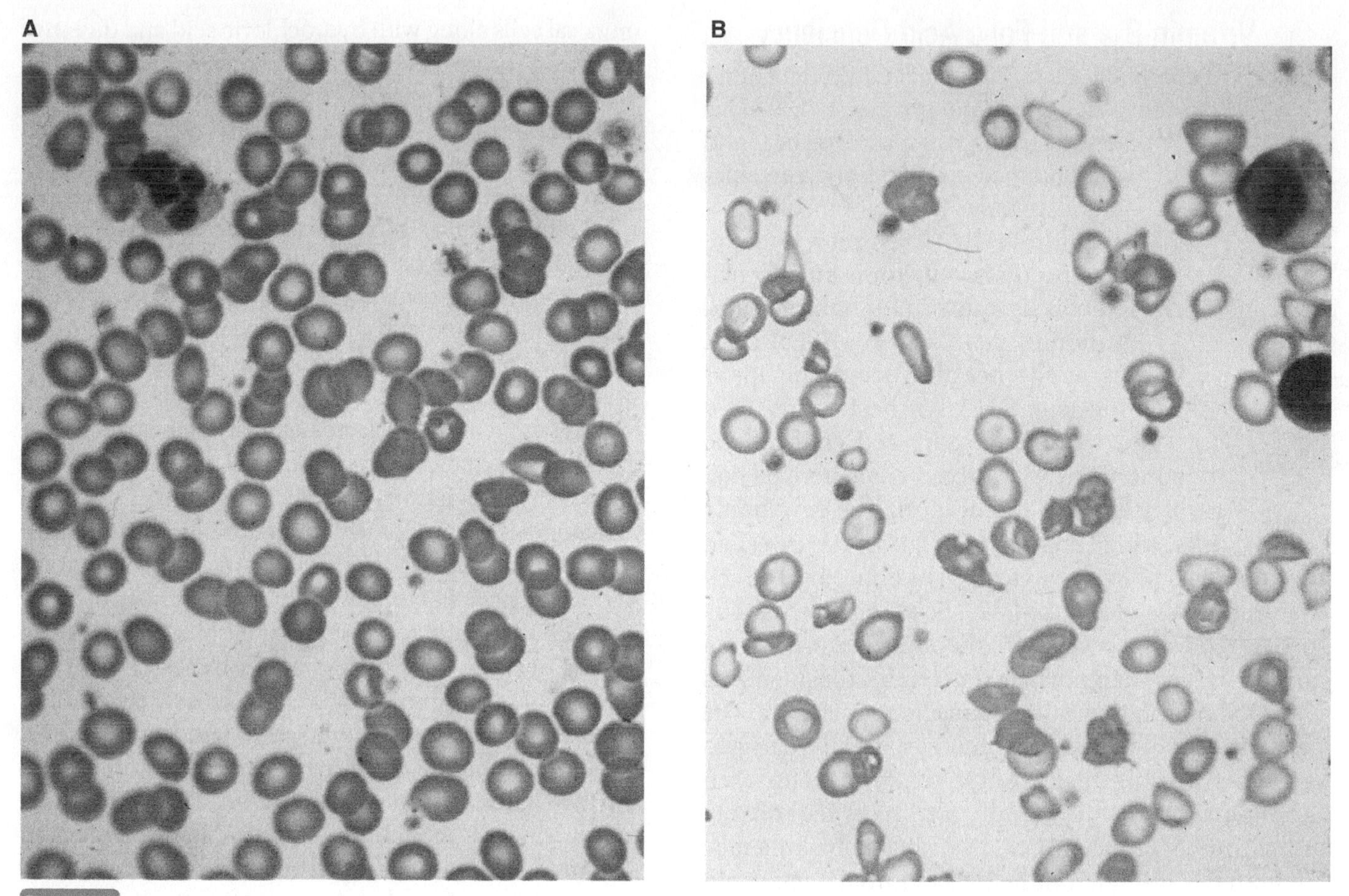

Figure 4 Comparison of normal red cells, A, with those of hypochromic microcytic anemia, B, caused by chronic iron deficiency (original magnification × 400).

Iron deficiency anemia is a hypochromic microcytic anemia (Figure 4). The cells are pale because they contain less hemoglobin than normal. The cells are also abnormally small because the body apparently attempts to "scale down" the size of the cell to conform to the reduced hemoglobin content.

Laboratory Tests to Evaluate Iron Metabolism in Iron Deficiency Anemia Various laboratory tests that measure iron stores, iron transport, and iron metabolism can be used as diagnostic tests in patients with suspected iron deficiency anemia. These include measurements of serum ferritin, serum iron, and serum iron-binding capacity.

In iron deficiency anemia, body iron stores are depleted and serum ferritin is low. Serum iron is also much lower than normal, but the amount of iron transport protein in the serum is much higher than normal, apparently reflecting the body's attempt to capture the meager iron available and transport it more efficiently. Consequently, the characteristic laboratory profile of iron deficiency anemia is low serum ferritin and serum iron, but a much higher than normal serum iron-binding protein with a much lower than normal percent of iron saturation.

Evaluation and Treatment of Iron Deficiency Anemia A physician treating a patient with iron deficiency anemia is primarily concerned with learning the cause of the anemia and then directing therapy toward the cause rather than the symptoms. In an infant with a history of a very poor diet, the cause may be obvious. In an adult, the anemia is usually a result of blood loss, and the physician must always be aware of this possibility and investigate to determine the reason for the blood loss. Chronic blood loss, for example, may be caused by a bleeding ulcer or an ulcerated carcinoma of the colon. In women, excessive menstrual bleeding is a common cause of iron deficiency anemia. Another sometimes overlooked cause of iron deficiency anemia in otherwise healthy young adults is too frequent blood donations. When the cause of the blood loss has been determined, proper treatment of the underlying cause can be instituted. In addition, the patient is given supplementary iron to replenish the body's depleted iron stores.

Vitamin B_{12} and Folic Acid Deficiency

mega-loblast (meg´al-ō-blast) An abnormal red cell precursor resulting from vitamin B_{12} or folic acid deficiency.

leukopenia (lōō-kō-pē´ni-uh) An abnormally small number of leukocytes in the peripheral blood.

thrombocytopenia (throm´bō-sī-tō-pē´ny-yuh) A deficiency of platelets.

Vitamin B_{12} is found in meat, liver, and other foods rich in animal protein. Folic acid is widely distributed in nature, being found in abundance in green leafy vegetables as well as many foods of animal origin.

Vitamin B_{12} and folic acid are required not only for normal hematopoiesis, but also for normal maturation of many other types of cells. In the absence of either vitamin B_{12} or folic acid, DNA synthesis is impaired and the developing red cells in the bone marrow exhibit a characteristic disturbance of cell maturation. The developing red cells, which are larger than normal, are called **megaloblasts** (*megalos* = large). The abnormal red cell maturation is called *megaloblastic erythropoiesis*. The mature red cells derived from the abnormal maturation also are larger than normal. Therefore, the anemia is classified morphologically as a macrocytic anemia. The development of white cell precursors and megakaryocytes is also abnormal. Consequently, patients with megaloblastic anemia usually also have **leukopenia** and **thrombocytopenia** as well as a macrocytic anemia. Vitamin B_{12}, but not folic acid, is required to maintain the structural and functional integrity of the nervous system; thus, a deficiency of this vitamin also may be associated with pronounced neurologic disturbances.

Anemia as a Result of Folic Acid Deficiency The body has very limited stores of folic acid, which rapidly become depleted if not replenished continually. As a result, folic acid–deficiency anemia is relatively common and may result from reduced dietary intake, impaired absorption, or increased folic acid requirements.

Deficiency caused by inadequate dietary intake is found in persons subsisting on inadequate diets and is encountered frequently in persons consuming excessive amounts of alcohol because of their typically deficient diet, and possibly also impaired absorption of folic acid compared with nondrinkers. Persons with chronic intestinal diseases may become folic acid deficient because of impaired ability to absorb the vitamin. Pregnant women also are at risk because pregnancy greatly increases folic acid requirements. Folic acid–deficiency anemia in pregnancy is uncommon because physicians routinely prescribe folic acid supplements to pregnant women.

Anemia as a Result of Vitamin B_{12} Deficiency Efficient absorption of vitamin B_{12} ingested in food requires a substance called intrinsic factor that is secreted by gastric mucosal cells along with hydrochloric acid and digestive enzymes. The intrinsic factor combines with the vitamin B_{12}, and the B_{12}–intrinsic factor complex is absorbed from the distal small intestine. The absorbed vitamin is stored in the liver and made available to the bone marrow and other tissues as required for cell growth and maturation.

A common cause of vitamin B_{12} deficiency is pernicious anemia. The basic defect in pernicious anemia is atrophy of the gastric mucosa, which sometimes develops in middle-age and older individuals and is often associated with autoantibodies directed against gastric mucosal cells and intrinsic factor. The atrophic mucosa fails to secrete intrinsic factor as well as gastric acid and digestive enzymes, and consequently, vitamin B_{12} is not absorbed. The vitamin B_{12} deficiency causes impaired hematopoiesis as well as various neurologic disturbances.

Pernicious anemia is not the only cause of vitamin B_{12} deficiency. Persons who have had most of their stomach surgically removed because of ulcer or gastric cancer or who have had a gastric bypass procedure to control obesity may not be able to secrete enough intrinsic factor. Persons who have had a small bowel resection of the distal ilium, where the vitamin B_{12}–intrinsic factor complex is absorbed, may not be able to absorb enough vitamin to supply their needs, and an individual with chronic intestinal disease affecting the vitamin B_{12}–absorbing area in the distal ileum (such as Crohn disease) also may be unable to absorb the vitamin adequately.

Pernicious anemia and other vitamin B_{12} deficiencies are treated with intramuscular administration of vitamin B_{12}. Parenteral administration avoids the problem of poor absorption of the vitamin.

Bone Marrow Suppression, Damage, or Infiltration Many conditions can depress bone marrow function. Chronic diseases of all types may impair hematopoiesis and lead to mild or moderate anemia, which is called *the anemia of chronic disease*. In this condition, iron and other "raw materials" supplied to the bone marrow are adequate, but they are not utilized efficiently to make red cells. White blood cell and platelet production are usually not disturbed. The most common cause of this type of anemia is chronic infection, but other chronic diseases and some malignant tumors also may be responsible.

The anemia of chronic disease usually causes only a relatively mild suppression of bone marrow function and improves when the disease that caused it is identified and treated. Chronic infections may respond to treatment, but unfortunately, it is often not possible to "cure" many of the other chronic diseases that lead to this type of anemia.

In contrast to the anemia of chronic disease, much more serious and sometimes irreversible damage to the bone marrow factory results from destruction of the bone marrow stem cells from which mature blood cells and platelets arise. This type of anemia is called **aplastic anemia** (*a* = without + *plasia* = growth), although this term is not strictly accurate because the stem cell damage leads to leukopenia and thrombocytopenia as well as anemia. The anemia is classified as a normocytic anemia because the red cells are normal in size and shape although inadequate in number. Many agents can cause aplastic anemia. Radiation, anticancer chemotherapy drugs, and various toxic chemicals may cause severe marrow damage. Other drugs, including some antibiotics, anti-inflammatory drugs, and anticonvulsant drugs, may damage marrow stem cells in susceptible individuals. In many cases, however, it is the body's own immune system that is responsible for the aplastic anemia, a manifestation of an autoimmune disease in which the body's own cytotoxic T lymphocytes attack and destroy the marrow stem cells.

Aplastic anemia is treated initially by blood and platelet transfusions to maintain an adequate volume of circulating blood cells while the cause of the bone marrow failure is being investigated. If the marrow damage is caused by a toxic drug or chemical and is not too severe, marrow function may recover; however, it is unlikely in severe aplastic anemia, and other methods of treatment are required to restore marrow function. Many patients respond to immunosuppressive agents that act against the destructive (cytotoxic) T lymphocytes responsible for stem cell destruction. Bone marrow transplantation is also effective and can be performed in highly selected patients using the same methods used to treat patients with leukemia.

An anemia similar to aplastic anemia involving white cells and platelets as well as red cells may also occur if bone marrow stem cells are crowded out and replaced by abnormal cells, such as leukemic cells or metastatic carcinoma. The term *bone marrow replacement anemia* is sometimes used to denote this type of anemia. Unfortunately, it may be difficult to restore marrow function after the marrow has been heavily infiltrated by leukemic cells or cancer cells, although adequate levels of hemoglobin and red cells can be maintained by blood transfusions.

Acute Blood Loss

A normocytic anemia may result from an episode of acute blood loss, as from a massive hemorrhage from the uterus or gastrointestinal tract. Provided that iron stores are adequate, the lost blood is rapidly replaced by the bone marrow, and the newly formed red cells are normal. This is in contrast with the anemia of chronic blood loss, in which the red cells are hypochromic and microcytic because prolonged bleeding has depleted the body's iron stores.

aplastic anemia (ā-plas′tik) An anemia caused by bone marrow failure.

hemolytic anemia An anemia caused by increased blood destruction.

hereditary spherocytosis A hereditary anemia caused by a defect affecting the red cell membrane that causes the biconcave disk-shaped red cells to change into small spherical cells that do not survive normally in the circulation.

Accelerated Blood Destruction

Normal red cells survive for about 4 months. Sometimes, however, their survival is considerably shortened, and anemia results because the regenerative capacity of the marrow is not sufficient to keep up with the accelerated destruction. This type of anemia is called a **hemolytic anemia** and may be a result of either defective red cells or a "hostile environment." Hemolytic anemias caused by defective red cells are called hereditary hemolytic anemias. Those resulting from damage to normal red cells by antibodies or other injurious agents are called acquired hemolytic anemias.

Hereditary Hemolytic Anemias

The genetically determined abnormalities of red cells that may shorten their survival fall into four major groups (Table 2):

1. Abnormally shaped cells
2. Abnormal hemoglobins
3. Defective hemoglobin synthesis
4. Enzyme deficiencies

Abnormally Shaped Cells The most common abnormality of shape is called **hereditary spherocytosis**. In hereditary spherocytosis, the structural framework (cytoskeleton) of the red cell membrane is defective, which reduces its stability and flexibility. New red cells produced by the bone marrow and released into the circulation have a normal biconcave disk configuration, but bits of their unstable cell membranes become detached from the cells as the red cells squeeze through extremely small capillaries during their travel through the bloodstream, which progressively reduces the surface area of the red cell membranes. The red cells adapt to their reduced surface area relative to their cell volume by gradually changing from biconcave disks to spherical cells, which is the only way that the smaller cell membrane can surround the comparatively large volume of the red cell (Figure 5). Unfortunately, the spherical shape puts the red cells at a disadvantage that greatly shortens their survival in the bloodstream. As blood flows through the spleen, normal flexible disk-shaped red cells can "work their way" through

Table 2 Inheritance and Manifestations of Some Hereditary Hemolytic Anemias			
Anemia	**Inheritance**	**Characteristics of Red Cells**	**Manifestations**
Hereditary spherocytosis	Dominant or recessive	Spherocytic	Mild to moderate chronic hemolytic anemia
Hereditary ovalocytosis	Dominant	Oval	Usually asymptomatic; may have mild anemia
Sickle cell anemia	Codominant	Normocytic; cells sickle under reduced oxygen tension	Marked anemia
Hemoglobin C disease	Codominant	Normocytic	Mild to moderate anemia
Sickle cell–hemoglobin C disease	Codominant	Normocytic; cells sickle under reduced oxygen tension	Moderate anemia
Thalassemia minor	Dominant (heterozygous)	Hypochromic-microcytic; total number of red cells usually increased	Mild anemia
Thalassemia major	Dominant (homozygous)	Hypochromic-microcytic	Severe anemia; usually fatal in childhood
Glucose-6-phosphate dehydrogenase deficiency	X-linked recessive	Normocytic; enzyme-deficient cells	Episodes of acute hemolytic anemia precipitated by drugs or infections

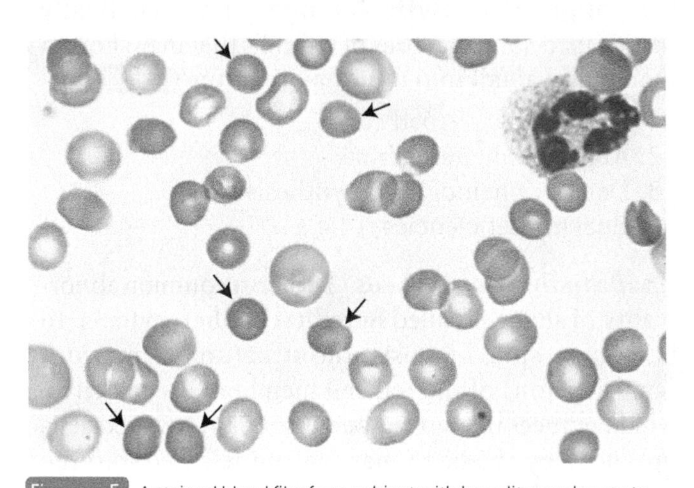

Figure 5 A stained blood film from subject with hereditary spherocytosis. The many small dark cells with little or no central pallor are spherocytes (*arrows*). The larger, more normal-appearing red cells are young red cells that have the same cell membrane defect but have not been circulating long enough to acquire a spherical shape. The relative large, faintly blue-staining red cell in the center of the field is a reticulocyte (original magnification × 400).

the splenic pulp and into the thin-walled veins (sinusoids) that carry the blood out of the spleen, but spherocytes are not thin enough or flexible enough to get through the spleen. They become trapped in the spleen where they are destroyed by the phagocytic cells in the splenic pulp. The bone marrow increases red cell production to compensate for the shortened survival of the spherocytes, resulting in a chronic hemolytic anemia. Splenectomy cures the anemia by removing the main site of red cell destruction but has no effect on the basic red cell defect.

Abnormal Hemoglobins The arrangement of amino acids in the globin chains of hemoglobin is controlled by genes. If the gene is abnormal, the amino acids forming the globin chains will be altered, leading to the formation of an abnormal hemoglobin. Genes directing the synthesis of the various types of hemoglobin are codominant. If an abnormal gene is present, the abnormal hemoglobin appears in the red cells. Many different abnormal hemoglobins can be identified and characterized by various laboratory tests. Some of the abnormal hemoglobins function normally, but others have unusual properties that impair their function. Hemoglobin S (sickle hemoglobin) is one of the more important abnormal hemoglobins. Its formation results from a change in only a single amino acid in the beta chain of hemoglobin. When the oxygen content (partial pressure) of the blood falls, as in venous blood, the hemoglobin S molecules aggregate and form rigid fibers, a process somewhat like crystallization (Figure 6). The "crystallization" is largely reversible, and the hemoglobin becomes soluble again when the oxygen tension rises as the blood is oxygenated in the lungs. About 8 percent of the black population are heterozygous carriers of the sickle cell gene. Their

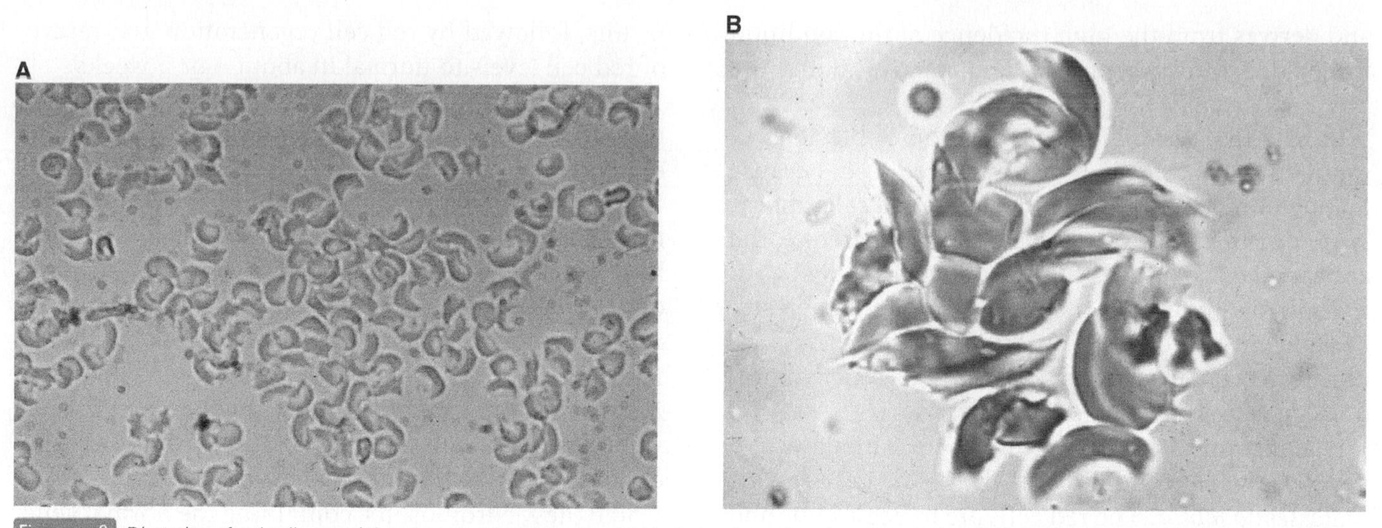

Figure 6 Distortion of red cells containing sickle hemoglobin when incubated under reduced oxygen tension. **A**, Overview of cells under low magnification (× 100). **B**, Higher magnification view (× 400) of red cell distortion caused by sickle hemoglobin.

erythrocytes contain both hemoglobin S and hemoglobin A. This condition is called *sickle cell trait*, and the hemoglobin S in their red cells can be demonstrated easily by a simple blood test. Persons with sickle cell trait normally do not experience any problems related to the sickle hemoglobin in their red cells unless they engage in vigorous activities at high altitude and the oxygen content of their blood falls to a very low level.

The homozygous state is called **sickle cell anemia** and is a serious disease that results when both parents have the sickle cell trait and each transmits the sickle cell gene to the infant. The cells of affected individuals contain no hemoglobin A and become sickled within the capillaries where the oxygen partial pressure is lower than in arterial blood. The clumps of sickled red cells plug blood vessels, which obstruct blood flow, causing progressive damage to the heart, kidneys, spleen, and other organs resulting from the impaired circulation. Anemia develops because the sickle-hemoglobin–containing cells have a shortened survival in the circulation. Consequently, the bone marrow must increase greatly its production of red cells, as demonstrated by an elevated peripheral blood reticulocyte count, in order to compensate for the shortened red cell survival.

Newborn infants with sickle cell anemia do not have problems initially because their red cells also contain a large amount of fetal hemoglobin, which "dilutes" the concentration of sickle hemoglobin in the red cells so that they function more like the red cells of a person with sickle cell trait. Symptoms usually don't appear until the infant is about 6 months old, when the red cells containing both fetal and sickle hemoglobin have been replaced by red cells containing almost entirely sickle hemoglobin.

Although there is no cure for sickle cell anemia, advances in treatment have improved survival, and many affected persons now live 40 to 50 years. They are quite susceptible to infections and should receive pneumococcal vaccine and other immunizing agents to reduce their infection risk. The hyperactive bone marrow requires abundant folic acid to promote red cell production, and folic acid supplements are recommended to ensure that supplies are adequate. A drug called hydroxyurea can be used to stimulate the bone marrow to produce fetal hemoglobin, thereby lowering the proportion of sickle hemoglobin in the red cells, but its long-term safety has not been determined.

sickle cell anemia A hereditary anemia characterized by formation of an abnormal hemoglobin that causes the red cells to become sickle shaped when the oxygen content of the blood is educed.

thalassemia (thal-uh-seem′-mia) A hereditary anemia characterized by defective production of globin chains required to produce normal hemoglobin, leading to a hypochronic microcytic anemia.

Simple, readily available tests can detect sickle cell trait in affected individuals, and genetic counseling is recommended for couples who are at risk of having a child with sickle cell anemia. DNA analysis of fetal cells obtained by amniocentesis can determine whether the fetus carries the sickle cell gene and, if present, whether the fetus is homozygous or heterozygous for the gene.

Defective Hemoglobin Synthesis Sometimes the globin chains of hemoglobin are normal, but their synthesis is defective. This genetically determined condition is called **thalassemia** and is transmitted as a Mendelian-dominant trait. Usually the defective synthesis involves the beta chains (*beta thalassemia*). This genetic abnormality is relatively common in persons of Greek and Italian ancestry. (The term *thalassemia* comes from the Greek word *thalassa*, meaning sea, and derives from the high incidence of the condition in persons who live in the regions surrounding the Mediterranean Sea.)

In beta thalassemia, the production of beta chains required to produce hemoglobin is reduced. Because hemoglobin synthesis is reduced, the red cells appear hypochromic and microcytic, somewhat like the appearance of the cells in iron deficiency anemia. In thalassemia, however, the hypochromia is the result of deficient hemoglobin production because of inadequate beta chain synthesis, rather than deficient production caused by iron deficiency.

If a person is heterozygous for the thalassemia gene, the anemia is mild and the condition is called *thalassemia minor*. The red cells are hypochromic and microcytic, and usually there is a compensatory overproduction of red cells; consequently, their numbers are greater than normal. The homozygous condition, which is called *thalassemia major*, occurs if both parents have thalassemia minor and each transmits the abnormal gene. The affected homozygous individual has a severe chronic hemolytic anemia that is usually fatal in childhood.

Red Cell Enzyme Deficiencies Red cells derive energy by metabolizing glucose by a series of chemical reactions that are catalyzed by various enzyme systems. These same energy-producing reactions also indirectly help prevent oxidation of the hemoglobin, thereby protecting the hemoglobin from the potentially harmful effects of oxidizing drugs or other agents that can damage it. This protective function is compromised if certain red cell enzymes are deficient. Under such circumstances, exposing the red cells to an oxidizing agent causes denaturation and precipitation of the protein chains of hemoglobin, as well as the cell-membrane proteins.

One of the most common red cell enzyme defects is a deficiency of an enzyme called *glucose-6-phosphate dehydrogenase*. In this condition, which is transmitted as an X-linked recessive trait, the enzyme is unstable and does not function normally. About 10 percent of black men are affected, and 30 percent of black women carry the abnormal gene on one of their X chromosomes. The abnormal gene occurs with high frequency in some white populations as well. The enzyme-deficient cells are highly susceptible to injury by drugs that do not affect normal red cells, and to various bacterial and viral infections. More than 40 drugs are known to induce an acute hemolytic anemia in susceptible subjects. Hemolysis begins soon after exposure to the drug or infectious agent and continues for about a week. Considerable red cell destruction results, followed by red cell regeneration and return of red cell levels to normal in about 4 or 5 weeks.

Because the mutant gene is carried on the X chromosome, affected males do not produce any normal enzyme, and all of their red cells are subject to hemolysis. Females who carry the mutant gene on one of their X chromosomes are also at risk of drug-induced hemolysis. However, because of random inactivation of one of the X chromosomes in the female, the red cells of the female contain two populations of red cells. Some are derived from red cell precursors in which the X chromosome containing the mutant gene is inactivated, and these cells will contain the normal enzyme. Other red cells will be derived from percursor cells in which the X chromosome containing the normal gene is inactivated, and these cells will contain a defective enzyme and will be susceptible to hemolysis. Usually the normal red cells and the enzyme-deficient red cells are present in approximately equal proportions; therefore, drug-induced hemolysis is less intense in a female carrier than in an affected male, as would be expected, because the proportion of hemolysis-susceptible red cells in the female carrier is always less than that of an affected male, in whom all the red cells contain the defective enzyme.

Acquired Hemolytic Anemia Sometimes the red cells are normally formed but are unable to survive normally because they are released into a "hostile environment." For example, antibodies that attack and destroy the red cells may be present in the circulation. Some of the autoimmune diseases, such as lupus erythematosus, and some diseases of the lymphatic system may be associated with a hemolytic anemia caused by autoantibodies. Some drugs also cause a hemolytic anemia by inducing formation of antibodies that damage red cells.

Diagnostic Evaluation of Anemia

After it is determined that a patient is anemic, the physician's function is to determine the cause so that proper, effective treatment can be instituted. A careful medical history and physical examination may provide important clues to the most likely cause. A complete blood count is essential in order to assess the degree of anemia and to determine whether leukopenia and thrombocytopenia also are present. Careful microscopic examination of a blood smear allows the physician to determine whether the anemia is hypochromic microcytic, normocytic, or macrocytic. This information helps identify the probable cause of the anemia. The rate of production of new red cells can be estimated by determining the percentage of reticulocytes in the circulation. This is called a reticulocyte count. An increased percentage of reticulocytes indicates rapid regeneration of red cells, as would be encountered after acute blood loss or hemolysis. In some patients, tests that measure iron stores, iron transport, and iron metabolism may be useful. In selected patients, examining the bone marrow provides very useful information. In this procedure, a small amount of bone marrow is removed from the pelvic bone, sternum, or other site and examined microscopically. Characteristic abnormalities in the maturation of the marrow cells are seen in pernicious anemia and in anemia caused by folic acid deficiency. Bone marrow examination also detects interference with bone marrow functions secondary to infiltration by leukemic cells or metastatic tumor. Aplastic anemia can generally be recognized by studying the bone marrow. Certain other tests are used when chronic blood loss from the gastrointestinal tract is suspected. Stools are examined for blood, and x-ray studies of the gastrointestinal tract are frequently performed to localize a site of bleeding. Other diagnostic procedures are performed in special circumstances.

Polycythemia

An increase of red cells and hemoglobin above normal levels is called **polycythemia**. Polycythemia may be secondary to an underlying disease that leads to decreased arterial oxygen saturation (secondary polycythemia), or it may be a manifestation of a leukemia-like overproduction of red cells for no apparent reason (primary polycythemia).

Secondary Polycythemia

Any condition associated with a reduced amount of oxygen transported in the bloodstream (low arterial PO_2) leads to increased erythropoietin production and hence to increased numbers of circulating red cells. The condition may accompany pulmonary emphysema, pulmonary fibrosis, or some other type of chronic lung disease that impairs the oxygenation of the blood. Persons with types of congenital heart disease associated with shunting of deoxygenated blood from the right cardiac chambers into the systemic circulation also develop secondary polycythemia. In these individuals, the amount of oxygen transported in the systemic circulation to supply the tissues is reduced (low arterial PO_2) by the admixture of shunted deoxygenated blood, which leads to cyanosis and a compensatory increase in red cell production.

Primary Polycythemia

Primary polycythemia, also called *polycythemia vera* (true polycythemia), is a manifestation of a diffuse hyperplasia of the bone marrow of unknown etiology. It is characterized by overproduction not only of red cells, but also of white blood cells and platelets. The disease has many features of a neoplastic process, and some patients with polycythemia vera eventually develop granulocytic leukemia.

polycythemia (päl-ē-sī-thē′mē-yuh) Increased number of red cells. May be caused by some types of chronic heart or lung disease (*secondary polycythemia*) or by marrow erythroid hyperplasia of unknown causes (*primary polycythemia*).

hemochromatosis (hemo-crow-mah-toe′-sis) A genetic disease characterized by excessive iron absorption, leading to accumulation of excessive amounts of iron in the body, causing organ damage.

Complications and Treatment of Polycythemia

The symptoms of polycythemia are related to the increased blood volume and increased blood viscosity. Many patients with polycythemia develop thromboses because of the increased blood viscosity and elevated platelet levels. Polycythemia vera is usually treated by drugs that suppress the bone marrow overactivity. Secondary polycythemia is sometimes treated by periodic removal of excess blood.

Iron Overload: Hemochromatosis

Although iron is essential for normal hematopoiesis and has other essential functions in the body, an excess of iron in the body is harmful.

Iron is absorbed with difficulty and excreted with difficulty. Iron uptake is very closely controlled by the body, and there are no normal pathways that allow for excretion of iron in excess of the body's needs. Men excrete only about 1 mg of iron per day, which reflects primarily small losses of iron contained in the cells that are being lost from the skin, intestinal tract, and other sites that are replaced by new cells. Premenopausal women excrete slightly more because of menstrual losses, as each milliliter of red cells contains about 0.5 mg of iron.

Because iron excretory pathways are lacking, any excess iron entering the body can't be eliminated, and the body becomes overloaded with iron, which accumulates in the body's tissues and organs. Eventually this leads to organ damage followed by scarring, leading to permanent derangement in the functions of the affected organs.

The usual cause of iron overload is a genetic disease called **hemochromatosis**, which is transmitted as an autosomal recessive trait. The gene occurs in about 10 percent of the population, but the disease only occurs in homozygous carriers of the gene, who absorb an excessive amount of iron, which leads to excessive accumulation of iron in the body.

Early recognition and treatment prevents progression of the disease and arrests organ damage. Treatment consists of repeated withdrawal of blood (phlebotomy) to remove iron from the body, as each 500 mL of blood withdrawn removes 250 mg of iron. Phlebotomies are repeated until iron stores are depleted, and then periodic phlebotomies are continued for the rest of the patient's life.

The excessive iron absorption and storage characteristic of hemochromatosis can be identified by the same type of laboratory tests used to measure iron storage and transport in subjects with iron deficiency anemia: serum ferritin, serum iron, and serum iron-binding capacity. When the body is overloaded with iron, serum ferritin is very high, reflecting the greatly increased iron stores that can be as much as 15 to 20 grams or more instead of the normal amount of about 1 gram. Serum iron is also much higher than normal and the iron-binding protein transferrin is completely loaded (saturated) with iron. These tests all point to increased uptake and storage of iron.

The following case illustrates the usefulness of screening studies for detecting this disease before irreparable organ damage occurs.

Case Study 1

A 40-year-old healthy woman was seen in consultation by a physician because routine screening laboratory tests had detected elevated serum iron.

Physical examination was normal, as were routine blood and urine tests, but tests measuring iron stores and iron metabolism were all abnormal. Serum iron was much higher than normal (234 mg per 100 mL), and serum iron-binding protein was completely saturated with iron. Serum ferritin was 1335 mg per liter, which is more than 10 times higher than normal. A diagnosis of hemochromatosis was made, and treatment consisting of periodic phlebotomies was begun in order to remove the excess iron from her body.

Thrombocytopenia

Blood platelets are fragments of the cytoplasm of megakaryocytes that are released into the bloodstream. These small structures serve a hemostatic function, sealing small breaks in capillaries and interacting with plasma factors in the initial stages of blood clotting. A significant reduction in the numbers of platelets in the blood leads to numerous small, pinpoint hemorrhages from capillaries in the skin and mucous membranes, called *petechiae*, and to larger areas of hemorrhage, called *ecchymoses*. This type of skin and mucous membrane bleeding is called **purpura**, and the disease entity is called *thrombocytopenic purpura*. This condition may result either from (1) inadequate production of platelets caused by damage to the bone marrow, or (2) shortened survival of platelets in the circulation caused by antiplatelet autoantibodies.

Thrombocytopenic purpura from bone marrow damage is often caused by drugs, chemicals, or other substances that disrupt platelet production, and may also result if the bone marrow is infiltrated by leukemic cells or metastatic carcinoma that "crowd out" the platelet-producing megakaryocytes. These conditions are called *secondary thrombocytopenic purpura* because the purpura results from an underlying disease of the bone marrow.

In thrombocytopenia caused by shortened platelet survival, the bone marrow produces platelets normally but the antiplatelet autoantibodies in the blood destroy the platelets, and the antibodies can be detected in the blood of the affected person. Cases of this type, in which no underlying bone marrow disease can be detected, are called primary thrombocytopenic purpura. This condition is often encountered in children, sometimes related to a recent viral infection, and subsides spontaneously within a short time. When the disease develops in adults, it tends to be more chronic.

The Lymphatic System

The lymphatic system consists of the lymph nodes and spleen, together with various organized masses of lymphoid tissue elsewhere throughout the body; these include the tonsils, the adenoids, the thymus, and lymphoid aggregates in the intestinal mucosa, respiratory tract, and bone marrow. The primary function of the lymphatic system is to provide immunologic defenses against foreign material by means of cell-mediated and humoral (antibody-mediated) defense mechanisms. The lymph nodes, which constitute a major part of the system, form an interconnected network linked by lymphatic channels.

Lymph nodes are small, bean-shaped structures that vary from a few millimeters to as much as 2 centimeters in diameter. They are interspersed along the course of lymphatic channels, where they act somewhat like filters. Frequently, they form groups at locations where many lymphatic channels converge, such as around the aorta and inferior vena cava, in the mesentery of the intestine, in the axillae (armpits) and groin, and at the base of the neck. Each node consists of a mass of lymphocytes supported by a meshwork of reticular fibers in which are scattered phagocytic cells of the mononuclear phagocyte system (reticuloendothelial system). As the lymph flows through the nodes, the phagocytic cells filter out and destroy any microorganisms or other foreign materials that have gotten into the lymphatic channels. The lymphocytes and mononuclear phagocytes within the node also interact with the foreign material and initiate an immune response.

The spleen is specialized to filter blood rather than lymph. Much larger than lymph nodes, it is about the size of a man's fist and is located under the ribs in the left upper part of the abdomen. It consists of compact masses of lymphocytes and a network of sinusoids (capillaries having wide lumens of variable width) within a supporting framework composed of reticular fibers and numerous phagocytic cells. As the blood flows through the spleen, worn-out red cells are removed from the circulation by the phagocytic cells, and the iron that they contain is salvaged for reuse. Abnormal red cells, such as those that are damaged by disease, are abnormal in shape, or contain a large amount of an abnormal hemoglobin, also are destroyed by the splenic phagocytes, which accounts for their shortened survival in the circulation.

The thymus is a bilobed lymphoid organ overlying the base of the heart. It is a large structure during infancy and childhood but gradually undergoes atrophy in adolescence. Only a remnant persists in the adult. The thymus plays an essential role in the prenatal development of the lymphoid system and in the formation of the body's immunologic defense mechanisms.

Diseases of the Lymphatic System

The principal diseases affecting the lymphatic system are infections and neoplasms.

Inflammation of the Lymph Nodes (Lymphadenitis)

Lymph nodes draining an area of infection may become enlarged and tender, resulting from spread of infection through the lymphatic channels and acute inflammation in the node. This is called lymphadenitis.

Infectious Mononucleosis

Infectious mononucleosis is a relatively common viral disease. The virus belongs to the same family as the herpesvirus that causes fever blisters. The virus has been named the **Epstein-Barr virus** (usually simply called *EB virus*). The disease is encountered most frequently in young adults and is transmitted by close contact, often by kissing. The virus causes an acute, debilitating, febrile illness associated with a diffuse hyperplasia of lymphoid tissue throughout the body. The lymphoid hyperplasia is manifested by a moderate increase of lymphocytes in the peripheral blood, enlargement and tenderness of lymph nodes, and some degree of splenic enlargement. The spleen, which normally weighs about 150 grams and is well protected under the rib cage in the upper abdomen, may double or triple in size and extend several centimeters below the left costal margin. The lymphocytes circulating in the peripheral blood show rather distinctive morphologic abnormalities, and the diagnosis can generally be made by the pathologist from a careful examination of the blood smear. The lymphocytes are larger than normal, with abundant deep blue cytoplasm and an irregularly shaped nucleus (Figure 7). Enlargement and ulceration of lymphoid tissue in the throat is responsible for the sore throat often accompanying the disease.

purpura (pur′pura) A condition characterized by hemorrhage in the skin and mucous membranes (petechiae and ecchymoses).

Epstein-Barr virus A virus that causes infectious mononucleosis.

The EB virus infects B lymphocytes, which proliferate actively during the first week of the infection. Then cytotoxic (CD8+) T lymphocytes and antibodies produced by plasma cells against the EB virus destroy the majority of the virus-infected cells, but some evade destruction and persist for life within the lymphatic system of the infected individual. The atypical lymphocytes seen in the blood are the activated cytotoxic T cells attacking the virus-infected cells. Many persons infected with EB virus never develop the clinical manifestations of

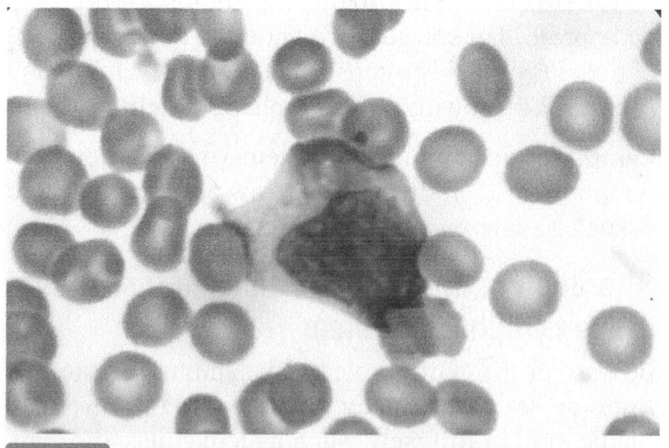

Figure 7 Large lymphocyte from subject with infectious mononucleosis, illustrating characteristic morphologic abnormalities, as described in text (original magnification × 1000).

infectious mononucleosis because the body's defenses destroy the virus-infected cells. Only a small proportion of infected persons develop the elevated temperature, sore throat, enlarged spleen, and enlarged lymph nodes that are characteristic of the disease.

Generally, the disease is self-limited, and no specific treatment is required; however, it may be several weeks before the patient feels well again. Young adults recovering from infectious mononucleosis should avoid contact sports such as basketball, as long as the spleen remains enlarged and extends below the ribs into the upper abdomen. Any athletic activities that expose the upper abdomen to possible trauma may rupture the enlarged spleen, which is a very serious injury. Individuals with an impaired or suppressed immune system, such as persons with AIDS or persons who have had a bone marrow or organ transplant and are receiving treatment to suppress the immune system, may face another problem. The surviving infected B cells, unrestrained by the nonfunctional immune system, may become activated and proliferate extensively, giving rise to a malignant B cell lymphoma.

Neoplasms Affecting Lymph Nodes

Metastatic Tumors Lymph nodes may be affected by the spread of metastatic tumor from malignant tumors arising in the breast, lung, colon, or other sites. The nodes first affected lie in the immediate drainage area of the tumor. The tumor may then spread to other, more distant lymph nodes through lymphatic channels and may eventually gain access to the circulatory system through the thoracic duct (Figure 8).

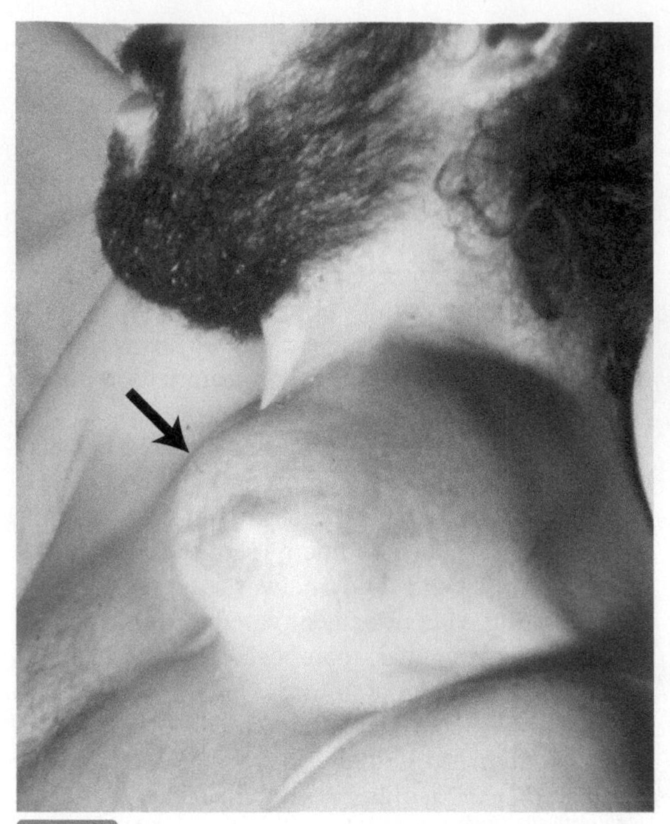

Figure 8 Large deposit of metastatic carcinoma in the supraclavicular lymph nodes of a young man with carcinoma of the testicle.

Malignant Lymphoma A lymphoma is a primary malignant neoplasm of lymphoid tissue. The two main types of lymphoma are Hodgkin's disease and non-Hodgkin's lymphoma. A lymphoma usually begins in a single lymph node or a small group of nodes but often spreads to other nodes; frequently, the disease becomes widespread. The spread of lymphoma to multiple groups of nodes is probably a consequence of the recirculation of lymphocytes within the lymphatic system.

Lymphocytic Leukemia Leukemia may develop from lymphoid cells in the bone marrow or from lymphoid tissue elsewhere in the body.

Alteration of Immune Reactions in Diseases of the Lymphatic System

Because of the central role of the lymphatic system in immune reactions, many diseases affecting the lymphatic system diffusely, such as leukemias and lymphomas, may be associated with abnormal immune responses. These responses may be manifested either by production of autoantibodies directed against the red cells, white cells, or platelets of the affected individual, or by a loss of normal cell-mediated and humoral defenses that leads to an increased susceptibility to infection.

The Enlarged Lymph Node as a Diagnostic Problem

The patient who visits a physician because one or more lymph nodes are enlarged may present a difficult diagnostic problem. Lymph node enlargement may be a manifestation of a localized infection in the area drained by the node. It may be caused by a systemic infection with initial manifestations in the node. It may be caused by metastatic tumor in the node, or it may be an early manifestation of leukemia or malignant lymphoma. Often the cause of the lymphadenopathy can be determined by the physician from the clinical evaluation of the patient in conjunction with laboratory studies, including an examination of the peripheral blood. Sometimes the cause cannot be established, however, and the physician must perform a lymph node biopsy to determine the reason for the enlargement. The enlarged lymph node is surgically excised and submitted to the pathologist for microscopic examination and microbiologic studies. In difficult cases, more elaborate and sophisticated studies may be required.

The Role of the Spleen in Protection Against Systemic Infection

The spleen is an efficient blood-filtration system. Any bacteria or other foreign material that gains access to the bloodstream are promptly removed by the splenic phagocytes as the blood flows through the spleen. In addition, the spleen manufactures antibodies that facilitate prompt elimination of pathogenic organisms.

Sometimes it is necessary to remove the spleen. Splenectomy may be required to prevent fatal hemorrhage if the spleen has been lacerated in an automobile accident or other injury. Splenectomy may be performed on patients with blood diseases characterized by excessive destruction of blood cells within the spleen, such as thrombocytopenic purpura and some types of hereditary hemolytic anemia.

Splenectomized persons are less able to eliminate bacteria that gain access to the bloodstream and do not produce antibodies as well as before removal of the spleen. Consequently, they are more likely to develop serious bloodstream infections caused by pathogenic bacteria. To reduce this risk, splenectomized patients are often immunized with bacterial vaccines because high levels of antibacterial antibodies facilitate removal of bacteria from the circulation, and this can substitute for splenic function to some extent. Many physicians also recommend that a splenectomized patient begin taking antibiotics at the first sign of a respiratory infection or other febrile illness.

CHAPTER REVIEW

Questions for Review

1. What types of cells are found in the circulating blood, and what are their major functions?
2. What is anemia? What is the difference between an etiologic and a morphologic classification of anemia? Outline a simple etiologic classification of anemia.
3. What is an iron deficiency anemia? How does it arise? How is it treated? What is the morphologic appearance of the red cells?
4. What is the effect of vitamin B_{12} and folic acid on blood cell maturation? What type of anemia results from deficiency of these vitamins?
5. What is the difference between an aplastic anemia and a hemolytic anemia? What is the difference between polycythemia and thrombocytopenia? What is hemochromatosis? What are its manifestations? How is the condition diagnosed and treated?
6. What is the lymphatic system? How is it organized? What are the major cells of the lymphatic system? What are the major functions of the lymphatic system?
7. What is the EB virus? What is its relationship to infectious mononucleosis? What are the clinical manifestations of infectious mononucleosis? How is the disease treated? What are some possible complications of the infection?
8. A patient has an enlarged lymph node. What types of diseases could produce lymph node enlargement? How does the physician arrive at a diagnosis when the patient presents with enlarged lymph nodes?
9. What types of altered immune reaction are sometimes encountered in diseases of the lymphatic system?
10. What are the functions of the spleen? What are the adverse effects of splenectomy?

Supplementary Reading

Bain, B. 2005. Diagnosis from the blood smear. *New England Journal of Medicine* 353:498–507.

Even in the "high-tech" era of medical practice, the blood smear remains a valuable diagnostic tool. Examination of a well-stained blood smear is essential whenever the results of a complete blood count indicate an abnormality. Methods are available to transmit photographs of atypical or abnormal blood smears to consultants for interpretation or second opinions.

Beers, M. H., Fletcher, A. J., Jones, T. V., and Porter, R. 2003. *The Merck Manual of Medical Information; Home Edition*. 2nd ed. New York: Simon & Schuster.

Good sections on blood coagulation and hematology.

Hoagland, H. C. 1995. Myelodysplastic (preleukemic) syndromes: The bone marrow factory failure problem. *Mayo Clinic Proceedings* 70:673–77.

A review article.

Kark, J. A., Posey, D. M., Schumacher, H. R., and Ruehle, C. J. 1987. Sickle-cell trait as a risk factor for sudden death in physical training. *Journal of the American Medical Association* 317:782–86.

The association between sudden death and exertion is not widely appreciated. The prevalence of sickle cell trait is about 8 percent in the black population, and the incidence of sudden death related to exertion may be about 40 times higher than in the general population.

Likhite, V. V. 1976. Immunologic impairment and susceptibility to infection after splenectomy. *Journal of the American Medical Association* 236:1376–77.

Describes the adverse effects of splenectomy on phagocytosis of bacteria and on antibody formation.

Looker, A. C., Dallman, P. R., Carroll, M. D., et al. 1997. Prevalence of iron deficiency in the United States. *Journal of the American Medical Association* 277:973–76.

Iron deficiency and iron deficiency anemia are still common in toddlers, adolescent girls, and women of childbearing age.

Pagano, J. S. 2002. Viruses and lymphomas. *New England Journal of Medicine* 347:78–9.

A survey of the viruses that cause various types of lymphoid neoplasms, emphasizing the role of EB virus in both B cell and T cell lymphomas.

Pietrangelo, A. 2004. Hereditary hemochromatosis: A new look at an old disease. *New England Journal of Medicine* 350:2383–97.

Several different gene mutations may cause hemochromatosis. The most common cause is a specific mutation of paired HFE genes, and transmission is as an autosomal recessive trait; however, it is not possible to predict how the mutations will be expressed (gene penetrance) in a person homozygous for the mutant gene. Methods for detecting and evaluating hemochromatosis are described. Treatment depends on the manifestations of the disease in an affected person.

Interactive Activities

Multiple Choice

1. The usual survival of red cells in the circulation is
   - A. 2 weeks
   - B. 2 months
   - C. 4 weeks
   - D. 4 months
2. Which of the following conditions is NOT associated with megaloblastic anemia?
   - A. Vitamin B_{12} deficiency
   - B. Folic acid deficiency
   - C. Iron deficiency
3. A patient has a blood disease characterized by a greatly increased white blood cell count consisting of mature lymphocytes, with anemia and thrombocytopenia. The most likely diagnosis is
   - A. Malignant lymphoma
   - B. Acute lymphocytic leukemia
   - C. Chronic lymphocytic leukemia
   - D. Infectious mononucleosis
4. Which of the following statements regarding iron deficiency anemia is NOT true?
   - A. May result from bleeding ulcer
   - B. May result from excessive blood donations
   - C. May result from deficiency of vitamins required for efficient iron absorption
   - D. May result from excessive menstrual blood loss

Critical Thinking

1. Mary Jones is a 23-year-old college student who has a moderate anemia. Her white count and platelets are normal. What possible causes of the anemia appear likely? What tests would you perform to confirm your initial impression?
2. An elderly man consulted his physician because of fatigue and enlarged lymph nodes. What possible conditions would you consider as diagnostic possibilities? What further studies would be helpful to make a diagnosis?

Answers

Multiple Choice: 1D; 3C

Critical Thinking:

1. Mary's white cells and platelets are normal, which suggests that the anemia is not caused by leukemia or some other disease that destroys or replaces the bone marrow with abnormal cells. She probably has an iron-deficiency anemia, possibly from excessive menstrual bleeding leading to iron deficiency. This can be confirmed by examination of a blood smear to see whether she has a hypochromic microcytic anemia, and laboratory tests to confirm an iron deficiency.

The Respiratory System

LEARNING OBJECTIVES

1. Explain the basic anatomic and physiologic principles of ventilation and gas exchange.
2. Describe the causes, clinical effects, complications, and treatment of pneumothorax and atelectasis.
3. Describe the histologic characteristics of a tuberculous infection. Explain the possible outcome of an infection. Describe methods of diagnosis and treatment.
4. Differentiate between bronchitis and bronchiectasis.
5. List the anatomic and physiologic derangements in chronic obstructive lung disease. Explain its pathogenesis. Describe the clinical manifestations and methods of treatment.
6. Describe the pathogenesis and manifestations of bronchial asthma and respiratory distress syndrome.
7. Explain the causes and effects of pulmonary fibrosis. Describe the special problems associated with asbestosis.
8. List the major types of lung carcinoma. Describe the clinical manifestations of lung carcinoma and explain the principles of treatment.

Oxygen Delivery: A Cooperative Effort

Normal life processes require that an adequate supply of oxygen be delivered to the tissues and that the waste products of cell metabolism be removed. These functions are carried out by a cooperative effort of the respiratory and circulatory systems. The respiratory system oxygenates the blood and removes carbon dioxide. The circulatory system transports these gases in the bloodstream.

Structure and Function of the Lungs

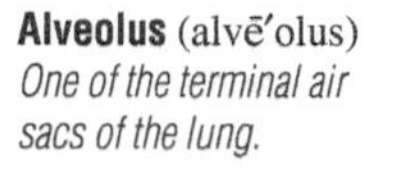

Alveolus (alvē′olus) *One of the terminal air sacs of the lung.*

The lungs consist of two distinct components: a system of tubes whose chief function is to conduct air into and out of the lungs and the **alveoli** (singular, alveolus), where oxygen and carbon dioxide are exchanged between air and the pulmonary capillaries. Just as a tree branches progressively and ends in a foliage of leaves, so the conducting tubes branch repeatedly and terminate in clusters of pulmonary alveoli. The lung is divided into several large segments called lobes. Each lobe in turn consists of a large number of smaller units called lobules. The architecture and structural features of a normal lung can be studied to best advantage when the lung is inflated and air dried (FIGURE 1A). The individual lobes, fissures, and pleural surfaces are well defined. The poorly defined cobblestonelike pattern of the pleural surface defines the location of the individual lung lobules, which frequently are accentuated by carbon pigment deposited in the connective tissue that surrounds and circumscribes the individual lobules. When sections of normal air-dried lung are examined against an illuminated background, one can appreciate the spongelike, fine structure of a normal lung, which is essential for normal gas exchange (FIGURE 1B).

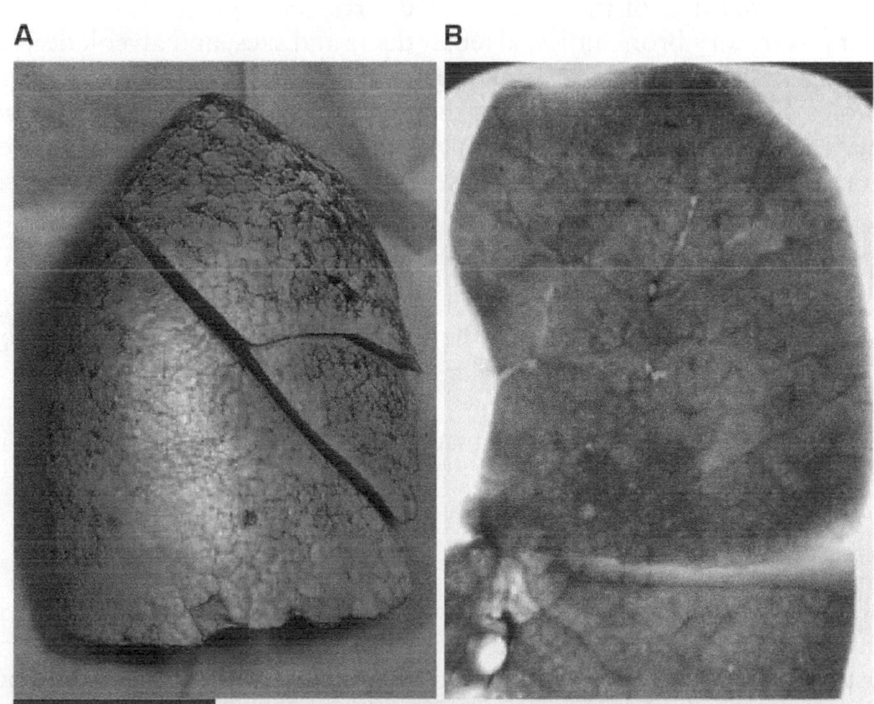

FIGURE 1 Normal lung that has been inflated and air dried so that the structure of the lobes and lobules can be visualized and the fine structure of the alveoli can be studied. **A**, External surface illustrating lobes and fissures. The faint cobblestonelike pattern of the pleural surface defines the individual lung lobules. **B**, A backlighted section of lung illustrating the fine, spongelike pattern produced by the respiratory units where gas exchange occurs.

BRONCHI, BRONCHIOLES, AND ALVEOLI

The largest conducting tubes are called **bronchi** (singular, bronchus). Tubes less than about 1 mm in diameter are called **bronchioles** (little bronchi), and the smallest bronchioles, which function only for conduction of air, are called terminal bronchioles. The tubes distal to the terminal bronchioles are called respiratory bronchioles because they have alveoli in their walls and not only transport air but also participate in gas exchange. Each terminal bronchiole gives rise to several respiratory bronchioles, which branch to form alveolar ducts. The alveolar ducts in turn subdivide into alveolar sacs, and multiple alveoli in turn open into each alveolar sac (FIGURE 2A AND B).

Bronchus
One of the large subdivisions of the trachea.

Bronchiole
(bron′ke-ōl)
One of the small terminal subdivisions of the branched bronchial tree.

Each alveolus is a small air space surrounded by a thin wall, the alveolar septum, which consists of thin-walled capillaries supported by a few connective tissue fibers and lined by a layer of epithelial cells (FIGURE 2B). Each alveolus contains a relatively small volume of air surrounded by a large network of capillaries, conditions that promote rapid diffusion of oxygen and carbon dioxide between alveolar air and pulmonary capillaries as the blood flows through the lung. Any condition that enlarges the pulmonary alveoli or reduces the number of pulmonary capillaries impedes the efficiency of pulmonary ventilation.

Two types of cells line the alveoli. Most are flat squamous cells. A few are larger secretory cells that produce a lipid material called **surfactant**, which reduces surface tension. Surface tension is the attraction between molecules of a fluid that cause the fluid to aggregate into droplets instead of spreading as a thin film. The surface tension of the molecules in the fluid lining the alveoli would normally tend to pull the alveolar walls together. This effect would hinder expansion of the lungs during inspiration and would cause the alveoli to collapse during expiration because of the cohesive force of the water molecules. Surfactant acts somewhat like a detergent by lowering the surface tension of the fluid and thereby facilitating respiration.

Surfactant
(sur-fak′tant)
A lipid material secreted by alveolar lining cells that facilitates respiration by decreasing the surface tension of the fluid lining the pulmonary alveoli.

The functional unit of the lung is called a **respiratory unit**. It is formed by the cluster of respiratory bronchioles, alveolar ducts and sacs, and alveoli derived from a single terminal bronchiole. A **lung lobule** consists of a small group of terminal bronchioles and the respiratory units that arise from them. Lobules are partially circumscribed by connective tissue septa and are easiest to identify just beneath the pleura, where the connective tissue septa defining the lobules can be easily seen (FIGURE 1A).

Respiratory unit
A functional unit of the lung consisting of a cluster of respiratory bronchioles, alveolar ducts, and alveoli derived from a single terminal bronchiole. Another term for acinus.

Lung lobule
A small group of terminal bronchioles and their subdivisions.

Respiration has two functions, corresponding to the two structural components of the lungs:

1. Ventilation, which concerns the movement of air into and out of the lungs
2. Gas exchange between alveolar air and pulmonary capillaries

Both ventilation and gas exchange must function normally if respiration is to be effective.

VENTILATION

Air is moved into and out of the lungs by the bellows action of the thoracic cage. During inspiration, the ribs become more horizontal because of the action of the intercostal muscles, and the diaphragm descends. Consequently, the volume of the thoracic cage increases. The lungs expand to fill the larger intrathoracic space, and air is drawn into the lungs through the trachea and bronchi. During expiration, the ribs become more vertical, and the diaphragm rises. The volume of the thoracic cage is reduced. The lungs, which conform to the size of the thorax, also decrease in volume, and air is expelled.

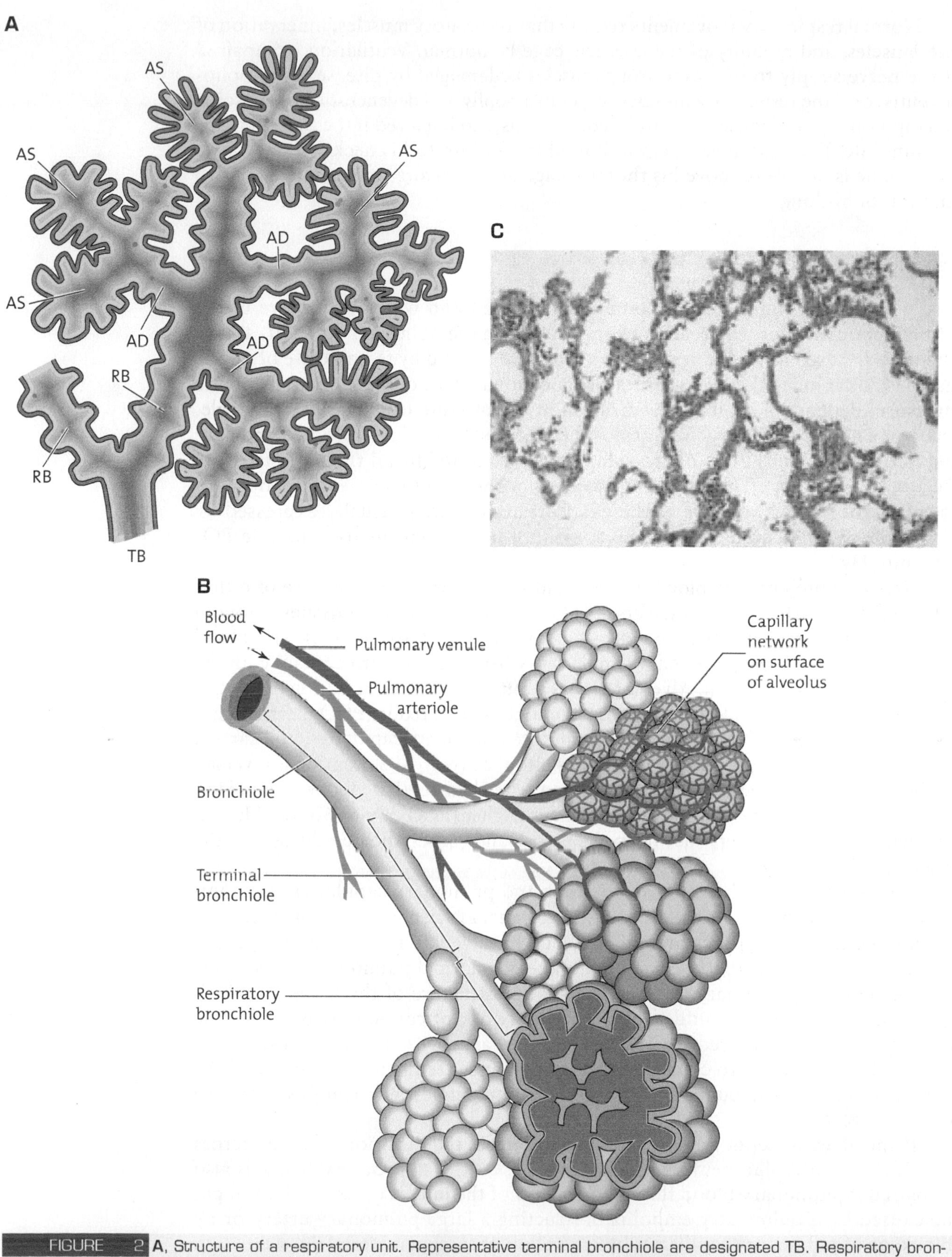

FIGURE 2 **A**, Structure of a respiratory unit. Representative terminal bronchiole are designated TB. Respiratory bronchiole (RB) has alveolar sacs projecting from the wall of the bronchiole. Alveolar ducts are designated AD, and alveolar sacs are designated AS. Multiple alveoli (not labeled) open into each alveolar sac. **B**, Structure of terminal air passages. The interior of one alveolar duct is illustrated in cutaway view. **C**, Histologic structure of the lung illustrating alveoli and thin alveolar septa containing pulmonary capillaries (original magnification × 100).

Normal respiratory movements require that respiratory muscles, innervation of the muscles, and mobility of the thoracic cage be normal. Ventilation is impaired if the nerve supply to the respiratory muscles is damaged by disease, as in poliomyelitis, or if the respiratory muscles undergo atrophy and degeneration, as in some uncommon types of muscle disease. Ventilation is also impaired if the thoracic cage is immobile. For example, a person buried in sand up to his neck will suffocate because he is unable to move his thoracic cage and therefore cannot move air into and out of his lungs.

GAS EXCHANGE

Oxygen and carbon dioxide, along with nitrogen and water vapor, are in the atmospheric air that we breathe, in the air within the pulmonary alveoli, and in the blood. At sea level, the atmospheric pressure exerted by the mixture of all the gases is 760 mm Hg. Each gas exerts a proportionate part of the total atmospheric pressure, depending on its concentration in the mixture of gases. For example, the concentration of oxygen in atmospheric air is 20%. Therefore, the pressure exerted by oxygen is 20% of the total pressure exerted by all the gases ($0.20 \times 760 = 152$ mm Hg). The part of the total atmospheric pressure exerted by a gas is called the partial pressure of the gas. Partial pressure is usually expressed by the letter "P" preceding the chemical symbol for the gas, as for example PO_2 152 mm Hg.

Gases diffuse between blood, tissues, and pulmonary alveoli because of differences in their partial pressures. Venous blood returning from the tissues is low in oxygen (PO_2 40 mm Hg) and high in carbon dioxide (PCO_2 47 mm Hg). This blood is pumped through the pulmonary capillaries, where it comes into contact with the air in the pulmonary alveoli. Alveolar air has a much higher concentration of oxygen (PO_2 105 mm Hg) but a lower concentration of carbon dioxide (PCO_2 35 mm Hg). Therefore, oxygen diffuses from alveolar air into pulmonary capillaries, and carbon dioxide diffuses from pulmonary capillaries into the aveoli. The situation is reversed in the tissues. The tissue oxygen concentration is much lower (PO_2 about 20 mm Hg), and the carbon dioxide concentration is much higher (PCO_2 about 60 mm Hg); so oxygen diffuses into the tissues from the blood, and carbon dioxide diffuses in the opposite direction.

Exchange of gases between alveolar air and pulmonary capillaries is accomplished by diffusion across the alveolar membrane. Efficient gas exchange requires (1) a large capillary surface area in contact with alveolar air, (2) unimpeded diffusion of gases across the alveolar membrane, (3) normal pulmonary blood flow, and (4) normal pulmonary alveoli. The spongy structure of the lungs, in which each tiny air sac is surrounded by a large network of capillaries, provides the large surface area required for efficient gas exchange (FIGURE 3A). Destruction of alveolar septa leads to coalescence of alveoli and a reduction in the size of the capillary network surrounding the alveoli, resulting in less efficient gas exchange (FIGURE 3B).

If the alveolar septa are thickened and scarred, the diffusion of gases across the thickened alveolar membranes is impeded (FIGURE 3C). Gas exchange is also impaired if pulmonary blood flow to a portion of the lung is obstructed, as might be caused by a pulmonary embolus obstructing a large pulmonary artery or by blockage of pulmonary capillaries by fat emboli or foreign material (FIGURE 3D). If the pulmonary alveoli become filled with fluid or inflammatory exudate, inspired air cannot enter the diseased alveoli, and pulmonary gas exchange is impeded (FIGURE 3E).

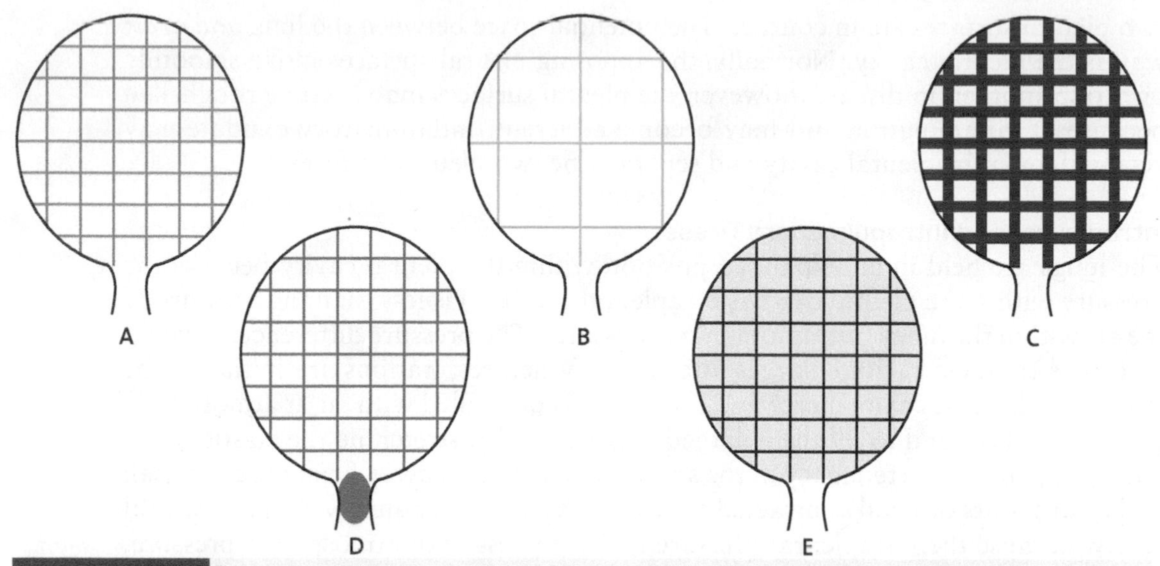

FIGURE 3 Types of structural and functional abnormalities that adversely affect pulmonary gas exchange. **A**, Normal alveoli and pulmonary blood flow. **B**, Destruction of alveolar septa, leading to coarsening of alveolar structure with corresponding reduction in size of pulmonary capillary bed. **C**, Fibrous thickening and scarring of alveolar septa, impeding diffusion of gasses across alveolar membrane. **D**, Obstruction of pulmonary blood flow to a part of the lung. **E**, Alveoli filled with fluid or inflammatory exudate.

PULMONARY FUNCTION TESTS

Vital capacity
The maximum volume of air that can be forcefully expelled after a maximum inspiration.

One-second forced expiratory volume (FEV_1)
The maximum volume of air that can be expelled from the lungs in 1 second.

Pulmonary function tests can be used to evaluate the efficiency of pulmonary ventilation and pulmonary gas exchange. Pulmonary ventilation is usually tested by measuring the volume of air that can be moved into and out of the lung under standard conditions. Two commonly used measurements are **vital capacity**, which measures the maximum volume of air that can be expelled after a deep inspiration, and the **one-second forced expiratory volume (FEV_1)**, which measures the maximum volume of air that can be expelled in 1 second. If the bronchioles are narrowed by inflammation or spasm, impeding the movement of air out of the lungs, FEV_1 is often reduced. Specialized tests can measure the total volume of air in the lungs and the volume of air remaining in the lungs after a maximum expiration.

The concentrations of oxygen and carbon dioxide (O_2 and CO_2) in the patient's arterial blood can also be measured in order to determine the efficiency of gas exchange in the lungs. In chronic pulmonary disease, oxygenation of the blood is inefficient. Oxygen concentration is reduced, and arterial oxygen saturation is decreased correspondingly. Often, the arterial PCO_2 also is higher than normal because carbon dioxide is inefficiently eliminated by the lungs. Arterial blood for analysis is usually collected by inserting a small needle into the radial artery in the wrist and withdrawing a small amount of blood. One can also determine how effectively the lungs are oxygenating the blood (arterial oxygen saturation) using a device called a pulse oximeter. A fingertip is inserted into the device, which measures photoelectrically the changes in light absorption of the hemoglobin in the fingertip capillaries at various wavelengths during systole and diastole. Then the data are used to calculate automatically the oxygen saturation of the arterial blood, and the device promptly displays the result.

Pleura
(plōōr'äh)
*The mesothelial covering of the lung (*visceral pleura*) and chest wall (*parietal pleura*).*

THE PLEURAL CAVITY

The lungs are covered by a thin membrane called the **pleura**, which also extends over the internal surface of the chest wall. Because the lungs fill the thoracic cavity, the two pleural surfaces are in contact. The potential space between the lung and chest wall is the pleural cavity. Normally, the apposing pleural surfaces move smoothly over one another. In disease, however, the pleural surfaces may become roughened because of inflammation and may become adherent. Inflammatory exudate may accumulate in the pleural cavity and separate the two pleural surfaces.

Intrapleural and Intrapulmonary Pressures

The lungs are held in an expanded position within the pleural cavity because the pressure within the pleural cavity (intrapleural pressure) is less than the pressure of the air within the lungs (intrapulmonary pressure). The pressure differences develop when the thoracic cavity enlarges after birth. When respirations are initiated, the size of the thoracic cavity increases. The lungs become filled with air at atmospheric pressure and expand to fill the enlarged thoracic cavity, stretching the elastic tissue within the lungs. The tendency of the stretched lung to pull away from the chest wall and return to its original contracted state creates a slight vacuum within the pleural cavity. Because the intrapleural pressure is slightly less than atmospheric pressure, it is often called "negative pressure."

Pneumothorax

Because the intrapleural pressure is subatmospheric, air flows into the pleural space if the lung or chest wall is punctured. When this occurs, the subatmospheric ("negative") pressure that holds the lung in the expanded position is lost, and the lung collapses because the elastic tissue within the lung contracts. This condition, which is called a **pneumothorax** (*pneumo* = air), may follow any type of lung injury or pulmonary disease that allows air to escape from the lungs into the pleural space. It may also result from a stab wound or some other penetrating injury to the chest wall that permits atmospheric air to enter the pleural space (FIGURE 4).

Pneumothorax
(nōō-mō-thor′ax)
Accumulation of air in the pleural cavity.

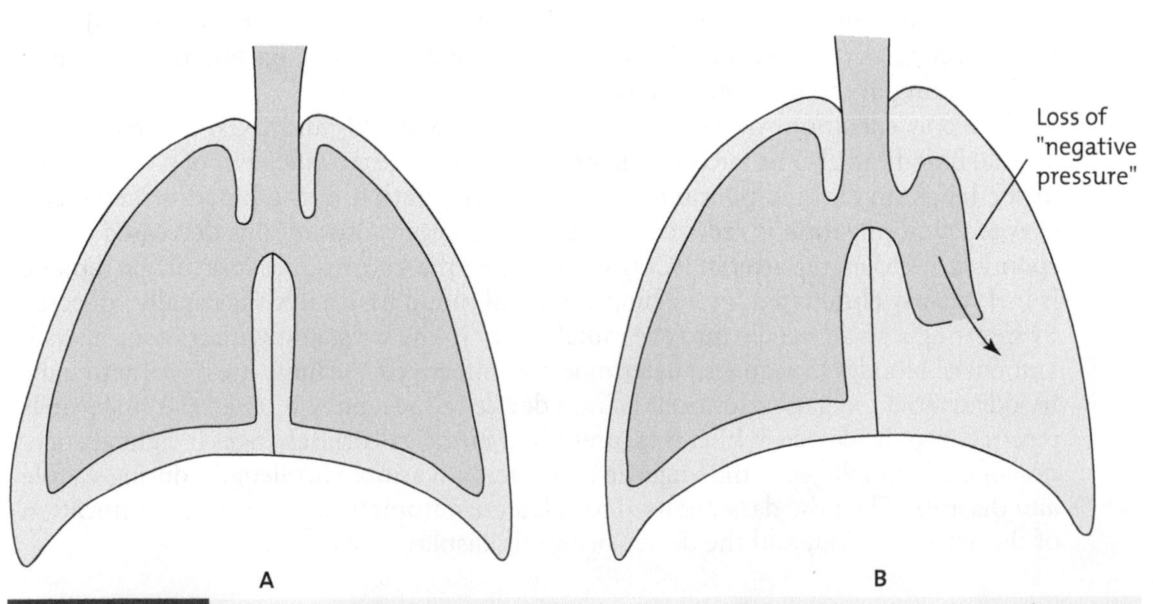

FIGURE 4 **A**, Normal relation of lung to chest wall. Pleural space is exaggerated, and surfaces are normally in contact. "Negative pressure" is primarily a result of the tendency of the stretched lung to pull away from the chest wall. **B**, Pneumothorax caused by a perforating injury of lung, allowing the air under atmospheric pressure to escape into the pleural cavity.

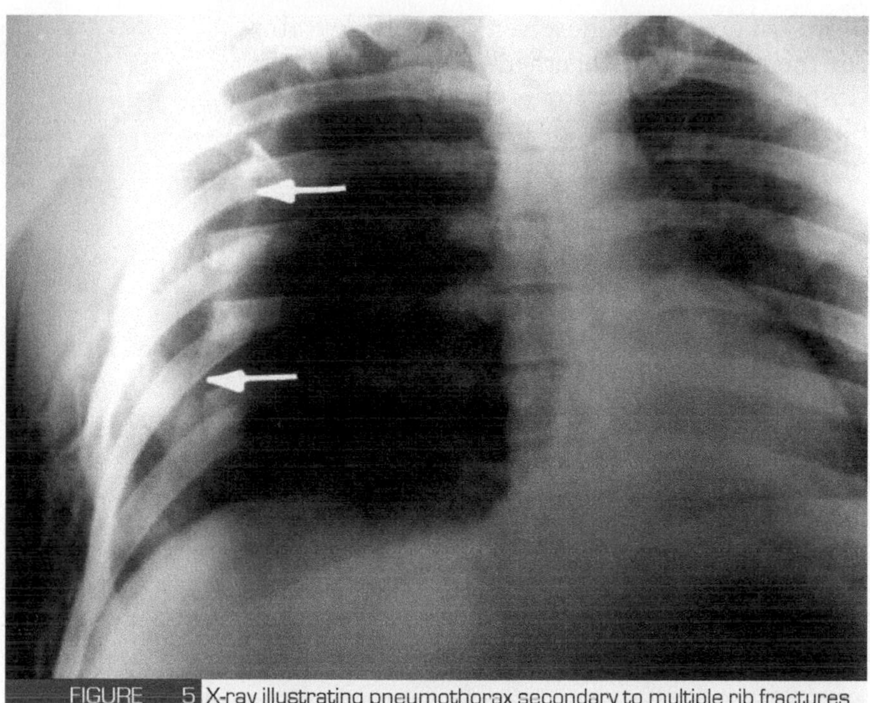

FIGURE 5 X-ray illustrating pneumothorax secondary to multiple rib fractures in which broken ends of fractured ribs have torn through the pleura and torn underlying lung. The *arrows* indicate the surface of lung that is no longer in contact with chest wall.

Occasionally, a pneumothorax occurs without apparent cause. This is called spontaneous pneumothorax. Most cases occur in young healthy persons, usually as a result of rupture of a small, air-filled, subpleural bleb at the apex of the lung.

The sudden escape of air into the pleural cavity that is associated with any type of pneumothorax usually causes chest pain and often some shortness of breath. The breath sounds, which normally can be heard with a stethoscope when the air moves in and out of the lung during respiration, are diminished on the affected side. A chest x-ray reveals partial or complete collapse of the lung and the presence of air in the pleural cavity (FIGURE 5).

The development of a positive (higher than atmospheric) pressure in the pleural cavity, called tension pneumothorax, may accompany any type of pneumothorax. This dangerous complication may occur if the lung has been perforated in such a way that the pleural tear acts as a one-way valve (FIGURE 6). In this circumstance, air flows through the perforation into the pleural cavity as the

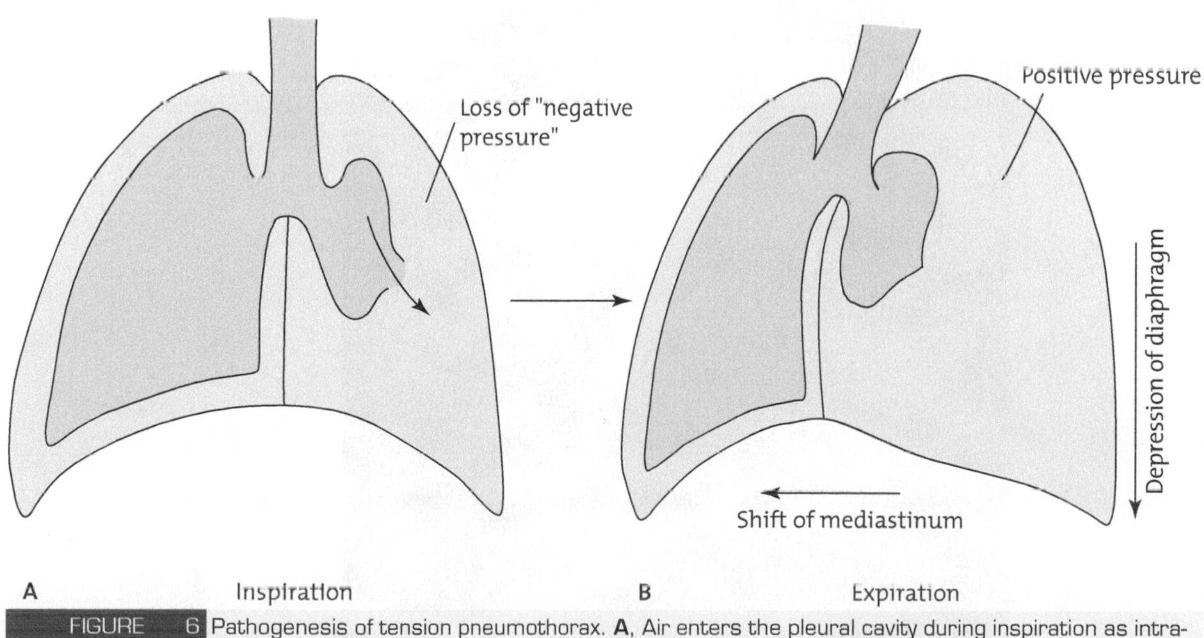

FIGURE 6 Pathogenesis of tension pneumothorax. **A**, Air enters the pleural cavity during inspiration as intrapleural pressure falls. **B**, Rising intrapleural pressure on expiration closes the pleural tear, trapping air within the pleural space. The diaphragm on affected side is displaced downward. The trachea and mediastinal structures are shifted away from side of pneumothorax and encroach on opposite pleural cavity.

intrapleural pressure falls on inspiration. On expiration, however, the intrapleural pressure rises and forces the edges of the pleural tear together, trapping the air within the pleural space. With each inspiration, more air enters the pleural cavity but cannot escape. Eventually, the pleural cavity becomes overdistended with air under pressure, and the affected lung collapses completely. As the pressure builds up in the pleural cavity, the heart and mediastinal structures are displaced away from the side of the pneumothorax and encroach on the opposite pleural cavity, impairing the expansion of the opposite lung (FIGURE 7). A tension pneumothorax can be fatal if it is not recognized and treated promptly by evacuating the trapped air to relieve the pressure.

A pneumothorax is usually treated by inserting a tube into the pleural cavity through an incision in the chest wall. The tube prevents accumulation of air in the pleural cavity and aids reexpansion of the lung. The tube is connected to an apparatus that permits the air to be expelled from the pleural cavity during expiration but prevents the air from being sucked back into the pleural cavity during inspiration. The tube is left in place until the tear in the lung heals and no more air escapes. Any air remaining in the pleural cavity is gradually reabsorbed into the bloodstream, and the lung reexpands as the air is absorbed. Sometimes a slight vacuum is applied to the tube in order to evacuate the air more rapidly and hasten reexpansion of the lung.

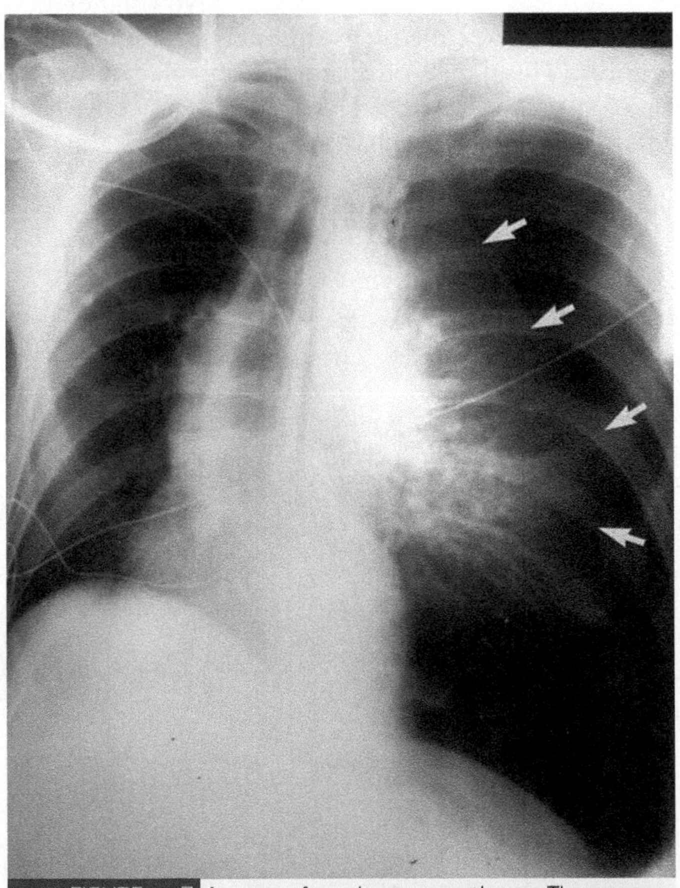

FIGURE 7 An x-ray of tension pneumothorax. The *arrows* indicate the surface of the collapsed lung. Note the low diaphragm on the affected side and displacement of mediastinal structures.

Atelectasis

Atelectasis
(ah-tel-ek′tuh-sis)
*Collapse of the lung, either caused by bronchial obstruction (*obstructive atelectasis*) or external compression (*compression atelectasis*).*

Atelectasis literally means incomplete expansion of the lung (*ateles* = incomplete + *ectasia* = expansion). It refers to a collapse of parts of the lung. There are two types:

1. Obstructive atelectasis, which results from bronchial obstruction
2. Compression atelectasis, which results from external compression of the lung

OBSTRUCTIVE ATELECTASIS

Complete blockage of a bronchus by thick mucous secretions, by a tumor, or by an aspirated foreign object prevents air from entering or leaving the alveoli supplied by the blocked bronchus, and the air already present is gradually absorbed into the blood flowing through the lungs. As a result, the part of the lung supplied by the blocked bronchus gradually collapses as the air is absorbed. The volume of the affected pleural cavity also decreases correspondingly, causing the mediastinal structures to shift toward the side of the atelectasis and the diaphragm to elevate on the affected side (FIGURE 8). If the bronchial obstruction is relieved promptly, the lung reexpands normally. This is illustrated by the following unusual case of obstructive atelectasis, which was initially thought to be secondary to an obstructing lung carcinoma.

CASE 1

A 66-year-old man with a long history of heavy smoking and excessive alcohol consumption consulted his physician because of shortness of breath. He was found to have an atelectasis of the left lung (FIGURE 9). An obstructing carcinoma was suspected, and a bronchoscopic examination was performed. A soft rubber stopper was found obstructing the left main bronchus. The subject apparently had been chewing the stopper while intoxicated and had accidentally inhaled it. The stopper was removed. An x-ray taken the following day revealed that the lung had reexpanded completely.

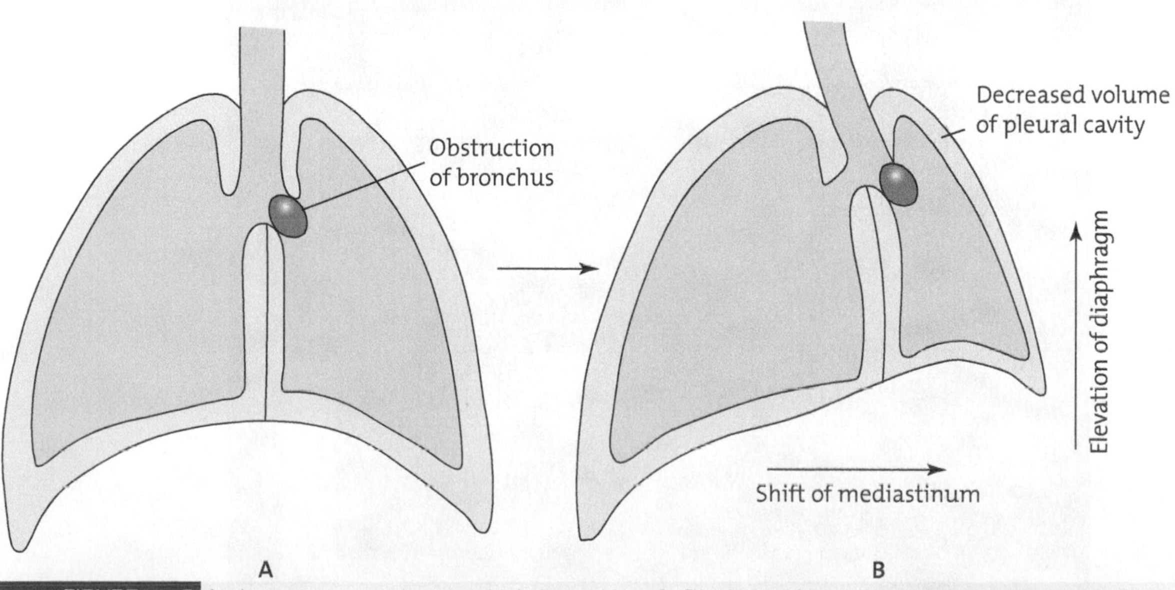

FIGURE 8 Atelectasis caused by bronchial obstruction. **A**, Blockage of bronchus prevents aeration of lung supplied by obstructed bronchus. **B**, Absorption of air causes collapse of the lung and a corresponding reduction in size of the pleural cavity. The diaphragm rises, and the mediastinum shifts toward the affected side.

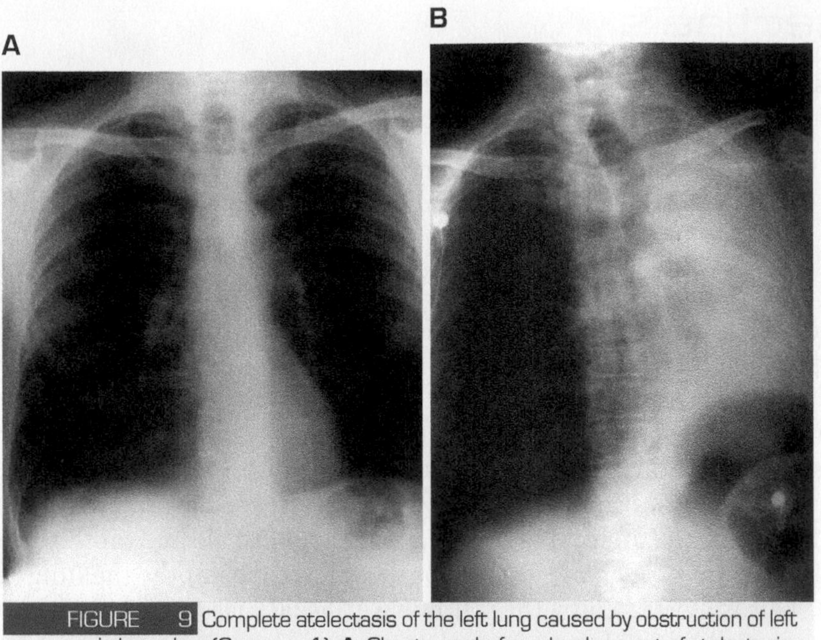

FIGURE 9 Complete atelectasis of the left lung caused by obstruction of left main bronchus (Case 1). **A**, Chest x-ray before development of atelectasis. **B**, Atelectasis of entire left lung. The collapsed lung appears dense because the air has been absorbed. The left half of diaphragm is elevated. Trachea and mediastinal structures are shifted toward the side of the collapse.

Atelectasis sometimes develops as a postoperative complication. Because of postoperative pain, the patient does not cough or breathe deeply, and mucous secretions accumulate in the bronchi (FIGURE 10). To prevent this problem, the physician encourages the postoperative patient to breathe deeply and cough frequently to keep the respiratory passages clear of secretions.

COMPRESSION ATELECTASIS

Compression atelectasis results when fluid, blood, or air accumulates in the pleural cavity, reducing its volume and thereby preventing full expansion of the lung.

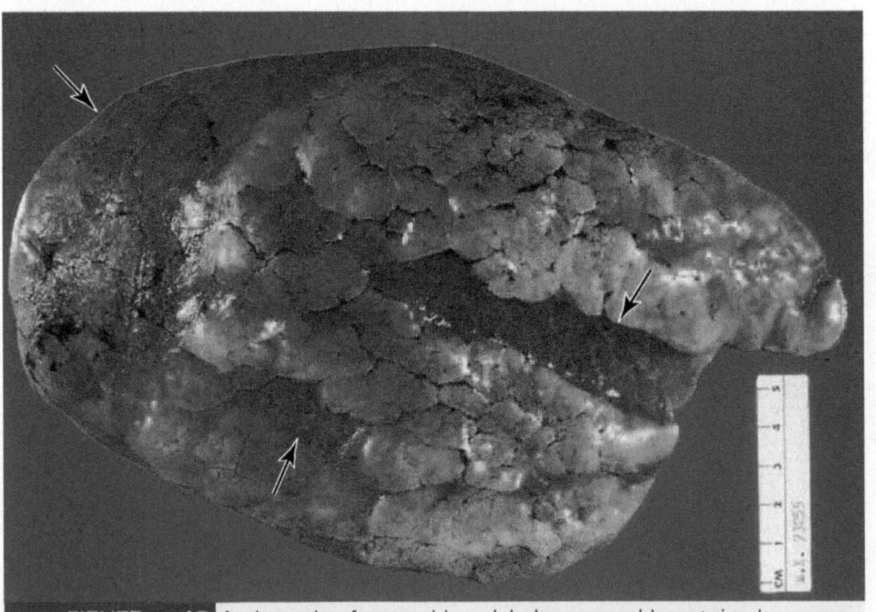

FIGURE 10 Atelectasis of several lung lobules caused by retained mucous secretions. Note the contrast between the pale normally aerated lung and the atelectatic areas (*arrows*), which appear dark and depressed.

Pneumonia

Pneumonia
(nōō-mōn yuh)
Inflammation of the lung.

Pneumonia is an inflammation of the lung characterized by the same type of vascular changes and exudation of fluid and cells as that of inflammation in any other location. However, the inflammatory process is influenced by the spongy character of the lungs. The inflammatory exudate spreads unimpeded through the lung, filling the alveoli, and the affected portions of lung becomes relatively solid (termed consolidation) (FIGURE 11A). The inflammatory exudate may reach the pleural surface in some areas, causing irritation and inflammation of the pleura; sometimes inflammatory exudate accumulates in the pleural space.

A

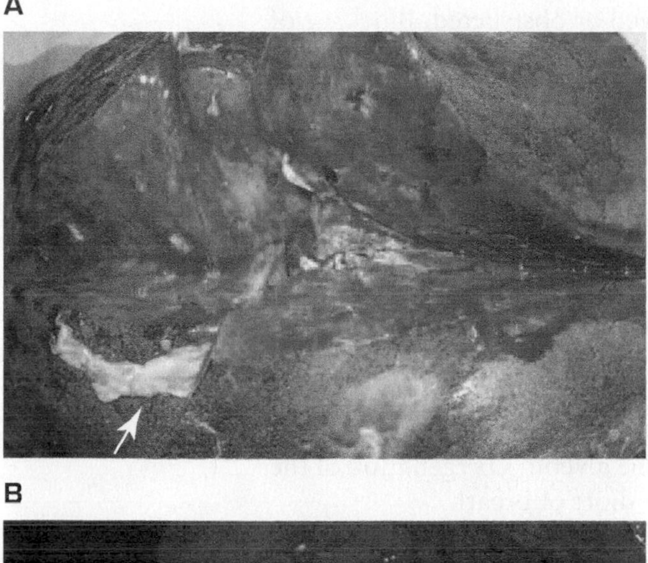

B

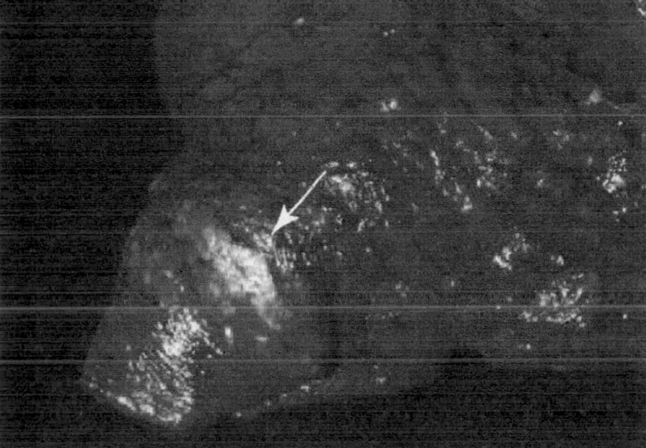

C

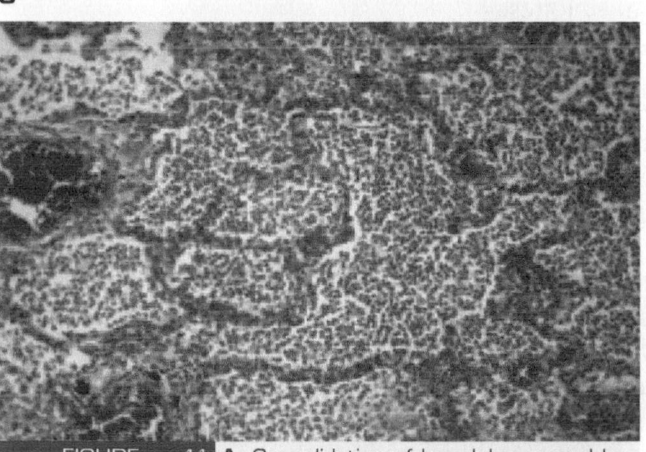

FIGURE 11 **A**, Consolidation of lung lobe caused by lobar pneumonia. The lung has been incised, and cut surfaces are exposed. An *arrow* indicates a deposit of fibrin on pleura. **B**, Bronchopneumonia. Inflammation involves lung lobules rather than an entire lobe. An *arrow* indicates most severely involved lobules. **C**, Histologic appearance of pneumonia. Alveoli are filled with neutrophils, and no air can enter the affected alveoli (original magnification × 100).

CLASSIFICATION OF PNEUMONIA

Pneumonia may be classified in several ways:

1. By etiology
2. By anatomic distribution of the inflammatory process
3. By predisposing factors that led to its development

The etiologic classification is the most important because it serves as a guide to treatment. Pneumonia may be caused by bacteria, chlamydiae, mycoplasmas, rickettsiae, viruses, or fungi. Whenever possible, the pneumonia is classified in greater detail by designating the exact organism responsible for the infection, such as the pneumococcus, staphylococcus, mycoplasma, or coronavirus.

The anatomic classification describes what part of the lung is involved (FIGURE 11). Lobar pneumonia refers to an infection of an entire lung lobe. Bronchopneumonia describes an infection involving only parts of one or more lobes (lung lobules) adjacent to the bronchi. Lobar pneumonia and bronchopneumonia are infections caused by pathogenic bacteria. A third anatomic classification is called interstitial pneumonia or primary atypical pneumonia and is usually caused by a virus or mycoplasma (*Mycoplasma pneumoniae*). This type of pulmonary infection involves the pulmonary alveolar septa rather than the alveoli, and the inflammatory cells infiltrating the septa are primarily lymphocytes, monocytes, and plasma cells rather than neutrophils.

Classification of pneumonia by predisposing factors is common. Any condition associated with poor lung ventilation and retention of bronchial secretions predisposes an individual to the development of pneumonia. Postoperative pneumonia is a pulmonary inflammation that develops in the postsurgical patient who is unable to cough or breathe deeply because of pain; the resultant poor ventilation and retention of secretions predisposes to atelectasis of lung lobules, which is followed by secondary bacterial invasion leading to bronchopneumonia. Aspiration pneumonia occurs when a foreign body, food, vomit, or other irritating substance is aspirated into the lung. Obstructive pneumonia develops in the lung distal to an area where a bronchus is narrowed or obstructed. Blockage of a bronchus by a tumor or foreign body leads to poor aeration and to retention of bronchial secretions in the obstructed part of the lung, which predisposes to infection.

CLINICAL FEATURES OF PNEUMONIA

The signs and symptoms of pneumonia are those of any systemic infection. The patient is ill and has an elevated temperature, and the number of white blood cells in the peripheral blood is frequently higher than normal. Bronchial inflammation is evident, manifested by cough and purulent sputum. If the inflammatory process involves the pleura, the patient experiences pain on respiration because the inflamed pleural surfaces rub against each other. The patient may also have symptoms related to partial loss of lung function caused by consolidation of part of the lung, resulting from the accumulation of inflammatory cells within the alveoli. Oxygenation of the blood is impaired, and the patient may become quite short of breath.

Pneumonia is treated by correcting any predisposing factors that contributed to the development of the pulmonary infection and administering appropriate antibiotic therapy.

Legionnaires' disease is a type of pneumonia caused by a gram-negative, rod-shaped bacterium called *Legionella pneumophila* that is widely distributed in the environment: in the soil and in freshwater ponds, lakes, and streams. The organism thrives in moist environments, such as air-conditioning ducts, shower heads, and humidifiers. People become infected by inhaling airborne organisms in aerosolized water droplets. The infection is not transmitted directly from person to person. The disease was first recognized in 1976 among people attending an American Legion convention in Philadelphia. After the infectious agent was identified, it was determined in retrospect that this same organism had in the past caused other outbreaks of pneumonia, but the infectious agent was not identified at the time. Clinically, the disease is characterized by the usual symptoms of a pulmonary infection, and the chest x-ray reveals evidence of pneumonia. The infection responds to appropriate antibiotics.

Legionnaires' disease
A type of pneumonia caused by an airborne bacterium called Legionella pneumophila.

SEVERE ACUTE RESPIRATORY SYNDROME (SARS)

This condition is a highly communicable serious pulmonary infection caused by an unusual coronavirus that has spread rapidly through several countries since it was first identified in late 2002. There are no effective antiviral drugs that can influence the course of the disease.

Coronaviruses are ribonucleic acid (RNA) viruses that received their name from the crownlike spikes projecting from the viruses as seen by electron microscopy (*corona* = crown). There are three major groups of coronaviruses that cause disease in animals and humans. Previously, most of the infections in humans caused by coronaviruses were common colds, not lower respiratory tract infections. The SARS-associated virus, however, is a unique virus that is not closely related to other known coronaviruses and is the first one known to cause severe disease in people. Precautions to prevent infection when dealing with patients include gloves, gowns, masks, and eye protection.

The illness begins with chills and fever, sometimes mild respiratory symptoms, and occasionally diarrhea. After 3–7 days, manifestations of lower respiratory tract infection appear: cough, shortness of breath, and evidence of pneumonia demonstrated by chest x-ray examination. The severity of the illness is quite variable. The lungs of severely affected patients show the characteristic features of the adult respiratory distress syndrome, and they require mechanical ventilation using an increased oxygen concentration to improve the diffusion of oxygen across the thickened edematous alveolar septa, as well as other measures to improve pulmonary function, as described in the section on the adult respiratory distress syndrome.

PNEUMOCYSTIS PNEUMONIA

Humans harbor *Pneumocystis jiroveci*, a small parasite of low pathogenicity now classified as a fungus, and many animals also harbor a similar parasite. The parasite does not affect normal persons but may cause serious pulmonary infections in susceptible individuals. Those at risk include adults whose immune defenses have been impaired by communicable disease, such as by AIDS, or by administration of immunosuppressive drugs, and premature infants in whom immune defenses are poorly developed.

The life cycle of the parasite is complex. The most easily recognized form is a round or cup-shaped cyst about the size of a red blood cell that cannot be identified by routine (hematoxylin and eosin) stains but can be demonstrated by means of special stains containing silver compounds. Within the cysts are small structures called sporozoites, which are released from the cyst and mature to form larger structures called trophozoites. Some trophozoites give rise to more cysts, repeating the cycle. Others attack and injure the cells lining the pulmonary alveoli, causing a mild inflammatory reaction within the alveolar septa, which leads to exudation of large amounts of protein-rich material that accumulates within the alveoli. The parasites, intermixed in the alveolar exudate but unstained by routine stains, appear as pale areas within the brightly stained exudate, imparting a foamy, "soap-bubble" appearance to the exudate. Special stains, however, demonstrate that the soap bubbles represent *Pneumocystis* cysts and may also reveal central clusters of sporozoites, which appear as dark dots within the centers of the cysts (FIGURE 12).

Clinically, pneumocystis pneumonia is characterized by progressive shortness of breath and cough in a person whose immunologic defenses are impaired and who is at high risk of developing the disease. Evidence of pulmonary consolidation caused by the alveolar exudate can be demonstrated by x ray. The diagnosis of pneumocystis pneumonia is established by biopsy of lung tissue obtained by bronchoscopy. Histologic study of the biopsy material reveals the characteristic foamy alveolar exudate containing large numbers of parasites, as demonstrated by special stains. Often, the parasite also can be demonstrated in material aspirated from the bronchi by bronchoscopy. It is much more difficult to demonstrate the organisms in sputum because they are enmeshed in the alveolar exudate and do not escape from the alveoli. The infection is always very serious and is often life threatening because it affects persons whose ability to respond to infection is greatly impaired. Treatment consists of administering drugs that inhibit the growth of the organism.

Tuberculosis

Pulmonary tuberculosis is a special type of pneumonia caused by an acid-fast bacterium, the tubercle bacillus *Mycobacterium tuberculosis*. Because the tubercle bacillus has a capsule composed of waxes and fatty substances, it is more resistant to destruction than many other organisms. The body's response to the tubercle bacillus also differs from the usual acute inflammatory reaction. Monocytes accumulate around the bacteria; many of them fuse, forming rather characteristic large multinucleated

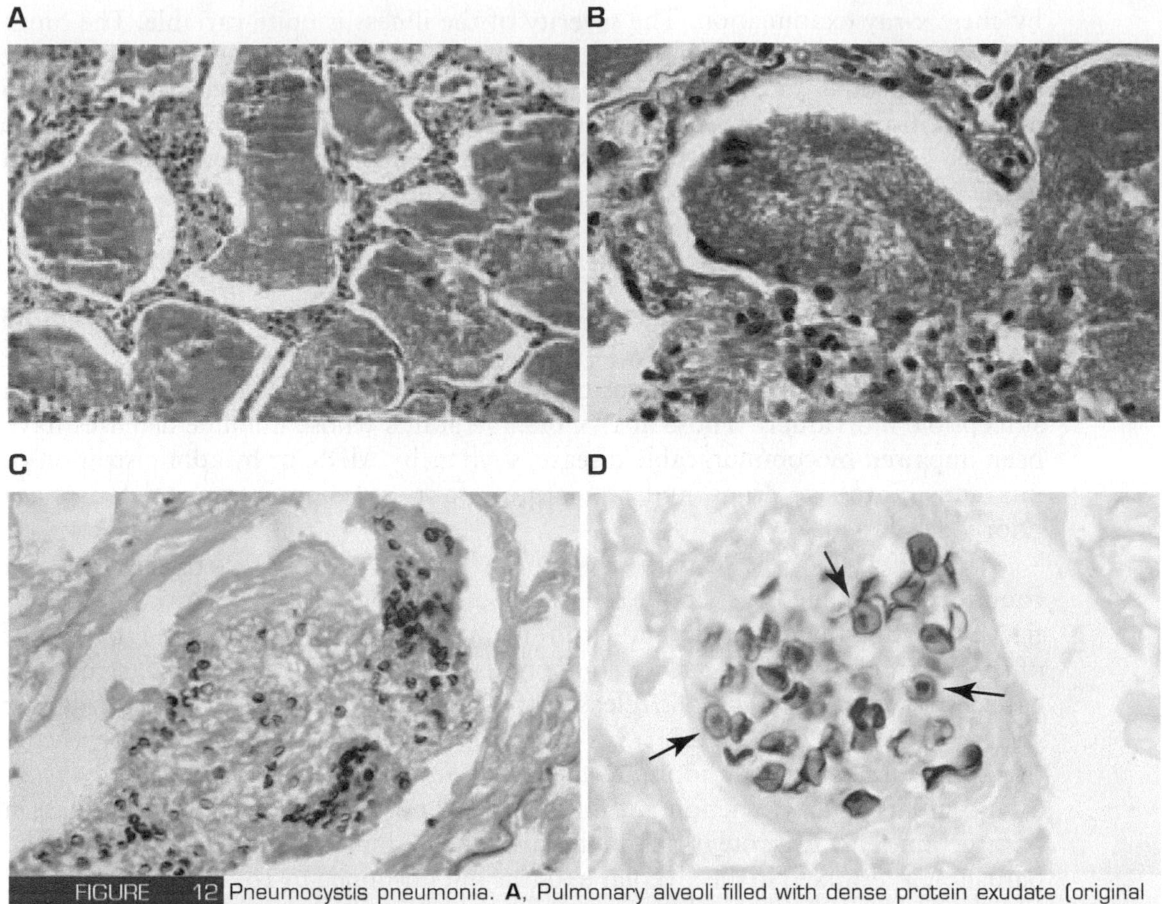

FIGURE 12 Pneumocystis pneumonia. **A**, Pulmonary alveoli filled with dense protein exudate (original magnification × 100). **B**, Higher magnification, illustrating the foamy "soap-bubble" appearance of the alveolar exudate. The clear areas in the alveolar exudate are *Pneumocystis* organisms that are not stained by routine stains (original magnification × 400). **C**, Demonstration of *Pneumocystis jiroveci* cysts within the alveolar exudate by means of silver-containing stains (original magnification × 400). **D**, High-magnification view of the organisms demonstrated by silver stains. Central dark dots within the cysts are clusters of sporozoites (original magnification × 1,000).

cells called giant cells. Lymphocytes and plasma cells also accumulate, and fibrous tissue proliferates around the central cluster of monocytes and giant cells. The central portion of the cellular aggregation usually becomes necrotic. This characteristic nodular mass of cells with central necrosis is called a granuloma, and the inflammatory process is called a granulomatous inflammation (FIGURE 13). The granulomatous response to the tubercle bacillus and the necrosis within the granulomas indicate the development of cell-mediated immunity against the organism, which is the primary immune defense against the tubercle bacillus.

COURSE OF A TUBERCULOUS INFECTION

The initial infection is acquired from organisms inhaled in airborne droplets that have been coughed or sneezed into the air by a person with active tuberculosis who is discharging organisms into the environment. The organisms lodge within the pulmonary alveoli, where they proceed to multiply. Initially, the organisms introduced into the lungs do not elicit a marked inflammatory reaction because they do not produce any toxins or destructive enzymes that damage the tissues. Macrophages phagocytose the bacteria but are unable to destroy them; they may even carry the organisms to other parts of the lung and into the regional lymph nodes. After several

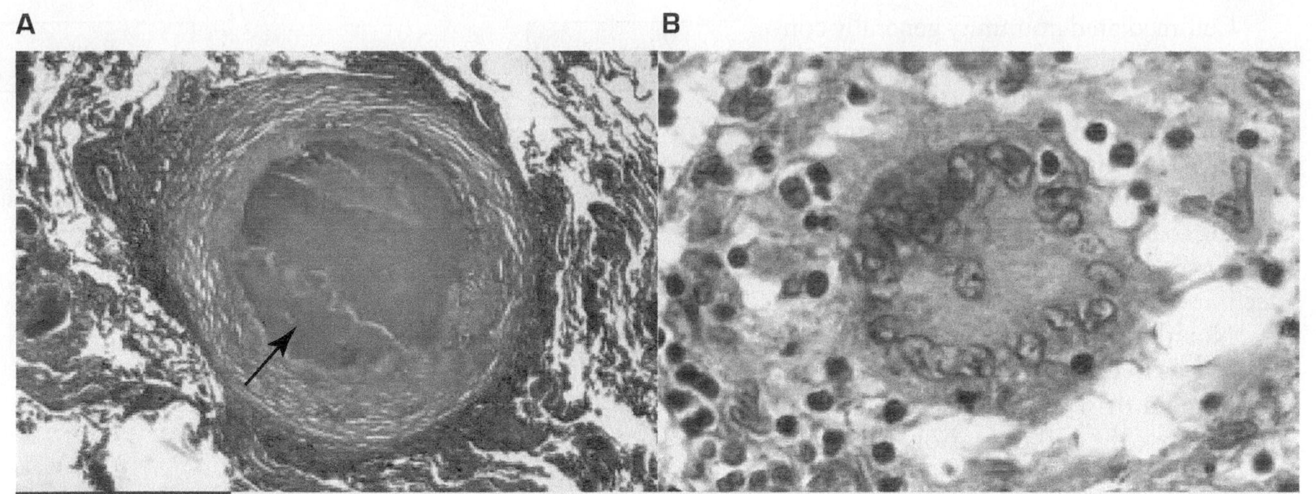

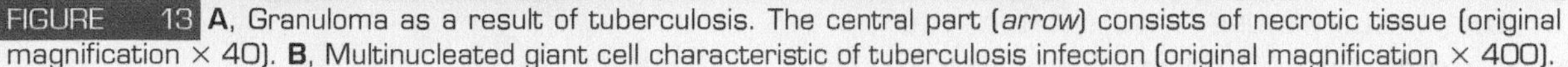

FIGURE 13 **A**, Granuloma as a result of tuberculosis. The central part (*arrow*) consists of necrotic tissue (original magnification × 40). **B**, Multinucleated giant cell characteristic of tuberculosis infection (original magnification × 400).

weeks, however, a cell-mediated immunity develops. Sensitized lymphocytes attract and activate macrophages, which acquire a greatly enhanced phagocytic and destructive capability. The activated macrophages attack and destroy many of the organisms, forming characteristic granulomas containing areas of necrosis and surrounded by a rim of fibrous tissue. In the majority of cases, the infection is arrested; the granulomas in the lung and regional lymph nodes heal with scarring, often followed by calcification of the granulomas. In most cases, the infection does not cause any symptoms, and the person may be unaware of the infection. Sometimes the granuloma in the lung is large enough to be identified in a chest x-ray (FIGURE 14), but often the area of infection is too small to be detected in an x-ray. The positive skin test (Mantoux test), which reveals a hypersensitivity to the proteins of the tubercle bacillus, may be the only evidence of recent infection.

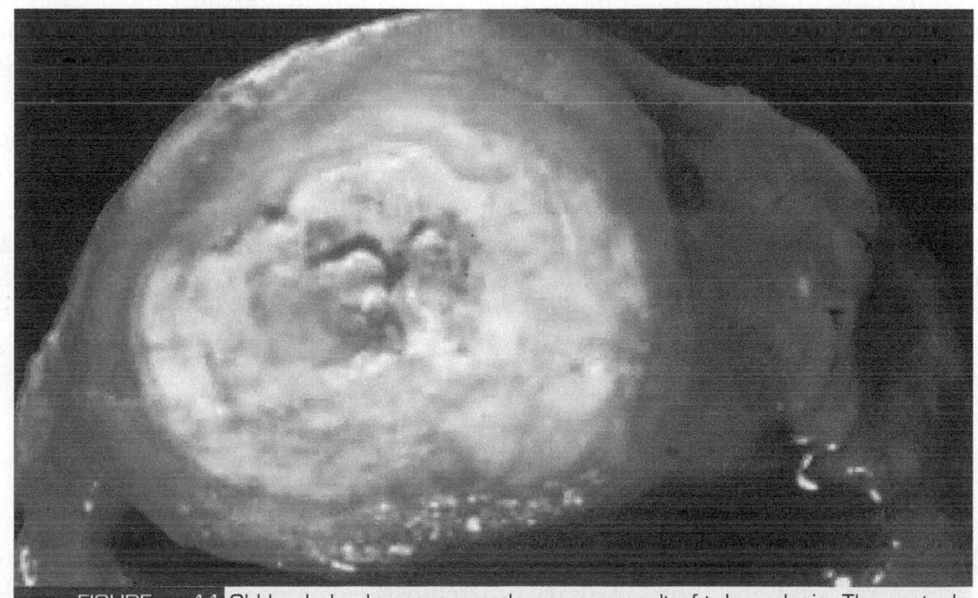

FIGURE 14 Old healed pulmonary granuloma as a result of tuberculosis. The central part consists of necrotic tissue containing calcium deposits surrounded by rim of dense fibrous tissue.

Cell-mediated immunity generally controls the infection, and the arrested infection may never cause any further problems. The healed granulomas, however, may contain small numbers of viable organisms, and the infection may become reactivated, leading to progressive pulmonary tuberculosis if the body's cell-mediated immunity declines.

Not all primary infections respond as favorably. If a large number of organisms are inhaled or if the body's defenses are inadequate, the inflammation will progress, causing more extensive destruction of lung tissue (FIGURE 15). Often, the granulomatous inflammatory process makes contact with a bronchus, and the necrotic inflammatory tissue is discharged into it. A cavity then forms within the lung, surrounded by granulomatous inflammatory tissue containing masses of tubercle bacilli (FIGURE 16). People who have active progressive tuberculosis with a tuberculous cavity can infect others because they discharge large numbers of tubercle bacilli in their sputum.

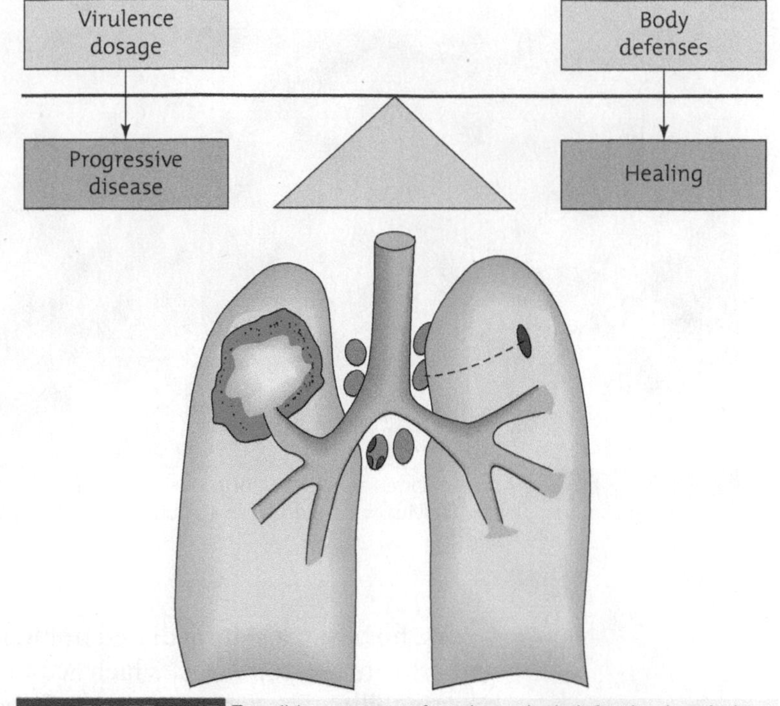

FIGURE 15 Possible outcome of a tuberculosis infection in relation to virulence and dosage of the organism and resistance of the body. The frequent involvement of the regional lymph nodes is indicated. *Left*, Progressive disease with formation of cavity within lung, caused by infection by a large number of organisms or inadequate body defenses. *Right*, Healing with scarring as a result of small numbers of organisms or a high degree of resistance to infection.

In a tuberculous infection of the lung, organisms are often carried in lymphatic channels from the lung into the peribronchial lymph nodes, leading to a tuberculous inflammation in the regional lymph nodes.

Many cases of active progressive pulmonary tuberculosis do not result from the initial infection. They develop in persons who have been infected at some time in the past and have developed a cell-mediated immunity directed against the organism. In the past, tuberculosis in previously infected persons was called reinfection tuberculosis because physicians believed that the active tuberculosis was caused by a new infection with the tubercle bacillus in a person who had been infected previously with the organism. Indeed, some cases of tuberculosis in previously infected persons are actually new infections. However, most cases of active tuberculosis in older patients result from a reactivation of an old infection rather than a new infection with the tubercle bacillus. It is well known that old tuberculous lesions that appear completely healed may harbor tubercle bacilli. If the resistance of the individual is lowered by AIDS or other debilitating diseases, by treatment with adrenal corticosteroids, or by other factors, an apparently healed focus of tuberculosis may flare up and lead to active progressive tuberculosis.

MILIARY TUBERCULOSIS AND TUBERCULOUS PNEUMONIA

Miliary tuberculosis
(mi'lē-air-ē)
Multiple foci of tuberculosis throughout the body as a result of bloodstream dissemination of tubercle bacilli from a primary focus in the lung or peribronchial lymph nodes.

Miliary tuberculosis and tuberculous pneumonia are two uncommon but extremely serious forms of tuberculosis. **Miliary tuberculosis** develops if a mass of tuberculous inflammatory tissue erodes into a large blood vessel, disseminating large numbers of organisms throughout the body through the bloodstream. The term miliary is derived

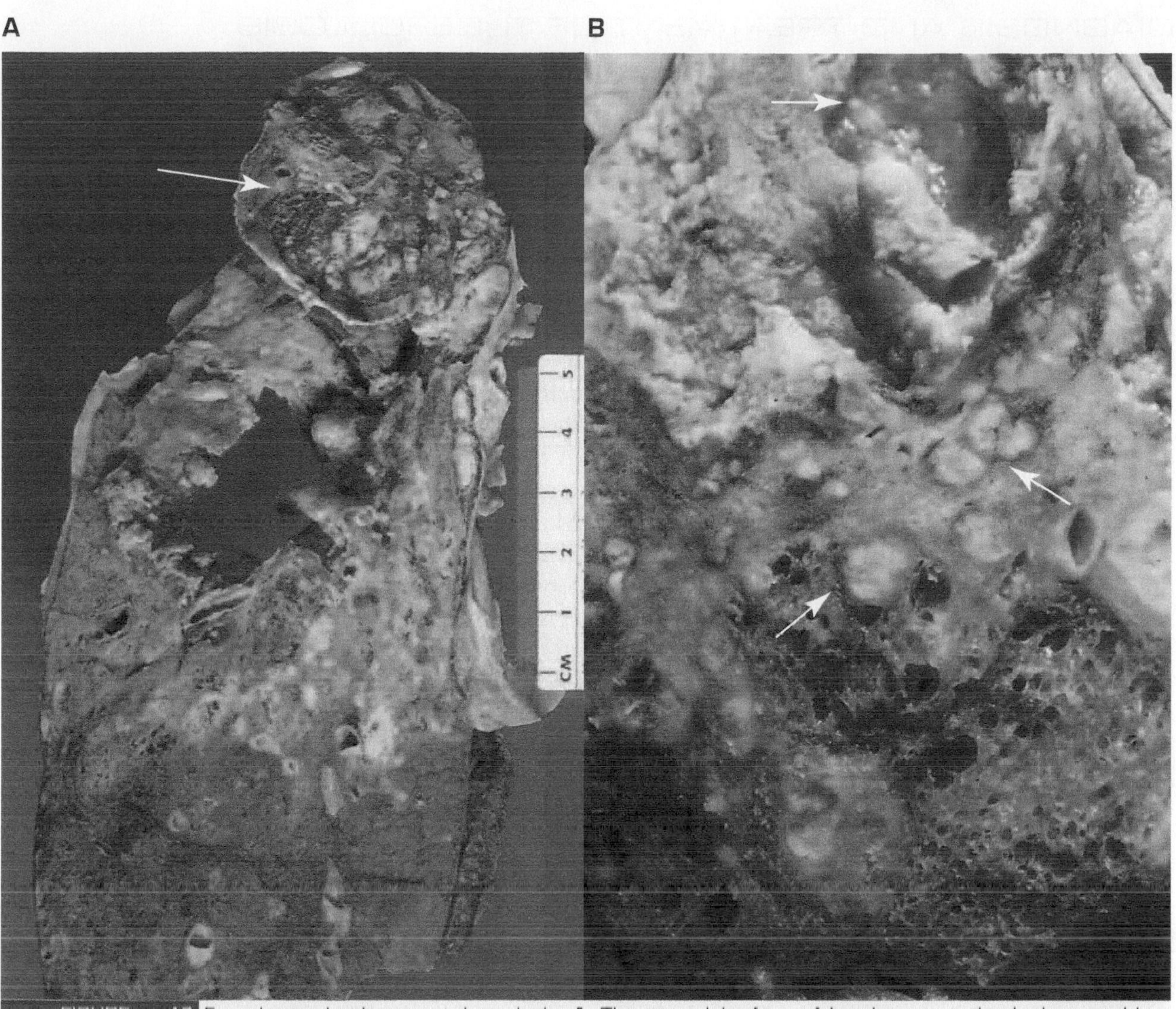

FIGURE 16 Far-advanced pulmonary tuberculosis. **A**. The upper lobe (*arrow*) has been completely destroyed by tuberculosis, and there is extensive tuberculosis in the lower lobe with a large cavity in the lung that communicates with a bronchus. Only the lower part of the lobe is free of disease (*extreme bottom* of photograph). **B**. A closer view of tuberculosis. A large cavity (*upper arrow*) surrounded by nodular and diffuse granulomatous inflammation. Several discrete granulomas (*lower arrows*) can be seen below the cavity.

from the resemblance of the multiple foci of disseminated tuberculosis (present in liver, spleen, kidney, and other tissues) to millet seeds. These foci are small white nodules from about 1 to 2 mm in diameter. Tuberculous pneumonia is an overwhelming infection characterized by extensive tuberculous consolidation of one or more lobes of the lung. Persons with AIDS and other immunocompromised persons are prone to this type of rapidly progressive infection.

EXTRAPULMONARY TUBERCULOSIS

Sometimes tuberculosis develops in the kidneys, bones, uterus, fallopian tubes, or other extrapulmonary location. The infection results from hematogenous spread of tubercle bacilli from a focus of tuberculosis in the lung. Sometimes, the secondary focus of infection may progress even though the pulmonary infection has healed, leading to an active extrapulmonary tuberculous infection without clinically apparent pulmonary tuberculosis.

DIAGNOSIS AND TREATMENT OF TUBERCULOSIS

Tuberculous infection is associated with the development of hypersensitivity to proteins in the tubercle bacillus, as discussed on immunity, hypersensitivity, allergy, and autoimmune diseases. A positive skin test (Mantoux test) indicates that the person was at one time infected with the tubercle bacillus; it does not necessarily indicate an active infection.

At present, many physicians recommend that persons who develop an infection with the tubercle bacillus, as manifested by conversion of a negative into a positive skin test reaction, be treated with antituberculosis drugs. Treatment is also recommended for patients with inactive tuberculosis who have an increased risk of developing a reactivation of an old, apparently healed tuberculous infection.

Unfortunately, the frequency of tuberculosis, which declined steadily from about 1950 to 1980, began to rise at an alarming rate in the United States, and a number of factors appear to be responsible for the increase. A large number of persons have immigrated to the United States from Asian, African, and Latin American countries, where the prevalence of tuberculosis is much higher. Many of these persons have been infected, although they do not have active tuberculosis. This group serves as a reservoir of infected persons in whom active tuberculosis can develop if immunity declines, which in turn may be followed by infection of other persons with whom they are in close contact. Social problems of poverty, drug abuse, alcoholism, and homelessness create conditions favoring transmission of tuberculosis from person to person. Many of these unfortunate persons with active tuberculosis do not receive adequate ongoing medical care; they may also not be motivated to complete the full course of treatment needed to arrest the disease. Failure to complete treatment leads to treatment failure, and premature cessation of treatment also promotes the emergence of drug-resistant strains of the organism.

DRUG-RESISTANT TUBERCULOSIS

Effective drug treatment of tuberculosis has transformed the infection from a potentially fatal chronic disease to one that could be treated effectively by a number of antibiotics and chemotherapeutic agents, but now drug-resistant tuberculosis (TB) is becoming a major problem. Tuberculosis caused by organisms resistant to at least two of the most commonly used antituberculosis drugs is designated multiple drug-resistant tuberculosis (MDR-TB), which is more difficult to treat. The course of treatment is more prolonged and the results of treatment are less satisfactory. Recently, the drug-resistance problem has become even more threatening. Some strains have become "super resistant." They no longer respond to a large number of antituberculosis drugs, and an infection by these organisms is designated extremely drug-resistant tuberculosis (XDR-TB). Were these strains to become widespread, tuberculosis would no longer be a potentially treatable infection. Instead, an XDR-TB infection would be a very serious disease having an outcome comparable to that of tuberculosis infections before antibiotic treatment had become available, and it is essential to prevent spread of this highly resistant strain. Persons with XDR-TB need to obtain treatment at a facility accustomed to dealing with these resistant organisms, and the patients' activities need to be restricted so they cannot spread the infection. The World Health Organization has become increasingly concerned about the spread of XDR-TB cases. Most have been concentrated in Eastern Europe, South Africa, and Asia, but cases are appearing in the United States, and control measures to prevent further spread are considered essential.

SPREAD OF TUBERCULOSIS

Tuberculosis remains a serious problem, and unrecognized cases such as that illustrated in Case 2 may expose many susceptible individuals. Infected individuals who take no precautions to prevent infecting others also may increase exposure, as illustrated by the case summarized in the Supplementary Readings article by Markel and others, which deals with extensively drug-resistant tuberculosis.

CASE 2

A 17-year-old female high school student developed a dry cough accompanied by weakness and fatigue, elevated temperature, chills, and a 15-lb weight loss. She had also recently noted that she became short of breath after climbing two flights of stairs. Previously, she had lived for a time with an uncle who had tuberculosis. Examination revealed extensive consolidation in the upper part of both lungs as a result of tuberculosis (FIGURE 17). Smears and cultures of sputum revealed tubercle bacilli. She was hospitalized and received a course of antituberculous drug therapy. Her school was contacted, and steps were taken to check other students with whom she had had contact for possible tuberculous infection. The infection slowly responded to therapy, and she was later released from the hospital to continue treatment as an outpatient.

Bronchiectasis (bron-kē-ek′tuh-sis) *Dilatation of bronchi caused by weakening of their walls as a result of infection.*

Bronchitis and Bronchiectasis

Acute inflammation of the tracheobronchial mucosa is common in many upper respiratory infections. The raw throat and cough associated with many respiratory infections are a result of the associated acute bronchitis. Chronic bronchitis also is common; often, it results from constant irritation of the respiratory mucosa by smoking cigarettes or breathing air containing large amounts of atmospheric pollution.

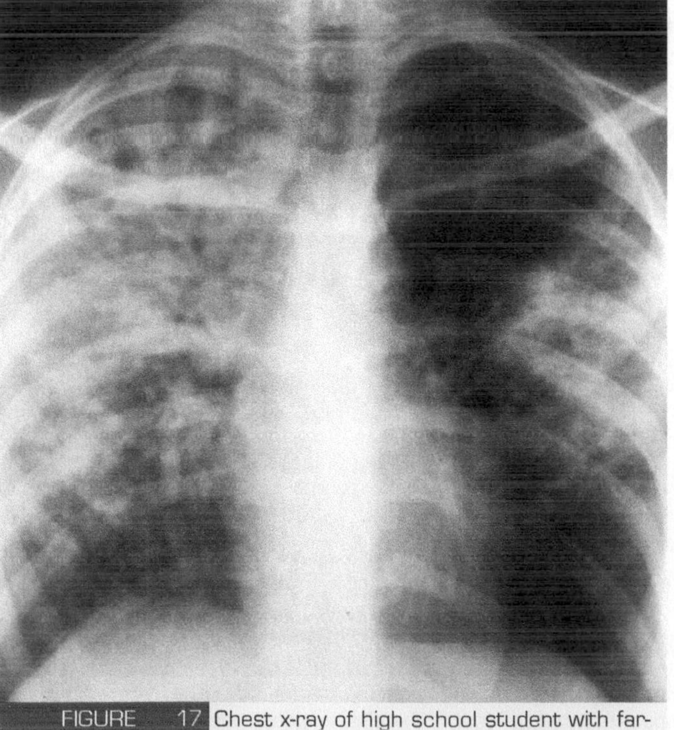

FIGURE 17 Chest x-ray of high school student with far-advanced pulmonary tuberculosis, illustrating extensive consolidation of both lungs (Case 2).

Sometimes the bronchial walls in parts of the lung become weakened as a result of severe inflammation or other factors, and the affected bronchi become markedly dilated. This condition is called **bronchiectasis** (*ectasis* = dilation). The distended bronchi tend to retain secretions. Consequently, patients with bronchiectasis frequently have a chronic cough associated with production of large amounts of purulent sputum. Often, they suffer repeated bouts of pulmonary infection. The only effective treatment of bronchiectasis is surgical resection of the affected segments of lung. Bronchiectasis can be recognized by means of a special type of radiologic examination called a bronchogram. The procedure consists of taking x-ray films after instilling a radiopaque oil into the trachea and bronchi. The oil covers the mucosa of the bronchi, and the abnormal bronchi can be recognized as dilated saccular or fusiform structures (FIGURE 18).

Chronic Obstructive Lung Disease

Pulmonary emphysema is a disease in which the air spaces distal to the terminal bronchioles are enlarged and their walls are destroyed. The disease is an important cause of disability and death, and its incidence is increasing at an alarming rate. In emphysema, the normally fine alveolar structure of the lung is destroyed, and large, cystic air spaces form throughout the lung (FIGURE 19). The destructive process usually begins in the upper lobes but eventually may affect all lobes of both lungs. Usually, there is an associated chronic inflammation of the terminal bronchioles. Emphysema and chronic bronchitis occur together so frequently that they are usually considered a single entity, designated chronic obstructive pulmonary disease (COPD). The chief clinical manifestations of any type of chronic pulmonary disease are dyspnea and cyanosis. Dyspnea is a sensation of shortness of breath. Cyanosis is a blue tinge of the skin and mucous membrane that results from an excessive amount of reduced hemoglobin in the blood. Reduced hemoglobin is dark purplish red, in contrast with normally oxygenated blood, which is bright red.

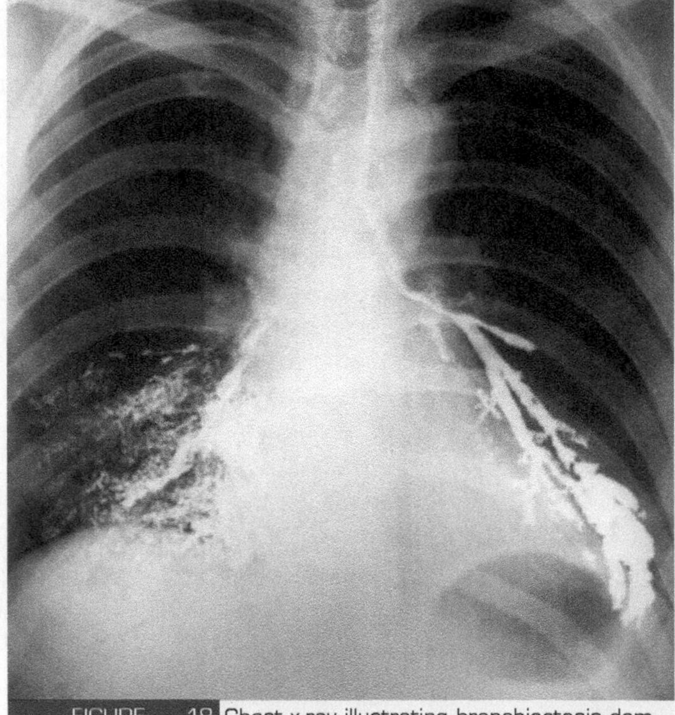

FIGURE 18 Chest x-ray illustrating bronchiectasis demonstrated by bronchogram. Right lower lobe bronchi (*left*) appear normal. Bronchi on the opposite side exhibit saclike and fusiform dilatation, as outlined by radiopaque contrast material within dilated bronchi.

The three main anatomic derangements in chronic obstructive pulmonary disease are (1) inflammation and narrowing of the terminal bronchioles, (2) dilatation and coalescence of pulmonary air spaces, and (3) loss of lung elasticity. These derangements in turn cause severe disturbances in pulmonary function.

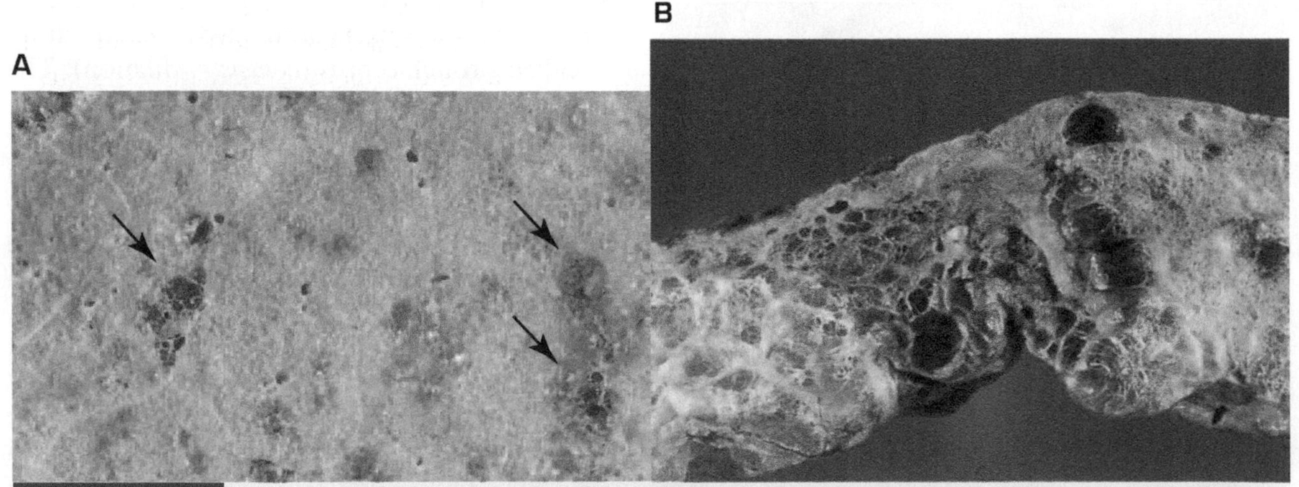

FIGURE 19 Sections of air-dried lung preparations illustrating the gross appearance of emphysema. **A**, Mild emphysema. Beginning breakdown of lung tissue to form cystic spaces (*arrows*). Most of the alveoli appear normal. **B**, Advanced emphysema with multiple confluent cystic spaces within lung. Very little normal lung tissue remains. The dark color is a result of accumulation of carbon pigment in the emphysematous lung from inhaling "dirty" air.

DERANGEMENTS OF PULMONARY STRUCTURE AND FUNCTION

Chronic inflammation of the bronchioles probably initiates the destructive process. Chronic inflammation causes swelling of the bronchial mucosa, which reduces the caliber of the bronchi and bronchioles and stimulates increased bronchial secretions. Because a tube's resistance to air flow varies with the fourth power of its diameter, a slight reduction in the caliber of the bronchioles greatly restricts the flow of air. Normally, the bronchi and bronchioles dilate slightly during inspiration and become smaller during expiration. Consequently, air can enter the lungs more readily than it can be expelled through the narrowed bronchioles; so air tends to become trapped in the lungs during expiration. The lungs cannot empty completely, and they become chronically overinflated. As a result, the amount of additional air that can be inspired when the subject takes a deep breath is much reduced, and the subject is unable to increase his or her ventilation adequately in response to increased demand.

The bronchiolar obstruction also disturbs pulmonary function by causing unequal air flow to various parts of the lung. Some alveoli are overventilated; others are inadequately supplied, reducing the overall efficiency of pulmonary ventilation. The excess air supplying the overventilated alveoli is "wasted" because more is provided than is needed to oxygenate completely the blood flowing through the surrounding pulmonary capillaries. Conversely, the blood flowing to the poorly ventilated alveoli does not become fully oxygenated. When it mixes with normally oxygenated blood flowing from other parts of the lungs, the oxygen content of the blood delivered to the tissues is reduced.

The destruction of the alveolar septa leads to enlargement of the air spaces and at the same time reduces the number of pulmonary capillaries available for gas exchange (FIGURE 20). Normally, there are about 400 million alveoli in both lungs, and the surface area of the pulmonary capillaries supplying the alveoli is about 30 times as great as the surface area of the body. Each alveolus contains a relatively small volume of air surrounded by a rich network of capillaries. This arrangement promotes optimal diffusion of gases between alveolar air and pulmonary capillaries. Diffusion of gases is much less efficient from large cystic spaces because the spaces contain a much larger volume of air than does a normal alveolus and are surrounded by a relatively sparse network of capillaries. Moreover, the movement of air into and out of the enlarged spaces is impeded by the bronchiolar obstruction.

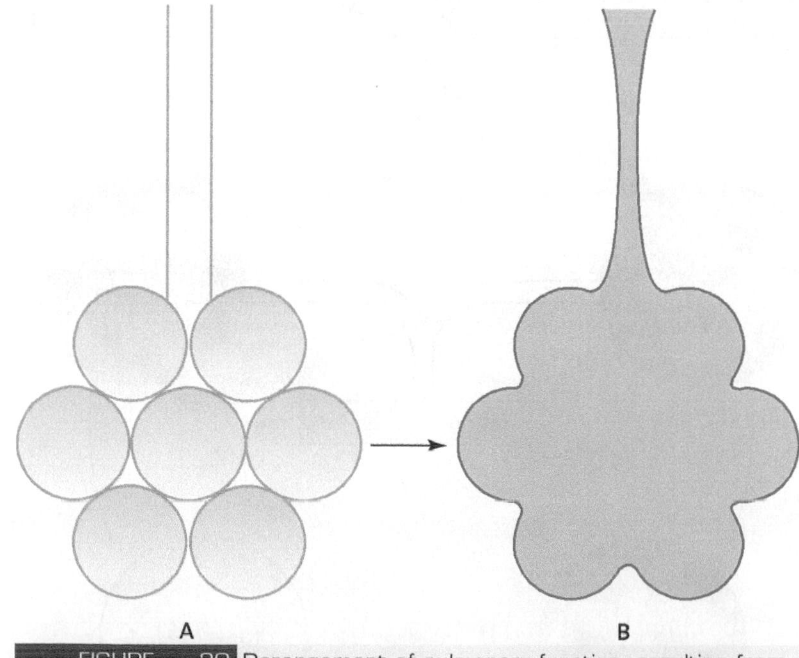

FIGURE 20 Derangement of pulmonary function, resulting from enlargement of air spaces and reduction of pulmonary capillary bed. **A**, Normal structure, illustrating schematically a cluster of alveoli surrounded by a rich capillary bed connected to normal bronchiole. **B**, Emphysema, illustrating coalescence of air spaces to form a large cystic space with greatly reduced capillary bed and narrowed bronchiole.

Destruction of the alveolar septa also leads to loss of the elastic tissue in the septa that forms the structural framework of the lungs, and so the lungs no longer "recoil" normally after they have been stretched during inspiration. Expiration is no longer a passive process. The air must be actively forced out of the lungs by contraction of the intercostal muscles. Breathing requires more effort that in turn requires a greater oxygen consumption. The pressure required to actively force air out of the lungs during expiration also raises the intrapleural pressure and compresses the lungs, which causes further problems with pulmonary ventilation. The bronchi and bronchioles have lost their normal structural support because of loss of lung elasticity and tend to collapse during expiration, obstructing the outflow of air and trapping more air within the lungs.

The chief symptom of emphysema is shortness of breath. Initially, this is noted only on exertion, but later it may be present even at rest. The patient usually also has a chronic cough with purulent sputum, owing to the associated chronic bronchitis. Eventually, severely affected patients may die because they lack enough functionally normal lung tissue to sustain life or because of a superimposed pulmonary infection. Emphysema is also a frequent cause of respiratory acidosis, one of the common disturbances of acid–base balance. This is discussed in water, electrolyte, and acid–base balance.

PATHOGENESIS OF CHRONIC OBSTRUCTIVE PULMONARY DISEASE

Cigarette smoking and atmospheric air pollution appear to be the major factors responsible for the rising incidence of emphysema. Exactly how they exert their destructive effect on the lung is not completely understood. FIGURE 21 summarizes one concept of the pathogenesis of this serious and disabling disease. Smoking and air pollution are considered to expose the bronchial mucosa to chronic irritation, eventually producing chronic bronchitis associated with a chronic cough and increased bronchial secretions. The inflammatory swelling of the mucosa narrows the smaller bronchioles, increasing their resistance to expiration and causing air to be trapped within the lung.

The leukocytes that accumulate in the bronchioles and alveoli may also contribute to the lung damage by releasing proteolytic (protein-digesting) enzymes that attack the elastic fibers making up part of the lung's structural framework. Moreover, the mechanisms that inactivate the leukocyte enzymes are less efficient in the emphysematous lung.

Repeated bouts of coughing, with consequent extreme elevations in intrabronchial pressure, cause the alveolar septa to rupture, gradually converting the alveoli into large, cystic air spaces. The lungs become overdistended and lose their normal elasticity. The patient cannot expel air normally from the overdistended lungs because normal lung elasticity is lost and the bronchioles are obstructed; difficulty expectorating the excessive bronchial secretions also is apparent. Retention of secretions and poor drainage of secretions from the bronchi tend to perpetuate the chronic bronchitis, and a vicious circle is created. The diseased lungs are also more susceptible to infection because of

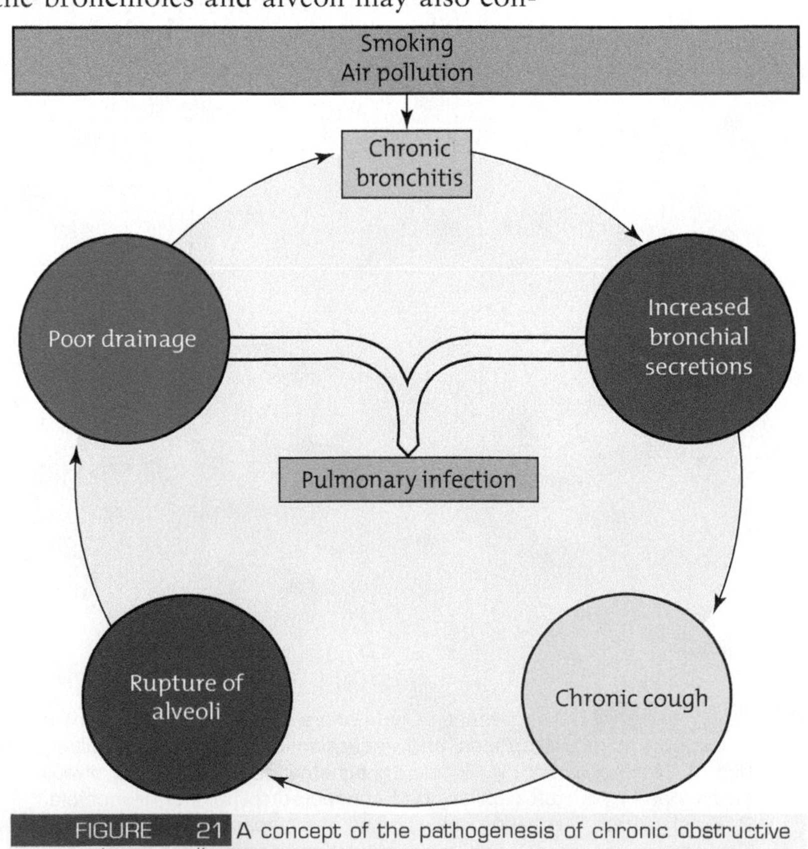

FIGURE 21 A concept of the pathogenesis of chronic obstructive pulmonary disease.

impaired pulmonary ventilation, bronchial inflammation, bronchiolar obstruction, and excessive bronchial secretions. Therefore, patients with emphysema frequently have repeated bouts of pneumonia, further damaging the lung tissue.

PREVENTION AND TREATMENT

For the most part, emphysema can be prevented by refraining from smoking and avoiding inhalation of other substances known to be injurious to the lungs. Atmospheric air pollution contributes to the increasing incidence of emphysema, and various measures are being undertaken to control this serious public health problem.

After emphysema has developed, the damaged lungs cannot be restored to normal. However, several measures can be employed to promote the drainage of bronchial secretions, to improve pulmonary ventilation, and to decrease the frequency of superimposed pulmonary infections. These measures, along with cessation of smoking, will retard or arrest further progression of the disease.

Surgical procedures called lung volume reduction surgery have also been investigated. These procedures excise the nonfunctional extremely emphysematous segments of the upper lobes, thereby reducing the size of the overinflated lungs so that the less severely involved lower lobes might be able to function more efficiently. A large recently completed U.S. government-sponsored clinical trial involving more than 1,000 patients (The National Emphysema Treatment Trial) compared the results of lung volume reduction surgery in one group of patients with medical treatment in a comparable group. In general, the overall mortality rates in both groups were similar, indicating that surgical treatment did not improve survival for most patients. One group, however, did benefit from surgery: patients who had a very limited capacity for exercise caused by the emphysema, in whom the emphysema was restricted to the upper lobes of the lungs. On the other hand, patients who did not meet these criteria had a higher mortality rate than medically treated patients and did not get any significant benefit from the surgical procedures. Unfortunately, even the initial benefit of surgery in the group who responded was of short duration, and 2 years later their pulmonary function had declined to the point where it was no better than it had been before surgery.

The following case illustrates the clinical features of a patient with chronic pulmonary emphysema who developed severe respiratory insufficiency that was precipitated by a bout of pneumonia.

CASE 3

A 70-year-old man entered the hospital because of severe, progressive shortness of breath for the previous 2 weeks. He had had chronic pulmonary emphysema for many years secondary to heavy cigarette smoking and had stopped smoking recently. On physical examination, he was very short of breath, and there was moderate cyanosis of the lips and nail beds. Lungs appeared overinflated, and respiratory excursions were poor. Laboratory studies revealed a low arterial oxygen content (PO_2 31 mm Hg) and oxygen saturation (53%), with elevated carbon dioxide tension (PCO_2 53 mm Hg) and plasma bicarbonate (40 mEq/liter). Blood pH was reduced to 7.29. These changes indicated severe pulmonary emphysema with respiratory acidosis. Chest x-ray revealed a pneumonia in the right lower lobe. Treatment consisted of supplementary oxygen, antibiotics, and various other measures to improve pulmonary function. The pneumonia slowly subsided, and the patient left the hospital 2 weeks later.

EMPHYSEMA AS A RESULT OF ALPHA1 ANTITRYPSIN DEFICIENCY

Blood and other body fluids contain a serum protein classified as an $alpha_1$ globulin that is capable of neutralizing trypsin and many other proteolytic (protein-digesting) enzymes such as fibrinolysins and thrombin. This specialized protein is called $alpha_1$ antitrypsin, and its concentration in the blood is genetically determined. Most individuals produce normal amounts of antitrypsin. Others are severely deficient, and a third group has subnormal levels of this protein.

Individuals with severe antitrypsin deficiency are prone to develop an unusual type of progressive pulmonary emphysema that usually becomes manifest in adolescence or early adulthood and tends to affect chiefly the lower lobes of the lungs. It is much less common than the usual type of emphysema described. Usually, there is no associated chronic bronchitis, so cough and excessive sputum production are absent. Persons with only moderately reduced antitrypsin levels do not develop severe emphysema at an early age but are quite susceptible to lung damage from cigarette smoking, atmospheric air pollution, or respiratory infections.

Low antitrypsin levels are correlated with lung disease because $alpha_1$ antitrypsin protects the lung from injury by leukocyte enzymes. Normally, polymorphonuclear leukocytes tend to accumulate in the pulmonary capillaries, and macrophages migrate from the bloodstream into the alveolar walls and pulmonary alveoli. Some of these leukocytes degenerate and release their proteolytic enzymes, but the enzymes are normally inactivated by antitrypsin so that they do not injure the alveolar septa. However, if antitrypsin is severely deficient, the leukocyte enzymes are not inactivated and can digest the connective tissues of the alveolar septa and terminal air passages, leading to pulmonary emphysema. The individual with a subnormal level of antitrypsin manifests an increased susceptibility to chronic pulmonary disease because pulmonary irritants (such as cigarette smoke and polluted air), and pulmonary infections cause leukocytes to accumulate within the lung. The liberated leukocyte enzymes are less efficiently neutralized than in normal individuals and may injure the lungs.

Bronchial Asthma

Bronchial asthma is a spasmodic contraction of the smooth muscle in the walls of the smaller bronchi and bronchioles. It is also associated with increased secretions by the bronchial mucous glands. Asthmatic attacks cause shortness of breath, and wheezing respirations occur caused by restricted movement of air through the tightly constricted air passages. The physiologic derangements in asthma result from narrowing of the bronchioles and are similar to those in patients with emphysema. Bronchiolar spasm exerts a greater effect on expiration than on inspiration because the caliber of the bronchioles varies with the phase of respiration. Consequently, air flow is impeded more on expiration than on inspiration, which leads to trapping of air within the lungs and overinflation of the lungs.

Many cases of asthma have an allergic basis. The attacks are precipitated by inhalation of dust, pollens, animal dander, or other allergens, which interact with mast cells coated with IgE antibody. This leads to release of chemical mediators that induce the bronchospasm. Acute attacks are treated by administering drugs such as epinephrine or theophylline, which relax the bronchospasm. Often, one can prevent attacks by administering drugs that block the release of mediators from mast cells. (Allergic diseases are considered in the discussion on immunity, hypersensitivity, allergy, and autoimmune diseases.)

Respiratory Distress Syndrome

RESPIRATORY DISTRESS SYNDROME OF NEWBORN INFANTS

The condition known as respiratory distress syndrome of newborn infants is characterized by progressive respiratory distress that occurs soon after birth, leading to serious problems in oxygenation of the blood. The condition occurs most often in premature infants, infants delivered by cesarean section, and infants born to mothers with diabetes. The basic cause is an inadequate quantity of surfactant in the lungs of the affected infants. As a result, the alveoli do not expand normally during inspiration and tend to collapse during expiration. The permeability of the pulmonary capillaries also is increased, and protein-rich fluid leaks from the pulmonary capillaries. The fluid, which is rich in fibrinogen, tends to clot and form adherent membranes that line the air passages. These membranes contribute to respiratory distress by impeding the diffusion of gases between the air passages and the pulmonary capillaries. The presence of these prominent acellular red-staining membranes lining the alveoli was the basis for the older name, hyaline membrane disease, which was given to this condition (FIGURE 22).

If delivery of a premature infant with immature lungs cannot be avoided, adrenal corticosteroid hormones administered to the mother within 24 hours of anticipated delivery will stimulate increased production of surfactant by the fetal lungs, thereby reducing the risk of respiratory distress syndrome. Infants who have developed respiratory distress syndrome after delivery are treated with supplementary oxygen and are also treated by instillation of a surfactant-type material that resembles natural surfactant. The material is instilled by means of a tube inserted into the infant's trachea (endotracheal tube), and the surfactant treatments are continued for several days

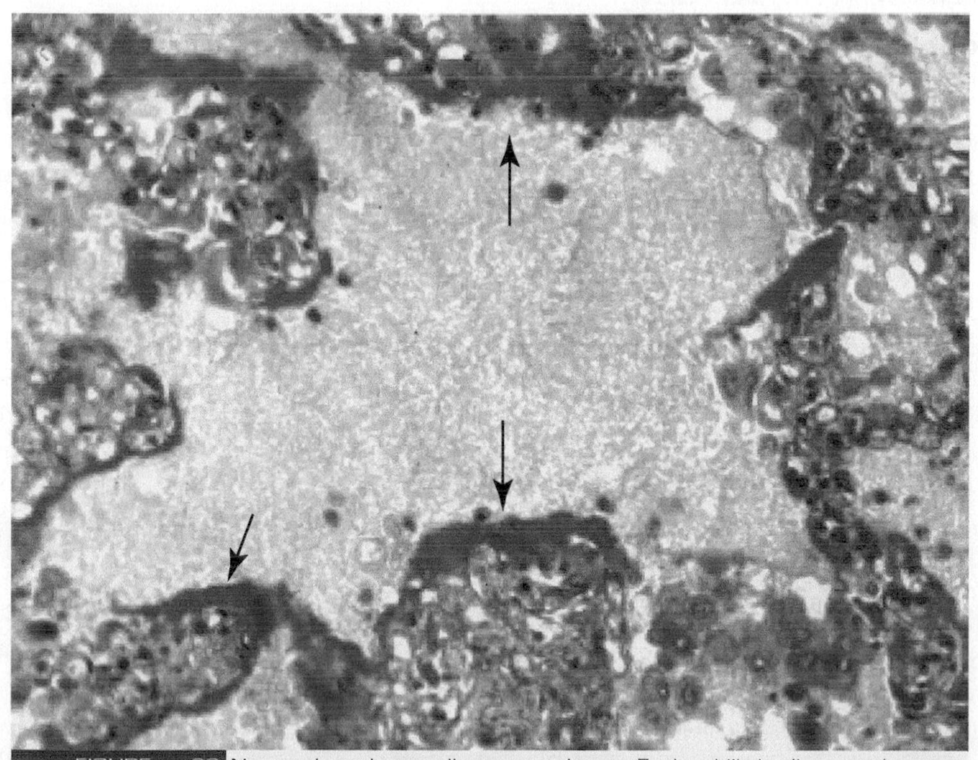

FIGURE 22 Neonatal respiratory distress syndrome. Eosinophilic hyaline membranes (*arrows*) composed of coagulated protein cover alveolar septa, impeding gas exchange between alveoli and pulmonary capillaries.

after delivery. TABLE 1 compares the respiratory distress syndrome in infants with a somewhat similar condition in adults, which has a different pathogenesis and method of treatment, although the histologic changes in both conditions are quite similar.

ADULT RESPIRATORY DISTRESS SYNDROME

The adult respiratory distress syndrome is often called by its initials ARDS, or sometimes by the term shock lung because shock is a major manifestation of the syndrome. The conditions causing this syndrome fall into two major groups. The first group contains many different conditions that cause shock with consequent fall in blood pressure and correspondingly reduced blood flow to the lungs. The shock may result from any type of severe injury (traumatic shock) or from a serious systemic infection (septic shock), and the pulmonary capillary and alveolar damage is an indirect result of the impaired pulmonary blood flow. The second group encompasses various conditions that directly damage the pulmonary capillaries and alveolar septa, including such conditions as aspiration of acid gastric contents, inhalation of irritant or toxic gasses, or lung damage caused by the SARS-associated coronavirus.

Whatever the predisposing cause of the alveolar damage, the pathophysiologic derangements are the same as in the neonatal respiratory distress syndrome: damage to alveolar capillaries and alveolar lining cells, impaired formation of surfactant, leakage of protein-rich fluid from the injured capillaries into the alveolar septa with formation of intra-alveolar hyaline membranes, and impaired diffusion of oxygen across the swollen, thickened alveolar septa.

Treatment is directed toward correcting the shock, treating the underlying condition that initiated the respiratory distress, and improving the oxygenation of the

TABLE 1

Comparison of neonatal and adult respiratory distress syndrome

	Neonatal	Adult
Groups affected	Premature infants Delivery by cesarean section* Infant born to diabetic mother**	Adults who have sustained direct or indirect lung damage
Pathogenesis	Inadequate surfactant	*Direct damage:* lung trauma, aspiration, irritant or toxic gasses *Indirect damage:* reduced pulmonary blood flow caused by shock or sepsis *Associated condition:* surfactant production reduced
Treatment	Corticosteroids to mother before delivery Endotracheal surfactant Oxygen	Support circulation and respiration Endotracheal tube and respirator Positive pressure oxygen

*Labor increases surfactant synthesis, which is lacking in cesarean delivery.
**High insulin blood level in the fetus of a mother with diabetes suppresses surfactant synthesis.

blood by means of a ventilator capable of delivering an increased concentration of oxygen to the lungs under slightly increased pressure, thereby facilitating diffusion of oxygen across the swollen alveolar septa.

Pulmonary Fibrosis

The lungs are continually exposed to a number of injurious substances, such as irritant gases discharged into the atmosphere and many kinds of airborne organic and inorganic particles. Severe pulmonary injury may lead to pulmonary fibrosis. Fibrous thickening of alveolar septa makes the lungs increasingly rigid, restricting normal respiratory excursions. Diffusion of oxygen and carbon dioxide between alveolar air and pulmonary capillaries also is hampered because of the increased thickness of the alveolar septa. Pulmonary fibrosis causes progressive respiratory disability similar to that encountered in pulmonary emphysema.

Some types of collagen diseases, characterized by injury to connective tissue, may have as their major manifestation injury to the connective tissue framework of the lung, leading to pulmonary fibrosis.

Pneumoconiosis
(nōō'mō-kō-nēēiō'sis)
An occupational lung disease caused by inhalation of injurious substances such as rock dust.

Silicosis
(sil-ik-ō'sis)
A type of occupational lung disease caused by inhalation of rock dust.

Asbestosis
(as-bes-tō'sis)
A type of pneumoconiosis caused by inhalation of asbestos fibers.

Certain occupational diseases are recognized as being caused by inhalation of injurious substances. The general term **pneumoconiosis** (*pneumo* = lung + *konis* = dust + *osis* = condition) is used to refer to lung injury produced by inhalation of injurious dust or other particulate material. The best known of the pneumoconioses are silicosis and asbestosis. **Silicosis** is a type of progressive nodular pulmonary fibrosis caused by inhalation of rock dust. **Asbestosis** is a diffuse pulmonary fibrosis caused by inhalation of asbestos fibers. Within the body, the fibers become coated with a protein having a high content of iron to form characteristic structures called asbestos bodies. Sometimes these can be identified in the sputum of patients with asbestosis (FIGURE 23). Inhalation of coal dust, cotton fibers, certain types of fungus spores, and many other substances attending certain occupations also may cause pulmonary fibrosis.

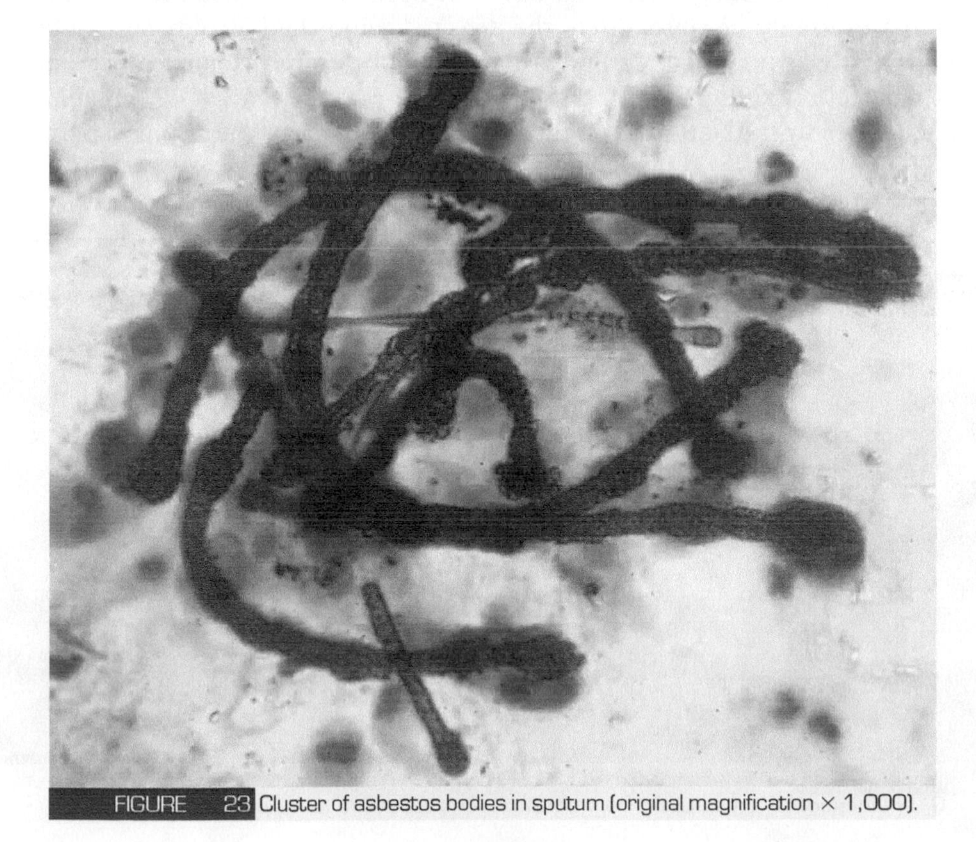

FIGURE 23 Cluster of asbestos bodies in sputum (original magnification × 1,000).

Patients with asbestosis have other problems as well because asbestos fibers appear to be carcinogenic. These patients have a higher incidence of lung carcinoma than the general population, and some develop an unusual type of malignant tumor arising from pleural mesothelial cells called a malignant mesothelioma.

Lung Carcinoma

Lung carcinoma is another important disease related to cigarette smoking. Lung carcinoma was once uncommon. Now lung cancer is the chief cause of cancer deaths, which kills 160,000 persons annually. It is a common malignant tumor in men, and the mortality in women caused by lung carcinoma now exceeds that of breast carcinoma. The tumor is uncommon in nonsmokers. Because the neoplasm usually arises from the bronchial mucosa, the term bronchogenic carcinoma is often used when referring to lung cancer. There are several different histologic types. Squamous cell carcinoma and adenocarcinoma are two of the more common (FIGURE 24). A third type composed of large, bizarre epithelial cells is called by the descriptive term large cell carcinoma. A fourth type is composed of small, irregular dark cells with scanty cytoplasm that look somewhat like lymphocytes. This type is called a small cell carcinoma and carries a very poor prognosis (FIGURE 25). Frequently, tumor cells can be identified in the sputum of patients with lung carcinoma (FIGURE 26).

Because of the rich lymphatic and vascular network in the lung, the neoplasm readily gains access to lymphatic channels and pulmonary blood vessels and soon spreads to regional lymph nodes and distant sites. Treatment usually consists of surgical resection of one or more lobes of the lung. Radiation therapy in combination with anticancer chemotherapy rather than surgery is used to treat small cell carcinoma and is also used to treat tumors that are too far advanced for surgical resection. Results of treatment are disappointing because the disease is often widespread by the time it is recognized.

Chest x-rays for lung carcinoma have not been very effective for reducing lung carcinoma mortality because, often, the detected tumor had already spread beyond the lungs and was no longer curable. In an attempt to improve lung cancer survival by early detection and prompt treatment of affected subjects, a lung screening trial was undertaken by the National Institutes of Health comparing the results of annual CT

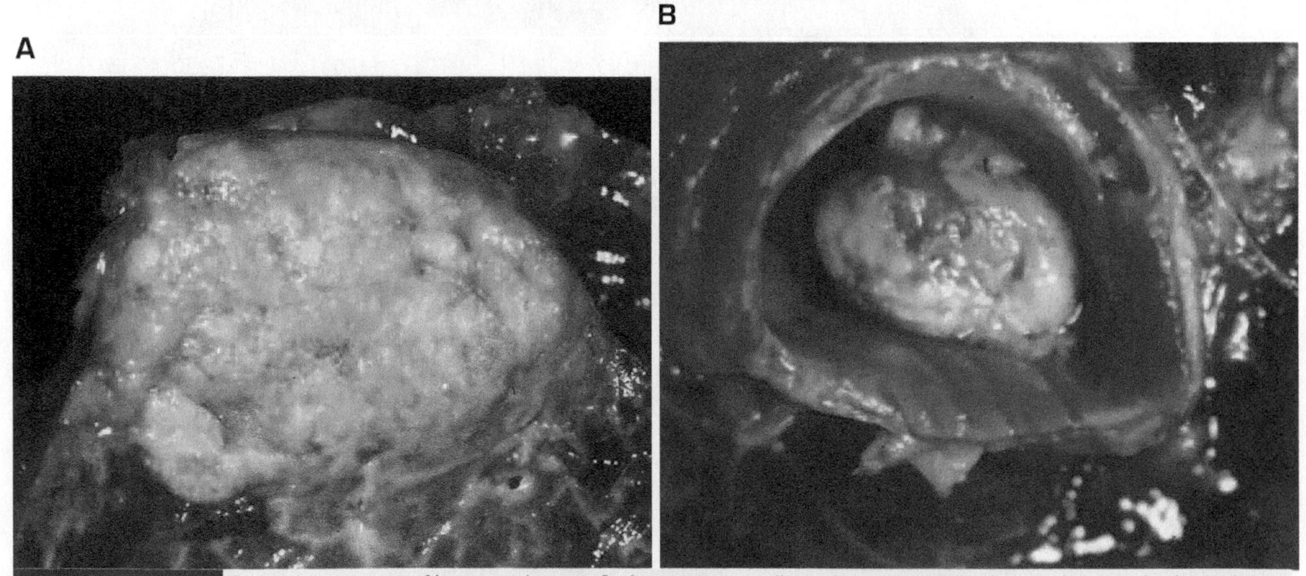

FIGURE 24 Gross appearance of lung carcinoma. **A**, A squamous cell carcinoma partially obstructing a major bronchus. **B**, An adenocarcinoma arising from smaller bronchus at the periphery of the lung.

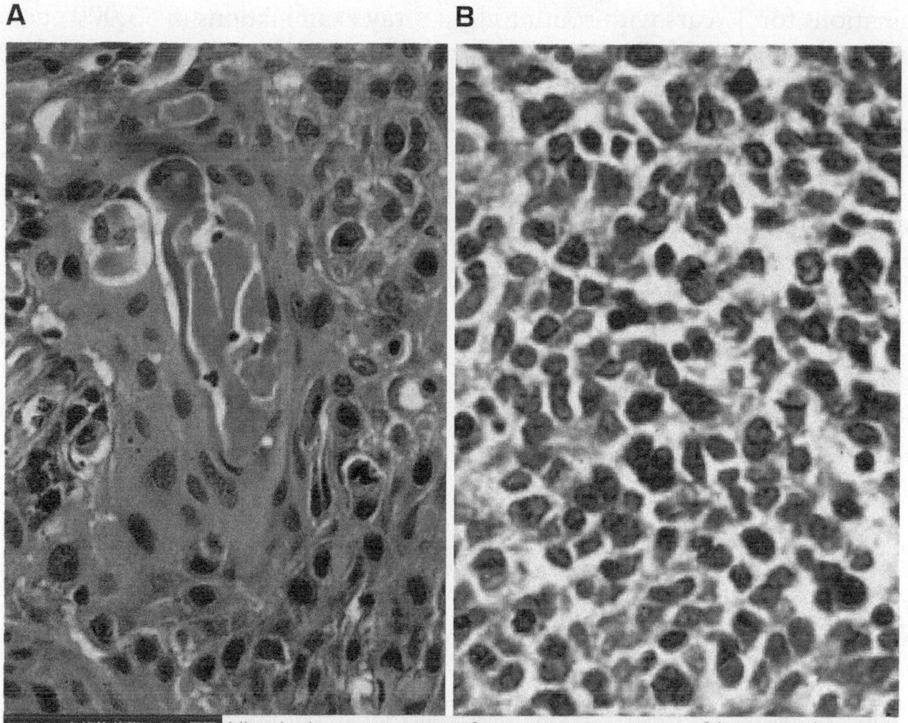

FIGURE 25 Histologic appearance of two common types of lung carcinoma. **A**, Moderately well-differentiated squamous cell carcinoma (original magnification × 200). **B**, Small cell carcinoma (original magnification × 200).

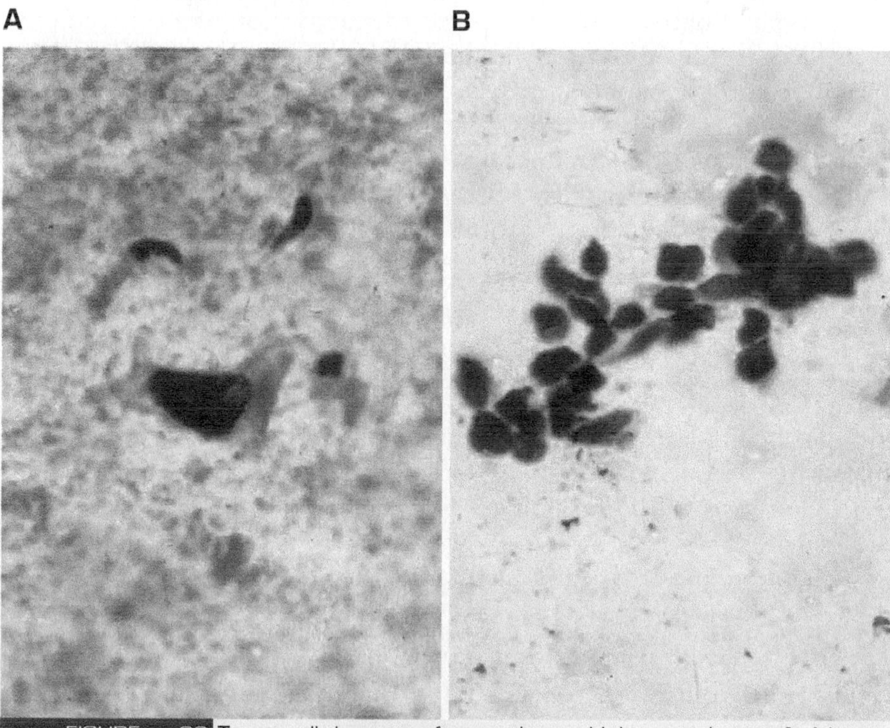

FIGURE 26 Tumor cells in sputum from patients with lung carcinoma. **A**, A large neoplastic squamous cell from a patient with squamous cell carcinoma of lung. **B**, A cluster of small, darkly stained cells from a patient with small cell carcinoma.

examinations for 3 years with routine chest x-ray examinations in 53,000 current and former smokers aged 55–74 years. Half the participants were screened by chest x-ray and half by CT. At the end of an 8-year follow-up, 364 CT-screened persons had died of lung carcinoma, compared with a significantly higher 442 deaths among the chest x-ray subjects. Presumably, the CT can pick up tumors earlier, which provides a better chance of survival. On the other hand, repeated CT procedures for screening are expensive and also expose the subject to significantly more radiation than chest x-ray exams. Many physicians believe that since 87% of lung cancers are caused by smoking, the longer term goal should be to eliminate the cause of most lung cancers by not smoking.

QUESTIONS FOR REVIEW

1. How do the lungs function? What is the difference between ventilation and gas exchange? How is pulmonary function disturbed if the alveolar septa are thickened and scarred?
2. What is pneumothorax? How does it develop? What is its effect on pulmonary function?
3. What is pneumonia? How is pneumonia classified? What are its major clinical features?
4. How does the tubercle bacillus differ in its staining reaction from other bacteria? What type of inflammatory reaction does it cause? What factors determine the outcome of a tuberculous infection? How does a cavity develop in lungs infected with tuberculosis? Is a person with a tuberculous cavity infectious to other persons? What is miliary tuberculosis?
5. A patient has tuberculosis of the kidney, but no evidence of pulmonary tuberculosis is detected by means of a chest x-ray. How did this happen?
6. What is meant by the term "inactive tuberculosis"? Under what circumstances may an old inactive tuberculous infection become activated? What type of patients are susceptible to reactivation of a tuberculous infection?
7. What is the difference between bronchitis and bronchiectasis?
8. What is pulmonary emphysema? What factors predispose to its development? How may it be prevented? What is the difference between pulmonary emphysema and pulmonary fibrosis?
9. What is the relationship between carcinoma of the lung and cigarette smoking? How is lung carcinoma treated?

SUPPLEMENTARY READINGS

Antonucci, G., Girardi, E., Raviglione, M. C., et al. 1995. Risk factors for tuberculosis in HIV-infected persons. A prospective study. The Gruppo Italiano di Studio Tubercolosis e AIDS (GISTA). *Journal of the American Medical Association* 274:143–8.

- TB is a big problem in HIV-infected persons and may progress rapidly. Methods for monitoring persons at risk are discussed.

Bach, P. B., Jett, J. R., Pastorino, U., et al. 2007. Computed tomography screening and lung cancer outcomes. *Journal of the American Medical Association* 297:953–61.

- Screening for lung cancer by computed tomography (CT) may detect cancers earlier but may not reduce the risk of advanced cancer or the lung cancer death rate.

Bernard, G. R., Luce, J. M., Sprung, C. L., et al. 1987. High-dose corticosteroids in patients with the adult respiratory distress syndrome. *The New England Journal of Medicine* 317:1565–70.

- High-dose corticosteroids are not beneficial in patients with ARDS as a result of sepsis, aspiration, or mixed causes.

Centers for Disease Control and Prevention. 1998. Recommendations for prevention and control of tuberculosis among foreign-born persons. *Morbidity and Mortality Weekly Report* (Supplement RR-16) 47:1–29.

- Most TB cases among foreign-born persons result from reactivation of previously acquired infections. The risk of reactivation is highest in the first years after U.S. arrival. Screening and preventive therapy are discussed.

Colditz, G. A., Brewer, T. F., Berkey, C. S., et al. 1994. Efficacy of BCG vaccine in the prevention of tuberculosis. Meta-analysis of the published literature. *Journal of the American Medical Association* 271:698–702.

- BCG vaccination reduces the risk of tuberculosis by about 50%.

Daley, C. L., Small, P. M., Schecter, G. F., et al. 1992. An outbreak of tuberculosis with accelerated progression among persons infected with the human immunodeficiency virus. *The New England Journal of Medicine* 326:231–5.

- HIV infection promotes rapid progression of tuberculosis.

Driver, C. R., Valway, S. E., Morgan, W. M., et al. 1994. Transmission of *Mycobacterium tuberculosis* associated with air travel. *Journal of the American Medical Association* 272:1031–5.

- A flight attendant became infected after exposure to a family member who died of tuberculosis. She did not receive prophylactic treatment and developed active tuberculosis 3 years later. She infected other airline crew members and may also have infected passengers before her disease was diagnosed and treated.

Dye, C. 2004. A booster for tuberculosis vaccines. *Journal of the American Medical Association* 291:2127–8.

- A large group of Alaska Eskimos who received BCG vaccination were followed for many years, and the vaccine appeared to be effective for as long as 60 years. BCG vaccination does provide some protection against infection.

Fraser, D. W., Tsai, T. R., Orenstein, W., et al. 1977. Legionnaires' disease: Description of an epidemic of pneumonia. *The New England Journal of Medicine* 297:1189–97.

- Describes the classic epidemic that occurred in Philadelphia in 1976.

Man, S. F., McAlister, F. A., Anthonisen, N. R., et al. 2003. Contemporary management of chronic obstructive pulmonary disease: Clinical applications. *Journal of the American Medical Association* 290:2313–6.

- Early evaluation and treatment are recommended for any patient suspected of having COPD. Principles of diagnosis and treatment are considered.

Markel, H., Gostin, L. O., and Fidler, D. P. 2007. Extensively drug-resistant tuberculosis: An isolation order, public health powers, and a global crisis. *Journal of the American Medical Association* 298:83–6.

- A very interesting article on extremely drug-resistant tuberculosis (XDR-TB) and its potential impact, including discussion of legal authority to quarantine in the United States and on travel restrictions when dealing with XDR-TB.

National Emphysema Treatment Trial Research Group. 2003. A randomized trial comparing lung-volume-reduction surgery with medical therapy for severe emphysema. *The New England Journal of Medicine* 348:2059–73.

- The definitive article analyzing the applications and limitations of this procedure.

Patel, J. D., Bach, P. B., and Kris, M. G. 2004. Lung cancer in US women: A contemporary epidemic. *Journal of the American Medical Association* 291:1763–8.

- As a result of increased smoking by women beginning in about 1930 and continuing to the present, lung cancer in women has increased by 600%, and lung cancer now causes as many deaths as all breast cancers and all gynecologic cancers combined. Women appear to be more susceptible than men to the carcinogenic properties of cigarette smoke.

Ryu, J. H., Colby, T. V., and Hartman, T. E. 1998. Idiopathic pulmonary fibrosis: Current concepts. *Mayo Clinic Proceedings* 73:1085–101.

- Pulmonary fibrosis results from many different causes, and proper classification allows more reliable prognosis and management.

Truong, D. H., Hedemark, L. L., Mickman, J. K., et al. 1997. Tuberculosis among Tibetan immigrants from India and Nepal in Minnesota, 1992–1995. *Journal of the American Medical Association* 277:735–8.

- Tuberculosis infection is nearly universal among Tibetans settling in Minnesota, and a single screening evaluation failed to detect most of the cases. Persons with a previous history of active TB require close follow-up even though sputum cultures are negative.

Voelker, R. 2007. Pattern of US tuberculosis cases shifting. *Journal of the American Medical Association* 297:685.

- Previously reported Centers for Disease Control and Prevention (CDC) data showed that from 1994 to 2004, TB cases among U.S.-born residents fell by 62%, while increasing in foreign-born persons to 54% of all U.S. cases. Twenty-four percent of the TB cases were in foreign-born persons who had been living in the United States for more than 5 years, and most of the cases resulted from reactivation of a latent infection that had been acquired in their country of origin many years ago. Tuberculin testing and treating of latent infections in foreign-born persons should be extended to include longer term foreign-born residents living in the United States.

OUTLINE SUMMARY

Structure and Function of the Lungs

THE STRUCTURE OF CONDUCTING TUBES AND ALVEOLI

Bronchi: larger conducting tubes.

Bronchioles: tubes less than 1 mm in diameter.

Respiratory bronchioles: bronchioles with alveoli in their walls.

Alveoli: small air sacs where gas exchange occurs.

VENTILATION

Air movement caused by movement of ribs and diaphragm.

Lungs change in volume in response to changes in size of thoracic cage.

GAS EXCHANGE

Gases diffuse owing to differences in partial pressures.

Efficient exchange in lungs requires large capillary surface area.

PULMONARY FUNCTION TESTS

Vital capacity: maximum volume of air expired after maximum inspiration.

One-second forced expiratory volume (FEV_1): maximum volume of air expelled in 1 second.

Arterial PO_2 and PCO_2 measure efficiency of gas exchange in lungs.

Pulse oximeter measures arterial oxygen saturation.

THE PLEURAL CAVITY

"Negative" intrapleural pressure is caused by the tendency of stretched lung to pull away from chest wall.

Release of vacuum in pleural cavity leads to collapse of lung.

Pneumothorax

PATHOGENESIS

Chest or lung injury permits air to escape into pleural cavity.

Spontaneous pneumothorax: no apparent cause.

MANIFESTATIONS

Subjective: chest pain and dyspnea.

Objective: air in pleural cavity demonstrated by x-ray and examination.

Tension pneumothorax: complication of pneumothorax when air can enter pleural cavity but cannot escape on expiration. Air under pressure displaces mediastinum and impairs expansion of opposite lung.

TREATMENT

Chest tube inserted in pleural cavity; vacuum sometimes applied.

Atelectasis

CLASSIFICATION

Obstructive: caused by bronchial obstruction.

Compression: caused by air or fluid in pleural cavity.

TREATMENT

Remove obstruction or material compressing lung.

Pneumonia

CLASSIFICATION

By etiologic agent.

By anatomic distribution of inflammation in lung.

By predisposing factors.

CLINICAL FEATURES

Manifestations of systemic infection.

Manifestations of lung inflammation: cough, chest pain.

Severe Acute Respiratory Syndrome (SARS)

A serious highly communicable pulmonary infection.

Caused by unique coronavirus.

Initial nonspecific manifestations followed by acute respiratory distress syndrome.

No antiviral therapy currently available.

Pneumocystis Pneumonia

Caused by protozoan parasite of low pathogenicity.

Affects immunocompromised persons.

Organisms injure alveoli, leading to exudation of protein-rich material into alveoli.

Cysts demonstrated by special stains.

Infection characterized by dyspnea, cough, pulmonary consolidation.

Diagnosis established by lung biopsy.

Treatment available, but infection has high mortality.

Tuberculosis

CHARACTERISTICS OF TUBERCULOSIS

A granulomatous inflammation characterized by necrosis and giant cells.

MANIFESTATIONS

Depends on dosage and resistance. May heal by scarring or progress to cavitation.

Miliary tuberculosis: dissemination of organisms by bloodstream.

Extrapulmonary tuberculosis: hematogenous dissemination from lungs to distant site.

DIAGNOSIS AND TREATMENT

Skin test: indicates previous exposure to organism.

Chest x-ray: indicates pulmonary infiltrate.

Culture: identifies organism in sputum.

Treatment by means of antibiotic and chemotherapeutic agents.

Bronchitis and Bronchiectasis

CLASSIFICATION

Acute bronchitis: common and self-limited.

Chronic bronchitis: secondary to chronic irritation.

Bronchiectasis: walls weakened by inflammation and dilate.

DIAGNOSIS AND TREATMENT

Acute bronchitis: self-limited.

Chronic bronchitis: cease irritation, as by cessation of smoking.

Bronchiectasis: bronchogram demonstrates dilation.

Diseased areas resected.

Chronic Obstructive Lung Disease

DEFINITION

Combined emphysema and chronic bronchitis.

DERANGEMENTS OF STRUCTURE AND FUNCTION

Chronic inflammation of bronchioles leads to trapped air in lungs.

Nonuniform ventilation of alveoli reduces efficiency of ventilation.

Enlargement of air spaces and reduction of capillary bed reduces efficiency of gas exchange.

Loss of lung elasticity requires active expiratory effort.

PREVENTION AND TREATMENT OF EMPHYSEMA

Refrain from smoking and inhalation of injurious agents.

Treatment cannot restore damaged lung but can prevent further progression and may improve pulmonary function.

EMPHYSEMA AS A RESULT OF ALPHA$_1$ ANTITRYPSIN DEFICIENCY

Antitrypsin prevents lung damage from lysosomal enzymes released from leukocytes in lung.

Deficiency permits enzymes to damage lung tissue.

Bronchial Asthma

PATHOGENESIS

Spasmodic contraction of bronchial smooth muscle narrows air passages.

TREATMENT

Drugs that relax bronchospasm or prevent release of mediators from mast cells.

Many cases caused by allergy.

Neonatal Respiratory Distress Syndrome

PATHOGENESIS

Inadequate surfactant impedes normal lung expansion and promotes collapse.

Premature infants, infants born by cesarean section, and infants by diabetic mothers predisposed to syndrome.

TREATMENT

Administering of corticosteroids to mother may stimulate lung maturation in fetus. Intratracheal surfactant installation to treat affected infants.

Adult Respiratory Distress Syndrome

PATHOGENESIS

Systemic disease with shock and impaired lung perfusion.

Direct lung damage: trauma, gastric aspiration, inhalation of irritants or toxic gases.

DERANGEMENT

Damaged alveolar capillaries leak fluid and protein.

Impaired surfactant production from damaged alveolar lining cells.

Formation of hyaline membranes.

TREATMENT

Correct predisposing conditions.

Administer oxygen under positive pressure.

Pulmonary Fibrosis

PATHOGENESIS

Collagen diseases.

Pneumoconioses:

- *Silicosis.*
- *Asbestosis (also predisposes to lung carcinoma and pleural mesothelioma).*
- *Various other injurious substances inhaled in course of occupations.*

TREATMENT

No specific treatment. Prevent occupational exposure.

Lung Carcinoma

PATHOGENESIS

A smoking-related neoplasm.

Mortality in women now exceeds breast carcinoma.

Arises from mucosa of bronchi and bronchioles.

CLASSIFICATION AND PROGNOSIS

Several histologic types, which differ in their prognosis.

Poor prognosis as a result of early spread to distant sites.

TREATMENT

Depends on histologic type. Generally by resection.

Small cell carcinoma treated by chemotherapy and radiation.

http://health.jbpub.com/humandisease/9e

Human Disease Online is a great source for supplementary human disease information for both students and instructors. Visit this website to find a variety of useful tools for learning, thinking, and teaching.

The Liver and the Biliary System

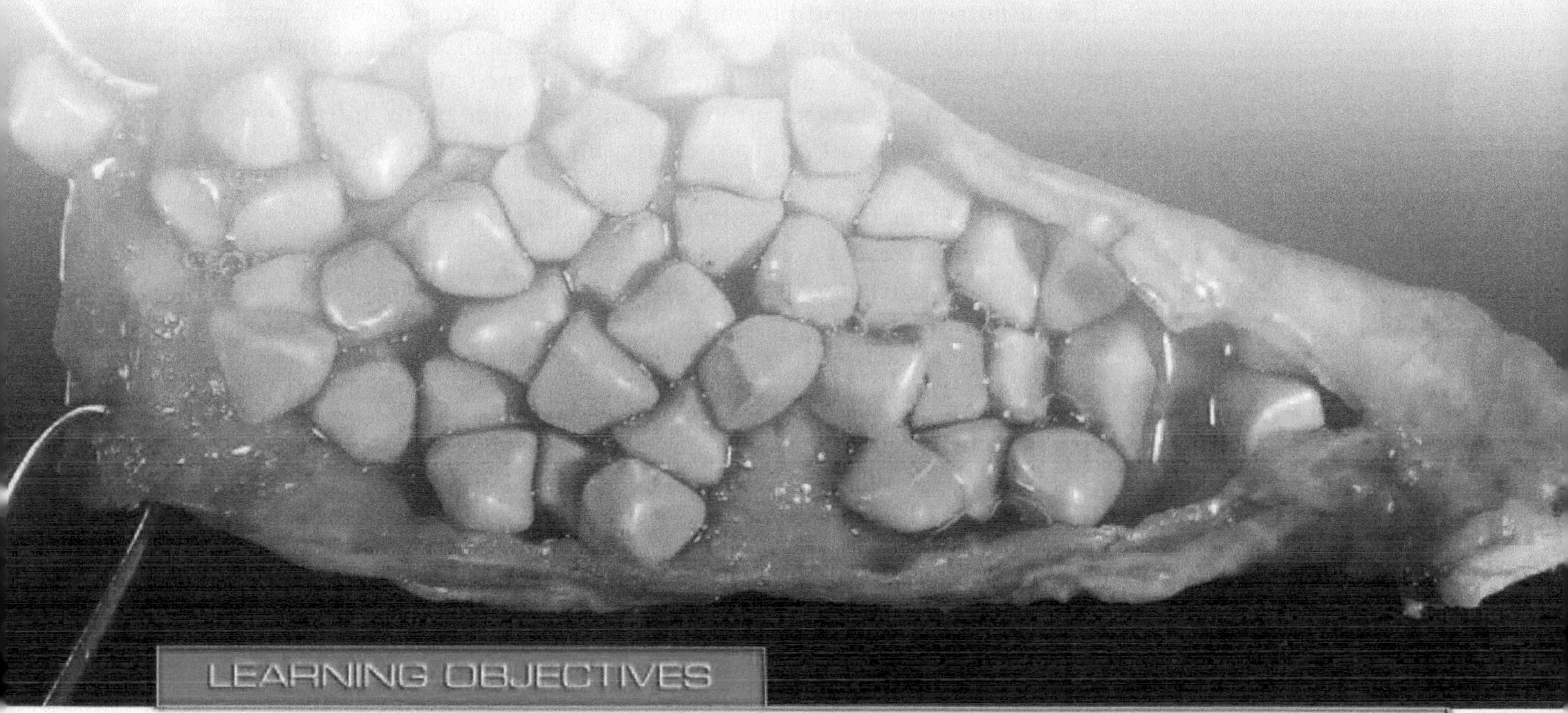

LEARNING OBJECTIVES

1. Describe the normal structure of the liver, and explain the functions of the liver as they relate to the major diseases of the liver.
2. List the major causes of liver injury, and describe their effects on hepatic function.
3. Compare the three major types of viral hepatitis in terms of their pathogenesis, incubation period, incidence of complications, and frequency of carriers. Explain the diagnostic tests used to identify each type of viral infection, and describe methods of prevention.
4. Explain the adverse effects of excess alcohol intake on liver structure and function.
5. Explain how gallstones are formed, and describe their causes and effects.
6. Compare the three major causes of jaundice.

Structure and Function of the Liver

The liver is the largest organ in the body. It has a roughly triangular shape and is located beneath the diaphragm in the upper abdomen (FIGURE 1). It is a complex organ with many functions. These are concerned mainly with the following:

1. Metabolism of ingested carbohydrates, protein, and fat delivered through the portal circulation
2. Synthesis of various substances, including plasma proteins and proteins taking part in blood clotting

3. Storage of vitamin B_{12} and other materials
4. Detoxification and excretion of various substances

The liver has a double blood supply. About three quarters of the blood flow is provided by the portal vein, which drains the spleen and gastrointestinal tract. Portal blood is rich in nutrients absorbed from the intestines but low in oxygen content. The rest of the blood, which comes from the hepatic artery, has a high oxygen content but is low in nutrients. Blood flowing from the hepatic artery and the portal vein mixes as the blood flows through the liver and is eventually collected into the right and left hepatic veins, which drain into the inferior vena cava.

The liver cells are arranged in the form of long, wide plates interconnected at various angles to form a lattice. The hepatic sinusoids occupy the spaces between the plates (FIGURE 2A).

Portal tract
Branch of hepatic artery, portal vein, and bile duct located at periphery of liver lobule.

Liver lobule
A histologic subdivision of the liver in which columns of liver cells converge toward a central vein and portal tracts are located at the periphery.

Bile canaliculus
(kan-al-ik′u-lus)
Small terminal bile channel located between liver cords.

Branches of the hepatic artery, portal vein, bile ducts, and lymphatic vessels travel together within the liver and are called the **portal tracts** (FIGURE 2B). The terminal branches of both the hepatic artery and the portal vein discharge their blood into the hepatic sinusoids (FIGURE 2C). In histologic sections, the liver plates appear as cords surrounded on each side by sinusoids that converge toward the central veins. The portal tracts appear at the periphery. This anatomic configuration, which is called a **liver lobule**, is illustrated diagrammatically in FIGURE 3A.

Blood flow in the liver is from portal tracts through the sinusoids into central veins (FIGURE 3B). Consequently, the liver cells nearest the portal tracts receive the most oxygen and nutrients, and those nearest the central veins are much less well supplied. Because of their relatively poor nutritional state, the liver cells nearest the central veins are more vulnerable to injury from toxic agents or circulatory disturbances, as occurs in shock and heart failure, than are the cells nearer the portal tracts.

The small terminal bile channels are called **bile canaliculi**. They are located between adjacent liver cords and drain into the bile ducts traveling in the portal tracts. The direction of the bile flow is opposite that of the blood flow in the sinusoids (FIGURE 3B). The bile ducts gradually converge to form larger ducts,

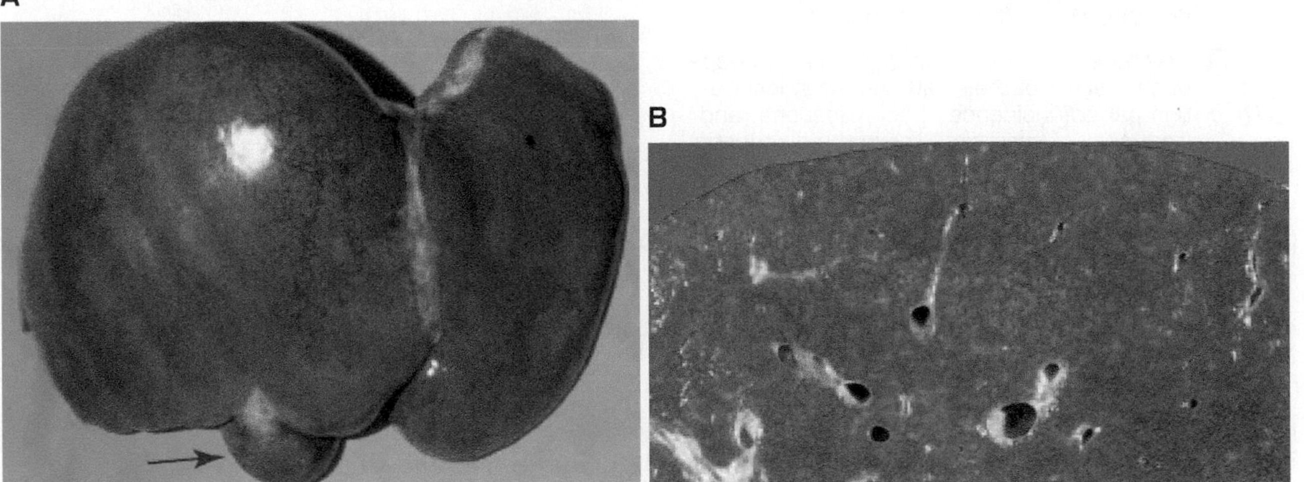

FIGURE 1 **A**, A normal liver viewed from above to show its superior and anterior surfaces. The gallbladder is located on the undersurface of the liver, and the fundus of the gallbladder projects slightly beyond the anterior edge of the liver (*arrow*). **B**, Section of liver illustrating the uniform appearance of the hepatic parenchyma and the large blood vessels (branches of the portal vein) transporting blood into the liver from the gastrointestinal tract.

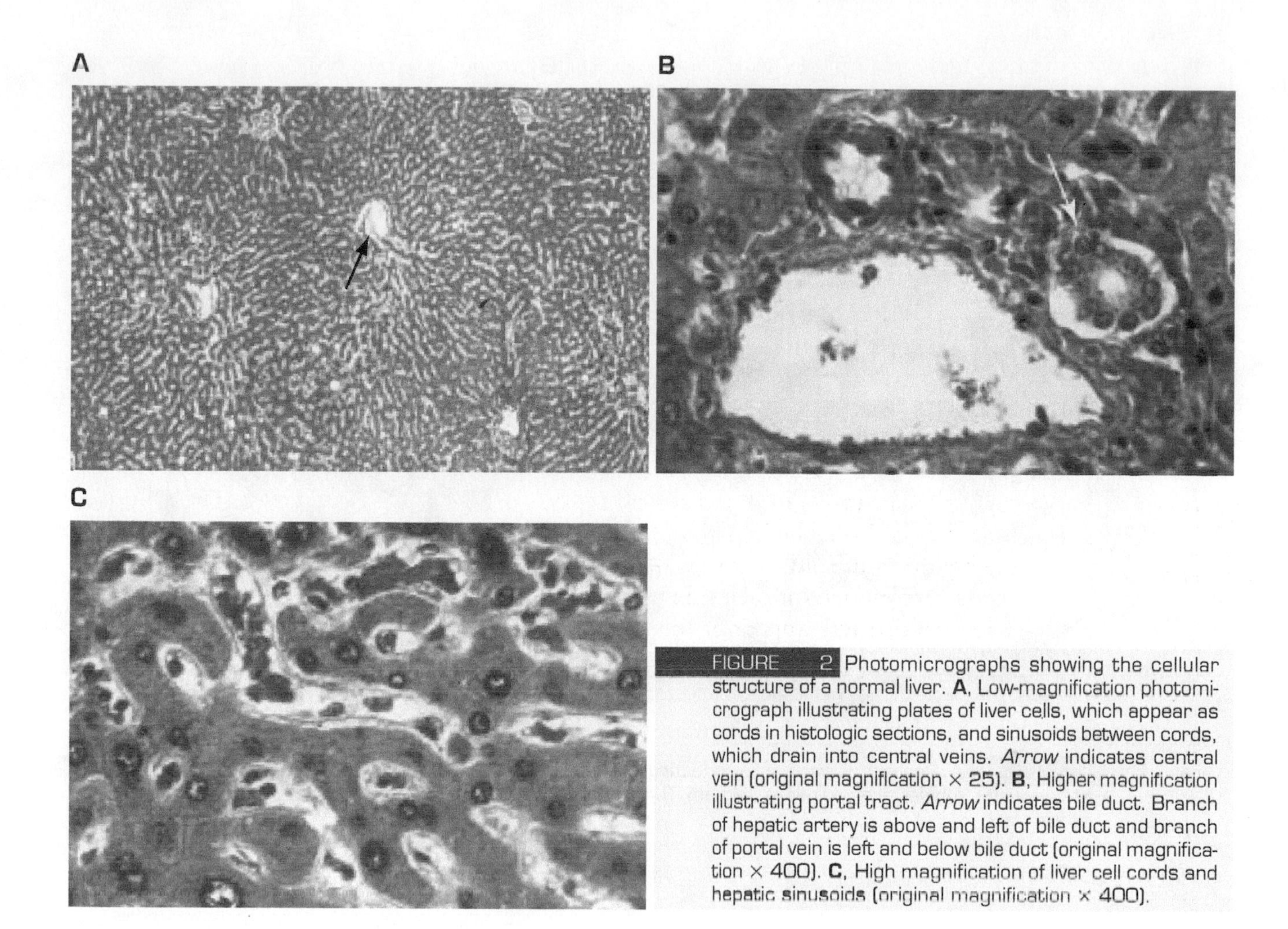

FIGURE 2 Photomicrographs showing the cellular structure of a normal liver. **A**, Low-magnification photomicrograph illustrating plates of liver cells, which appear as cords in histologic sections, and sinusoids between cords, which drain into central veins. *Arrow* indicates central vein (original magnification × 25). **B**, Higher magnification illustrating portal tract. *Arrow* indicates bile duct. Branch of hepatic artery is above and left of bile duct and branch of portal vein is left and below bile duct (original magnification × 400). **C**, High magnification of liver cell cords and hepatic sinusoids (original magnification × 400).

which finally unite as the large right and left hepatic ducts. The two hepatic ducts join to form the common hepatic duct. The gallbladder joins the common hepatic duct by means of the cystic duct to form the common bile duct that enters the duodenum.

Bile

FORMATION AND EXCRETION

Bile pigment is a product of the breakdown of red blood cells. Red cells normally survive for about 4 months. The worn-out erythrocytes are broken down by the mononuclear phagocytes (reticuloendothelial cells) throughout the body. The iron derived from the hemoglobin is conserved by the body and reused to synthesize new hemoglobin. The iron-free heme pigment forms **bilirubin**. Because the breakdown of red cells proceeds in mononuclear phagocytes throughout the body, small quantities of bile pigment are continually present in the blood. When the blood passes through the liver, the bilirubin is removed by the liver cells. Excretion is accomplished by combining the bilirubin with other substances, a process called conjugation, which requires certain specific enzymes. Most of the bilirubin is conjugated with glucuronic acid and excreted

Bilirubin
(bil-i-rū′bin)
One of the bile pigments derived from breakdown of hemoglobin.

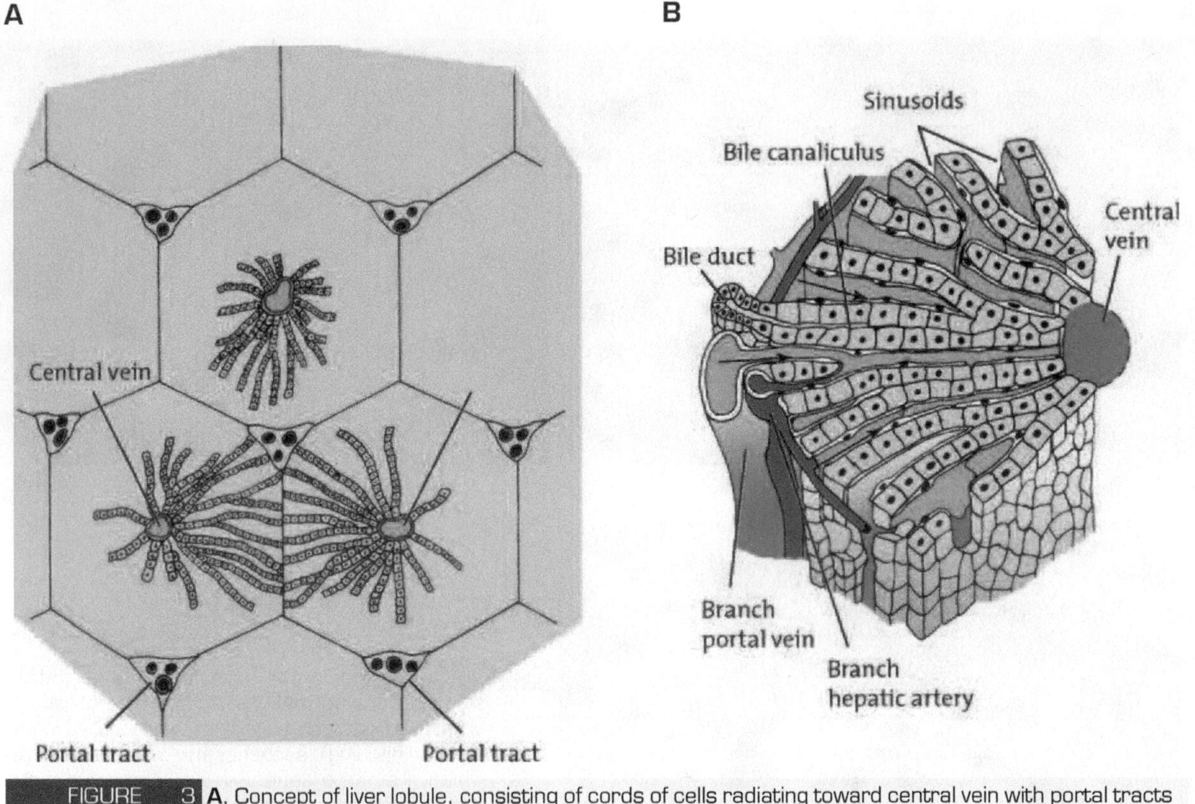

FIGURE 3 **A**, Concept of liver lobule, consisting of cords of cells radiating toward central vein with portal tracts at periphery. Lobules are outlined in diagram. **B**, Blood flow in sinusoids toward central vein; flow of bile toward portal tract.

Conjugated bilirubin
A more soluble form of bilirubin produced by the addition of two molecules of glucuronic acid to the bilirubin molecule.

Bile
A secretion of the liver containing bile salts, cholesterol, and other substances.

Cholesterol (kō-les′ter-ol)
A complex compound (sterol) *containing several ring structures.*

Bile salts
Derivatives of bile acids present in bile that act as emulsifiers to promote fat digestion and absorption.

Lecithin (les′ith-in)
A phosphorus-containing lipid (phospholipid) *having detergent properties similar to bile salts.*

as bilirubin glucuronide. The **conjugated bilirubin** is much more soluble and less toxic than the unconjugated material. The bile pigment is excreted into the small bile channels between the liver cell cords; it is collected into large ducts at the periphery of the lobules that eventually unite to form the major bile ducts. FIGURE 4 summarizes the basic anatomy of the biliary duct system.

COMPOSITION AND PROPERTIES

Bile is an aqueous solution containing various dissolved substances excreted by the liver. In addition to conjugated bilirubin, it contains bile salts, lecithin, cholesterol, water, minerals, and other materials that have been detoxified by liver cells and excreted. **Cholesterol** is a lipid with a complex ring structure that is classified as a sterol. **Bile salts**, the major constituent of bile, are derivatives of cholesterol and certain amino acids. They function as detergents because of their molecular structure, which contains both a lipid-soluble (hydrophobic) and a water-soluble (hydrophilic) part. **Lecithin** is a phosphorous-containing lipid (phospholipid) that has detergent properties similar to bile salts. Bile is secreted continually and is concentrated and stored in the gallbladder. During digestion, the gallbladder contracts, squirting bile into the duodenum. Bile does not contain digestive enzymes but functions as a biologic detergent. Bile salts emulsify fat into small globules, increasing the surface area so that the fat can be acted on more readily by pancreatic enzymes. Digestion of fat is much less efficient in the absence of bile.

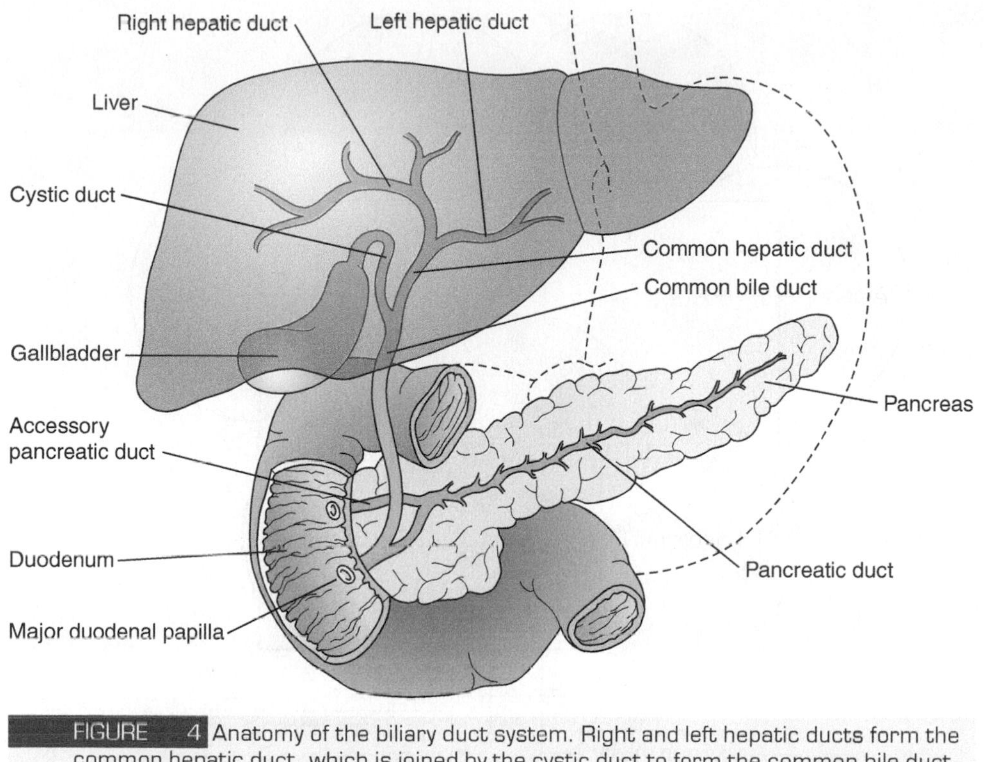

FIGURE 4 Anatomy of the biliary duct system. Right and left hepatic ducts form the common hepatic duct, which is joined by the cystic duct to form the common bile duct, which opens into the duodenum along with the pancreatic duct through a common channel.

Causes and Effects of Liver Injury

The liver is vulnerable to injury by many agents. Histologically, liver injury may be manifested by necrosis of liver cells, by accumulation of fat within the liver cell cytoplasm, or by a combination of the two. Some injurious agents primarily cause cell necrosis, whereas others chiefly induce fatty change in liver cells.

The effect of hepatic injury depends on the extent of damage induced by the injurious agent. If liver injury is mild, the liver cells will completely recover, restoring liver function to normal. Fortunately, this is the usual outcome. If the injury is extremely severe, large amounts of liver tissue are completely destroyed, and not enough liver may remain to sustain life. If the patient does survive, healing of the severe injury may be associated with severe scarring (postnecrotic scarring), and liver function may never return to normal. Multiple episodes of relatively mild liver injury may have a cumulative effect, leading to scarring and permanent impairment of liver function. Similarly, any chronic or progressive injury may cause scarring and impairment of function.

Liver cell injury caused by drugs, chemicals, alcohol, or toxins can produce fatty change in liver cells rather than necrosis. FIGURE 5 diagrams the general causes and possible effects of various degrees of liver injury.

Clinically, the most common types of liver disease characterized by injury to liver cells are viral hepatitis, and liver cell injury associated with consuming excessive amounts of alcoholic beverages, which is called alcoholic liver disease. Chronic liver cell injury from any cause may in turn be followed by diffuse scarring throughout the liver, which is called cirrhosis of the liver.

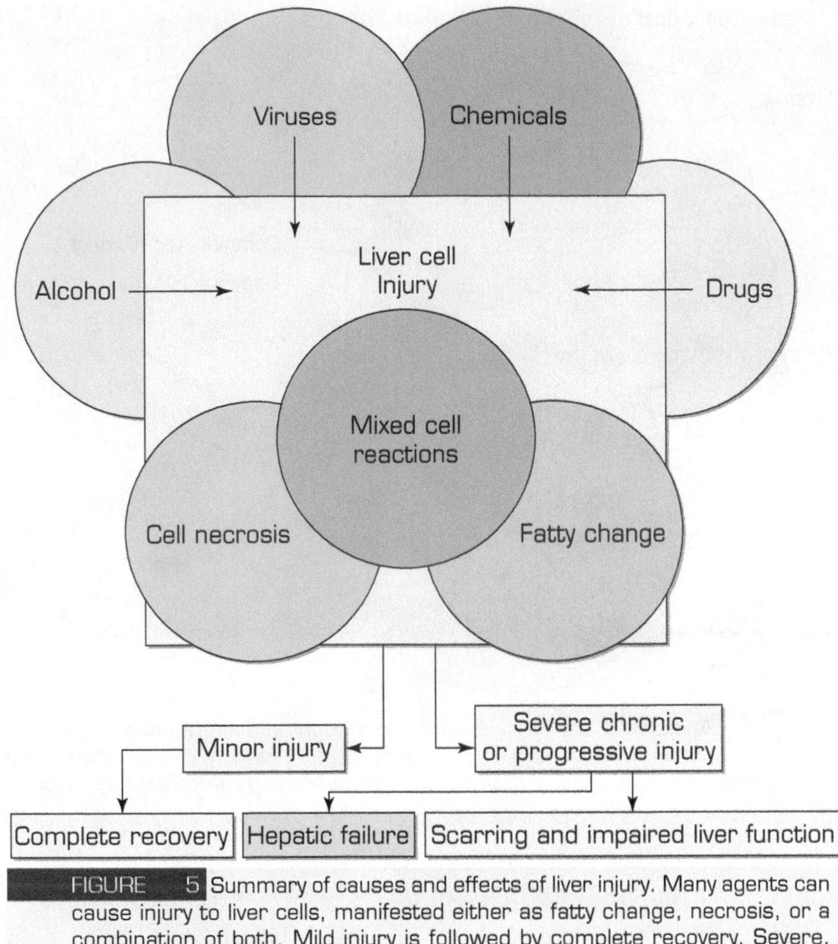

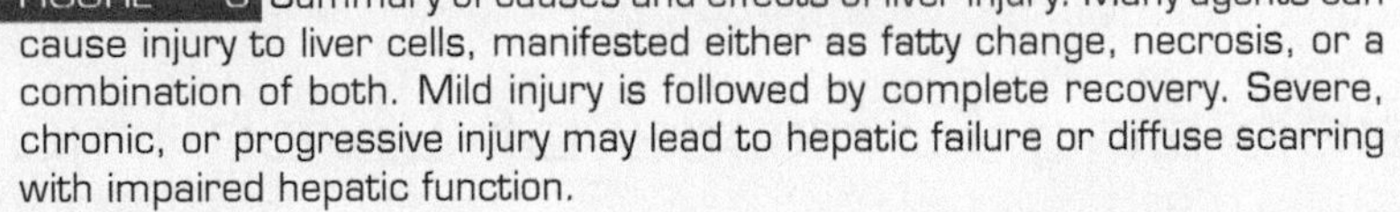

FIGURE 5 Summary of causes and effects of liver injury. Many agents can cause injury to liver cells, manifested either as fatty change, necrosis, or a combination of both. Mild injury is followed by complete recovery. Severe, chronic, or progressive injury may lead to hepatic failure or diffuse scarring with impaired hepatic function.

Viral Hepatitis

Within recent years, much new information has become available about the hepatitis viruses. The term viral hepatitis applies to several clinically similar infections. Two of these diseases, hepatitis *A* (formerly called infectious hepatitis) and hepatitis B (formerly called serum hepatitis), have been recognized as separate diseases since the early 1940s. Subsequently, a third type of viral hepatitis, originally designated non-A, non-B hepatitis, and later called hepatitis C, was recognized as a separate entity. These three types account for most cases of viral hepatitis. Two additional types of viral hepatitis also have been identified. One type, called hepatitis D or delta hepatitis, occurs in persons already infected with the hepatitis B virus. Another type, called hepatitis E, is found primarily in third world countries and is infrequently encountered in North America.

CLINICAL MANIFESTATIONS AND COURSE

Hepatitis
Inflammation of the liver.

Viral **hepatitis** is a type of liver injury, and the comments regarding the course and outcome of any liver injury also apply to viral hepatitis. All of the hepatitis viruses produce similar histologic changes in the liver that are characterized by diffuse inflammation throughout the liver lobules associated with liver cell swelling and necrosis of individual liver cells, as illustrated in FIGURE 6. The clinical manifestations of

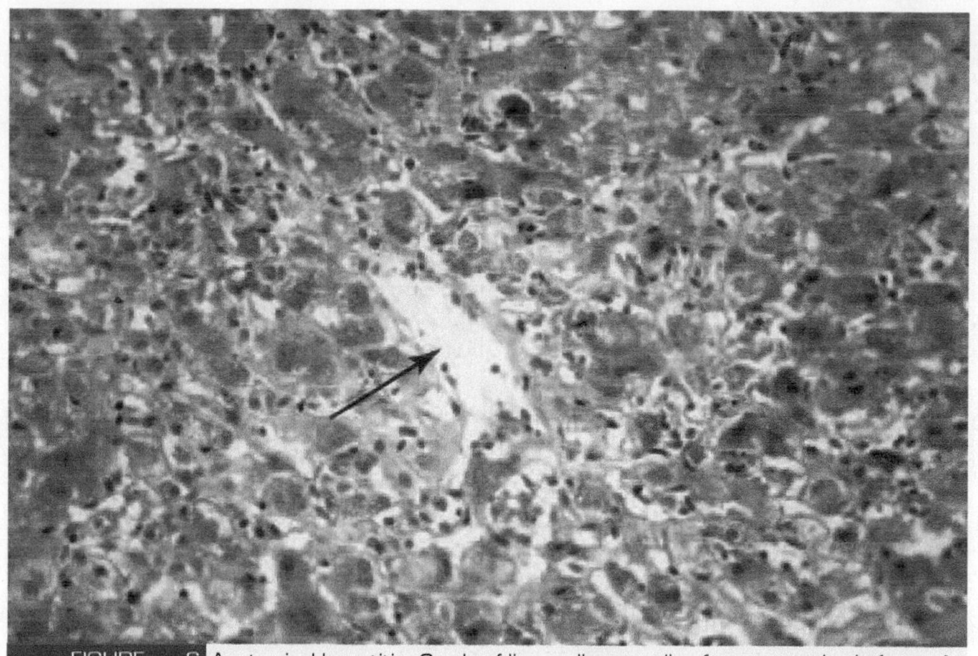

FIGURE 6 Acute viral hepatitis. Cords of liver cells extending from central vein (*arrow*) have lost their orderly arrangement and appear disrupted by swelling of liver cells, necrosis of individual cells, and scattered aggregates of inflammatory cells throughout the liver lobules (original magnification × 100).

viral hepatitis are quite variable and correlate with the degree of liver cell injury and associated inflammation. Some affected subjects experience loss of appetite, feel ill, become jaundiced, and laboratory tests are abnormal. Others become ill, and their laboratory tests are abnormal, but they never become jaundiced. This condition is called anicteric hepatitis (*ana* = without + *icterus* = jaundice). Still, others have few symptoms and do not seek medical attention, but laboratory tests reveal liver injury. Their infection, which could easily escape detection, is sometimes called subclinical hepatitis. Despite the absence of symptoms, these subjects can transmit the infection to others.

The outcome of viral hepatitis depends primarily on which virus caused the infection. Most cases of hepatitis caused by the hepatitis A virus (HAV) are quite mild, and patients recover completely without complications. An unfavorable outcome occurs in only a very small percentage of cases. In contrast, persons infected with hepatitis B virus (HBV) or the hepatitis C virus (HCV) may become chronic carriers of the virus and develop chronic progressive hepatitis that eventually leads to cirrhosis and liver failure. TABLE 1 summarizes the salient features of the three major types of viral hepatitis.

HEPATITIS A

Hepatitis A virus (HAV) is an RNA-containing virus measuring 27 nm (1 nanometer, abbreviated nm, equals 1 billionth of a meter). Hepatitis A has a relatively short incubation period that varies from 2 to 6 weeks. The virus is excreted in oropharyngeal (nose and throat) secretions and in the stools during the late-incubation period and for about 2 weeks after the onset of symptoms. Transmission is by direct person-to-person contact or by fecal contamination of food or water. Food- or water-borne infections frequently occur in epidemics. One epidemic of 107 cases, which occurred in a large city, was traced to a food-service employee who had

TABLE 1

Comparison of three major types of viral hepatitis

	Hepatitis A	Hepatitis B	Hepatitis C
Type of virus	RNA	DNA	RNA
Incubation period	2–6 weeks	6 weeks to 4 months	3–12 weeks
Method of transmission	Fecal–oral contaminated food or water	Blood or body fluids	Blood or body fluids
Antigen–antibody test results	Anti-HAV (confers immunity)	Infected persons are HBsAg positive and lack anti-HBs	HCV RNA in blood indicates virus in blood and active infection
		Immune persons lack HBsAg and have anti-HBs	Anti-HCV denotes infection (does not confer immunity)
Complications	No carriers or chronic liver disease	10% become chronic carriers and may develop chronic liver disease	75% become carriers and many develop chronic liver disease
Prevention of disease after exposure	Gamma globulin	Hepatitis B immune globulin	None available
Immunization available	Yes	Yes	No

contracted hepatitis A from her grandson and contaminated the food that she was preparing. In another epidemic, 240 persons developed hepatitis from eating raw oysters grown in virus-contaminated water.

The infection is self-limited, and there are no chronic carriers of the virus. Antibody to hepatitis A virus, which appears in the blood after recovery, provides immunity against hepatitis A virus but not against other hepatitis viruses. Hepatitis A is a common infection in the United States, and almost half the adult population has antibodies against the virus. If a susceptible person is exposed to hepatitis A, gamma globulin provides protection if administered within 14 days of exposure. An inactivated hepatitis A vaccine is available. It is recommended for immunizing persons who are at relatively high risk of becoming infected, such as healthcare workers who have frequent contact with infected persons and persons traveling in foreign countries where there is a high incidence of hepatitis A in the population. Currently, many physicians also recommend routine immunization of children living in states or communities where there is a high incidence of hepatitis A, which not only prevents childhood infections but also reduces the spread of hepatitis A from infected children to other members of the community.

HEPATITIS B

Hepatitis B virus (HBV) is a DNA-containing virus measuring 42 nm, which is somewhat larger than the hepatitis A virus. It is composed of an inner core and an outer

Figure has been removed due to copyright issues

coat. The core consists of a double strand of DNA and an enzyme (DNA polymerase) enclosed within a protein shell. The DNA strand and its inner protein shell together are called the **hepatitis B core antigen (HBcAg)**. The outer coat composed of lipid and protein is called the **hepatitis B surface antigen (HBsAg)**. The core antigen and surface antigen together form the complete virus particle, which is often called the Dane particle after the pathologist who first described it.

Hepatitis B core antigen
The antigen contained in the core of the hepatitis B virus.

Hepatitis B surface antigen
The coating of the hepatitis B virus that is also found in great excess in the blood of infected patients.

In contrast to hepatitis A, hepatitis B has a much longer incubation period, which varies from 6 weeks to 4 months. When an individual becomes infected, the virus invades the liver and multiplies within the hepatic cells. The core of the virus is produced in the nucleus, and the surface antigen is produced in the cytoplasm. For some unexplained reason, much more surface antigen is produced within the infected cells than is necessary to coat the virus particles, and the large excess is released into the bloodstream, where it can be detected by special laboratory tests (FIGURE 7). Such blood is called surface-antigen (HBsAg) positive. Although the laboratory tests detect only the surface antigen, HBsAg-positive blood is infectious because it also contains complete virus particles (FIGURE 7).

In the course of an infection, the surface antigen first appears during the incubation period and can be detected during the first few weeks of the infection. Normally, it does not persist in the blood for more than 2 or 3 weeks. Then antibodies begin to appear, both to the core of the virus (anti-HBc) and to the surface antigen (anti-HBs). Various other antigens and antibodies also appear in the blood of persons with HBV infection. One is a soluble protein called the e antigen (HBeAg), which appears along with HBsAg. The corresponding antibody, anti-HBe, often appears along with anti-HBs during recovery (FIGURE 8). Many people possess antibodies against the virus as a result of prior infection or as a result of immunization against the virus.

Most infected individuals eliminate the virus from the bloodstream in a few weeks and recover completely, but about 10% become chronic carriers of the virus. Some of the carriers develop chronic hepatitis, which causes progressive liver damage. About 1% of the US population are asymptomatic chronic carriers of the virus, and

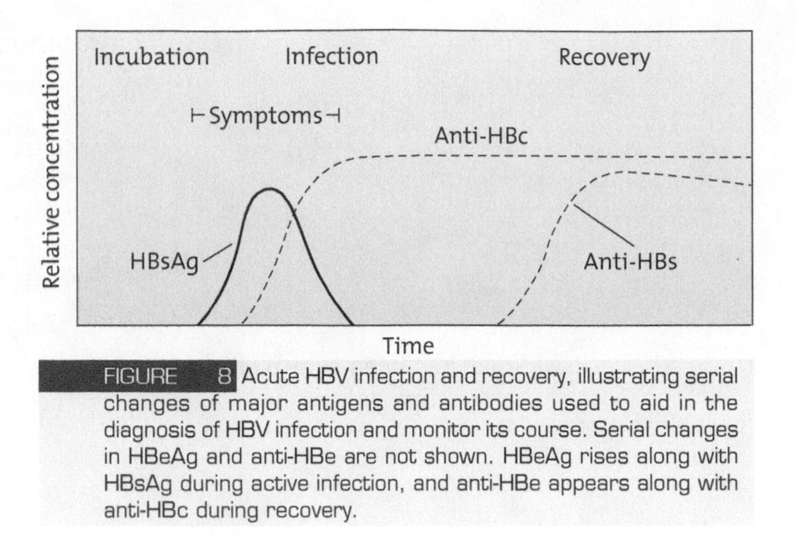

FIGURE 8 Acute HBV infection and recovery, illustrating serial changes of major antigens and antibodies used to aid in the diagnosis of HBV infection and monitor its course. Serial changes in HBeAg and anti-HBe are not shown. HBeAg rises along with HBsAg during active infection, and anti-HBe appears along with anti-HBc during recovery.

their blood is infectious. The carrier rate is much higher among drug abusers and male homosexuals. In the Vietnamese and some other population groups, the carrier rate may approach 20%.

Worldwide, more than 350 million people are infected with the hepatitis B virus, and about one million people each year die of the complications of the disease. Some antiviral drugs are available that can suppress viral multiplication and slow disease progression in persons who have active hepatitis and circulating virus in their bloodstream.

Hepatitis B virus is not excreted in the stool. Consequently, transmission does not occur by means of contaminated food or water. Most HBV infections result from contact with the blood or secretions of HBsAg-positive individuals. Drug abusers may transmit the virus by sharing needles and syringes. Physicians, dentists, nurses, laboratory personnel, and other health professionals may become infected from contact with blood of HBsAg-positive patients. Contaminated dental instruments or instruments used for ear piercing also may transmit HBV. Because HBV is also present in saliva, vaginal secretions, and seminal fluid, infection may also be spread by close family contacts or sexual contacts. An HBsAg-positive mother may transmit the virus to her newborn infant, who usually acquires the infection from maternal blood and vaginal secretions at the time of delivery. Unfortunately, infected infants are often unable to eliminate the virus and frequently become chronic carriers of the virus. Formerly, many cases followed blood transfusions; however, this is no longer true because all blood collected for transfusion is now tested routinely for HBsAg, and antigen-positive blood is not used for transfusion.

Hepatitis B immune globulin provides some protection if administered promptly after exposure to the virus and is given routinely to newborn infants born to HBsAg-positive mothers. A vaccine is available to immunize against HBV. The vaccine induces the formation of anti-HBs and provides a high degree of immunity against HBV infection. Universal vaccination is recommended, and HBV vaccination is included in vaccination schedules recommended for infants and children.

HEPATITIS C

The hepatitis C virus is an 80-nm RNA virus that is transmitted by infected blood and body fluids, as is HBV. There are six serologic types, which differ in their response to treatment. Type 1 is the most common type and, unfortunately, is the type most resistant to treatment. In many ways, HCV infection is an even more serious problem than HBV infection for several reasons:

1. HCV is a frequent cause of chronic hepatitis in the United States, accounting for almost half of the reported cases.
2. Most HCV-infected persons are unable to eliminate the virus and become chronic carriers. About 1 to 2% of the population are chronic carriers of the virus, and their blood and body fluids are infectious. Many of the chronic carriers will develop chronic hepatitis, which in turn is followed by cirrhosis in many of the infected persons.
3. There are no agents like gamma globulin that can protect an uninfected person who has been exposed to the virus, as by an accidental needle stick when drawing blood from an infected person.
4. There is no available immunizing agent that can be used to establish an active immunity against the virus, and none is likely to be developed in the foreseeable future.

HCV-infected persons may experience symptoms of hepatitis, as previously described, but many infected persons have few symptoms of infections, and some may not even know that they have become infected. Infected persons develop antibodies against HCV, but antibodies may not appear for several months after the infection. Viral RNA, a measure of virus particles in the circulation, is an indication of active infection, and the amount of viral RNA can be measured in the blood of infected persons to monitor the course of the infection.

In the past, many HCV infections followed blood transfusion of HCV-infected blood or use of blood products such as antihemophilic globulin prepared from infected blood. However, in 1992, a screening test to identify anti-HCV antibody became available as a diagnostic test for HCV infection. As soon as the test became available, it was used routinely by blood banks as a screening test. HCV-antibody–positive blood could be identified and not be used for transfusion. As a result, infections acquired by blood transfusion or use of blood products are no longer a problem.

Currently, most HCV infections are acquired from infected blood or body fluids in much the same ways that HBV and HIV infections are acquired. The Centers for Disease Control and Prevention, which monitors HBV infections, estimates that about 60% of HCV infections occur in injection drug users who share virus-contaminated needles. In 20% of cases, the infection was acquired by sexual contact, although HCV is not as easily transmitted by sexual practices as is HBV. About 10% of cases result from other types of blood and body fluid exposures, such as household contacts, infections associated with hemodialysis treatment, occupational exposures of healthcare workers, and virus transmission from mother to infant during childbirth. In another 10% of cases, the source of infection could not be determined.

Many people may have become infected by virus-contaminated blood or blood products before routine HCV blood testing procedures were available, but have no symptoms. Nevertheless, they are at risk of developing chronic hepatitis and its associated complications. Other persons in the past may have engaged in practices that put them at risk of becoming infected, such as injecting drugs, but they were unaware of the risks at the time. Most infected individuals cannot rid themselves of the virus and the HCV infection becomes chronic, although they may not have symptoms of active infection. Although an unfavorable outcome occurs in only a small percentage of infected persons, this is still a large number of people at risk of serious liver disease because HCV infection is so prevalent. Liver failure resulting from severe chronic liver disease caused by HCV is now the main indication for liver transplantation, and usually the virus also infects the transplanted liver just as it infected and destroyed the person's own liver.

Because of the serious late complications that can occur in some infected persons, the Centers for Disease Control and Prevention recommends that the following groups of high-risk individuals be tested for possible asymptomatic HCV infection:

1. Persons who have ever injected illegal drugs, even persons who injected drugs only once or a few times and do not consider themselves drug users.
2. Persons who received antihemophilic globulin or other clotting factor concentrates before 1987, when the manufacturing processes used were not adequate to eliminate the virus from the concentrates.
3. Persons who received blood transfusions before 1992, when screening blood for HCV was not available, or who had other contacts with blood before 1992, such as hemodialysis or organ transplants.
4. Health care personnel who had been exposed to blood or body fluids, as might have occurred following an accidental needle stick while drawing blood.
5. Children born to HCV-infected mothers because about 5% of infants born to infected mothers become infected.

Because of the potential late complications of HCV infection, all HCV-positive persons should be referred for further medical evaluation. Those who have chronic hepatitis, as demonstrated by abnormal liver function tests, viral RNA in their blood, and a liver biopsy demonstrating chronic inflammation in the liver, should be treated by drugs that inhibit viral multiplication. The preferred treatment is an antiviral compound called ribavirin combined with interferon or a modification of interferon (called pegylated interferon) that has a more prolonged antiviral action and appears to be more effective than interferon. Fortunately, treatment has improved recently with the addition of a protease inhibitor drug (boceprevir), which is given along with ribavirin and interferon. This new combination has improved greatly the response to treatment of type 1 HCV. It is hoped that other new drugs will follow to continue the progress being made against this disease.

HEPATITIS D (DELTA HEPATITIS)

This type of hepatitis is caused by a small defective RNA virus that can only infect persons who are already infected with the hepatitis B virus, either chronic carriers of HBV or those with an acute HBV infection. The delta virus is always associated with an HBV infection because the virus is unable to produce its own outer viral coat and can reproduce itself only by coating itself with HBsAg produced by HBV, thereby forming complete but hybrid virus particles composed of a delta virus core and an HBsAg outer layer. Delta hepatitis is less common than other types of viral hepatitis, and most cases in the United States are found among intravenous drug abusers who became infected by sharing contaminated needles.

HEPATITIS E

Hepatitis E is caused by an RNA virus that is transmitted by the fecal–oral route, like the hepatitis A virus; most of the cases are in third world countries, where outbreaks have been traced to contaminated water supplies. Only a few cases have been reported in North America, and the infected persons acquired the disease while traveling outside the United States. A diagnostic test has been developed to detect anti-HEV antibodies as an indication of HEV infection. Gamma globulin does not provide protection against HEV infection because gamma globulin preparations do not contain anti-HEV antibodies.

OTHER HEPATITIS VIRUSES

Other viruses may, at times, cause a mild hepatitis. These include the **Epstein-Barr (EB) virus**, which causes infectious mononucleosis (see the hematopoietic and lymphatic systems), and another somewhat similar virus called **cytomegalovirus**, which may also cause an infection resembling infectious mononucleosis.

Epstein-Barr virus
A virus that causes infectious mononucleosis.

Cytomegalovirus
(sī-tō-meg′u-lō-vī-rus) *One of the herpes viruses. Causes an infectious mononucleosislike syndrome in adults; may cause congenital malformation in fetus.*

HEPATITIS AMONG MALE HOMOSEXUALS

All types of viral hepatitis are common in male homosexuals and are transmitted by sexual contact. The hepatitis A virus is excreted in the stool of infected subjects and may also contaminate the anal–genital skin. Consequently, the virus is readily transmitted by anal–oral and oral–genital sexual activity. Hepatitis B virus, which is present in the blood and secretions of infected individuals, is transmitted among male homosexuals primarily by anal intercourse, and hepatitis C also may be transmitted in this way. Minor abrasions of the anal, rectal, and genital mucosa of sexual partners permits transfer of virus-infected blood and body fluids between partners.

The following case illustrates the usual clinical and laboratory features of viral hepatitis as a result of HBV infection:

CASE 1

A 22-year-old man was seen by a physician because of upper abdominal discomfort, nausea, loss of appetite, and jaundice. The patient had noted that his urine had become darker in color. He was homosexual and stated that a sexual partner had suffered a similar illness recently. Physical examination revealed a jaundiced young man with a slightly enlarged, tender liver. There were no findings to suggest chronic liver disease. Laboratory studies revealed a slight elevation of bilirubin and abnormalities of several liver function tests. Tests for hepatitis B surface antigen were positive. The patient was considered to have hepatitis B, probably contracted through sexual activities with a partner who either had active hepatitis or was a chronic carrier of the virus. The patient made an uneventful recovery. Hepatitis B surface antigen was no longer detected in the blood 3 weeks later, and antibody to hepatitis B surface antigen appeared during convalescence.

Fatty Liver

The liver performs many important functions related to the metabolism of food, including an important role in fat metabolism, and conditions that disturb liver functions can lead to accumulation of fat in liver cells. Fatty liver is a special type of liver injury (FIGURE 9). A number of injurious agents are capable of disrupting the metabolic processes within the liver cell, leading to an accumulation of fat globules within the liver cell cytoplasm (FIGURE 10). Diffuse fatty change within the liver can be demonstrated by ultrasound examination, by computed tomography (CT) scans, or by magnetic resonance imaging (MRI). Liver biopsy can determine whether there is any liver cell damage associated with the fatty change. In the United States, the most common cause of fatty liver is excessive alcohol ingestion, but a number of volatile solvents, drugs, chemicals, and some poisons can cause fat accumulation in liver cells. Obese persons and many persons with diabetes also accumulate excess fat in the liver unrelated to excess alcohol consumption. Usually, the affected persons

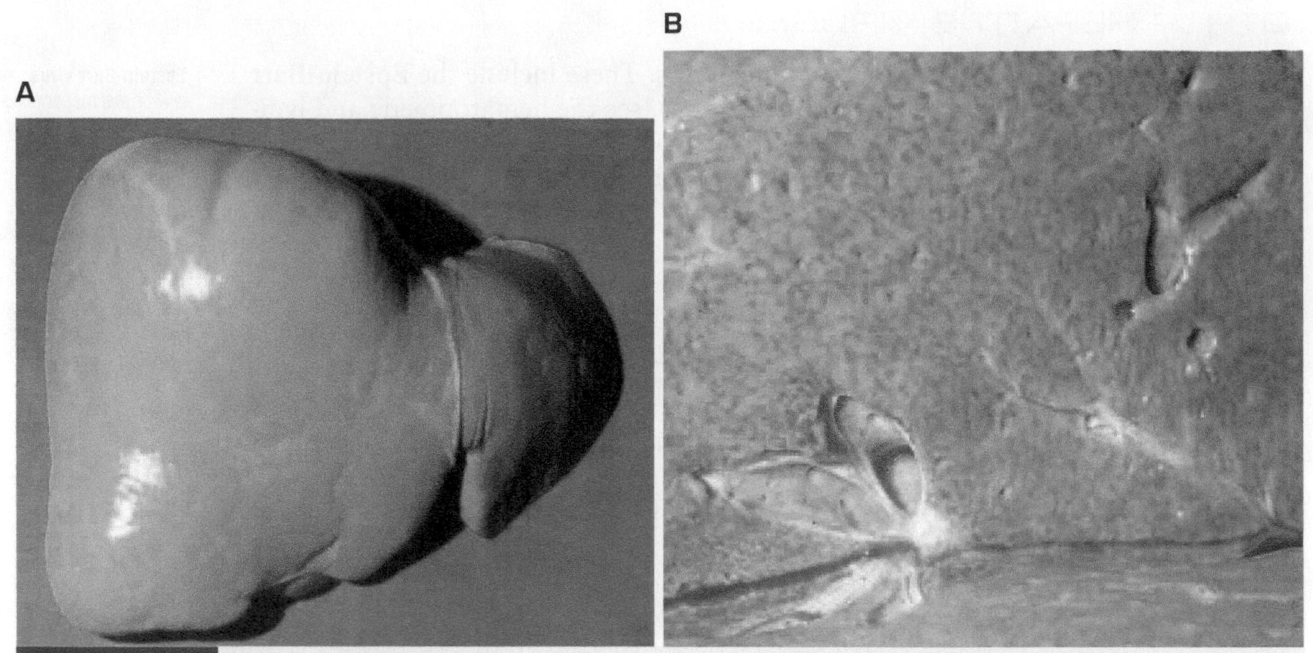

FIGURE 9 Fatty liver. **A**, The liver appears yellow because of a large amount of fat within liver cells, but otherwise appears normal. **B**, A section of liver that appears normal except for the yellow color caused by the fat.

have a higher than normal blood glucose or diabetes caused by obesity, which causes the body cells to become less responsive to insulin. The fatty change in the liver cells is called **nonalcoholic fatty liver** to distinguish it from the fatty liver of alcoholic subjects. Usually, heavy fat infiltration impairs liver function and may cause mild liver injury, but the liver cell damage usually is reversible. However, prolonged and severe fatty infiltration can cause significant liver cell damage associated with inflammation and scarring similar to the liver cell damage encountered in alcoholic subjects. This condition is called **nonalcoholic steatohepatitis** (*steatos* = fat), which can progress to cirrhosis

Nonalcoholic fatty liver
Fatty liver without significant inflammation or scarring within the liver, which usually occurs in insulin-resistant obese subjects with lipid abnormalities.

Nonalcoholic steatohepatitis
Fat-associated liver damage associated with inflammation and scarring similar to the features seen in alcohol-related liver disease.

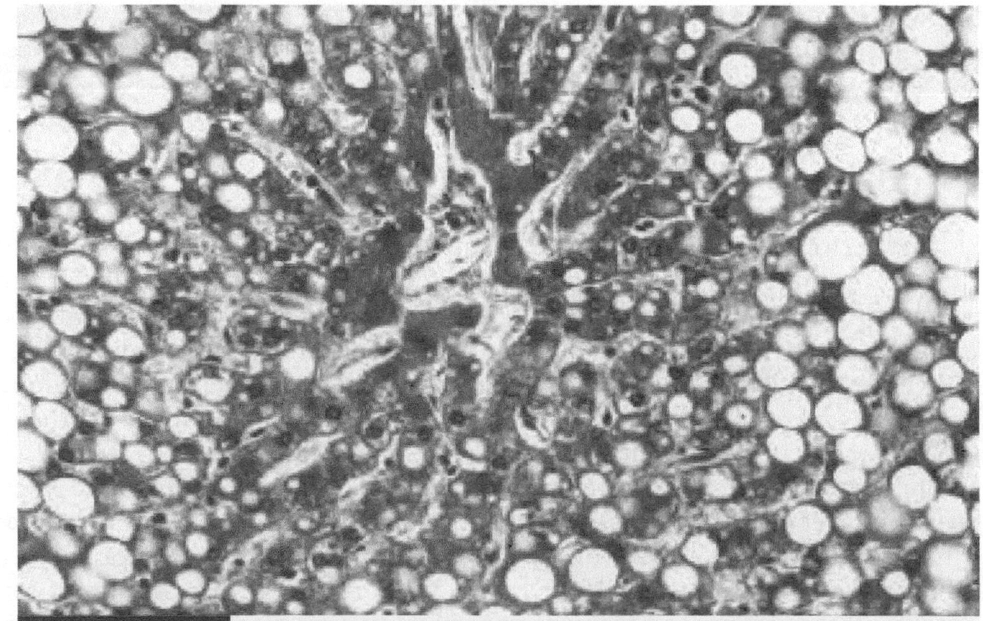

FIGURE 10 Photomicrograph of fatty liver. Liver cord cells in center of photograph appear relatively normal. Other cells contain large fat globules that appear as clear spherical vacuoles within liver cells in photograph (original magnification × 100).

and eventually to liver failure, like the similar condition that occurs in alcoholic liver disease. Unfortunately, nonalcoholic steatohepatitis and its complications are becoming more frequent because of the increasing obesity and diabetes in our population.

Fatty liver is also a characteristic feature of a condition called Reye's syndrome, which is described later in this chapter.

ALCOHOLIC LIVER DISEASE

The term alcoholic liver disease refers to a group of structural and functional changes in the liver resulting from excessive alcohol consumption. The severity of the liver injury and its rate of progression are determined not only by how much alcohol is consumed, but also how long the person has been drinking excessively.

It is convenient to subdivide alcoholic liver disease into three stages of progressively increasing severity: (1) alcoholic fatty liver, (2) alcoholic hepatitis, and (3) alcoholic cirrhosis.

Alcoholic Fatty Liver

This is the mildest form of alcoholic liver disease. If the subject stops drinking, the liver function gradually returns to normal, and the fat globules in the liver cells disappear as the liver cells process the accumulated fat.

Alcoholic Hepatitis

This is the next stage in the progressive liver injury caused by alcohol. Heavy alcohol intake not only promotes fatty change in liver cells, but causes other degenerative changes as well and may actually induce liver cell necrosis. A rather characteristic feature of severe alcoholic liver injury is the accumulation of irregularly shaped, pink deposits within the cytoplasm of the liver cells. These structures, which are called **Mallory bodies** or alcoholic hyalin, indicate that the cell has been irreparably damaged. Neutrophilic leukocytes also accumulate in response to the liver cell necrosis, and the injury is followed by progressive fibrous scarring throughout the liver. The term alcoholic hepatitis is used to refer to this type of liver injury, which is characterized not only by fatty change, but also by liver cell degeneration with Mallory bodies and leukocyte infiltration (FIGURE 11).

Mallory body
An irregular rod staining structure in the cytoplasm of injured liver cells, usually resulting from alcohol-induced liver injury.

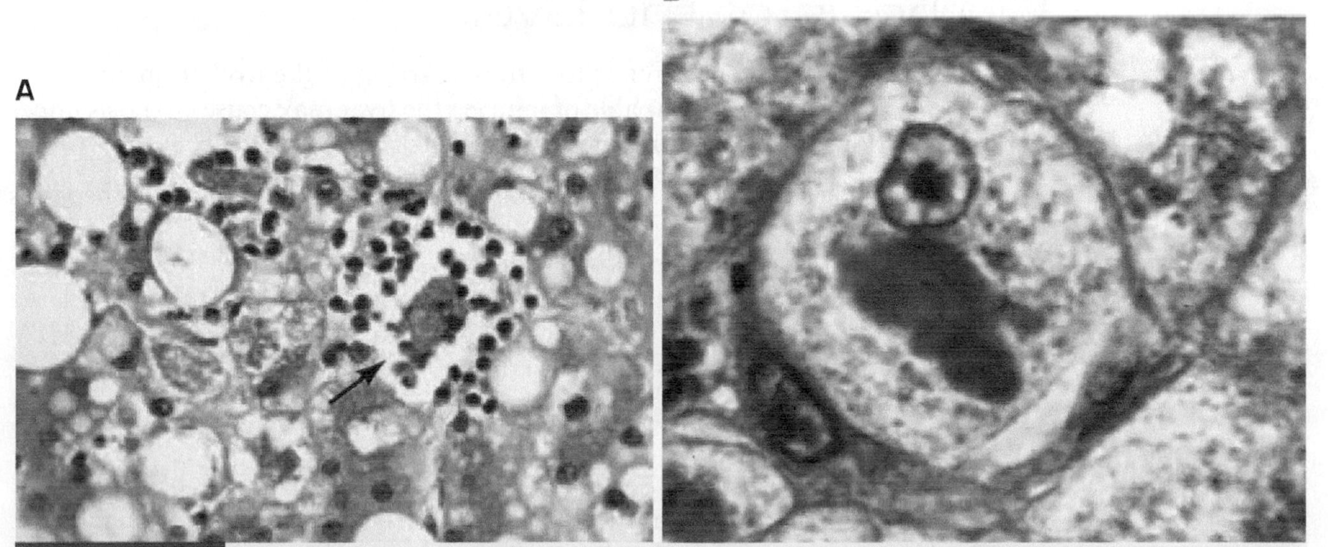

FIGURE 11 A photomicrograph illustrating hepatic cellular structure in alcoholic hepatitis. **A**, Many cells contain fat vacuoles. Others are swollen and contain Mallory bodies. One necrotic cell (*arrow*) is surrounded by cluster of neutrophils (original magnification × 400). **B**, A high-magnification photomicrograph of Mallory body in swollen liver cell (original magnification × 1,000).

In this case, the term "hepatitis" refers to the inflammatory cell infiltration secondary to liver cell necrosis and does not imply an infection, as in viral hepatitis.

Alcoholic Cirrhosis

This is the third and most advanced stage of alcoholic liver injury. It is characterized by diffuse scarring throughout the liver, which disturbs liver function and also impedes blood flow through the liver. Cirrhosis and its complications are described in the following section. In the United States, a large number of cases of cirrhosis are related to heavy alcohol ingestion and follow repeated episodes of alcoholic hepatitis. It is generally considered that a person must drink more than 1 pint of whiskey daily, or its equivalent in other alcoholic beverages, for 10 to 15 years in order to develop alcoholic cirrhosis. However, there is considerable individual variation in susceptibility to alcoholic liver injury. Occasionally, the disease develops more rapidly, and it has been seen in teenagers and young adults.

The following clinical summary illustrates the clinical features seen in a young man who died of severe alcoholic liver disease.

CASE 2

A 33-year-old man had been drinking heavily for many years and was in the habit of consuming about 1 qt. of liquor per day. Recently, he had noticed weakness and loss of appetite. The physical examination revealed that he was slightly jaundiced. His liver was enlarged, and there was moderate ascites. Laboratory studies revealed a reduced serum albumin and a moderate elevation of serum bilirubin.

Other tests of liver function were abnormal. The clinical impression was severe alcoholic liver disease. Despite intensive therapy, the patient's condition did not improve, and he eventually died of chronic liver failure. The autopsy revealed fatty change in liver cells and active alcoholic hepatitis with many Mallory bodies in the cytoplasm of the liver cells and the early stages of cirrhosis.

Cirrhosis of the Liver

Cirrhosis of the liver
(si-rō′sis)
A disease characterized by diffuse intrahepatic scarring and liver cell degeneration.

The term **cirrhosis of the liver** refers to diffuse scarring of the liver from any cause (FIGURE 12). Any substance capable of injuring the liver may cause cirrhosis under certain conditions. The two most common causes of cirrhosis are

1. Alcoholic liver disease, resulting from repeated episodes of alcoholic hepatitis followed by scarring.
2. Chronic hepatitis caused by HBV or HCV infections, which eventually leads to diffuse liver scarring. In many parts of Asia and Africa, where a large proportion of the population are chronic carriers of HBV, chronic HBV infection is the major cause of cirrhosis.

Less common causes of cirrhosis include

1. An episode of severe liver necrosis, such as after an attack of severe viral hepatitis (sometimes called posthepatitic cirrhosis or postnecrotic cirrhosis).
2. Various other drugs and chemicals that damage liver cells.
3. Various genetic diseases that directly or indirectly lead to liver damage such as hemochromatosis (discussion on the hematopoietic and lymphatic

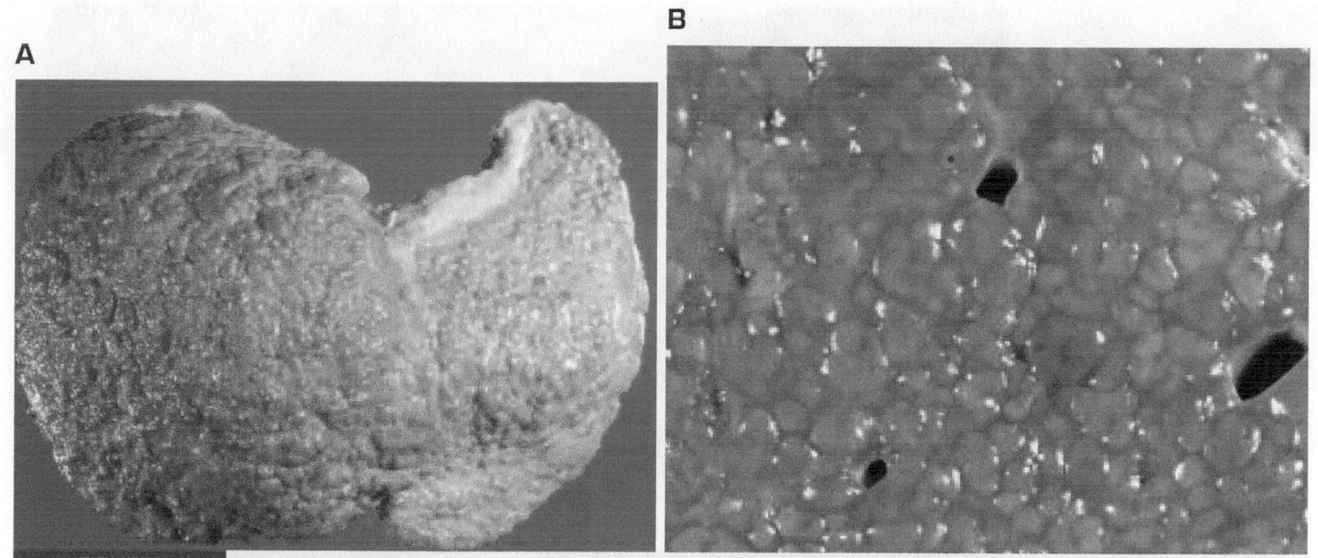

FIGURE 12 Advanced hepatic cirrhosis illustrating elevated nodules of liver tissue surrounded by depressed areas of scar tissue. **A**, Exterior of liver. **B**, A closer view of the liver in cross section.

systems) and $alpha_1$ antitrypsin deficiency, which also causes some types of pulmonary emphysema (discussion on the respiratory system).

4. Long-standing bile duct obstruction, which causes a special type of cirrhosis called **biliary cirrhosis**.

DERANGEMENTS OF LIVER STRUCTURE AND FUNCTION

In cirrhosis, the liver is converted into a mass of scar tissue containing nodules of degenerating and regenerating liver cells, proliferating bile ducts, and inflammatory cells (FIGURE 13). The normal architectural pattern of the liver is completely disorganized, and the intrahepatic branches of the hepatic artery and portal vein are constricted by scar tissue.

The two major functional disturbances in cirrhosis are impaired liver function and portal hypertension.

Impaired Liver Function

As a result of liver cell damage, scarring, and impairment of blood supply to the liver caused by scarring, the number of functioning liver cells is greatly reduced. Eventually, a patient with cirrhosis may die of liver failure. Clinical manifestations commonly found in men with advanced cirrhosis are testicular atrophy, loss of sex drive, and breast hypertrophy. These manifestations result from impaired liver function and appear to be the result of an excess of estrogen. Normally, men produce not only male sex hormone (testosterone), but small amounts of estrogen as well. The estrogen is normally inactivated by the liver and exerts little effect. The cirrhotic liver, however, is unable to accomplish this function efficiently; consequently, estrogen accumulates and produces these associated clinical manifestations.

Portal Hypertension

Normally, the portal vein blood passes through sinusoids into the hepatic veins and then into the inferior vena cava. In cirrhosis, venous return through the portal system is impaired, and the pressure in the portal vein rises because the blood flow is obstructed by scar tissue. The high pressure affects the portal capillaries, and this contributes to

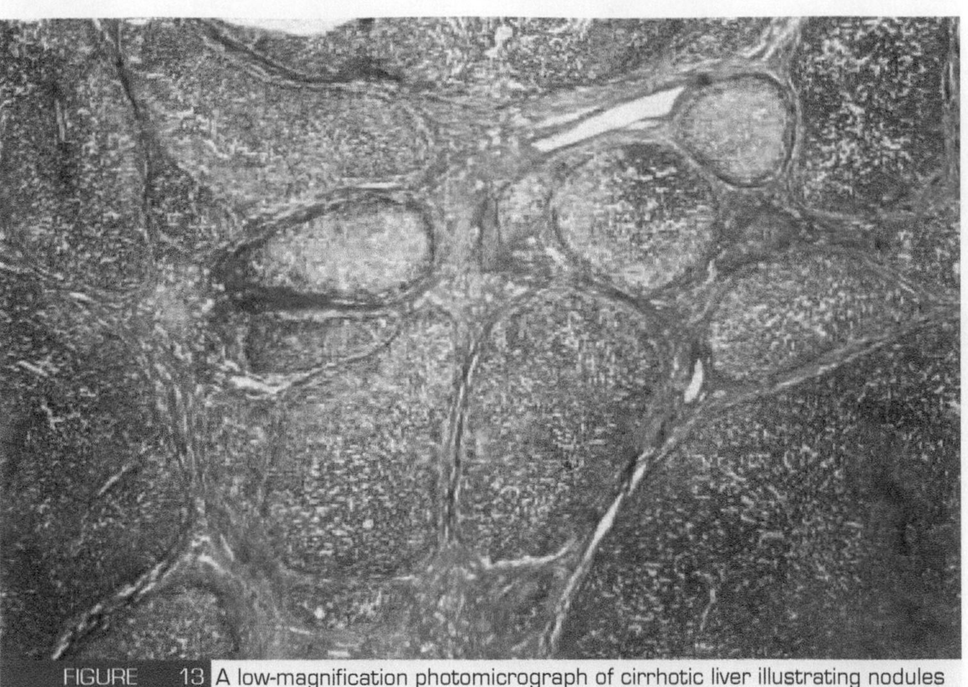

FIGURE 13 A low-magnification photomicrograph of cirrhotic liver illustrating nodules of liver cells circumscribed by dense scar tissue (blue-green stain). The normal architectural pattern is lost. The number of functioning liver cells is reduced and replaced by scar tissue, and the scar tissue disrupts blood flow through the liver. Compare with FIGURE 2 (original magnification × 25).

excessive leakage of fluid from the capillaries. Eventually, the abdomen becomes distended by fluids that accumulate within the abdominal cavity (ascites) (FIGURE 14).

A reduced concentration of albumin in the blood also contributes to ascites because albumin is crucial to maintaining the normal colloid osmotic pressure of the blood, which is the force that tends to hold fluid in the capillaries (discussion on circulatory disturbances). Albumin, which is produced by the liver, is reduced in

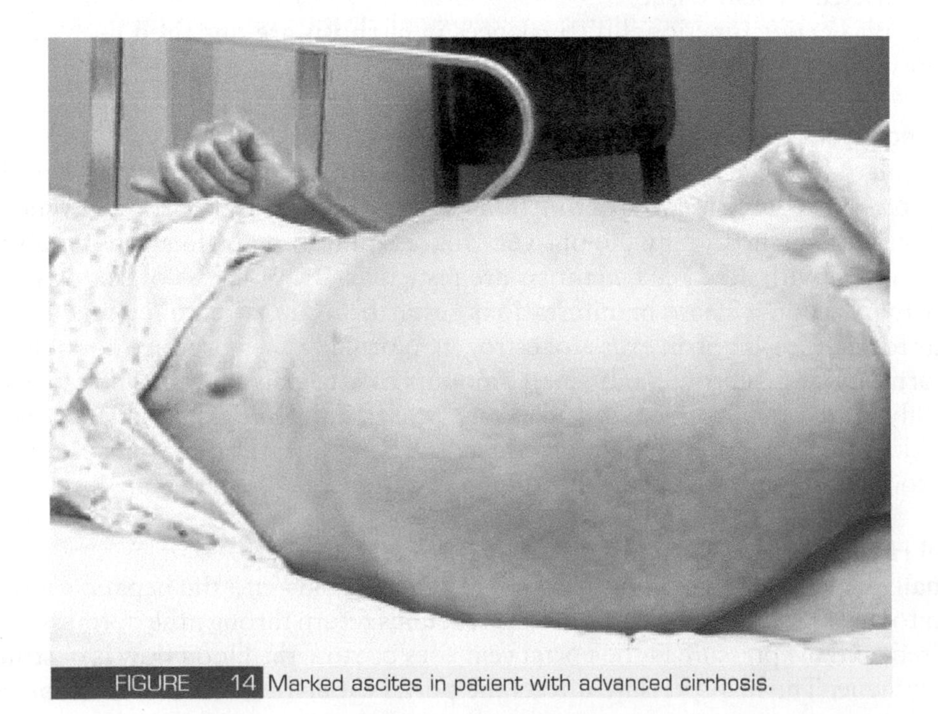

FIGURE 14 Marked ascites in patient with advanced cirrhosis.

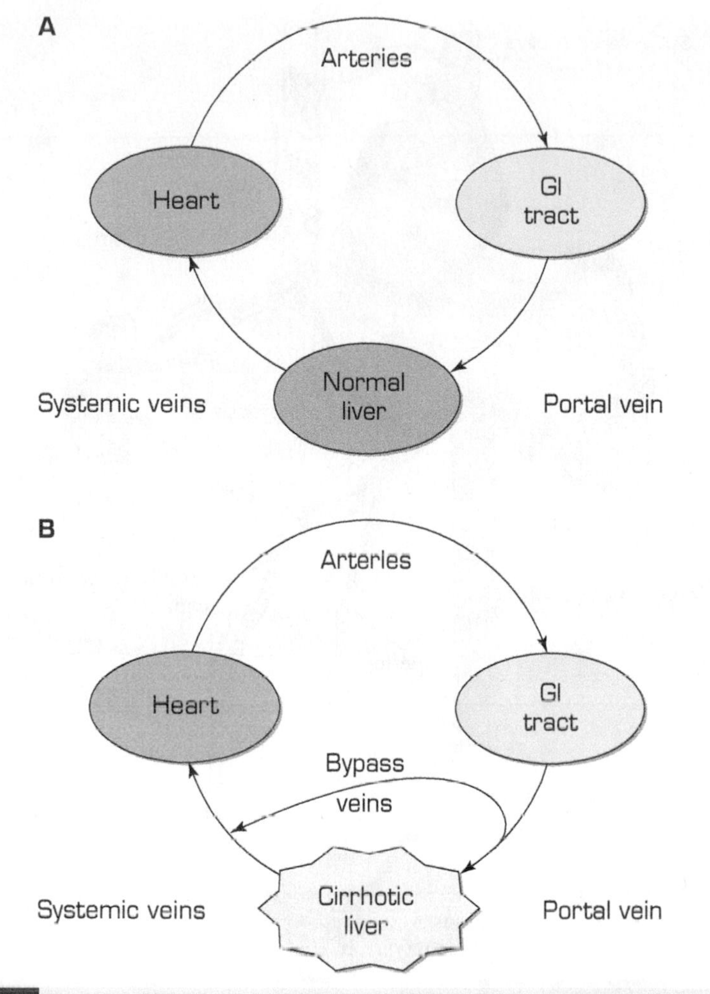

FIGURE 15 A comparison of normal blood flow pathways with those in cirrhosis. **A**, Normal flow pattern. The heart pumps blood through the aorta to the gastrointestinal tract from which blood collects in portal vein and flows through hepatic sinusoids into hepatic veins, then into vena cava, and finally, back to heart to be repumped. **B**, The flow pattern in cirrhosis. Blood pumped to gastrointestinal tract is collected in portal vein; however, flow through hepatic sinusoids is interrupted by intrahepatic scarring, and portal vein pressure rises. Bypass channels shunt blood into superior or inferior vena cava in order to return blood to the heart. Bypass veins cannot handle increased blood flow under increased pressure and become dilated.

cirrhosis because the cirrhotic liver is unable to manufacture this protein in sufficient quantities; consequently, the colloid osmotic pressure of the blood is lower than normal, and fluid leaks from the portal capillary bed.

Because of the obstruction of portal venous return, a collateral circulation develops in an attempt to bypass the intrahepatic obstruction and deliver portal blood directly into the systemic circulation. Anastomoses develop where tributaries of portal and systemic veins are closely associated, and they shunt blood from the portal system of veins where the pressure is high into the veins of the systemic circulation where the pressure is much lower (FIGURE 15). The communications that are most important clinically are the anastomoses developing between veins around the stomach and spleen, which drain into the portal vein, and the esophageal veins that eventually drain into the superior vena cava by way of the intercostal veins and azygos veins (FIGURE 16). The esophageal veins are not equipped to handle the increased blood flow and high pressure. They become dilated and form varicose veins, which are called esophageal varices (plural of varix). Esophageal varices are thin-walled

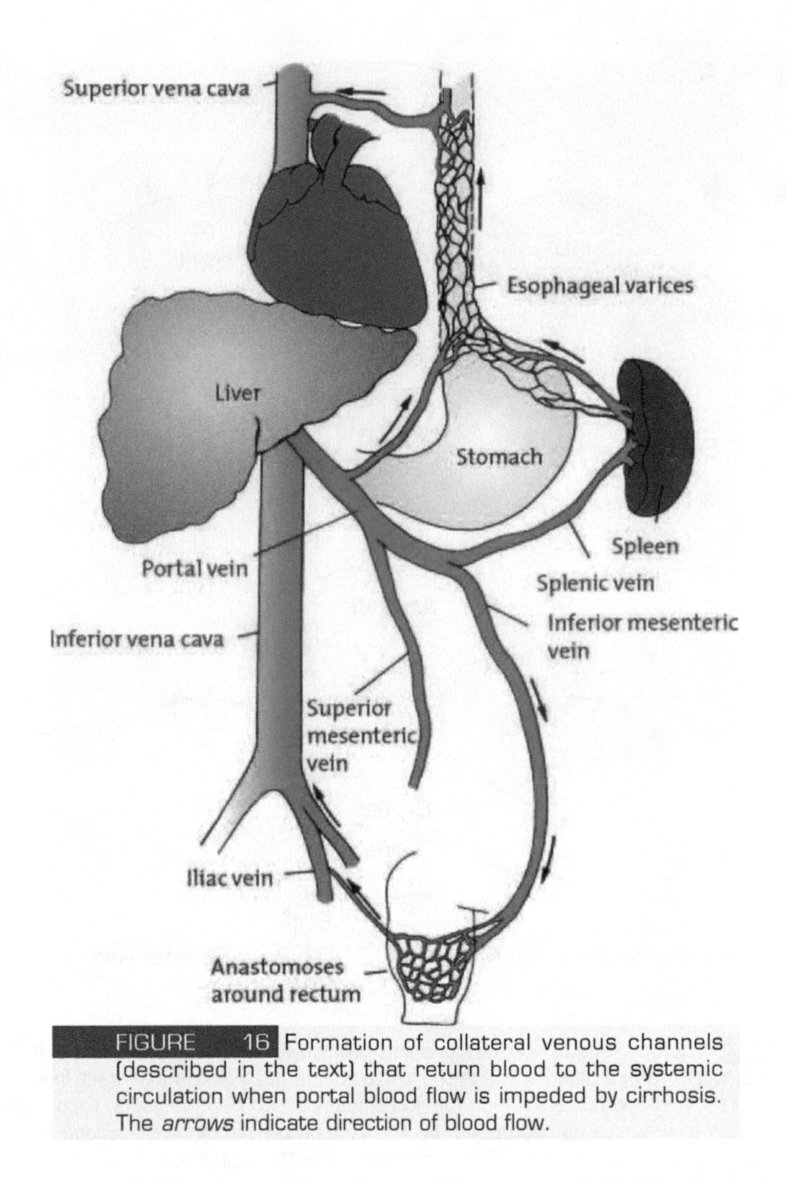

FIGURE 16 Formation of collateral venous channels (described in the text) that return blood to the systemic circulation when portal blood flow is impeded by cirrhosis. The *arrows* indicate direction of blood flow.

vessels covered by a thin layer of esophageal epithelium (FIGURE 17) and frequently rupture, leading to profuse and sometimes fatal hemorrhage.

Other anastomoses develop between branches of the portal vein and the veins draining the abdominal wall that eventually flow into either the superior or the inferior vena cava. Still, other anastomoses develop around the rectum between branches of the inferior mesenteric veins and the iliac veins, permitting blood to flow through the iliac veins into the inferior vena cava. The extent of the communications between the portal and systemic vein branches in patients with advanced cirrhosis is not always obvious. Special photographic techniques, however, can demonstrate the dilated veins extending in the subcutaneous tissues of the chest and abdominal wall that are shunting blood around the scarred liver (FIGURE 18).

The blood flow through the collateral channels reduces the engorgement of the abdominal organs that has resulted from overdistention of the portal circulation. The elevated portal pressure also declines somewhat but does not return to normal.

Hepatic Encephalopathy

Hepatic encephalopathy (*encephalon* = brain + *pathy* = disease) is a deterioration of brain function characterized by impaired consciousness, confusion, disorientation,

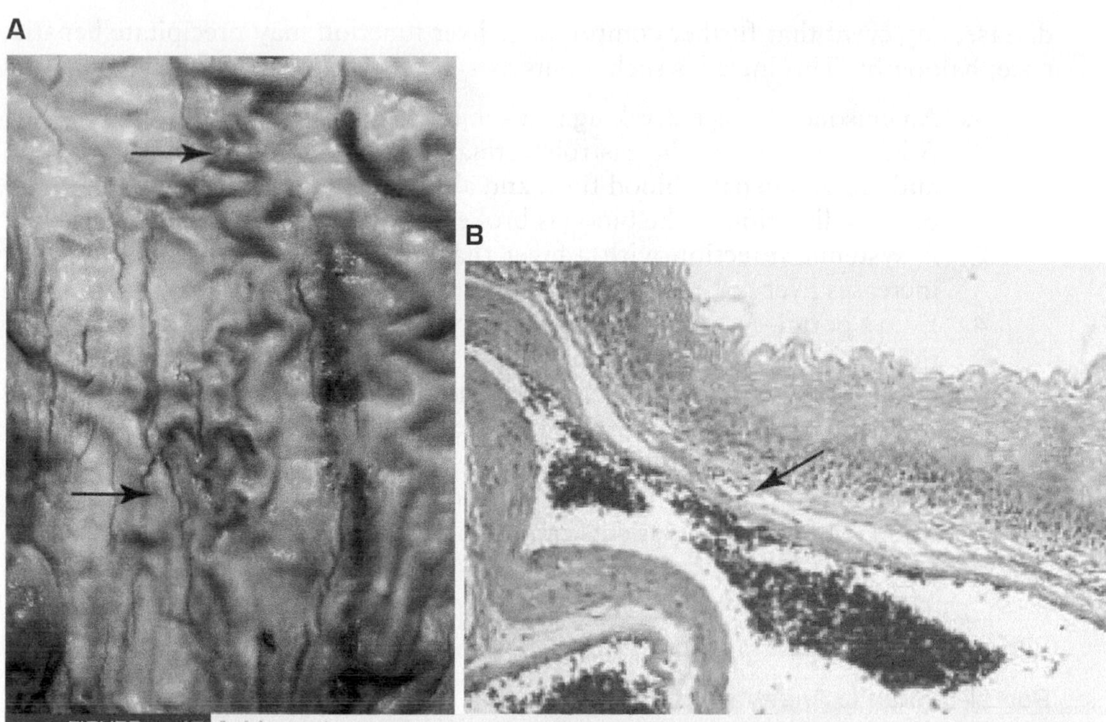

FIGURE 17 **A**, Mucosal surface of esophagus illustrating varices, which appear as tortuous elevations of the mucosa (*arrows*). **B**, A photomicrograph of a varix. The very thin vein wall (*arrow*) is covered only by a thin layer of esophageal squamous epithelium and is very susceptible to rupture (original magnification × 40).

and eventually coma. The condition results from toxic substances that accumulate in the bloodstream and are normally detoxified and excreted by the liver, a task that the cirrhotic liver is unable to accomplish efficiently. Not all of the toxic products have been identified, but many of them are products of protein digestion, especially ammonia, which comes from deamination of amino acids, and other products derived from bacterial decomposition of material in the colon. In a person with advanced liver

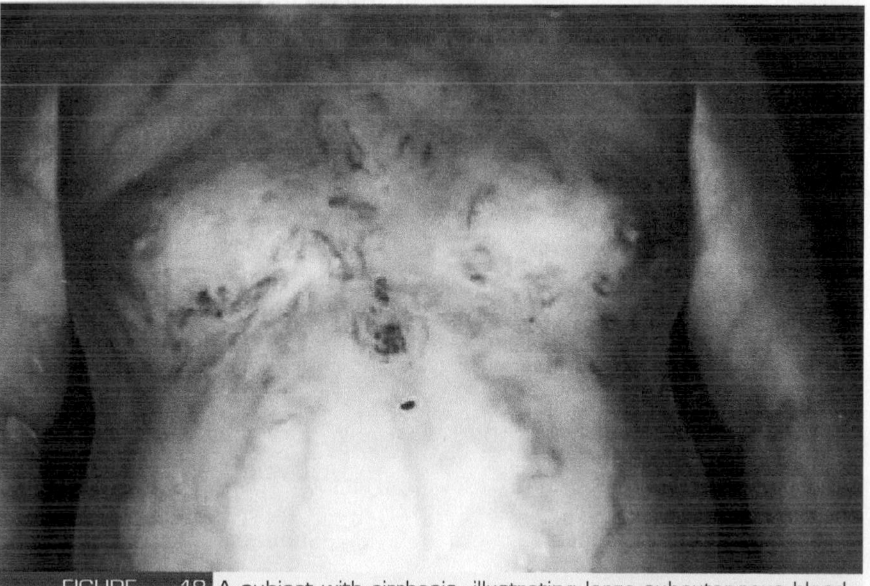

FIGURE 18 A subject with cirrhosis, illustrating large subcutaneous blood vessels that are part of the collateral circulation shunting blood around the cirrhotic liver, as demonstrated by an infrared-sensitive film technique.

disease, any event that further compromises liver function may precipitate hepatic encephalopathy. This includes such events as

1. An episode of binge drinking in a subject with alcoholic liver disease.
2. A hemorrhage into the gastrointestinal tract, which drops blood pressure and reduces hepatic blood flow, and also provides more toxic products of protein digestion as the blood is broken down within the intestinal tract.
3. A systemic infection with a fever that reduces hepatic blood flow and increases liver cell metabolism.
4. Even a portal–systemic vein bypass procedure, described in the following sections, which diverts some of the portal vein blood directly into the systemic circulation, may precipitate hepatic encephalopathy in some patients. The bypassed portal vein blood also bypasses whatever remaining detoxification function the diseased liver still possesses and delivers the bypassed blood and its toxins directly into the systemic venous circulation and then to the brain. Many bypass patients can tolerate the diversion, but some cannot.

PROCEDURES TO TREAT MANIFESTATIONS OF CIRRHOSIS

Portal–Systemic Anastomoses

If a patient has developed esophageal varices and is at risk of hemorrhage, it is possible to lower the pressure in the portal system by surgically connecting the splenic vein to the renal vein side-to-side (**splenorenal shunt**) or making a side-to-side connection between the portal vein and inferior vena cava (**portacaval shunt**). A shunt decompresses the portal system by permitting portal blood to flow directly into the inferior vena cava (FIGURE 19). Blood no longer is forced to circumvent the scarred

Splenorenal shunt
(splē′no-rē′nul)
Surgically created anastomosis between splenic vein and renal vein, performed to lower portal pressure in the treatment of esophageal varices.

Portacaval shunt
(por′tuh-kay′vul)
Surgically created anastomosis between the portal vein and the vena cava, performed to lower portal pressure in the treatment of esophageal varices.

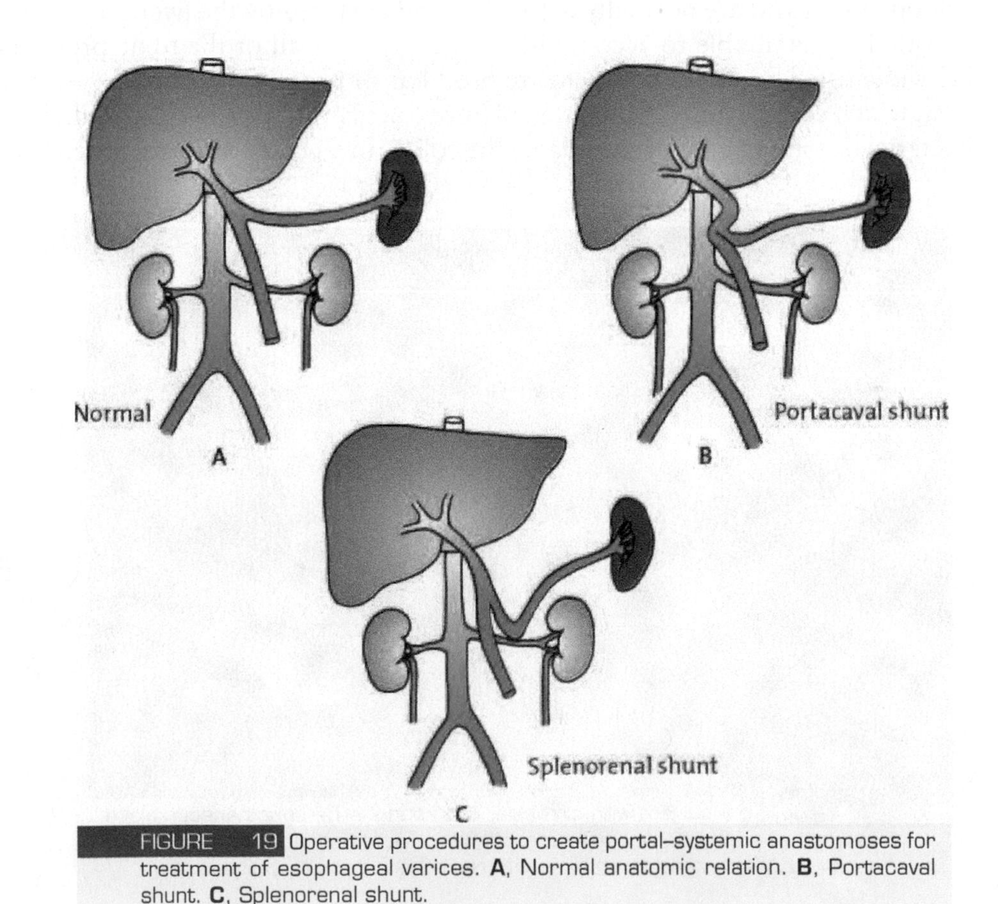

FIGURE 19 Operative procedures to create portal–systemic anastomoses for treatment of esophageal varices. **A**, Normal anatomic relation. **B**, Portacaval shunt. **C**, Splenorenal shunt.

liver by collateral channels. The dilated esophageal veins decrease in size, and the risk of hemorrhage from varices is greatly reduced.

Intrahepatic Portosystemic Shunts

In selected patients, a nonsurgical portal–systemic communication can be accomplished by means of a procedure called a **transjugular intrahepatic portosystemic shunt**, which is often called simply the TIPS procedure. Under x-ray guidance, a catheter is introduced into the right internal jugular vein and passed retrograde into the inferior vena cava and then into one of the hepatic veins (which drain blood from the liver into the inferior vena cava). Then a guide wire is passed through the catheter, which penetrates the hepatic vein wall and passes through the liver tissue to connect with a large intrahepatic branch of the portal vein. The procedure creates a tract between portal vein and hepatic vein within the liver. The tract is dilated, and a device (called a stent) is inserted to keep the tract open. When the procedure has been completed, much of the portal blood flows directly from a portal vein branch directly into one of the hepatic veins and then into the inferior vena cava, without flowing through the hepatic sinusoids (FIGURE 20). As a result, the high pressure in the portal vein falls toward normal. The shunt may also improve the patient's ascites because the lower portal pressure resulting from the shunt lowers the venous pressure in the capillaries draining into the portal system, and less fluid is forced from the capillaries to accumulate in the abdominal cavity.

Transjugular intrahepatic portosystemic shunt
A nonsurgical method used to lower portal vein pressure in a person with cirrhosis by connecting an intrahepatic branch of the portal vein to a hepatic vein branch.

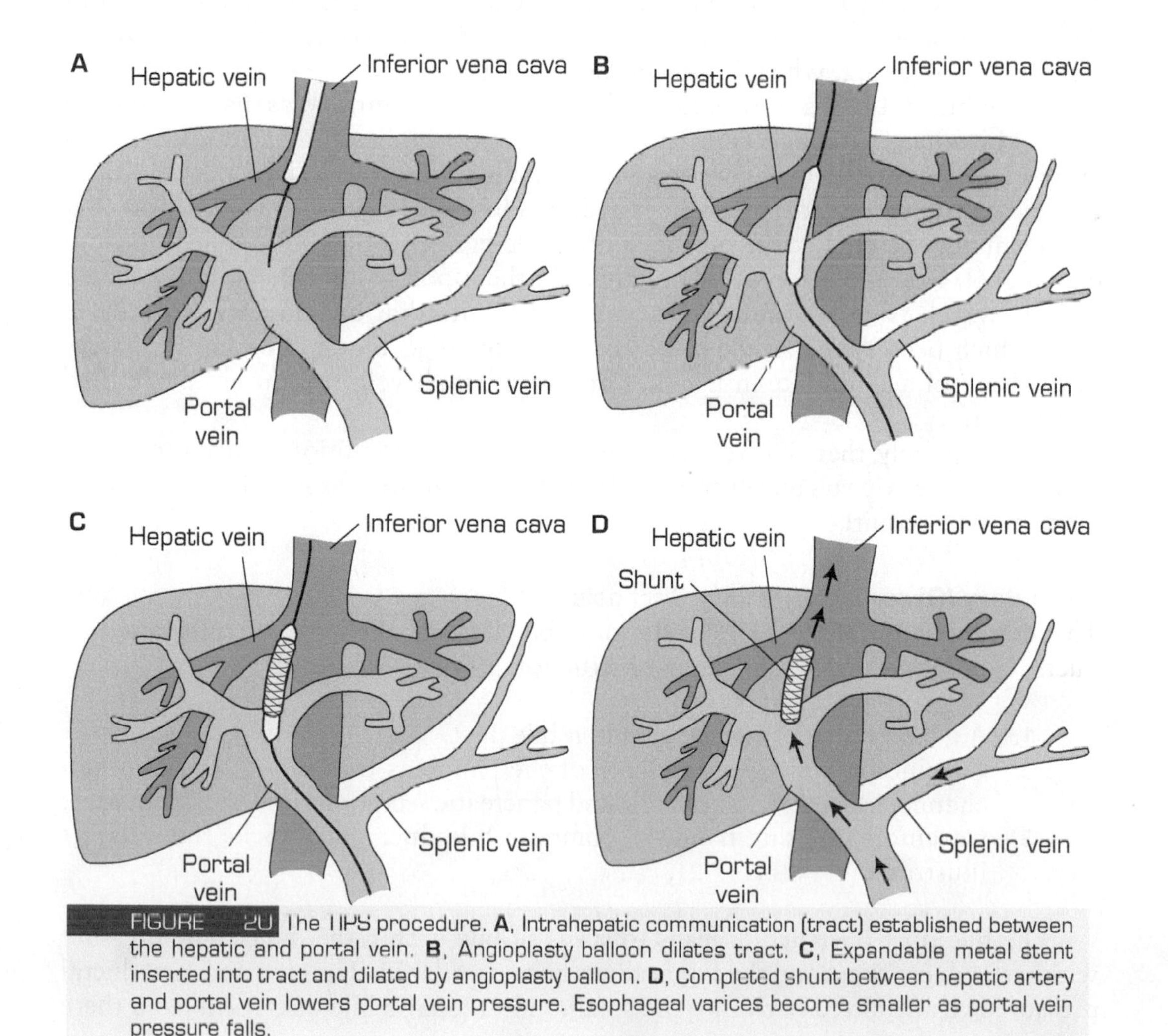

FIGURE 20 The TIPS procedure. **A**, Intrahepatic communication (tract) established between the hepatic and portal vein. **B**, Angioplasty balloon dilates tract. **C**, Expandable metal stent inserted into tract and dilated by angioplasty balloon. **D**, Completed shunt between hepatic artery and portal vein lowers portal vein pressure. Esophageal varices become smaller as portal vein pressure falls.

Obliteration of Varices by Sclerosing Solution

Another way to treat varices is to obliterate them by injecting them with a sclerosing solution. The procedure is performed by first visualizing the lining of the esophagus and the location of the varices by means of an esophagoscope. The sclerosing solution is then injected directly into the dilated veins and connective tissue around the vein. The solution, which is very irritating, causes an inflammation in and around the dilated veins, which is followed by scarring and eventual obliteration of the varices. Multiple injections over a period of several months are usually required.

BILIARY CIRRHOSIS

Biliary cirrhosis
Diffuse liver cell damage and scarring with distortion of liver cell structure and function (cirrhosis) caused by obstruction of bile ducts.

In some types of cirrhosis, the primary target of the liver damage is the epithelium of the bile ducts rather than the functional cells (hepatocytes) of the liver lobules. This type of cirrhosis is called **biliary cirrhosis** to distinguish it from the more common type of cirrhosis in which liver cell injury involves primarily the hepatocytes. There are two main types of biliary cirrhosis. The first, which is called primary biliary cirrhosis, is an autoimmune disease that targets the small intrahepatic bile ducts. The second, called secondary biliary cirrhosis or obstructive biliary cirrhosis, results from long-standing obstruction of the large extrahepatic bile ducts.

Primary Biliary Cirrhosis

This is a slowly progressive chronic disease characterized by inflammation and destruction of the small intrahepatic bile ducts. Bile excretion is disrupted and is followed by scarring, which begins in the portal tracts and eventually spreads into the liver lobules. The disease appears to be caused by autoantibodies that are directed against bile duct epithelial cells. Antinuclear autoantibodies and antimitochondrial antibodies can usually be demonstrated in the blood of affected patients.

Because excretion of bile is impeded, products accumulate in the blood that are normally excreted in the bile, including bile pigment (bilirubin), bile salts, and cholesterol. Accumulation of bile pigment in the blood causes the skin to become yellow, which is called jaundice, and the bile salts that accumulate irritate the skin, which becomes very itchy. As a result of the high blood cholesterol, masses of cholesterol accumulate in the skin and form small yellow skin nodules called xanthomas.

Unfortunately, there is no effective treatment for this condition, which progresses slowly over many years and eventually leads to liver failure. Ultimately, a liver transplant may be required.

Secondary (Obstructive) Biliary Cirrhosis

This condition is caused by long-standing blockage of the large extrahepatic bile ducts. Common causes of bile duct obstruction are

1. A gallstone blocking the common bile duct.
2. Carcinoma arising in the head of the pancreas that blocks the common channel transporting both bile and pancreatic secretions into the duodenum.
3. Carcinoma arising from the common bile duct that blocks the duct, as illustrated in FIGURE 21.

The bile duct obstruction leads to stasis of bile within the ducts. The pressure within the ducts rises, and the larger ducts become dilated. The elevated intraductal pressure is transmitted back into the smaller intrahepatic bile ducts and from there

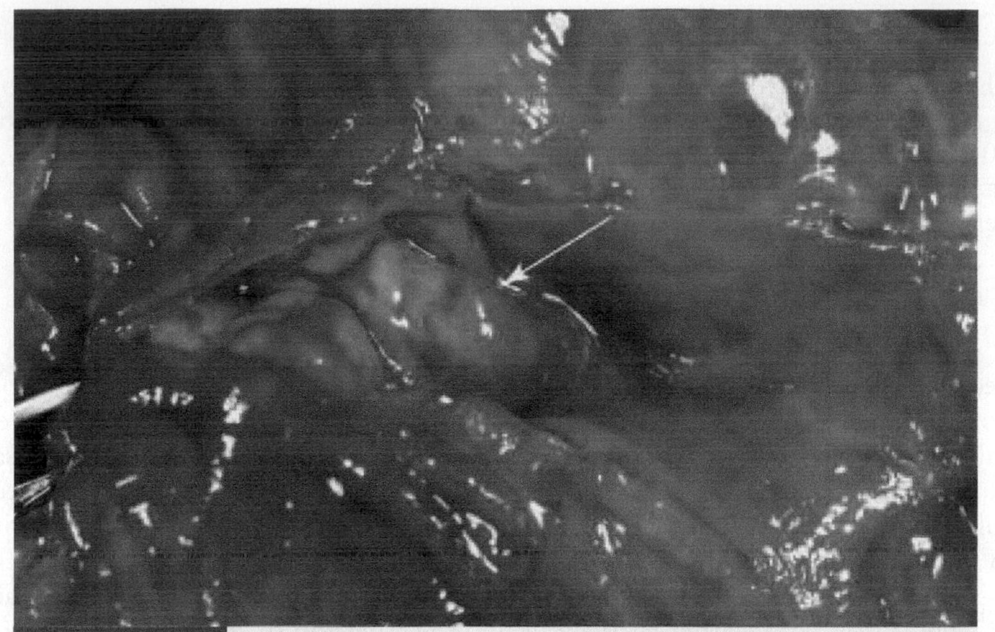

FIGURE 21 Carcinoma arising from common bile duct (*arrow*) blocking outflow of bile into duodenum. Common bile duct has been opened and is distended, a result of the increased pressure of the bile within the common duct caused by the duct obstruction.

into the small bile channels (bile canaliculi) that carry bile from the liver lobules into the bile ducts within the portal tracts at the periphery of the lobules. The elevated intraductal pressure and bile stasis damage the intrahepatic bile ducts, which is followed by portal tract inflammation and scarring.

The clinical manifestations of the extrahepatic bile duct obstruction are much the same as those caused by primary biliary cirrhosis. Treatment consists of various surgical procedures to unblock the obstructed bile duct. If this is not possible, some type of surgical procedure is used to bypass the obstruction and reestablish bile flow into the duodenum.

Reye's Syndrome

Reye's syndrome (rhymes with "eye") is a relatively uncommon acute illness that develops in infants and children after a mild viral infection and is characterized by both marked swelling of the brain with neurologic dysfunction and accumulation of fat within the cytoplasm of liver cells associated with impaired liver function. Clinically, the illness manifests as a sudden onset of vomiting and impaired consciousness, which may progress to delirium and coma. Laboratory tests reveal the disturbed liver function that is related to the accumulation of fat in the liver cells, and some patients become jaundiced. In severely affected patients, the mortality rate is about 25%, and some of the survivors may be left with neurologic abnormalities or psychiatric disturbances. There is no specific treatment.

Current evidence suggests that Reye's syndrome is related in some way to acetylsalicylic acid (aspirin) given to treat the fever and discomfort associated with the viral infection. The aspirin may increase the injurious effects of the virus or interact with the virus to cause the liver and brain injury. Therefore, acetaminophen (for example, Tylenol) is recommended to treat symptoms of viral infections in infants and children.

Cholelithiasis

Cholelithiasis
(kō′lē-lith-ī′uh-sis)
Formation of gallstones.

The formation of stones within the gallbladder is called **cholelithiasis** (*chole* = bile + *lith* = stone). Gallstones are very common and are estimated to develop in about 20% of the population. Most gallstones are composed entirely or predominantly of cholesterol, and they form because the bile contains more cholesterol than can be held in solution by the available bile salts and lecithin (FIGURE 22).

FACTORS AFFECTING THE SOLUBILITY OF CHOLESTEROL IN BILE

Micelle
(mi-sell′)
An aggregate of bile salt and lecithin molecules by which cholesterol is brought into solution in bile.

Because cholesterol is a lipid, it is not soluble in an aqueous solution such as bile but is brought into solution by bile salts and lecithin, which aggregate in clusters called **micelles.** In a micelle, the lipid-soluble (hydrophobic) parts of the bile salt molecules are oriented toward the center of the cluster, and the opposite water-soluble (hydrophilic) ends face outward. Cholesterol becomes soluble by dissolving in the hydrophobic center of the micelles, and the cholesterol-containing micelles dissolve in the bile because the peripheral hydrophilic parts of the bile salt molecules are water soluble. Lecithin participates in the formation of the micelles by fitting between the molecules of the bile salts (FIGURE 23).

Approximately seven molecules of bile salts interspersed between lecithin molecules in a micelle are required to dissolve one molecule of cholesterol. Consequently, the solubility of cholesterol in bile depends not only on its cholesterol content, but also on its content of bile salts and lecithin, because these substances are needed to hold the cholesterol in solution. Cholesterol remains soluble provided its concentration is not excessive in relationship to the amounts of available bile salts and lecithin. If there is an excess of cholesterol relative to bile salts and lecithin, the bile becomes supersaturated with cholesterol and cholesterol crystals may precipitate. On the other hand, if there is an excess of bile salts and lecithin relative to cholesterol, more cholesterol can dissolve in the bile. These relationships can be conceptualized by a board on a fulcrum, one end of the board being weighted by cholesterol and

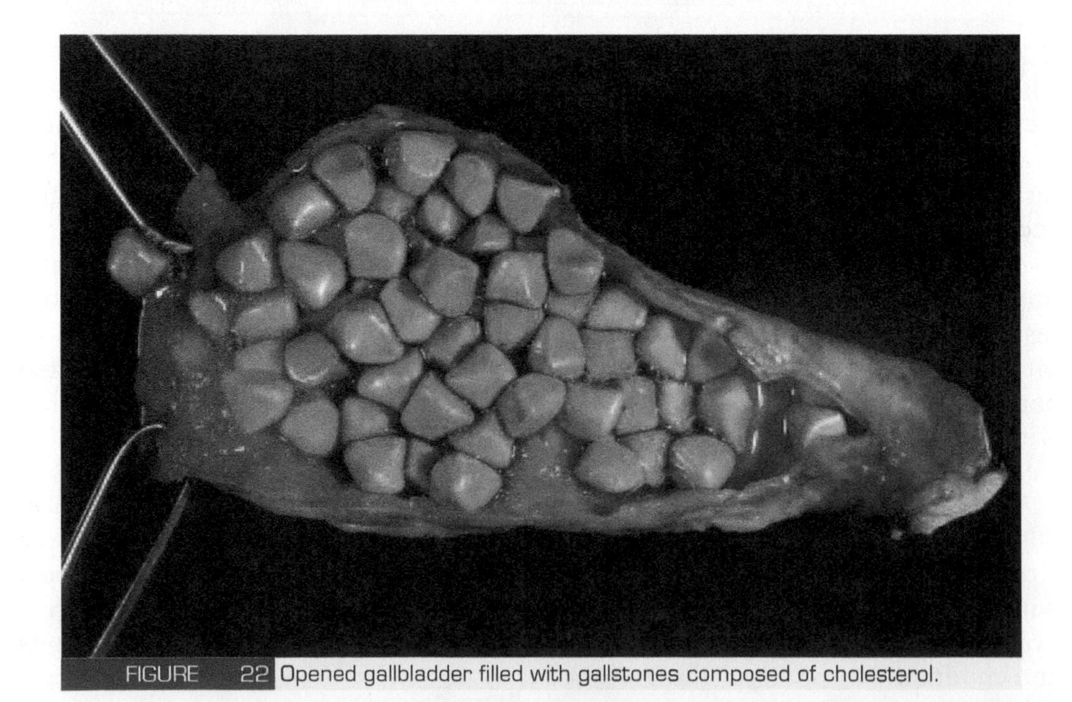

FIGURE 22 Opened gallbladder filled with gallstones composed of cholesterol.

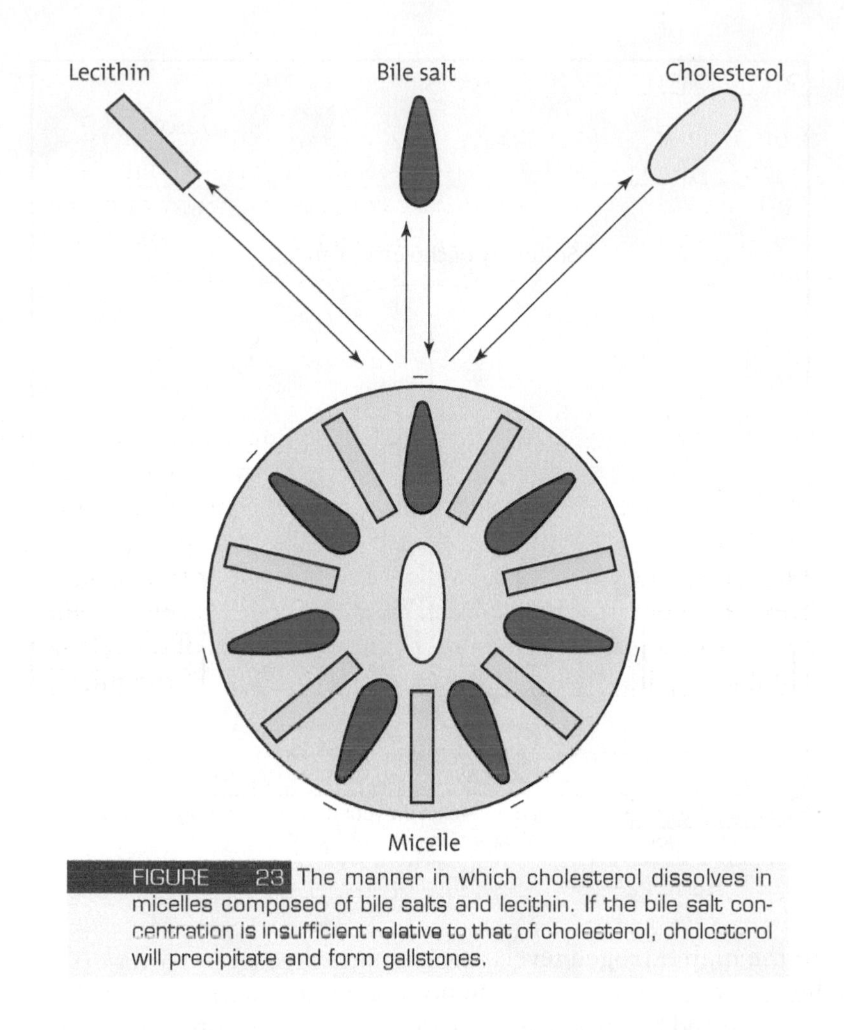

FIGURE 23 The manner in which cholesterol dissolves in micelles composed of bile salts and lecithin. If the bile salt concentration is insufficient relative to that of cholesterol, cholesterol will precipitate and form gallstones.

the other end by bile salts and lecithin. Variations in the "weight" on either end of the board cause corresponding changes in the solubility of the cholesterol in the bile (FIGURE 24).

Whenever bile contains a relative excess of cholesterol, it becomes supersaturated with cholesterol, and under proper conditions, the cholesterol may precipitate to form the beginnings of gallstones. This situation may arise because of an increased excretion of cholesterol in the bile, a reduced excretion of bile salts and lecithin, or a combination of both factors. As long as the bile remains supersaturated, cholesterol crystals continue to accumulate around those that have already precipitated, and the gallstones slowly increase in size. Eventually, the gallbladder may become filled with gallstones, the end stage of a process that began several years earlier.

Some people are known to have an increased risk of forming gallstones. The incidence of gallstones is

1. Higher in women than in men.
2. Higher in women who have borne several children than in childless women.
3. Twice as high in women who use contraceptive pills as in women who use other types of contraception.
4. Higher in obese women than in women of normal weight.

The incidence of gallstones is higher in these groups because their bile is more highly saturated with cholesterol. The incidence is higher in women than in men because estrogen promotes increased excretion of cholesterol in the bile while decreasing excretion of bile salts. The correlation of gallstones with multiple pregnancies

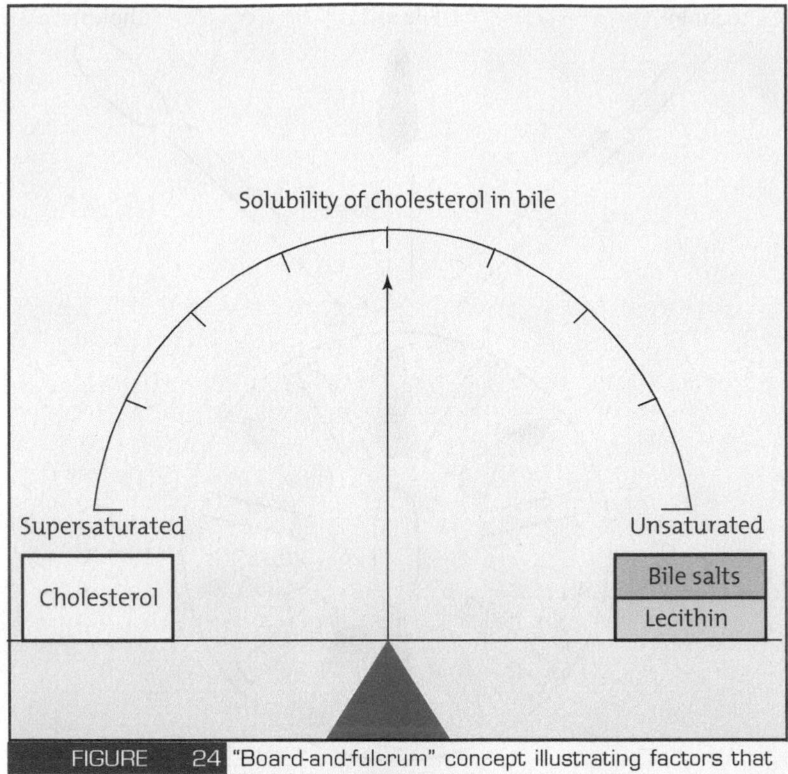

FIGURE 24 "Board-and-fulcrum" concept illustrating factors that affect solubility of cholesterol in bile.

is related to the high estrogen levels associated with pregnancy. (Estrogen levels are much higher in pregnancy than in the nonpregnant state because large amounts of estrogen are produced by the placenta.) Contraceptive pills predispose to cholelithiasis because they contain synthetic estrogens that, like natural estrogens, increase the saturation of gallbladder bile. Obesity predisposes to gallstones because extremely overweight persons have a higher blood cholesterol and excrete more cholesterol in their bile than do persons of normal weight.

Less commonly, gallstones form as a result of infection of the gallbladder. Infection predisposes to gallstones by reducing the solubility of cholesterol and other constituents in the bile.

COMPLICATIONS OF GALLSTONES

Biliary colic
Abdominal pain that results when a gallstone enters the biliary duct system.

Cholecystitis
(ko′lē-sis-tī′-tis)
An inflammation of the gallbladder.

Gallstones that remain in the gallbladder do not cause symptoms. Unfortunately, gallstones are sometimes extruded into the cystic duct or common bile duct when the gallbladder contracts after a fatty meal, and they may become impacted within the biliary ducts. This event causes severe abdominal pain called **biliary colic**. The pain results from spasm of the smooth muscle in the ducts combined with forceful contractions of the gallbladder that attempt to propel the stone through the ducts. Sometimes a stone can be passed through the ducts into the duodenum, but often it becomes impacted. If the stone lodges in the cystic duct, bile can neither enter nor leave the gallbladder, but flow of bile from the liver into the duodenum is not disturbed even though storage of bile in the gallbladder is no longer possible. If the gallbladder is the site of a chronic infection, the impaction of the stone may precipitate a flare-up of the infection in the gallbladder called **cholecystitis** (FIGURE 25). If there is no underlying gallbladder infection, the bile trapped within the gallbladder by the impacted stone is gradually absorbed into the bloodstream, and eventually the contents

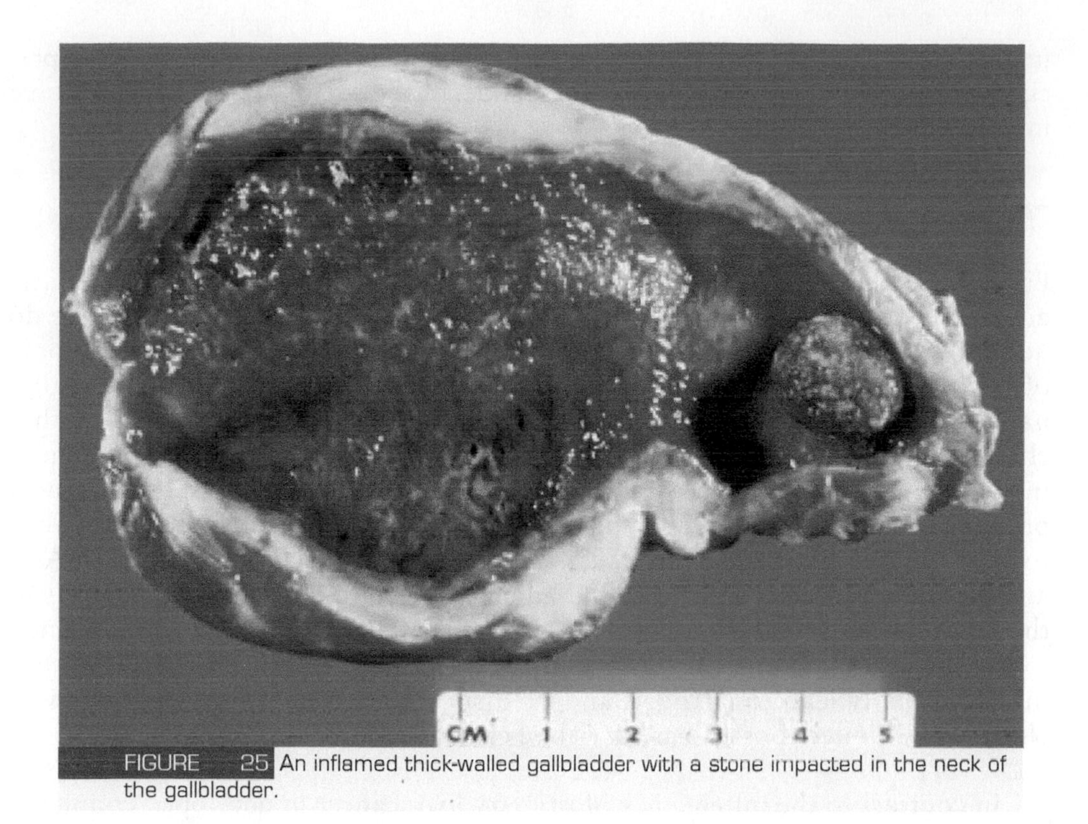

FIGURE 25 An inflamed thick-walled gallbladder with a stone impacted in the neck of the gallbladder.

of the gallbladder consist only of mucus that has been secreted by the epithelial cells lining the gallbladder.

If the stone blocks the common duct, bile can no longer be excreted into the duodenum, and it accumulates in the bloodstream. This condition is called obstructive jaundice.

TREATMENT OF GALLSTONES

The standard treatment of gallstones producing symptoms is surgical removal of the diseased gallbladder. In the past, it was necessary to perform a major surgical operation to remove the gallbladder. Now, most cholecystectomies can be performed by means of a laparoscopic procedure through a very small incision in the abdomen. It is possible, however, to dissolve cholesterol gallstones in some carefully selected patients who want to avoid a surgical procedure. This is accomplished by administering a bile salt (either ursodeoxycholic acid or chenodeoxycholic acid or a combination of both), which decreases the amount of cholesterol excreted in the bile. As the cholesterol content of the bile decreases, the bile becomes more unsaturated with cholesterol, and more cholesterol can be dissolved in the bile. As a result, the cholesterol contained within the gallstones becomes soluble in the unsaturated bile, and the gallstones slowly dissolve. Unfortunately, even if the stones are dissolved successfully, new stones often form within the gallbladder after the treatment is discontinued.

Cholecystitis

Inflammation of the gallbladder is called **cholecystitis** (*chole* = bile + *cyst* = bladder + *itis* = inflammation). It is a relatively common disease. Chronic cholecystitis appears to predispose an individual to develop gallstones. As previously described,

Cholecystitis
(ko′lē-sis-tī′-tis)
An inflammation of the gallbladder.

impaction of a gallstone in the neck of the gallbladder or the cystic duct may precipitate an acute cholecystitis if the gallbladder is the site of a preexisting chronic inflammation.

Tumors of the Liver and Gallbladder

Adenoma
A benign tumor arising from glands.

Primary tumors of the liver and gallbladder are uncommon. Benign hepatic **adenomas** develop occasionally in women taking contraceptive pills, but we do not know why the pills predispose to tumors in some women. Primary carcinoma of the liver is quite rare in the United States and Canada but is a common malignant tumor in Asian and African countries. The current evidence indicates that chronic carriers of the hepatitis B virus (HBV) not only have a relatively high incidence of chronic liver disease, but also carry an increased risk of developing a primary liver carcinoma, suggesting that chronic HBV infection predisposes both to liver injury and to liver cancer. The frequency of primary liver cancer in Asia and Africa is probably related to the high incidence of chronic HBV carriers in these populations. Failure of the body's immune defenses to destroy the infected liver cells and eliminate the virus leads to a smoldering chronic infection that may eventually lead to cirrhosis and predisposes to liver cancer. Patients with chronic HCV infections also are at risk of cirrhosis and liver cancer (FIGURES 26 AND 27).

In contrast to the infrequency of primary liver cancer in developed countries, the liver is a common site of metastatic carcinoma (FIGURE 28). Carcinoma arising in the gastrointestinal tract may spread to the liver, bits of tumor being carried to the liver in the portal venous blood. Tumors from the breast, lung, and other sites also often spread to the liver. The tumor cells are carried in the blood delivered to the liver by the hepatic artery. Sometimes, enlargement of the liver

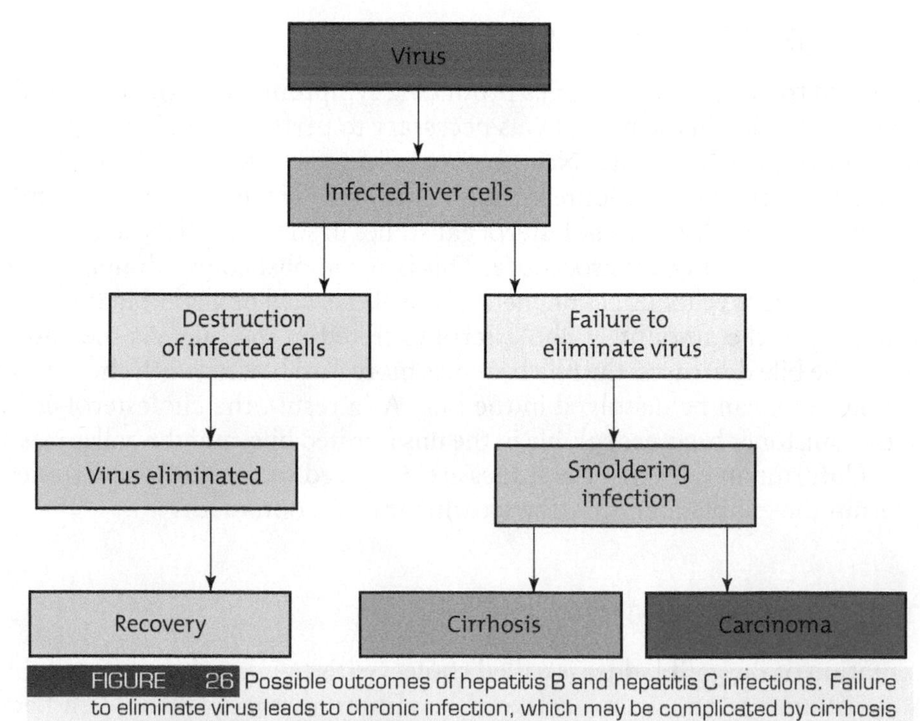

FIGURE 26 Possible outcomes of hepatitis B and hepatitis C infections. Failure to eliminate virus leads to chronic infection, which may be complicated by cirrhosis and liver cancer.

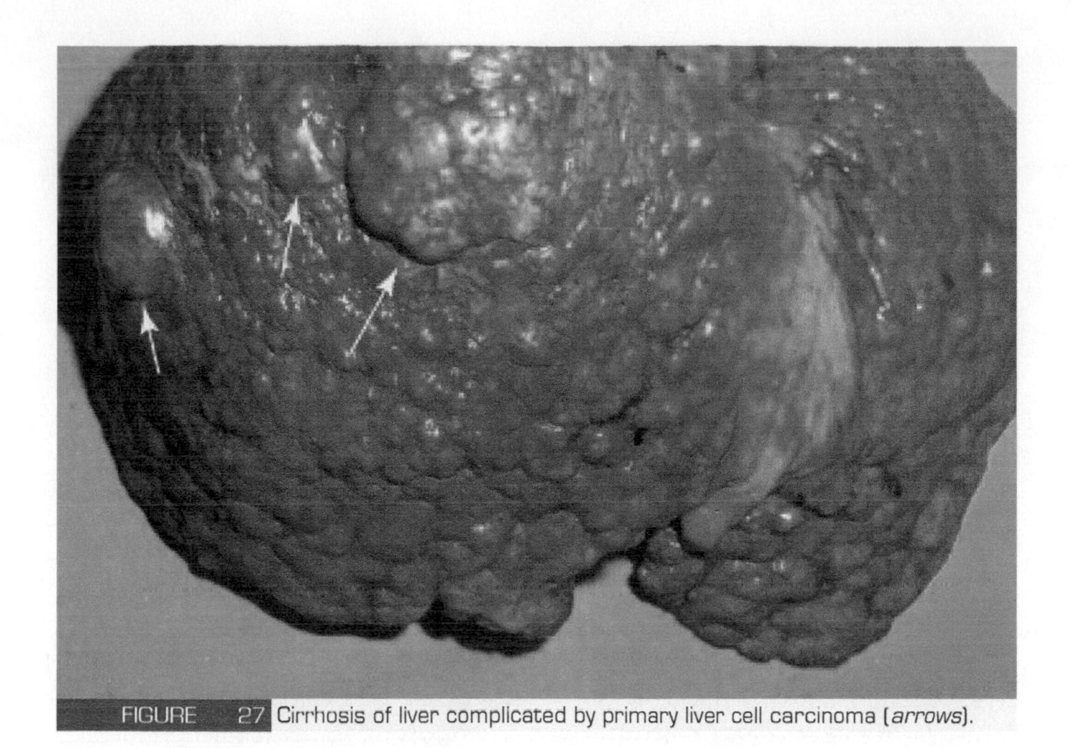

FIGURE 27 Cirrhosis of liver complicated by primary liver cell carcinoma (*arrows*).

as the result of metastatic carcinoma may be the first sign of a malignant tumor that originated in some other part of the body. Various diagnostic procedures can be used to identify tumors in the liver. The computed tomographic (CT) scan described in the discussion on general concepts of disease: principles of diagnosis is a very effective means of detecting cysts and tumors in the liver (FIGURE 29).

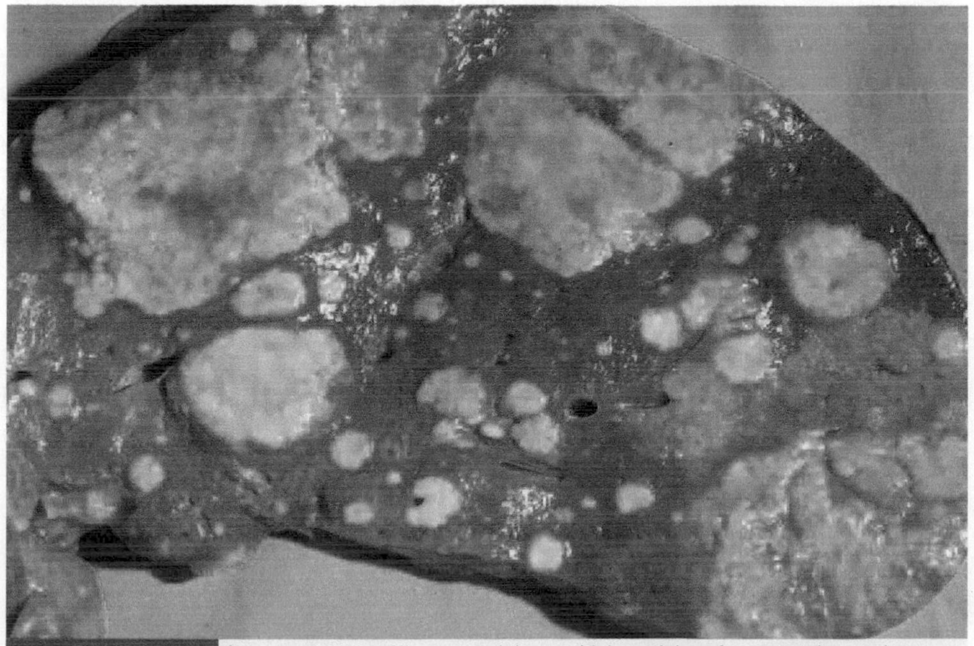

FIGURE 28 A cross section of liver containing multiple nodules of metastatic carcinoma.

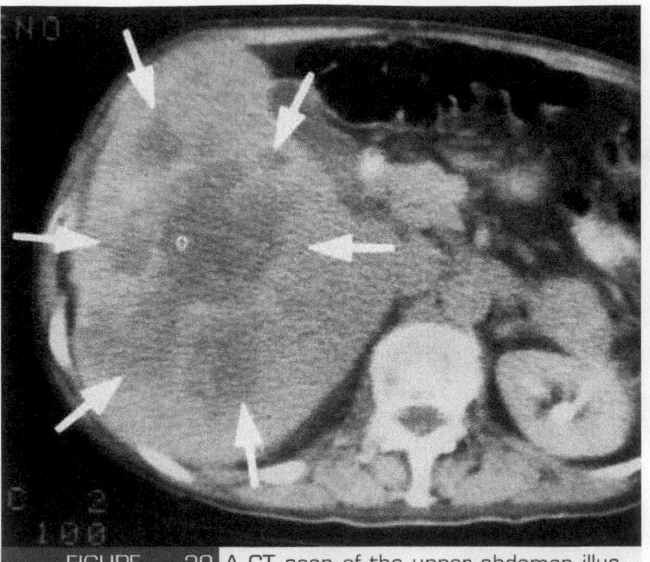

FIGURE 29 A CT scan of the upper abdomen illustrating the liver and upper abdominal organs. A large irregular area in the liver (*arrows*) is caused by deposit of metastatic carcinoma.

Jaundice

Jaundice
(jawn'dis)
Yellow color of the skin that results from accumulation of bile pigment within the blood.

Jaundice is a yellow discoloration of the skin and the sclerae (whites of the eyes) that results from accumulation of bile pigment (bilirubin) in the tissues and body fluids. This accumulation can have several causes. Bile pigment is derived from the breakdown of red cells, as described elsewhere in this text. The pigment is extracted from the blood by the liver cells, conjugated, and excreted into the biliary ducts. It is convenient to classify jaundice on the basis of the disturbance responsible for the retention of bile pigment. On this basis, jaundice is classified as hemolytic, hepatocellular, or obstructive. Jaundice can usually be classified correctly on the basis of certain laboratory tests in conjunction with the clinical features.

HEMOLYTIC JAUNDICE

In conditions associated with accelerated breakdown of red cells, excessive bile pigment is delivered to the liver, beyond the liver's ability to conjugate and excrete the pigment. Therefore, unconjugated bile pigment accumulates in the blood. Hemolytic jaundice is sometimes seen in adults with hemolytic anemia, but it is encountered most frequently in newborn infants with hemolytic disease as a result of blood group incompatibility between mother and infant (discussion on prenatal development and diseases associated with pregnancy).

HEPATOCELLULAR JAUNDICE

If the liver is severely damaged, as in hepatitis or cirrhosis, conjugation of bilirubin is impaired. Moreover, the excretion of conjugated bilirubin is extremely hampered because of injury to liver cells and disruption of small bile channels that lie between liver cell cords. As a result, conjugated bilirubin leaks back into the blood through the ruptured intrahepatic bile channels.

OBSTRUCTIVE JAUNDICE

In obstructive jaundice, the extraction and conjugation of bilirubin by liver cells are not impaired, but jaundice develops because the bile duct is obstructed, preventing delivery of bile into the duodenum. Often, the obstruction is caused by an impacted stone in the common duct. Carcinoma of the head of the pancreas is another common cause of common bile duct obstruction. As indicated in Figure 4, the common duct passes very close to the head of the pancreas as it enters the duodenum. Therefore, a pancreatic tumor frequently compresses and invades the common duct. As previously described, long-standing common bile duct obstruction leads to obstructive biliary cirrhosis.

Biopsy of the Liver

Many times, the exact cause and extent of liver disease in a given patient is difficult to determine. In such cases, a biopsy of the liver can be performed by inserting a needle through the skin directly into the liver and extracting a small bit of liver tissue. This can be examined microscopically by the pathologist, and generally, an exact diagnosis of the nature and severity of the liver disease can be made. This information can provide a basis for proper treatment.

QUESTIONS FOR REVIEW

1. What are some of the principal functions of the liver? How does the blood supply to the liver differ from that to the other organs? Why does severe liver disease cause disturbances in blood clotting?
2. What is the difference between hemoglobin and bilirubin? How does conjugated bilirubin differ from unconjugated bilirubin? What is the difference between bilirubin and bile? What role does bile play in digestion?
3. What are the possible causes and effects of liver injury (see Figure 5)? What is the usual outcome of a liver injury?
4. What is viral hepatitis? What are its major symptoms? How is hepatitis transmitted?
5. What is the difference between hepatitis A and hepatitis B? What is anicteric hepatitis? What is subclinical hepatitis?
6. What effect does alcohol have on the liver? What types of liver disease are associated with excessive alcohol ingestion?
7. What is cirrhosis? What liver diseases may lead to cirrhosis? Why does portal hypertension develop in patients with cirrhosis? Why does ascites develop in patients with cirrhosis? Why do esophageal varices develop?
8. What is jaundice? How is jaundice classified? Under what circumstances do gallstones cause jaundice?
9. What factors predispose to the development of gallstones?
10. What is the difference between viral hepatitis and alcoholic hepatitis?

SUPPLEMENTARY READINGS

Angulo, P. 2002. Nonalcoholic fatty liver disease. *The New England Journal of Medicine* 346:1221–31.

► Nonalcoholic fatty liver disease affects from 20 to 24% of the population and also occurs in 57–74% of obese subjects. Pathogenesis of the disease is described. Most affected persons have no symptoms of liver disease, but laboratory tests reveal abnormal liver function tests. Diffuse fatty change within the liver can be demonstrated by ultrasound examination, by computed tomography (CT) scans, or by magnetic resonance imaging (MRI). Liver biopsy can assess the extent of the liver cell damage caused by the fatty change. Advanced liver cell damage with associated scarring and inflammation cannot be differentiated from alcohol-related liver disease.

Bleich, H. L., and Boro, E. S. 1977. Metabolic and hepatic effects of alcohol. *The New England Journal of Medicine* 296:612–6.

- Describes the metabolism of alcohol by the liver and effects of alcohol on carbohydrate, protein, and fat metabolism. Describes alcohol-related disorders.

Centers for Disease Control and Prevention. 1993. Hepatitis E among U.S. travelers. *Morbidity and Mortality Weekly Report* 42:1–4.

- Hepatitis E outbreaks in third world countries are related to contaminated water supplies. Although the infection is not established in the United States, a few cases have been reported, and cases of hepatitis E may become more frequent among residents of states at the US–Mexico border. Gamma globulin does not contain anti-HEV antibodies; thus, gamma globulin does not provide protection against infection.

Galperin, C., and Gershwin, E. 1997. Immunopathogenesis of gastrointestinal and hepatobiliary diseases. *Journal of the American Medical Association* 278:1946–55.

- Discusses viral hepatitis, autoimmune hepatitis, and primary biliary cirrhosis.

Gross, J. B., Jr. 1998. Clinician's guide to hepatitis C. *Mayo Clinic Proceedings* 73:355–60.

- A review article dealing with epidemiology, diagnosis, prognosis, and treatment.

Hoofnagel, J. H., and Seeff, L. B. 2006. Peginterferon and ribavirin for chronic hepatitis C. *New England Journal of Medicine* 355:2444–51.

- Hepatitis C is often silent, and most infected patients have few symptoms of infection. Persisting infection leads to cirrhosis in 20–30% of infected patients, and from 1–4% of patients with cirrhosis also develop hepatocellular carcinoma each year. Liver cell injury in infected patients results from activation of the immune system in which natural killer cells and cytotoxic T cells attempt to eliminate the virus-infected liver cells. Hepatitis C progresses more rapidly in HIV-infected persons. Treatment is recommended for all subjects with detectable hepatitis C viral RNA in their bloodstream, elevation of serum enzyme levels indicating liver damage, and a positive liver biopsy indicating the characteristics and the severity of the liver cell injury. A 48-week course of treatment consists of weekly subcutaneous injection of pegylated interferon (a long-acting interferon produced by attaching polyethylene glycol to the interferon molecule) and twice daily oral doses of ribavirin. Unfortunately, the course of therapy has a high rate of side effects.

Jensen, D. M. 2011. A new era of hepatitis C therapy begins. *The New England Journal of Medicine* 364:1272–74.

- Boceprevir inhibits the protease complex of type 1 HCV when given along with interferon and ribavirin but has no significant effect against other HCV types. Side effects include anemia and neutropenia.

Kaplan, M. M., and Gershwin, M. E. 2005. Primary biliary cirrhosis. *The New England Journal of Medicine* 353:1261–73.

- Long-term outcome of this autoimmune disease has improved in recent years. Autoimmune damage to the liver appears to be related to antibodies directed against a bacterial or viral antigen that cross-reacts with similar antigens within liver cell mitochondria, and such antibodies are considered diagnostic of the disease. Treatment with a bile acid (ursodeoxycholic acid) appears promising.

Krawitt, E. L. 2006. Autoimmune hepatitis. *The New England Journal of Medicine* 354:54–66.

- Another autoimmune disease that appears to be caused by antibodies formed as a result of a viral infection in which antiviral antibodies cross-react with similar antigens in liver cells. Has many features similar to primary biliary cirrhosis, and the two conditions may be related.

Lauer, G. M., and Walker, B. 2001. Hepatitis C virus infection. *The New England Journal of Medicine* 345:41–52.

- A review of the current status of the disease and methods of treatment. In the United States, 1.8% of the population is positive for HCV antibodies, and 75% of seropositive persons have circulating virus in their bloodstream, indicating active HCV infection.

Navarro, V. J., and Senior, J. R. 2006. Drug-related hepatotoxicity. *New England Journal of Medicine* 354:731–39.

- Describes and classifies hepatotoxic drugs based on their clinical presentation and approaches to treatment. Acetaminophen is a commonly encountered hepatotoxin.

Poordad, F., McCone, J., Jr., Bacon, B. R., et al. 2011. Boceprevir for untreated chronic HCV genotype 1 infection. *The New England Journal of Medicine* 364:1195–206.

- Boceprivir is a potent protease inhibitor of HCV type 1 in conjunction with ribavirin and interferon is effective against type 1 HCV in whom previous treatment has been ineffective.

Scott, J. D., and Gretch, D. R. 2007. Molecular diagnostics of hepatitis C virus infection: A systematic review. *Journal of the American Medical Association* 297:724–32.

- Hepatitis C is a serious disease and is not always detected because many infected persons do not have symptoms of infection, anti-HCV antibodies may not be detected in their blood, and liver function tests indicating liver injury may not be abnormal. The conclusive test of infection is a nucleic acid test to identify viral RNA (HCV RNA) in the blood of the infected person. The test can also be used to monitor changes in the amount of circulating viral RNA in response to treatment. There are six different strains of virus designated genotypes 1 through 6, which respond differently to treatment, and genotype identification helps the physician select the type and duration of treatment.

Seef, L. B., et al. 2000. 45-year follow-up of hepatitis C virus infection in healthy young adults. *Annals of Internal Medicine* 132:105–11.

- The rate of HCV infection was determined from reexamination of frozen serum specimens collected from military recruits between 1948 and 1954 and revealed 0.1% infection rate in whites and 1.8% infection rate in African Americans. A 45-year follow-up revealed that liver disease occurred in 11.8% of HCV-positive persons and 2.4% of HCV-negative persons. One HCV-positive person died of liver disease. Healthy HCV-positive persons are at low risk of progressing to end-stage chronic liver disease.

Steffen, R., Kane, M. A., Shapiro, C. N., et al. 1994. Epidemiology and prevention of hepatitis A in travelers. *Journal of the American Medical Association* 272:885–89.

- Hepatitis A vaccine (or gamma globulin if vaccine not available) is recommended for all nonimmune travelers visiting developing countries.

Zemel, G., Katzen, B. T., Becker, G. J., et al. 1991. Percutaneous transjugular portosystemic shunt. *Journal of the American Medical Association* 266:390–93.

- An intrahepatic shunt between a branch of the hepatic and portal veins can decompress the portal venous pressure effectively.

OUTLINE SUMMARY

Structure and Function of the Liver

IMPORTANT FEATURES

Complex metabolic functions.
Double blood supply from hepatic artery and portal vein.
Liver lobule is basic structural unit.
Branches of hepatic artery, portal vein, and bile duct travel in portal tracts.
Blood flow in lobule is from portal tract to central vein.
Bile flow in canaliculi is from central vein toward portal tract.

Bile

FORMATION AND EXCRETION OF BILIRUBIN

Bile pigment derived from breakdown of red blood cells in reticuloendothelial system.
Conjugation and excretion by liver.

COMPOSITION AND PROPERTIES

Contains bile pigment, cholesterol, bile salts, lecithin, and other materials.
Functions as biologic detergent: no digestive enzymes.

Causes and Effects of Liver Injury

MANIFESTATIONS

Cell necrosis.
Fatty change.
Mixed necrosis and fatty change.

CLINICAL EFFECTS

Mild injury with complete recovery.
Severe injury with hepatic failure.
Chronic or progressive injury causes scarring with impaired liver function.

COMMON TYPES OF LIVER INJURY

Viral hepatitis.
Fatty liver.
Alcoholic liver disease.
Cirrhosis.

Viral Hepatitis

CLINICAL MANIFESTATIONS AND COURSE

One third become sick and jaundiced.
One third become sick but not jaundiced.
One third asymptomatic but liver function abnormal.

HEPATITIS A

RNA virus.
Short incubation period.
Virus in secretions and stools during early phases.
Transmitted by direct contact or contaminated food or water.
Self-limited, low mortality, no carriers.
Gamma globulin provides protection.
Immunization available.

HEPATITIS B

DNA virus.
Long incubation.
Large amount of surface antigen produced by virus can be detected in blood of carriers and infected persons.
Ten percent of infected persons become chronic carriers of virus.
High carrier rate in some populations.
Transmitted by blood or secretions of infected persons.
Gamma globulin provides some protection.
Immunizing vaccine provides protection against infection.

HEPATITIS C

Transmitted like hepatitis B.
Incubation period intermediate between HAV and HBV.
Many persons become chronic carriers.
No immunization available.
Gamma globulin does not provide protection.

HEPATITIS D (DELTA HEPATITIS)

Virus only infects persons with acute or chronic HBV infection.
Delta virus unable to produce own virus coat and uses HBsAg produced by HBV.

HEPATITIS E

OTHER HEPATITIS VIRUSES

Epstein-Barr (EB) virus.
Cytomegalovirus.

HEPATITIS AMONG MALE HOMOSEXUALS

Spread by sexual practices.

ALCOHOLIC LIVER DISEASE

Fatty Liver

PATHOGENESIS

Fat accumulates in liver cells owing to liver injury.
Common in heavy drinkers and alcoholics.
Sometimes caused by other chemicals and solvents.
Impaired liver function but injury reversible.
May also occur in obese subjects with insulin resistance and other manifestations of metabolic syndrome.

Alcoholic Liver Disease

MANIFESTATIONS

Three stages of progressively increasing severity.
Related to amount and duration of alcohol consumption.
Fatty liver: cells accumulate fat.
Alcoholic hepatitis: cell necrosis with Mallory bodies and inflammation.
Cirrhosis: diffuse scarring throughout liver.

Cirrhosis of the Liver

DEFINITION

Scarring in liver from any cause.

Repeated bouts of alcoholic hepatitis.

Massive liver necrosis.

Repeated episodes of liver injury.

Associated derangements of liver cell regeneration and liver function.

MANIFESTATIONS

Impaired liver function.

Portal hypertension.

Bypass routes connect systemic-portal venous systems.

Risk of fatal hemorrhage from esophageal varices.

PROCEDURES TO TREAT CIRRHOSIS

Portal–systemic anastomoses to control varices.

Splenorenal shunt.

Portacaval shunt.

Intrahepatic portosystemic shunt.

BILIARY CIRRHOSIS

Primary

An autoimmune disease attacking small intrahepatic bile ducts.

No specific treatment. May lead to liver failure and require liver transplant.

Secondary

Obstruction of large extrahepatic bile ducts.

Treated by relieving duct obstruction or bypassing obstruction.

Reye's Syndrome

PATHOGENESIS

Probably related to combined effect of viral illness and aspirin.

Acetaminophen recommended rather than aspirin to reduce risk.

CHARACTERISTICS

Affects primarily infants and children.

Fatty liver with liver dysfunction.

Cerebral edema with neurologic dysfunction.

No specific treatment available.

Cholelithiasis

FACTORS AFFECTING SOLUBILITY OF CHOLESTEROL IN BILE

Cholesterol insoluble in aqueous solution.

Dissolved in micelles composed of bile salts and lecithin.

Solubility of cholesterol depends on ratio of cholesterol to bile salts and lecithin.

Supersaturated bile promotes calculi.

COMPLICATIONS OF GALLSTONES

Asymptomatic in gallbladder.

Biliary colic results if stone extruded into ducts.

Common duct obstruction: obstructive jaundice.

Cystic duct obstruction: no jaundice, but acute cholecystitis may occur if preexisting infection of gallbladder.

TREATMENT OF GALLSTONES

Cholecystectomy.

Chenodeoxycholic acid dissolves gallstones.

Cholecystitis

Chronic infection common.

Gallstones may predispose to infection.

Impaction of stone in neck of gallbladder may precipitate acute cholecystitis.

Tumors of the Liver and Gallbladder

INCIDENCE

Benign adenomas uncommon: occur in women taking oral contraceptives.

Primary carcinoma uncommon: occurs in patients with cirrhosis.

Metastatic carcinoma common.

Spread from gastrointestinal tract, breast, lung, or other sites.

CT scan aids in recognition.

Jaundice

CLASSIFICATION

Hemolytic: excessive red cell breakdown.

Hepatocellular: liver cell injury.

Obstructive: common duct obstruction by tumor or stone.

Biopsy of the Liver

INDICATIONS AND METHOD

Indicated when cause of liver disease undetermined after clinical and laboratory evaluation.

Needle inserted through skin directly into liver.

Biopsy specimen examined histologically by pathologist.

http://health.jbpub.com/humandisease/9e

Human Disease Online is a great source for supplementary human disease information for both students and instructors. Visit this website to find a variety of useful tools for learning, thinking, and teaching.

The Pancreas and Diabetes Mellitus

LEARNING OBJECTIVES

1. Describe the pathogenesis and treatment of acute pancreatitis.
2. Describe the pathogenesis, manifestations, complications, and prognosis of pancreatic cystic fibrosis.
3. Differentiate between the two principal types of diabetes mellitus with respect to pathogenesis, incidence, manifestations, complications, and treatment.

Structure and Function of the Pancreas

The pancreas is actually two glands in one: a digestive gland and an endocrine gland. The exocrine tissue of the pancreas, which is concerned solely with digestion, secretes an alkaline pancreatic juice rich in digestive enzymes into the duodenum through the pancreatic duct. The powerful digestive enzymes break down proteins (trypsin and chymotrypsin), carbohydrates (amylase), and fats (lipase). The protein-digesting (proteolytic) enzymes are secreted in an inactive form and are activated after they are discharged into the duodenum. The endocrine tissue of the pancreas consists of multiple small clusters of cells scattered throughout the gland called the pancreatic islets or **islets of Langerhans**, which discharge their secretions directly into the bloodstream. Each islet is composed of several different types of cells. The three main types are alpha cells, beta cells, and delta cells. Alpha cells secrete a hormone called glucagon. The more numerous beta cells secrete insulin in response to a rise in blood glucose after eating, which restores blood glucose to normal. Both glucagon and insulin regulate the level of glucose in the blood but have opposing effects. Glucagon raises blood glucose; insulin lowers it. Delta cells produce a hormone called somatostatin, which inhibits secretion of both glucagon and insulin. Three other relatively rare cell types also have been described, and they produce hormones concerned primarily with regulating gastrointestinal functions. FIGURE 1 shows the anatomy and cellular structure of the pancreas.

Islets of Langerhans (län′ger-hänz) *Cluster of endocrine cells in the pancreas.*

Pancreatitis

ACUTE PANCREATITIS

Acute pancreatitis is caused by escape of pancreatic juice from the ducts into the substance of the pancreas, which leads to destruction of pancreatic acinar and islet tissue by activated pancreatic enzymes, accompanied by acute inflammation of the affected pancreatic tissue. Some of the enzymes leak from the damaged tissue into the bloodstream, where elevated levels of amylase and lipase can be detected by appropriate laboratory tests. The clinical manifestations of acute pancreatitis depend on how much pancreatic tissue has been damaged. Mild episodes are accompanied by abdominal pain together with elevated pancreatic enzymes detected by blood tests; however, the pain subsides, and the patient recovers. Patients with severe acute pancreatitis have marked abdominal pain and tenderness, and they are seriously ill. The activated pancreatic enzymes not only destroy much of the pancreas but also damage pancreatic blood vessels, which lead to marked hemorrhage in the damaged tissues. This condition is often called **acute hemorrhagic pancreatitis** (FIGURE 2).

Acute hemorrhagic pancreatitis *Severe pancreatic inflammation with necrosis of pancreatic ducts and release of pancreatic enzymes that damage the pancreas*

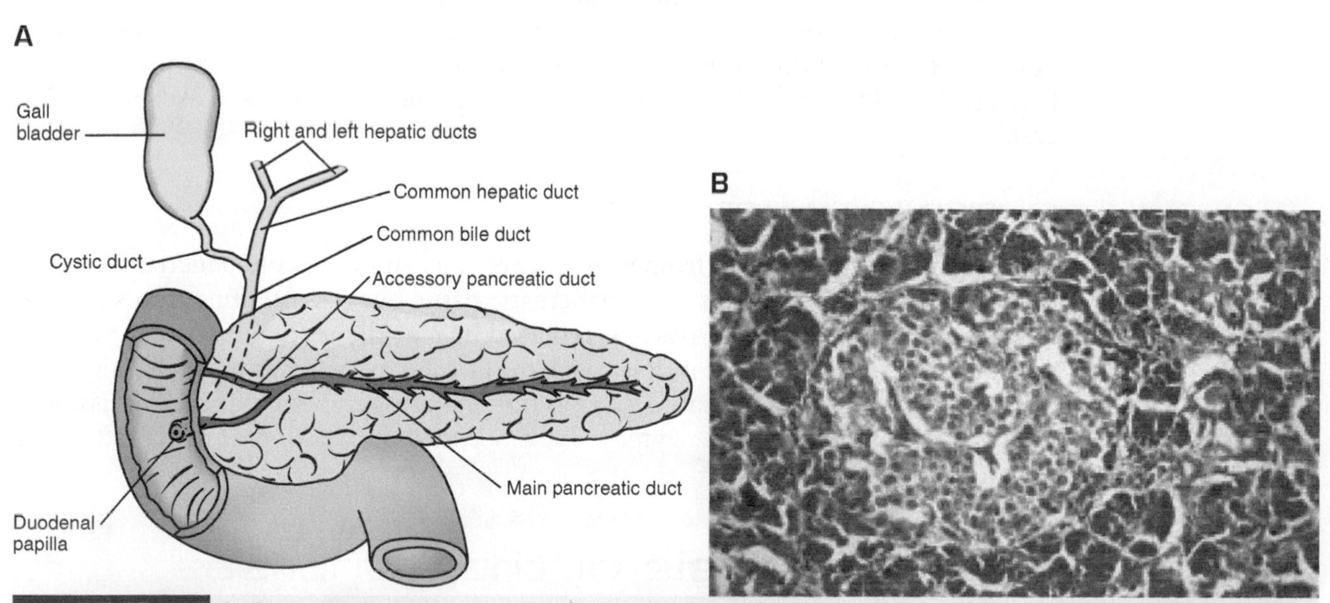

FIGURE 1 **A**, Duct system of pancreas. The main pancreatic duct usually joins the common bile duct to form a common channel that enters the duodenum by a single opening at the apex of a nipplelike projection called the duodenal papilla (ampulla of Vater). A much smaller accessory pancreatic duct, illustrated in the diagram, is frequently present and opens into the duodenum by a separate opening proximal to the duodenal papilla. **B**, A photomicrograph of pancreatic islet surrounded by exocrine pancreatic tissue.

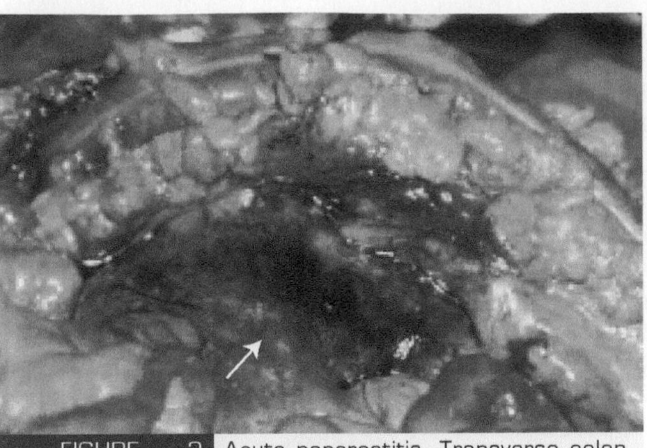

FIGURE 2 Acute pancreatitis. Transverse colon (*upper part of photograph*) has been elevated to reveal pancreas (*arrow*), which is inflamed and contains large areas of hemorrhage.

The pathogenesis of acute pancreatitis usually involves active secretion of pancreatic juice while the pancreatic duct is obstructed at its entrance into the duodenum. The buildup of obstructed secretions greatly increases the pressure within the duct system, causing the ducts to rupture and the pancreatic juice to escape. Two factors predispose to acute pancreatitis: disease of the gallbladder and excessive alcohol consumption.

Pancreatitis often develops in patients with gallstones because in most individuals, the common bile duct and common pancreatic duct usually enter the duodenum through a common channel (the ampulla of Vater). If a stone becomes impacted in the ampulla, it can obstruct the pancreatic duct and precipitate pancreatitis.

Patients who drink excessive amounts of alcohol also are prone to pancreatitis. Alcohol is a potent stimulus of pancreatic secretions, and it may also induce edema and spasm of the pancreatic sphincter in the ampulla of Vater. Pancreatitis develops because alcohol-induced hypersecretion combined with sphincter spasm leads to high intraductal pressure, followed by duct necrosis and escape of pancreatic juice.

CHRONIC PANCREATITIS

Chronic pancreatitis results from repeated episodes of mild acute pancreatitis. Each bout of pancreatitis destroys some pancreatic tissue but the inflammation subsides, and the damaged pancreatic tissue is replaced by scar tissue. Eventually, as progressively more pancreatic tissue is destroyed, the affected person has difficulty digesting and absorbing nutrients because there is not enough surviving pancreatic tissue to produce adequate digestive enzymes. The associated destruction of pancreatic islets may also lead to diabetes.

Cystic Fibrosis of the Pancreas

Cystic fibrosis is a relatively common, serious hereditary disease that is transmitted as an autosomal recessive trait and first becomes manifest in infancy and childhood. The disease has an incidence of about 1 per 3,000 whites but is quite rare in blacks and other races. The abnormal gene involved in the disease results from a mutation of a normal gene called the *CFTR* gene, which stands for cystic fibrosis transmembrane conductance regulator, a rather formidable term meaning that the gene regulates the movement of salt and water in and out of epithelial cells by means of ion channels located on the cell membranes. The gene has been localized to the long arm of chromosome 7, and a very large number of *CFTR* gene mutations have been identified. Tests have been developed to identify carriers of the more common gene mutations that are responsible for most cases of cystic fibrosis. The functions of the defective gene also appear to be modified by other genes that influence expression of the gene and the manifestations of the disease. In some individuals, the disease is relatively mild and compatible with survival into adolescence or adult life. Others, with more severe disease, die in childhood. Modern therapy has improved survival, but nevertheless, the average (median) life expectancy is only about 35 years.

As a result of the gene mutation, there is defective transport across cell membranes of chloride, sodium, and the water molecules in which they are dissolved. Electrolyte and water secretion is deficient in the mucus secreted by the epithelial cells of the pancreas, bile ducts, mucosa of respiratory tract, and other mucus-secreting cells throughout the body. As a result, the mucus becomes abnormally thick and tends to coagulate, forming dense plugs that obstruct the pancreatic ducts, bronchi and bronchioles, and bile ducts.

The most characteristic structural abnormalities are usually in the pancreas. Mucous plugs in the small pancreatic ducts block the secretion of pancreatic juice, which accumulates under increased pressure within the obstructed ducts. Eventually, the ducts become cystically dilated. The pancreatic secretory cells, unable to discharge their secretions into the duodenum, undergo atrophy and are replaced by fibrous tissue, but the pancreatic islets are unaffected because they discharge their hormones directly into the bloodstream. Eventually, the pancreas becomes converted into a mass of cystically dilated ducts surrounded by dense fibrous tissue (FIGURE 3). The name of the disease derives from these characteristic structural abnormalities.

In the lungs, the small bronchi and bronchioles become obstructed by the thick mucous secretions of the epithelial cells lining the respiratory tract. Bronchial obstruction predisposes to pulmonary infection, leading to bronchitis, bronchiectasis, and repeated bouts of pneumonia in the lung distal to the blocked bronchi. Eventually, the lungs are severely damaged by the repeated infections.

The function of sweat glands also is abnormal in cystic fibrosis. The sweat glands are unable to conserve sodium and chloride, and the sweat of affected individuals contains an excessively high salt concentration. This biochemical abnormality has served as the basis of a diagnostic test for cystic fibrosis called a sweat test. A small quantity of sweat is collected, and the sodium and chloride concentrations are determined. The salt concentration of the sweat is low in normal persons and high in persons with cystic fibrosis.

Many cystic fibrosis patients need to take capsules containing pancreatic enzymes in order to digest and absorb food properly because their own pancreas has been destroyed by the disease. Various types of treatment are also used to preserve as much pulmonary function as possible. Pulmonary infections caused by antibiotic-resistant bacteria are a serious problem and are difficult to deal with. Lungs so severely damaged by repeated infections that they can no longer function effectively can be treated by lung transplants.

The discovery of the *CFTR* gene and its defective counterpart have stimulated active research efforts that have led recently to the development of a drug that improved *CFTR* gene function, as demonstrated by more efficient chloride transport

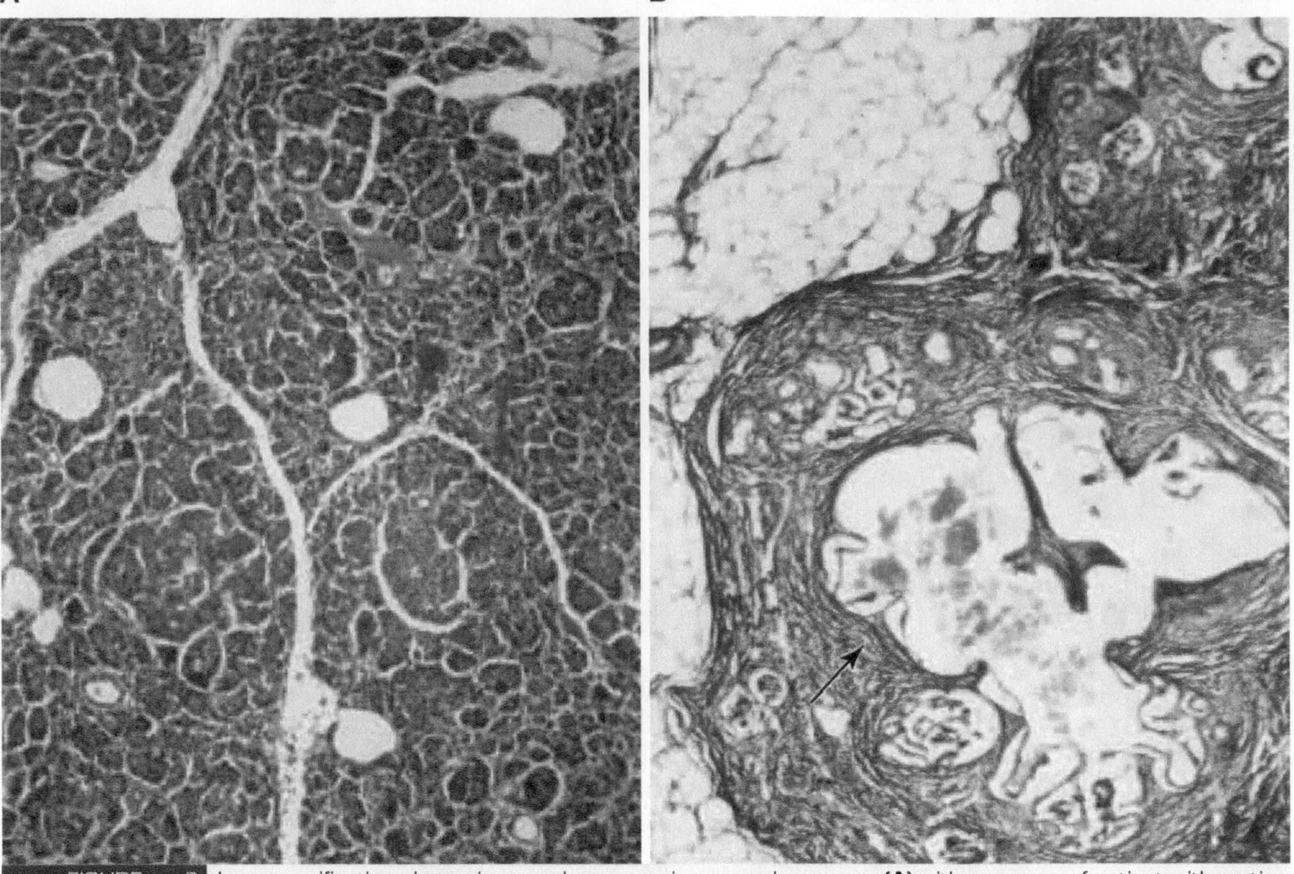

FIGURE 3 Low magnification photomicrographs comparing normal pancreas (**A**) with pancreas of patient with cystic fibrosis (**B**). Duct in center of field (*arrow*) exhibits cystic dilatation. Most of pancreatic glandular tissue has undergone atrophy and has been replaced by fibrous tissue (original magnification × 25).

across the cell membrane, which was associated with improved pulmonary function. These encouraging results have stimulated further pharmacologic studies designed to correct the biochemical disturbances resulting from the genetic defects responsible for cystic fibrosis.

Diabetes mellitus
(dī-u-bē′tēz mel′lit-is)
A metabolic disease characterized by hyperglycemia and caused by insufficient insulin secretion or inefficient utilization of insulin.

Hyperglycemia
(hī-per-glī-sē′mi-uh)
Excessively high blood glucose concentration.

Glycated hemoglobin test (Hemoglobin A_{1C} test)
A test that measures the amount of glucose permanently attached to hemoglobin, which is higher than normal in many persons with diabetes.

Diabetes Mellitus

Diabetes mellitus is a very common and important metabolic disease that results either because the pancreatic islets are incapable of secreting sufficient insulin or because the insulin is not being utilized efficiently. One of its major manifestations is an elevated level of glucose in the blood, which is called **hyperglycemia** (*hyper* = excess + *glyc* = sweet + *heme* = blood). A normal fasting blood glucose concentration is considered to be 60–100 mg per 100 ml of plasma, abbreviated 60–100 mg/dl. A diagnosis of diabetes requires a fasting glucose of 126 mg/dl or higher, which must be confirmed by repeat testing, or a glucose concentration over 200 mg/dl determined by an oral glucose tolerance test. Recently, another test called a **glycated hemoglobin test** also called the **hemoglobin A_{1C} test** is also acceptable, but with some reservations described later in this section.

Diabetes is divided into two major groups, depending on whether the diabetes results primarily from insulin deficiency, which is called type 1 diabetes, or from an inadequate response to insulin, which is called type 2 diabetes. Previously, type 1 diabetes was called insulin-dependent diabetes or juvenile-onset diabetes because it

TABLE 1

Comparison of two major types of diabetes mellitus

	Type 1	Type 2
Usual age of onset	Childhood Young adulthood	Middle age or later
Body build	Normal	Overweight
Plasma insulin	Absent or low	Normal or high
Complications	Ketoacidosis	Hyperosmolar coma
Response to insulin	Normal	Reduced
Response to oral antidiabetic drugs	Unresponsive	Responsive

resulted from insulin deficiency and often occurred in children and teenagers. Type 2 diabetes was called non-insulin–dependent diabetes or adult-onset diabetes because the islets produced insulin and the diabetes typically occurred in older adults. The two types of diabetes are not restricted to the age groups implied by this terminology, however, and these terms are used less frequently now.

TABLE 1 compares the major features of the two types.

TYPE 1 DIABETES MELLITUS

Type 1 diabetes is an autoimmune disease in which cytotoxic and delayed hypersensitivity T lymphocytes attack and destroy the pancreatic islets, assisted by antoantibodies directed against islet cells. The rate at which islets are destroyed by the immune system and the rate at which insulin secretion declines vary among affected subjects. In some, islet cell destruction proceeds rapidly, and in others, the destruction occurs more slowly. In some cases, onset of diabetes follows a viral infection, suggesting that the virus may have induced the disease by injuring or destroying the islets. Type 1 diabetes occurs primarily in children and young adults, and affected subjects are prone to develop a condition called **diabetic ketosis** caused by a lack of insulin. There is a hereditary predisposition to type 1 diabetes. Persons who inherit certain HLA-D types are at increased risk of acquiring this type of diabetes. (HLA types and predisposition to disease were considered in the discussion on chromosomes, genes, and cell division.)

Diabetic ketosis
A disturbance of the body's acid–base balance (acidosis) caused by an inability to utilize glucose, which requires the body to use fat as an energy source. Fat metabolism generates excessive amounts of acid ketone bodies, which disrupts the normal alkalinity of body fluids.

TYPE 2 DIABETES MELLITUS

Type 2 diabetes is by far the more common type and is a more complex metabolic defect. The pancreatic islets secrete normal or increased amounts of insulin, but the tissues are relatively insensitive to the action of insulin and are unable to respond appropriately. (Inadequate response to insulin is called *insulin resistance*.) The condition develops most frequently in older overweight and obese adults. The reason for the impaired response to insulin is not completely understood, but it seems to be related in some way to obesity because weight reduction restores insulin responsiveness and frequently controls the diabetes. Ketosis does not usually occur as a complication of type 2 diabetes, but affected persons may develop another complication called **hyperosmolar coma**, which results from the marked hyperglycemia.

Hyperosmolar coma
(hī-per-oz-mō′lär)
Coma resulting from neurologic dysfunction caused by hyperosmolarity of body fluids as a consequence of severe hyperglycemia.

Although insulin resistance plays an important role in the pathogenesis of type 2 diabetes, islet cell function is not completely normal either because the pancreas is unable to increase insulin output sufficiently to compensate for the insulin resistance.

Type 2 diabetes is a hereditary disease in which genetic factors play an even greater role than in type 1 diabetes, although in most cases we do not know the exact mode of inheritance or the genes that predispose to this type of diabetes. Children of parents who have type 2 diabetes are at significant risk of also eventually becoming diabetic. In some population groups, such as the Pima Indians of Arizona, as many as 40% of adults are diabetic.

PREDIABETES

Prediabetes
Higher than normal blood glucose but not high enough to establish diagnosis of diabetes.

In many people who eventually develop diabetes, blood glucose is higher than normal but not high enough to establish a diagnosis of diabetes. This condition was called impaired carbohydrate tolerance, later renamed **prediabetes**, to indicate that the number of insulin-producing beta cells is beginning to decline, and a further loss of islet cell function can lead to more marked hyperglycemia characteristic of diabetes. Often, a further reduction of functioning beta cells can be prevented or at least slowed by measures that make less demand on the pancreatic beta cells so that they do not have to "work as hard" to produce the amount of insulin required to return an elevated blood glucose to normal. Reducing the demands on the pancreas can be accomplished by weight loss if overweight, which reduces the insulin resistance of body cells so that less insulin is required; by moderate exercise, which uses the glucose as an energy source as it is being absorbed so less insulin is required; and by healthy eating habits emphasizing more slowly absorbed complex carbohydrates over sugar-rich foods that are absorbed quickly and raise blood glucose rapidly. All these measures help preserve beta cell function and promote more efficient utilization of glucose so that blood glucose does not rise as high after eating.

α-glucosidase (glu-ko-si-das) **inhibitor**
Inhibitor of an enzyme required to break down a glucose-containing disaccharide so glucose can be absorbed from the small intestine.

If diet and weight reduction are unable to lower postprandial (after eating) glucose elevations adequately, a drug can be added to improve glucose tolerance, which is called pharmacologic treatment. A frequently used type of glucose-lowering drug acts by inhibiting the absorption of glucose. Drugs of this type are called **α-glucosidase inhibitors** because they inhibit an enzyme required to absorb glucose from the small intestine. During the initial stages of carbohydrate digestion, complex carbohydrates are broken down into disaccharides, but only monosaccharides such as glucose and fructose can be absorbed and transported into the bloodstream. Breakdown of the disaccharides into glucose and other monosaccharides so they can be absorbed into the bloodstream is accomplished by an enzyme called **α-glucosidase** present on the absorbing surface (brush border) of intestinal epithelial cells, which breaks down disaccharides into glucose and other monosaccharides for absorption and transport into the bloodstream. An α-glucosidase inhibitor drug interferes with the disaccharide breakdown by inhibiting the α-glucosidase enzyme. Consequently, less glucose is available for absorption, which can help prevent progression to diabetes by reducing the glucose load presented to the overworked pancreatic beta cells. The effectiveness of this approach was demonstrated by a recent study involved two large groups of persons with prediabetes. One group was treated by weight reduction and diet; the other group received in addition an α-glucosidase inhibitor. After 2 years of observation, only 3.6% of the subjects receiving an α-glucosidase inhibitor had progressed to type 2 diabetes, in contrast to 9.6% of the other group who developed diabetes. Other drugs can also prevent progression of impaired carbohydrate tolerance to type 2 diabetes by reducing the demands on the less efficiently functioning pancreas. The same drugs used also to treat persons who have already developed type 2 diabetes are useful to slow the progression of prediabetes to diabetes.

PREGNANCY-ASSOCIATED DIABETES

As described in prenatal development and diseases associated with pregnancy, the high levels of placental hormones in pregnancy cause the pregnant woman to become less responsive to insulin (develop insulin resistance) but most women can compensate by secreting more insulin, and the blood glucose does not rise excessively. However, some women are unable to secrete enough additional insulin, and they develop pregnancy-related diabetes caused by their insulin resistance. The condition is called **gestational diabetes**, and is treated by diet along with supplementary insulin if necessary because hyperglycemia is harmful to the developing fetus. Although blood glucose returns to normal after delivery, a woman who has demonstrated significant insulin resistance during pregnancy is at risk of developing permanent diabetes in later years. Pregnancy-related diabetes serves as a "wake-up call" to begin taking steps that may avoid later permanent hyperglycemia: eating a healthy diet, controlling her weight, being active, and exercising moderately. A program of this type helps maintain normal blood glucose without promoting excessive insulin secretion, which helps preserve pancreatic beta cell function.

Gestational diabetes
Elevated blood glucose caused by insulin resistance resulting from elevated hormones related to the pregnancy. Blood glucose returns to normal postpartum, but woman has increased risk of diabetes later in life.

DIABETES AND THE METABOLIC SYNDROME

The term metabolic syndrome, also called the insulin resistance syndrome, is a group of conditions that often are identified in persons with impaired glucose tolerance or type 2 diabetes, and which can progress to diabetes-associated complications as well as cardiovascular disease and its complications. The metabolic syndrome components include

1. Obesity, especially when much of the excess fat accumulates in the abdomen
2. Insulin resistance, characterized by high normal or elevated blood glucose
3. Blood lipid abnormalities that predispose to cardiovascular disease (described in the discussion on the cardiovascular system), which is called dyslipidemia
4. Hypertension

Overweight people with excess abdominal fat, as indicated by their waist circumference (over 40 in. in men or 35 in. in women), should be screened for the other conditions associated with the syndrome by measuring blood pressure, blood glucose, and blood lipids. If other metabolic syndrome-associated abnormalities are detected, treatment to correct or improve the associated conditions can be undertaken.

ACTIONS OF INSULIN

Insulin has multiple effects that influence not only carbohydrate metabolism, but protein and fat metabolism as well. The chief sites of insulin action are on liver cells, muscle, and adipose tissue (fat). Insulin promotes entry of glucose into cells and favors utilization of glucose as a source of energy. In muscle and liver cells, it promotes storage of glucose as **glycogen**. In adipose tissue, insulin favors the conversion of glucose into fat (triglyceride) and storage of the newly formed triglyceride within the fat cells. Insulin also promotes entry of amino acids into the cells and stimulates protein synthesis. The main stimulus for insulin release is elevation of the level of glucose in the blood, as occurs after a meal.

Glycogen (glī'kō-jen)
A storage form of glucose present chiefly in liver and muscle.

FAT METABOLISM AND FORMATION OF KETONE BODIES

Fatty acid
A long, straight-chain carbon compound that contains a terminal carboxyl group, which enters into the formation of a triglyceride.

Acetyl coenzyme A
(acetyl-CoA)
A combination of a two-carbon acetate fragment with a complex organic compound called coenzyme A.

Ketone bodies
Various derivatives of acetyl-CoA, resulting from excessive mobilization of fat as an energy source.

Hyperglycemia
(hī-per-glī-sē'mi-ah)
Excessively high blood glucose concentration.

When fat is metabolized as a source of energy, it is split first into **fatty acids** and glycerol. The fatty acids are broken down into two carbon fragments, which are combined with a large carrier molecule called coenzyme A (CoA). The combination is called **acetyl coenzyme A** or acetyl-CoA. Some of the acetyl-CoA molecules are normally converted by the liver into compounds called **ketone bodies:** acetoacetic acid, beta-hydroxybutyric acid, and acetone. Acetoacetic acid is formed by condensation of two acetyl-CoA molecules, with loss of coenzyme A. Beta-hydroxybutyric acid is formed by the addition of a hydrogen atom to an oxygen atom, which becomes converted into a hydroxyl (OH) group. The term beta designates the carbon atom to which the hydroxyl group is attached. The first carbon after the carboxyl (COOH) group is called the alpha carbon, and the second is the beta carbon. Acetone is formed by removal of the carboxyl group of acetoacetic acid (FIGURE 4).

BIOCHEMICAL DISTURBANCES IN DIABETES

In diabetes mellitus, glucose is absorbed normally. However, because of lack of insulin or insulin insensitivity, it is not used normally for energy and is not stored normally as glycogen. Consequently, it accumulates in the bloodstream, resulting in a high level of blood glucose (hyperglycemia). The excessive glucose "spills over" in the urine and is excreted. Because glucose must be excreted in the urine in solution, the body loses excessive amounts of water and electrolytes along with the glucose. This may lead to disturbance in water balance and acid–base balance. (Water and electrolyte balance is discussed in water, electrolyte, and acid–base balance.)

Protein synthesis is also compromised, and body protein is broken down into amino acids. The liver converts these amino acids into glucose, augmenting the hyperglycemia and leading to additional losses of glucose, water, and electrolytes in the urine.

Diabetic Ketoacidosis

The person with type 1 diabetes, lacking insulin, is unable to use carbohydrates because insulin is required to promote entry of glucose into the cells where the glucose can be metabolized to yield energy. So the body turns to fat as an energy source.

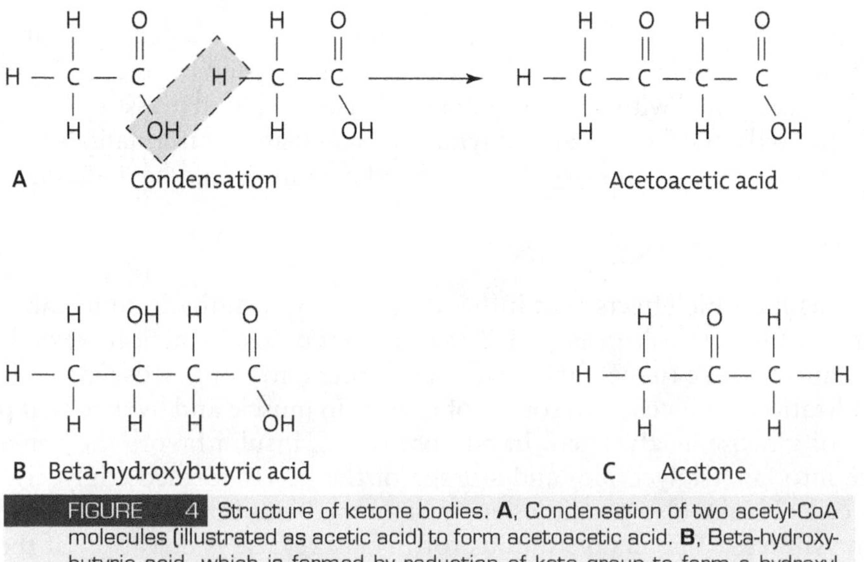

FIGURE 4 Structure of ketone bodies. **A**, Condensation of two acetyl-CoA molecules (illustrated as acetic acid) to form acetoacetic acid. **B**, Beta-hydroxybutyric acid, which is formed by reduction of keto group to form a hydroxyl group. **C**, Acetone formed by decarboxylation of acetoacetic acid.

Body fat is split into long-chain fatty acid molecules and glycerol. The fatty acids are broken down by enzymes into two carbon (acetyl) fragments, which are joined to coenzyme A to form acetyl coenzyme A (acetyl-CoA), but the acetyl-CoA molecules are produced in such large quantities that they cannot be oxidized efficiently to yield energy. Many of the acetyl CoA molecules condense to form ketone bodies, which can be used as an energy source, but so many ketone bodies are produced that the body cannot deal effectively with the excess. This condition is called **ketosis**. The ketone bodies accumulate in the blood and are excreted in the urine, carrying with them more water and electrolytes. The acid-ketone bodies can be buffered to some extent by the bicarbonate buffer systems in the bloodstream. If the diabetes is extremely severe, however, so many ketone bodies may be produced that the buffer systems cannot maintain a normal blood pH, and diabetic acidosis develops. The term ketoacidosis is often used for this type of acidosis because of its relationship to overproduction of ketone bodies. Severe acidosis may lead to coma because acidosis has an adverse effect on cerebral function.

Ketosis
An excess of ketone bodies in the blood resulting from utilization of fat as the primary source of energy.

All these effects can be reversed by supplying insulin, which promotes normal utilization of glucose and storage of glycogen. The disturbances of fat and protein metabolism also are reversed by the action of insulin. FIGURE 5 summarizes the major metabolic disturbances in type 1 diabetes.

The following case illustrates the clinical and biochemical disturbances in severe diabetic ketoacidosis.

CASE 1

A middle-aged woman with diabetes became unconscious while babysitting and was brought to the hospital by ambulance. Her temperature was moderately elevated. Respirations were rapid and deep. Blood pressure was normal. The patient was comatose but responded to painful stimuli. The skin was warm and dry. The remainder of the physical signs were normal. The patient's urine contained large amounts of glucose and a small amount of albumin. There was a strongly positive reaction for acetone and other ketone bodies. Blood glucose was 865 mg/dl (normal range 60–100 mg/dl). Other laboratory studies revealed a low blood pH and reduced plasma bicarbonate of 8 mEq/liter (normal range 24–28 mEq/liter). The patient was considered to have severe diabetic acidosis probably precipitated by a respiratory infection. She received intensive treatment with intravenous fluids, insulin, and antibiotics. Her condition gradually improved. The following day she was conscious and oriented and was able to take fluids orally. She continued to improve and was eventually discharged from the hospital on a diabetic diet and supplementary insulin therapy.

Hyperosmolar Hyperglycemic Nonketotic Coma

Persons with type 2 diabetes mellitus may become comatose as a result of the extreme hyperosmolarity of body fluids that results from severe hyperglycemia in the absence of ketosis. (Osmotic pressure and osmolarity are considered in the discussion on cells and tissues in connection with movement of materials into and out of cells.)

Although individuals with type 2 diabetes exhibit a reduced responsiveness to insulin, much less insulin is required to inhibit fat mobilization than is needed to promote entry of glucose into cells. In these subjects, the response to insulin is usually sufficient to prevent ketosis but inadequate to prevent hyperglycemia. Consequently,

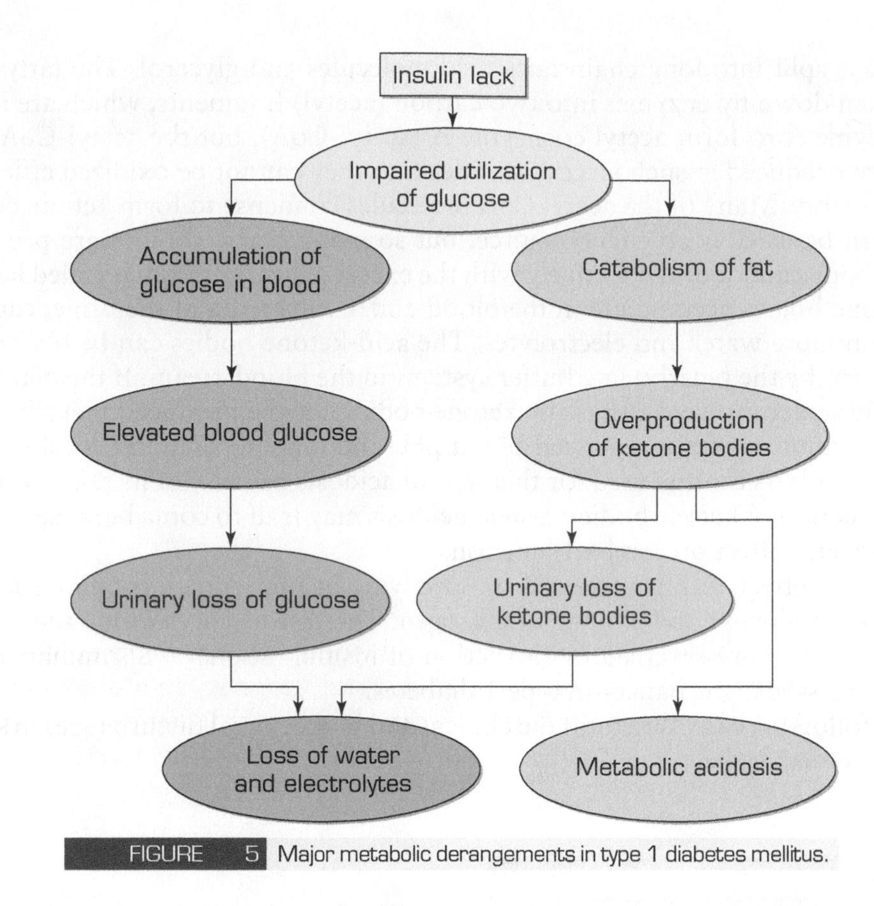

FIGURE 5 Major metabolic derangements in type 1 diabetes mellitus.

blood glucose rises, often to levels that are from 10 to 20 times normal. The extreme hyperglycemia causes the osmolarity of the body fluids to rise significantly, and water moves by osmosis from the cells into the more concentrated extracellular fluids. The cells become dehydrated, which disturbs the function of neurons and causes coma. Treatment consists of supplying insulin to reduce the hyperglycemia and administering hypotonic fluids to help reduce the hyperosmolarity of the body fluids, as illustrated by the following case.

CASE 2

A 52-year-old woman who was not previously known to be diabetic had experienced increased urinary output and thirst for the previous 2 weeks and had consumed large quantities of sugar-containing soft drinks. She became progressively more confused and eventually lapsed into coma. She was found by a neighbor and was brought to the hospital by ambulance. On admission, she was comatose and dehydrated. Her respiratory rate was not increased. Blood pressure was normal. The urine contained a large amount of glucose but no ketone bodies. Blood pH and bicarbonate were normal. Blood glucose was 1,750 mg/dl (normal range 60–100 mg/dl), and the osmolarity of the plasma was 396 mOsm/liter (normal range 280–295 mOsm/liter). A diagnosis of hyperosmolar nonketotic coma was made, and she was treated with large volumes of hypotonic (0.45%) saline solution and with insulin. Her condition gradually improved over the succeeding several days. Her blood glucose gradually fell toward normal and eventually reached 150 mg/dl on the fourth day. Plasma osmolarity also returned to normal as the elevated blood glucose declined.

MONITORING CONTROL OF DIABETES

The current goal of treatment is to achieve control of blood glucose that is as close as possible to normal, as close control of hyperglycemia reduces the long-term complications caused by diabetes. Tests used to monitor control of diabetes include

1. Frequent periodic measurements of blood glucose.
2. Measurement of a compound in the blood called **glycated hemoglobin** (also called hemoglobin A_{1C} and often abbreviated as HbA_{1C}) as an index of long-term control of hyperglycemia.
3. Urine tests for glucose used to be performed frequently to monitor blood glucose indirectly by detecting glucose spilling into the urine when blood glucose was too high, but are not used very often now because they have been replaced by frequent blood glucose tests. However, urine tests are still used in special situations, such as to check for ketone bodies as an indication of diabetic ketosis in persons with type 1 diabetes.

Glycated hemoglobin *Hemoglobin to which glucose molecules have become permanently attached. Concentration is related to concentration of glucose in the blood.*

Blood tests can be performed by the diabetic at home or at work. Blood testing products permit diabetics to monitor their own blood glucose at frequent intervals. A drop of blood is drawn by a sterile disposable lancet, collected on a specially treated strip of paper, and inserted into an instrument that displays the glucose concentration. Simple urine test strips are also available that can be dipped into a urine specimen and record a color change that is proportional to the amount of glucose in the urine.

The glycated hemoglobin test is a more complex test that must be done by a medical laboratory but is only necessary every 3–6 months. The test monitors how well the blood glucose is being controlled by treatment. Normally, a small amount of blood glucose becomes permanently attached to hemoglobin. This glucose–hemoglobin combination is called glycated hemoglobin, and its concentration is directly proportional to the average blood glucose concentration over the preceding 6–12 weeks, unlike the blood glucose test, which only indicates the concentration of blood glucose at the time the sample was collected. In normal persons, up to 6% of hemoglobin is glycated. In persons with very poorly controlled diabetes, the concentration may be much higher than normal. A value exceeding 6.5% indicates abnormally high blood glucose over the previous several weeks. Diabetics in whom blood glucose levels have been closely controlled can achieve glycated hemoglobin levels that are close to normal. Higher levels indicate less satisfactory control of blood glucose and indicate a need for more intensive treatment. In general, the better the long-term control of blood glucose, as indicated by a close to normal glycated hemoglobin value, the less likely the development of long-term late diabetic complications.

Currently, the glycated hemoglobin test is recommended by the American Diabetes Association as a diagnostic test for diabetes in nonpregnant adults. However, confirmation by blood glucose test results is recommended because the glycated hemoglobin test has some limitations and the results do not always correlate with blood glucose tests. To obtain a reliable glycated hemoglobin test result, the hemoglobin concentration must be normal and the hemoglobin must be hemoglobin A. The test will not be reliable if the hemoglobin is an abnormal hemoglobin, such as hemoglobin S or hemoglobin C, if the subject is anemic, or if the survival of the subject's red cells is shorter than normal.

TREATMENT OF DIABETES

Type 1 diabetics require insulin, and the dose should be adjusted in order to control the level of blood glucose as closely as possible because this appears to reduce late complications. Most type 1 diabetics require several insulin injections spaced throughout the day in order to maintain blood glucose within reasonably normal limits. Frequent measurements of blood glucose permit better regulation of insulin dosage and improve control of the diabetes.

Insulin pumps are sometimes useful for type 1 diabetics who are difficult to treat because of their need for frequent insulin injections. An insulin pump is a small battery-operated device that can be attached to the patient's belt. A short length of tubing extends from the pump to a fine (27 gauge) needle that is inserted into the subcutaneous tissue of the abdominal wall and secured with tape. The pump is programmed to deliver a small constant infusion of insulin, supplemented by larger doses just before meals, simulating the release of insulin by the pancreas. Despite the convenience, use of an insulin pump requires very close medical supervision because complications can arise from pump malfunction or infections at the site of needle placement. Many other devices are available to simplify insulin injections, and many different insulin preparations having different durations of activity are available. Human insulin produced by genetic engineering has almost completely replaced insulin from animal sources.

Type 1 diabetic patients are treated with insulin. Insulin dose, type of insulin used, and times of administration are adjusted to maintain blood glucose within a reasonably normal range.

Type 2 diabetic patients can often be managed by diet and weight reduction alone. If they do not respond adequately, oral hypoglycemic drugs are added. Several groups of drugs called oral hypoglycemic agents are available to treat type 2 diabetes. The four major groups are (1) sulfonurea drugs, (2) biguanide drugs, (3) α-glucosidase inhibitors, and (4) thiazolidinedione drugs. Sulfonurea drugs stimulate the pancreas to release insulin, which lowers blood glucose by stimulating the pancreas to work harder, even though the islets are already having difficulty supplying enough insulin. Biguanides do not stimulate insulin secretion. Instead they lower blood glucose by inhibiting the production of glucose from other nutrients primarily in the liver, which is called gluconeogenesis (*gluco* + glucose + *neo* = new + *genesis* = formation). The drug is not metabolized in the body and is excreted in the urine. α-Glucosidase inhibitor drugs lower blood glucose by inhibiting the enzyme that breaks down disaccharides into monosaccharides, a step required in order to absorb glucose from the small intestine. Thiazolidinedione drugs decrease insulin resistance so the secreted insulin is more effective. If diet, weight reduction, and hypoglycemic drugs do not control the hyperglycemia, insulin is used to regulate blood glucose in the same way that it is used in type 1 diabetes.

COMPLICATIONS OF DIABETES

Diabetics are liable to develop a number of complications that can be reduced to some extent by proper adherence to diet and other prescribed treatments. They have an increased susceptibility to infection, apparently related to the high levels of blood glucose. Pathogenic bacteria seem to grow more readily in the presence of elevated blood glucose levels. They may develop diabetic coma, as a result either of ketoacidosis or of the greatly increased osmolarity of body fluids resulting from hyperglycemia. They have a greater incidence of arteriosclerosis and its associated vascular complications such as strokes, heart attacks, and gangrene of the legs and feet as a result of poor circulation. The vascular problems probably result both from abnormalities in fat metabolism associated with diabetes and from the elevated blood lipids frequently found in diabetics. They are also subject to other late complications, which increase in frequency with the duration of the disease. The small blood vessels supplying the retina of the eye often undergo degenerative changes, which may eventually lead to blindness in some subjects. The glomerular arterioles and capillaries within the kidneys also undergo degenerative changes, which impair renal function and may result in renal failure (discussed in the section on the urinary system). The peripheral nerves may undergo degenerative changes, called peripheral neuritis, which cause pain and disturbed sensation in the extremities.

How high glucose leads to organ damage is not completely understood, but the organ damage is related either directly or indirectly to the hyperglycemia. One concept proposes that the hyperglycemia causes the proteins in the retina, peripheral nerves, and capillary basement membranes to undergo the same type of glycation as hemoglobin, and that the glycated proteins undergo further interactions with other cell components, leading eventually to the blood vessel and organ damage characteristic of long-standing poorly controlled diabetes.

OTHER CAUSES OF HYPERGLYCEMIA

Other conditions at times may lead to impaired glucose utilization and hyperglycemia, but they are much less common than true diabetes mellitus. These conditions include the following:

1. Chronic pancreatic disease, in which the hyperglycemia results from damage or destruction of pancreatic islets
2. Endocrine diseases associated with overproduction of pituitary or adrenal hormones because these hormones act in various ways to raise blood glucose
3. Ingestion of many different drugs, such as diuretics or antihypertensive drugs, in which glucose utilization is impaired as a side effect of the drug
4. A few rare hereditary diseases in which carbohydrate metabolism is disturbed

Hypoglycemia

The normal pancreas continually monitors the blood glucose and automatically adjusts its output of insulin to maintain the blood glucose level within the normal range. The type 1 diabetic patient, however, must adjust the dose of insulin to match the amount of carbohydrate to be metabolized. If there is insufficient insulin, the blood glucose is too high. If there is too much insulin, the blood glucose is too low, a condition called **hypoglycemia** (*hypo* = under). Two conditions predispose to hypoglycemia in a diabetic patient taking insulin. The first is a reduced intake of food, such as skipping a meal; blood glucose falls because carbohydrate intake is insufficient in relation to the amount of insulin injected. The second condition is increased activity, such as vigorous exercise, which lowers blood glucose by increasing glucose utilization. As a result, there is a relative excess of insulin. Too much insulin causes a precipitous drop in the level of glucose in the blood and initiates a chain of events called an insulin reaction or insulin shock. The adrenal medulla responds to the hypoglycemia by discharging epinephrine (adrenaline), which tends to raise blood glucose by converting liver glycogen into glucose. Epinephrine exerts widespread systemic effects as well: rapid heart rate, rise in blood pressure, constriction of cutaneous blood vessels causing the skin to appear pale, stimulation of sweat glands causing a cold sweat, and stimulation of the nervous system leading to increased excitability, anxiousness, hyperactive reflexes, and tremors.

Hypoglycemia (hī-pō-glī-sē′mē-ah) *Lower than normal concentration of glucose in the blood.*

Neurologic manifestations appear if the blood glucose continues to fall because the nervous system requires glucose to carry out its metabolic processes and begins to malfunction when deprived of its energy source. The subject becomes confused, loses consciousness, may have convulsions, and soon lapses into a deep coma. Prolonged severe hypoglycemia may cause permanent brain damage.

If the patient is still conscious and able to swallow, the insulin reaction can be stopped by ingesting a quick-acting carbohydrate, such as a piece of candy or a

TABLE 2

Differentiation of insulin shock from ketoacidosis and hyperosmolar coma

Diagnostic feature	Insulin shock	Ketoacidosis	Hyperosmolar coma
Food intake	May be insufficient	Normal or excessive	Normal or excessive
Insulin	Excessive	Insufficient	Normal or increased
Onset of symptoms	Rapid	Gradual (several days)	Gradual (several days)
Skin	Cold sweat, pale	Dry and flushed	Dry and flushed
Respirations	Normal or shallow	Slow and deep	Usually normal
Reflexes	Hyperactive	Depressed	Normal
Heart rate	Rapid	Rapid	Usually normal
Blood pressure	Normal or slightly elevated	Low	Usually normal
Glucose in urine	Absent	Large amount	Large amount
Blood glucose	Very low	High	Extremely high
Blood bicarbonate and pH	Normal	Low	Normal
Acetone in blood and urine	Absent	Present	Absent

glucose tablet. The diabetic patient should always have a quick-acting carbohydrate available for such emergencies. If the patient is unconscious, an injection of glucagon can be given; this raises blood glucose by mobilizing glucose from liver glycogen. A concentrated glucose solution may also be given intravenously.

TABLE 2 compares the clinical manifestations of insulin shock with those of diabetic ketoacidosis and hyperosmolar nonketotic coma, two other conditions to which the diabetic patient is predisposed.

Severe hypoglycemic reactions can also be caused by oral hypoglycemic drugs. Rarely, nondiabetic persons with emotional problems may deliberately ingest oral hypoglycemic drugs or inject themselves with insulin. They then consult a physician or enter a hospital emergency room with manifestations of severe hypoglycemia. If the possibility of self-induced hypoglycemia is suspected, special laboratory tests can determine the level of insulin in the blood. Tests can also determine whether the insulin in the patient's blood was secreted by the patient's own pancreas or is the type of insulin that is used by diabetic patients.

Tumors of the Pancreas

Carcinoma of the pancreas is relatively common and develops most often in the head of the pancreas. In this location, the neoplasm blocks the common bile duct, resulting in obstructive jaundice. Carcinoma elsewhere in the pancreas is usually far advanced when first detected and produces no specific symptoms.

Sometimes, benign tumors arise from the islet cells and produce symptoms as a result of overproduction of hormones. Beta cells give rise to insulin-secreting tumors that cause episodes of severe hypoglycemia similar to those experienced by a diabetic who receives too much insulin.

QUESTIONS FOR REVIEW

1. What is the difference between acute and chronic pancreatitis?
2. What are the major metabolic disturbances in type 1 diabetes? How does insulin correct these disturbances?
3. What are the major complications of diabetes?
4. Which type of diabetes can be treated by diet alone?
5. What is meant by the following terms: *sweat test*, *hyperosmolar nonketotic hyperglycemic coma*, *ketoacidosis*, and *ketone bodies*?
6. What is cystic fibrosis of the pancreas? What are its clinical manifestations? What is its pattern of inheritance?
7. What is hypoglycemia? What are its clinical manifestations? How is it treated?
8. What are the major differences between diabetic ketoacidosis and insulin shock?
9. What is gestation diabetes? Why does it occur?

SUPPLEMENTARY READINGS

Abrahamson, M. J. 2007. A 74-year-old woman with diabetes. *Journal of the American Medical Association* 297:196–204.

- A case-based discussion emphasizing that the metabolic disorder affects over 20 million people in the United States, of which 90% have type 2 diabetes. The basic disturbance is insulin resistance associated with impaired beta cell insulin production. In most persons who develop diabetes, the insulin resistance progresses for many years before type 2 diabetes finally results. Treatment with oral medications that stimulate insulin secretion by beta cells is effective, but supplementary insulin is needed by many patients to control the hyperglycemia. Oral drugs that act by promoting insulin secretion may hasten the failure of beta cell function.

American Diabetes Association. 2000. Type 2 diabetes in children and adolescents. *Pediatrics* 105:671–80.

- A review of current concepts. Type 2 diabetes is becoming more frequent in this age group, related primarily to obesity. Children with type 2 diabetes usually have a family history of diabetes, and those of non-European ancestry are disproportionately represented.

Beckman, J. A., Creager, M. A., and Libby, P. 2002. Diabetes and atherosclerosis: Epidemiology, pathophysiology, and management. *Journal of the American Medical Association* 287:2570–81.

- The prevalence of type 2 diabetes in children and in the developing nations is rising substantially. Most patients with diabetes die of the complications of atherosclerosis.

Bode, B. W., Sabbah, H., and Davidson, P. C. 2001. What's ahead in glucose monitoring? New techniques hold promise for improved ease and accuracy. *Postgraduate Medicine* 109:41–9.

► A review of the technologic advances in glucose monitoring, including easy-to-use meters and development of continuous glucose monitoring systems.

Boyle, M. P. 2007. Adult cystic fibrosis. *Journal of the American Medical Association* 298:1787–93.

► New methods of treatment and emphasis on nutritional support have greatly increased the survival of patients with cystic fibrosis and have also documented a number of mild cases that survive into middle age. The article describes principles of diagnosis and treatment, and describes the various complications resulting from the disease. The author suggests that the disease should be considered in adult patients presenting with any one of three conditions: bronchiectasis, chronic sinusitis with nasal polyps, or infertility in males. The value of the sweat test for screening is emphasized. The effectiveness of current treatment is illustrated by a 52-year-old man with cystic fibrosis who had few health or activity-limiting problems until his 40s.

Callery, M. P., and Freedman, S. D. 2008. A 21-year-old man with chronic pancreatitis. *Journal of the American Medical Association* 299:2589–94.

► Evaluation and treatment of chronic pancreatitis are considered based on the case history of a young man with pancreatitis having its onset at age 11 and recurring periodically. Causes and methods of treatment are discussed, including a rather limited role of surgical treatment. Some uncommon cases are caused by gene mutations, one of which is a different mutation of the same gene responsible for cystic fibrosis. Pancreatitis may also be a manifestation of an autoimmune disease targeting pancreatic tissue.

Ludwig, D. S., and Ebbeling, C. B. 2001. Type 2 diabetes mellitus in children: Primary care and public health considerations. *Journal of the American Medical Association* 286:1427–30.

► In prior years, type 2 diabetes occurred primarily in older overweight adults, and type 1 diabetes occurred in children and young adults. Now as many as half the new cases of diabetes in children are classified as type 2, which is related to the increasing prevalence of overweight children. Insulin resistance related to overweight causes the pancreas to secrete more insulin, eventually leading to failure of beta cell function. Many factors have contributed to childhood obesity and its most serious complication, which is type 2 diabetes.

McMahon, G. T., and Arky, R. A. 2007. Inhaled insulin for diabetes mellitus. *New England Journal of Medicine* 356:497–502.

► A review of the applications and limitations of a method for using insulin that does not require subcutaneous injection. A dry powder form of insulin was developed that can be inhaled using a specially designed inhaler to deliver the insulin into the pulmonary alveoli. However, there were several problems and potential complications associated with its use. It was not well received by diabetic patients, and the manufacturer discontinued the preparation, which is no longer available.

Mokdad, A. H., Bowman, B. A., Ford, E. S., et al. 2001. The continuing epidemic of obesity and diabetes in the United States. *Journal of the American Medical Association* 286:1195–200.

► As body mass index rises, so does the prevalence of type 2 diabetes.

Rosenbloom, A. L., Young, R. S., Joe, J. R., et al. 1999. The emerging epidemic of type 2 diabetes in youth. *Diabetes Care* 22:345–53.

► A review of the problem. Nonautoimmune forms of youth-onset diabetes are becoming more prevalent as rate of obesity in children and adolescents accelerates.

Rubinow, K. B., and Hirsch, I. B. 2011. Reexamining metrics for glucose control. *Journal of the American Medical Association* 305:1132–3.

- Glycated hemoglobin has assumed greater importance recently because a higher than normal concentration predicts vascular complications in persons with both type 1 and type 2 diabetes and has been promoted as the primary diagnostic test for diabetes and for making treatment decisions in diabetic patients. However, the test can be very unreliable and can provide misleading results because it is influenced by many factors, many of which are often encountered in ethnic groups prone to diabetes. For an individual patient, these limitations limit its usefulness for diagnosing diabetes, assessing the care of the diabetic patient and predicting diabetes-associated complications.

Weir, G. C. 1995. Which comes first in non-insulin-dependent diabetes mellitus: Insulin resistance or beta-cell failure? Both come first (Editorial). *Journal of the American Medical Association* 273:1878–9.

- This type of diabetes results from a mix of genetic and environmental factors that vary among different racial and ethnic groups.

Welsh, M. J. 2010. Targeting the basic defect in cystic fibrosis. *New England Journal of Medicine* 363:2056–57.

- The favorable results of this study indicate that drugs targeting the functions of *CFTR* can improve gene function and the patient's clinical condition.

Yoon, J. W., Austin, M., Onodera T., et al. 1979. Isolation of a virus from the pancreas of a child with diabetic ketoacidosis. *New England Journal of Medicine* 300:1173–9.

- A detailed investigative study.

OUTLINE SUMMARY

Structure and Function of the Pancreas

EXOCRINE FUNCTION

Secretes digestive enzymes.

ENDOCRINE FUNCTION

Islet alpha cells secrete glucagon: raise blood glucose.
Islet beta cells secrete insulin: lower blood glucose.
Islet delta cells secrete somatostatin, which inhibits insulin and glucagon secretion.

Pancreatitis

ACUTE PANCREATITIS

Pancreatic juice escapes from ducts and digests pancreas.
Serious illness with high mortality.

CHRONIC PANCREATITIS

Mild inflammation leading to progressive destruction of pancreatic tissue.

Cystic Fibrosis of the Pancreas

INCIDENCE

One in 3,000 whites, transmitted as autosomal recessive.
Rare in blacks and other races.

PATHOGENESIS

Responsible gene identified.
Tests available to identify carrier.
Cell dysfunction leads to thick mucus that plugs ducts.
Obstruction of pancreatic ducts causes atrophy and fibrosis of pancreas.
Obstruction of bronchi causes lung injury.
Obstruction of biliary ducts causes liver scarring.

SWEAT TEST IN CYSTIC FIBROSIS

Sweat gland function abnormal.
High concentration of sodium and chloride in sweat is basis of diagnostic test.

Diabetes Mellitus

TYPE 1 DIABETES

As a result of damage or destruction of islets.
Insulin secretion reduced or absent.
Develops chiefly in children and young adults.
Ketosis prone.

TYPE 2 DIABETES

More common type.
Insulin secretion normal or increased.
Tissues insensitive to insulin.
Not associated with ketosis.

PREDIABETES

Higher than normal glucose but not high enough to diagnose diabetes.

Progression to diabetes can be slowed or possibly prevented by diet, and exercise.

Some drugs are useful.

PREGNANCY-ASSOCIATED DIABETES

Hormones in pregnancy cause insulin resistance.

Some women unable to secrete enough insulin to compensate, and glucose rises.

Treatment by diet and insulin if needed.

Glucose returns to normal postpartum.

Increased long-term risk of permanent diabetes.

DIABETES AND THE METABOLIC SYNDROME

A group of conditions associated with insulin resistance.

Includes obesity, insulin resistance, abnormal blood lipids, and hypertension.

Screen overweight persons with abdominal obesity by checking blood pressure, blood glucose, and blood lipids.

Treat associated conditions when appropriate.

FAT METABOLISM AND FORMATION OF KETONE BODIES

Catabolism of fat yields acetate fragments (acetyl-CoA).

Converted by liver into ketone bodies.

BIOCHEMICAL DISTURBANCES IN DIABETES

Glucose absorbed but not utilized normally and accumulates in blood.

Excreted in urine with water and electrolytes.

Protein catabolism yields more glucose.

Ketoacidosis in type 1 diabetics.

Hyperosmolar nonketotic coma in type 2 diabetics.

Amount of insulin sufficient to prevent ketosis but not enough to prevent hyperglycemia.

Hyperosmolarity of extracellular fluid as a result of hyperglycemia causes cellular dehydration.

COMPLICATIONS OF DIABETES

Increased susceptibility to infection.

Diabetic coma.

Ketoacidosis.

Hyperosmolar coma.

Arteriosclerosis.

Blindness.

Renal failure.

Peripheral neuritis.

TREATMENT

Diet.

Insulin required for type 1 diabetes.

Oral hypoglycemic drugs or insulin for type 2 diabetes not controlled adequately by diet alone.

Hypoglycemia

PATHOGENESIS AND MANIFESTATIONS IN TYPE 1 DIABETIC SUBJECTS

Excessive insulin in relation to food intake.

As glucose falls, epinephrine is released by adrenal medulla, which mobilizes glucose from hepatic glycogen and exerts widespread systemic effects.

Neurologic manifestations occur because neurons are deprived of glucose, which is required for normal function.

Prolonged hypoglycemia causes permanent brain damage.

TREATMENT

Give oral carbohydrate if subject is conscious and able to swallow.

Inject glucagon or intravenous glucose solution if subject is unconscious.

OTHER CAUSES OF HYPOGLYCEMIA

Oral hypoglycemic drugs in type 2 diabetic patients.

Self-administration of oral hypoglycemic drugs or insulin by emotionally disturbed persons.

Rarely, islet cell tumor of pancreas.

Tumors of the Pancreas

CARCINOMA OF PANCREAS

Usually develops in head of pancreas.

Blockage of common bile duct causes obstructive jaundice.

ISLET CELL TUMORS

Beta cell tumors produce hyperinsulinism.

http://health.jbpub.com/humandisease/9e

Human Disease Online is a great source for supplementary human disease information for both students and instructors. Visit this website to find a variety of useful tools for learning, thinking, and teaching.

The Gastrointestinal Tract

LEARNING OBJECTIVES

1. Identify the major types of cleft lip and cleft palate deformity.
2. Explain the pathogenesis of dental caries and periodontal disease, and describe prevention and treatment.
3. Name the common congenital abnormalities of the gastrointestinal tract. Describe their clinical manifestations, and explain the methods of diagnosis and treatment.
4. Name and describe the three most common lesions of the esophagus that lead to esophageal obstruction.
5. Explain the pathogenesis of peptic ulcer. Describe the three major complications of peptic ulcer and their treatment. Name the methods of treatment.
6. Describe the common types of chronic and acute enteritis and their clinical manifestations.
7. Differentiate between appendicitis and Meckel diverticulitis in terms of pathogenesis, clinical manifestations, and treatment.
8. Describe the pathogenesis of diverticulitis, and explain the role of diet in the development of lesion.
9. Name the causes, clinical manifestations, and complications of intestinal obstruction, carcinoma of the colon, and diverticulosis of the colon. Explain their treatment.
10. Understand the major eating disturbances and their effects.

Structure and Functions

The gastrointestinal tract, which is concerned with the digestion and absorption of food, comprises the oral cavity and related parts of the face, the esophagus, the stomach, the small and large intestines, and the anus.

Cleft Lip and Cleft Palate

Embryologically, the face and palate are formed by coalescence of proliferating masses of cells that merge to form the facial structures and to separate the nasal cavity from the mouth. In the upper part of the face, the areas of coalescence are located on either side of the midline in a line that passes through the upper lip and jaw and extends into each nostril. The palate is formed by two shelflike masses of tissue that grow medially and fuse in the midline to close the communication between nose and mouth. If these developmental processes are disturbed, defects may result in the upper lip and jaw (**cleft lip**) or in the palate (**cleft palate**).

Cleft lip
Defect in the upper lip of variable degree, as a result of a developmental disturbance.

Cleft palate
Defect in hard palate allowing communication between oral cavity and nasal cavity, as a result of a developmental disturbance.

Cleft lip and palate are common abnormalities that frequently occur in combination. The incidence of these abnormalities is about 1 per 1,000 births.

Both cleft lip and cleft palate follow a multifactorial pattern of inheritance, as discussed in congenital and hereditary diseases. The incidence is significantly higher among the children of parents who have previously given birth to an infant with a cleft lip or palate and among the children of parents who themselves have a cleft lip or palate.

Cleft lip may be unilateral or bilateral and may range in severity from a relatively minor defect in the mucosa of the lip to a large cleft extending deeply into the upper jaw. In the most severe deformity, the cleft extends completely through the upper jaw into the floor of the nose (complete cleft) and may also extend posteriorly into the palate (FIGURE 1). Large bilateral clefts extending into the palate completely separate the hard palate from the midline tissue that forms part of the upper jaw, and the separated tissue is often displaced forward (FIGURE 2). Midline cleft palate may occur as an isolated abnormality, but it is usually associated with unilateral or bilateral cleft lip. FIGURE 3 illustrates the various types of cleft lip and palate that are encountered clinically.

TREATMENT

Although cleft lip and palate frequently occur together, they are corrected surgically at different times. Generally, cleft lip is repaired very soon after birth. Repair of

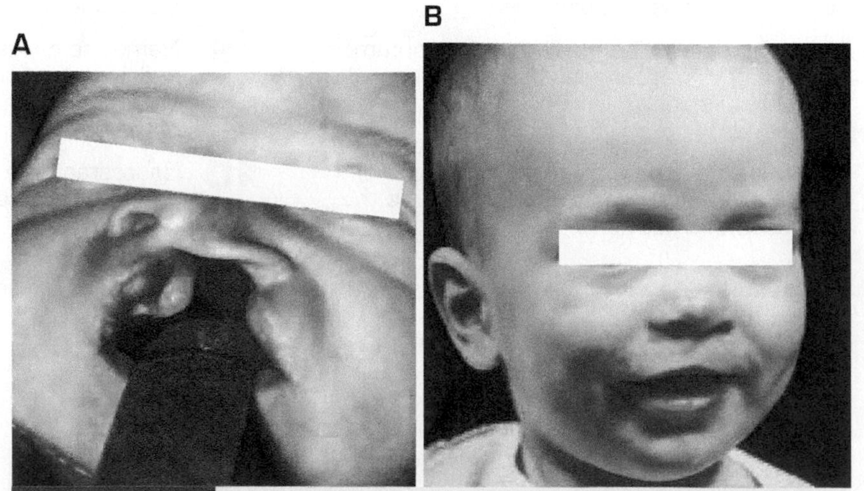

FIGURE 1 **A**, Widely cleft lip and palate in a 2-week-old infant. **B**, The same child at 14 months of age after surgical correction of the defect.

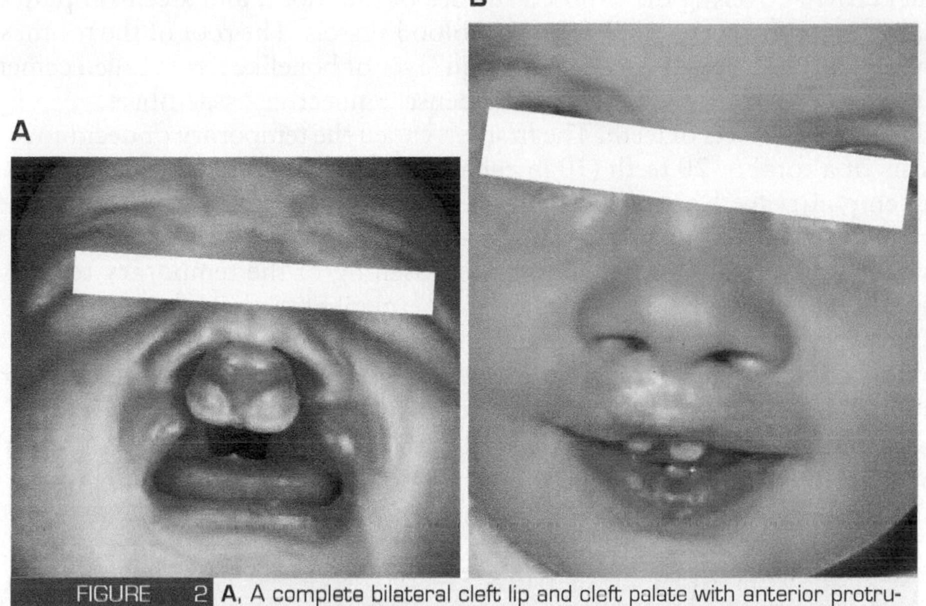

FIGURE 2 **A**, A complete bilateral cleft lip and cleft palate with anterior protrusion of tissues between clefts. **B**, The same child at 18 months of age after surgical correction of the defect.

cleft palate is generally deferred until the child is between 1 and 2 years old. After the cleft palate is repaired, speech therapy is begun in early childhood to correct the nasal quality that often results from abnormal palatal function.

Abnormalities of Tooth Development

The teeth are specialized structures developed in the tissues of the jaws. Each tooth consists of a solid portion called **dentine**, which forms the bulk of the tooth; an

Dentine
(den'tēn)
Bony structure of the tooth.

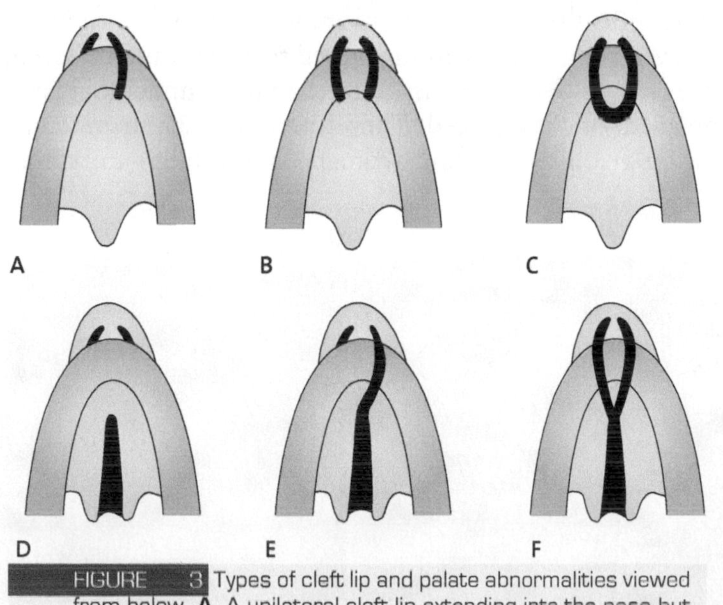

FIGURE 3 Types of cleft lip and palate abnormalities viewed from below. **A**, A unilateral cleft lip extending into the nose but not extending posteriorly into the palate. **B**, A bilateral cleft lip extending into the nose but not extending into the palate. **C**, A bilateral cleft lip extending into the nose and palate. **D**, A midline cleft palate. **E**, A cleft palate with unilateral cleft lip extending into the nose. **F**, A cleft palate with bilateral cleft lip extending into the nose.

enamel crown covering the exposed surface of the tooth; and a central pulp cavity containing nerve fibers, lymphatics, and blood vessels. The root of the tooth, which is embedded in the jaw, is covered by a thin layer of bonelike tissue called cementum, and the tooth is anchored in the jaw by dense connective tissue fibers.

There are two sets of teeth. The first set, called the temporary or deciduous teeth, consists of a total of 20 teeth (10 in each jaw) that erupt in childhood. Eventually, these temporary teeth are replaced by a second, permanent set of 32 teeth. When the permanent teeth begin to grow, they press against the roots of the temporary teeth. This causes resorption of the roots and loosening of the temporary teeth, which eventually fall out and are replaced by the permanent teeth.

Each deciduous and permanent tooth develops from a separate tooth bud, which is composed of two parts: one that forms the crown and a second that gives rise to the remainder of the tooth. The deciduous teeth are formed before birth and erupt during childhood. The permanent teeth do not begin to develop until after birth and erupt at various times in late childhood and adolescence. Calcium is deposited in the dentine and enamel of the tooth as it is being formed.

MISSING TEETH AND EXTRA TEETH

The absence of one or more teeth is relatively common and is often a familial trait that follows a multifactorial pattern of inheritance (FIGURE 4). It results from failure of one or more tooth buds to develop. Sometimes an extra tooth bud forms, resulting in an extra tooth.

ABNORMALITIES OF TOOTH ENAMEL CAUSED BY TETRACYCLINE

Enamel forms within the developing teeth at specific times. If the antibiotic tetracycline is administered while enamel is being formed in the teeth, the antibiotic is deposited with calcium in the enamel and causes permanent yellow-gray to brown discoloration in the crowns. The antibiotic may also disturb the formation of the enamel. If a tetracycline antibiotic is taken by a pregnant woman, the drug crosses the placenta and enters the fetal circulation, where it becomes incorporated in the enamel of the developing teeth. If administered to infants and children, tetracycline is deposited in the crowns of the permanent teeth that are undergoing enamel formation at the time the antibiotic is ingested. Therefore, it is recommended that tetracycline antibiotics not be given to pregnant women or to infants and children during the

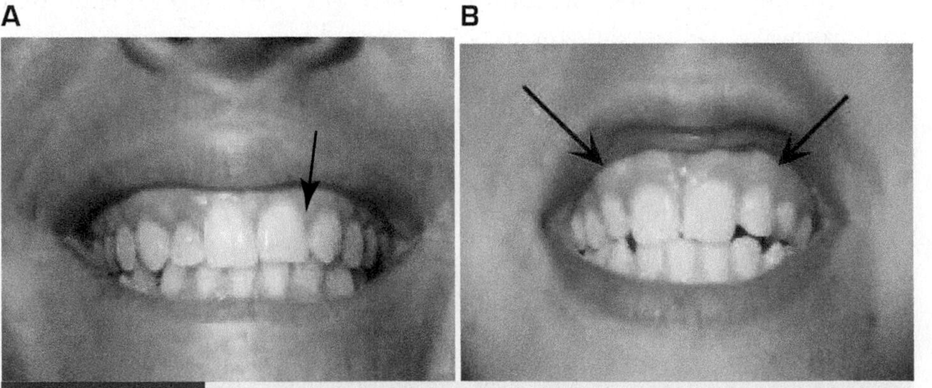

FIGURE 4 Congenital absence of teeth. **A**, Mother lacks the left lateral incisor (*arrow*). Left canine (cuspid) tooth is located lateral to left central incisor. Compare the appearance of the left side with the opposite side in which all teeth are present. **B**, Daughter lacks both lateral incisors. The canine teeth (*arrows*) are adjacent to the central incisors.

time when enamel is forming in the developing permanent teeth. This period extends through infancy and childhood to about the age of 8 years.

Dental Caries and Its Complications

The oral cavity contains a diverse collection of both aerobic and anaerobic bacteria. Masses of these bacteria intermixed with bacterial products and proteins from saliva form aggregates called **dental plaque** that adhere to the teeth and predispose to tooth decay.

Caries, the term for tooth decay, is a Latin word meaning dry rot. The condition is a decalcification of the tooth structure caused by mouth bacteria acting on bits of retained food material, such as sugar and highly refined, starchy foods. Bacterial fermentation liberates organic acids that erode the covering enamel, exposing the underlying dentine, which is attacked by the acids and invaded by mouth bacteria. The loss of tooth structure that results from the combined acid and bacterial action is called a dental **cavity**. The affected area appears discolored and is quite soft when probed with a dental instrument. Dental x-rays reveal the cavity as an area of decreased density in the affected tooth.

If the cavity is not treated and continues to enlarge, the decay eventually reaches the dental pulp. The bacteria invade the pulp and incite an inflammation that causes the throbbing pain characteristic of a toothache. Unchecked, the infection may spread to the apex of the tooth root, which is embedded in the jawbone, and from there spread to the bone surrounding the dental root. The result may be an abscess surrounding the apex of the tooth, which is called a periapical abscess (*peri* = around).

Dental plaque
Masses of bacteria, bacterial products, and salivary proteins adherent to teeth, which predisposes to tooth decay.

Caries
(ka′rēz)
Tooth decay.

Cavity (dental)
A loss of tooth structure caused by the combined action of mouth bacteria and organic acids derived from bacterial fermentation of retained food particles.

PREVENTION AND TREATMENT

The incidence of tooth decay can be reduced by proper mouth hygiene, including frequent brushing of the teeth and use of dental floss to remove food particles that promote bacterial growth. Fluoride added to water supplies and toothpaste helps to prevent cavities by promoting formation of a more acid-resistant tooth structure that resists decay. Dental caries is treated by removing the decayed area and packing the defect with some type of dental filling material. After infection of the pulp and dental root has occurred, more extensive treatment is required. Antibiotics may be needed if there is an acute infection or abscess at the apex of the tooth. After the infection is under control, the entire pulp cavity must be cleaned out and packed with dental filling material, a procedure called a root canal treatment. Sometimes the tooth cannot be salvaged and must be extracted.

Periodontal Disease

Masses of bacteria and debris accumulating around the base of the teeth may incite an inflammation. Initially, the inflammation affects only the gums surrounding the roots of the teeth, which is called gingivitis (*gingiva* = gum). Later, the inflammation extends between the teeth and the adjacent gums, leading to the formation of small pockets of infection between the teeth and gums. This condition is called periodontal disease (*peri* = around + *dens* = tooth). If pus is discharged from the margins of the infected gums, the descriptive term pyorrhea (*pyo* = pus + *rhea* = flow) is often used. The infection may spread into the tooth sockets that anchor the teeth in the jawbone, causing the teeth to loosen and eventually fall out. Various methods of treatment to the gums and teeth may control or arrest the condition, which is an important cause of loss of teeth.

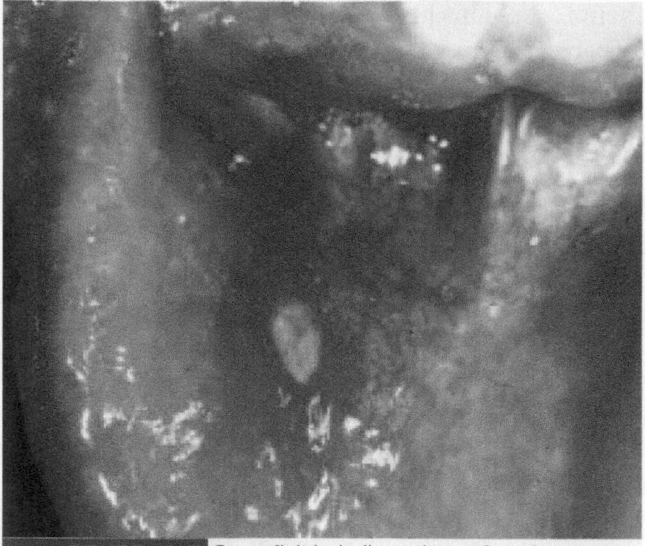
FIGURE 5 Superficial shallow ulcer of oral mucosa caused by canker sore.

Inflammation of the Oral Cavity

An inflammation of the oral cavity is called **stomatitis** (*stoma* = mouth). It may be caused by a number of irritants and infectious agents. Common irritants are alcohol, tobacco, and hot or spicy foods. Infectious agents include the herpes virus and some other viruses, the fungus *Candida albicans* (which also causes vaginal infections), and certain bacteria that cause a type of infection called trench mouth or Vincent infection.

Canker sores are another relatively common inflammatory disease involving the oral cavity. A canker sore appears as a small painful superficial ulcer of the oral mucosa surrounded by a narrow zone of inflammation that appears as a red border surrounding the ulcer (FIGURE 5). We do not know what causes canker sores, and there is no specific treatment for this condition, although various measures can reduce the discomfort caused by the ulcers.

Stomatitis
(stō-mäh-tī'tis)
Inflammation of the oral cavity.

Tumors of the Oral Cavity

Carcinoma of the oral cavity, which may arise from the squamous epithelium of the lips, cheek, tongue, palate, or back of the throat, is relatively common (FIGURE 6). It is treated by surgical resection or by radiation therapy.

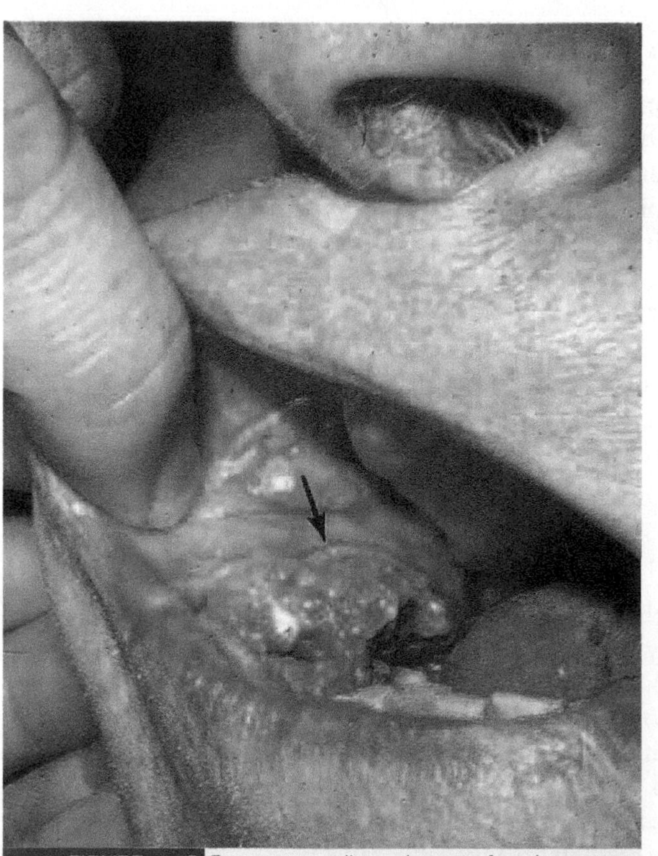
FIGURE 6 Squamous cell carcinoma of oral mucosa (*arrow*), which appears as an irregular overgrowth of tissue arising from the mucosa of the cheek.

Diseases of the Esophagus

The esophagus is a muscular tube extending from the pharynx to the stomach with sphincters at both upper and lower ends. The upper sphincter relaxes to allow passage of swallowed food, which is propelled down the esophagus by rhythmic peristaltic contractions. The lower esophageal sphincter (called the gastroesophageal or cardiac sphincter) relaxes when the food reaches the lower end of the esophagus and allows the food to pass into the stomach. Some of the more important conditions affecting the esophagus include the following:

1. Failure of the lower (cardiac) sphincter to function properly
2. Tears in the lining of the esophagus from retching and vomiting
3. Esophageal obstruction as a result of carcinoma, food impaction, or stricture

Symptoms of esophageal disease include difficulty in swallowing (dysphagia) together with variable degrees of substernal discomfort or pain. Complete obstruction of the esophagus leads to inability to swallow, which is often associated with regurgitation of food into the trachea, causing episodes of choking and coughing.

CARDIAC SPHINCTER DYSFUNCTION

The two major disturbances of cardiac sphincter function are failure of the cardiac sphincter to open properly, which is called cardiospasm, and inability of the sphincter to remain closed properly, which is called an incompetent cardiac sphincter, and leads to a condition called reflux esophagitis.

Cardiospasm

Sometimes the cardiac sphincter fails to open properly, caused by a malfunction of the nerve plexuses in the esophagus that control its functions. As a result, food cannot pass normally into the stomach, and the smooth muscle in the wall of the esophagus must contract more vigorously to force the food past the constricted sphincter. Eventually the esophageal muscle undergoes marked hypertrophy, and the esophagus becomes dilated proximal to the constricted sphincter because of food retention. Treatment consists of periodic stretching of the sphincter by means of an instrument introduced into the esophagus or by surgically cutting the muscle fibers in the constricted area. An alternative treatment in selected cases consists of injecting botulinum toxin into the sphincter through an esophagoscope. The toxin blocks the transmission of nerve impulses from the nerve plexuses to the muscle fibers for several months, which relaxes the sphincter and relieves the patient's symptoms.

Incompetent Cardiac Sphincter and Its Complications

In this relatively common condition, acid gastric juice leaks back into the esophagus through the improperly closed incompetent lower esophageal sphincter. The squamous epithelial lining of the esophagus, which was not "designed" to tolerate high-acid secretions, becomes irritated and inflamed, which is called **reflux esophagitis.** In some patients, the squamous mucosal lining may actually become ulcerated and scarred. Sometimes the squamous lining responds to the acidity by undergoing a change (metaplasia) into a more acid-resistant columnar gastric type mucosa. This condition, which is called Barrett esophagus after the person who first described it, may lead to additional problems. Unfortunately, the metaplastic columnar epithelium is frequently abnormal and poses an increased risk of developing adenocarcinoma arising in the abnormal columnar epithelium. Treatment of reflux esophagitis consists of avoiding lying down soon after eating because the recumbent position promotes reflux, sleeping with the head of the bed elevated to minimize reflux, and avoiding alcoholic beverages because alcohol not only stimulates gastric acid secretion but also tends to relax the lower esophageal sphincter, which facilitates reflux. Drugs that reduce secretion of gastric acid and antacids that neutralize gastric acid are helpful.

Reflux esophagitis
Inflammation of the lining of the esophagus caused by reflux of acidic gastric secretions through an incompetent lower gastroesophageal sphincter.

GASTRIC MUCOSAL TEARS

Retching and vomiting may cause tears in the mucosa of the gastroesophageal junction where the esophagus passes through the diaphragm or in the lining of the distal esophagus, and these tears can bleed profusely (FIGURE 7). The repetitive, intermittent, vigorous contractions of the abdominal muscles associated with vomiting raise intra-abdominal pressure and forcefully jam the upper part (cardia) of the stomach against the opening in the diaphragm through which the esophagus passes, causing tears in the mucosa. The additional stresses resulting from vigorous contractions of the muscular walls of the stomach and esophagus associated with vomiting probably place

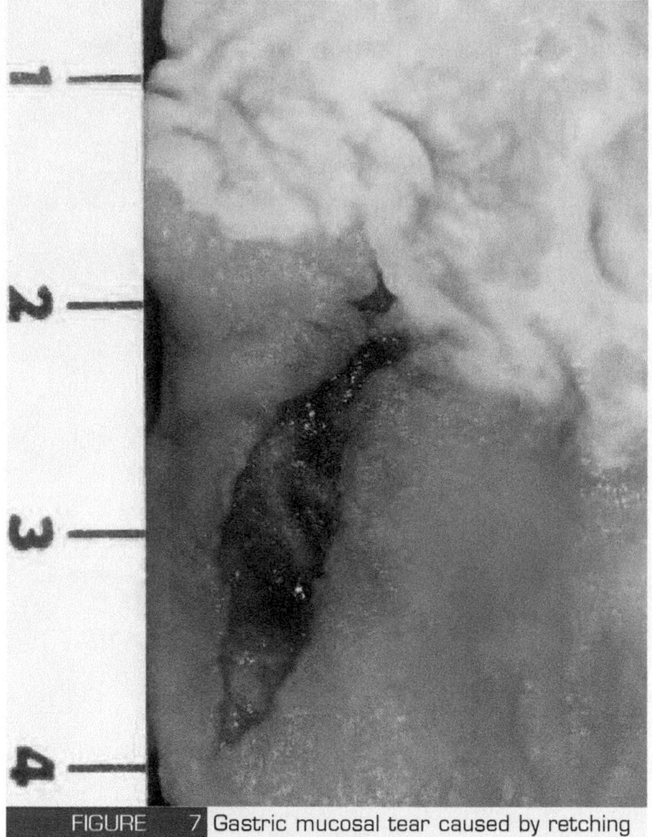

FIGURE 7 Gastric mucosal tear caused by retching and vomiting. The opaque mucosa in the upper part of the photograph is the normal stratified squamomus mucosa of the esophagus. The 2 cm long tear extends distally from the gastroesophageal junction and caused a fatal gastric hemorrhage.

additional stress on the mucosa, which also plays a role in causing the laceration. This vomiting-related complication most often follows the retching and vomiting related to excess alcohol intake but may follow vomiting from any cause, including self-induced vomiting to control weight.

ESOPHAGEAL OBSTRUCTION

Carcinoma of the Esophagus

Carcinoma may arise anywhere in the esophagus, either from the squamous epithelium or from the columnar epithelium associated with Barrett esophagus. The tumor gradually narrows the lumen of the esophagus, frequently infiltrates the surrounding tissues, and may invade the trachea. Necrosis of the tumor extending between the esophagus and trachea may lead to the formation of an abnormal communication between these two structures called a tracheoesophageal fistula (*fistula* = tube).

Food Impaction

Obstruction of the esophagus may be caused by impaction of poorly chewed meat in the distal part of the esophagus. This is sometimes encountered in persons who are unable to chew their food properly because they have poor teeth or improperly fitting dentures or who have poor eating habits.

Stricture

A stricture is a narrowing caused by scar tissue. Reflux esophagitis with ulceration and scarring may lead to a stricture. Esophageal scarring may also result from accidentally or deliberately swallowing a corrosive chemical that causes necrosis and inflammation. Severe scarring eventually follows. A common cause of esophageal stricture in children is accidental swallowing of commercial lye solutions (used for cleaning clogged drains).

Gastritis

Inflammation of the stomach is called gastritis, and the inflammation may be either acute or chronic. Many patients with gastritis have few symptoms, but some experience abdominal discomfort and nausea.

ACUTE GASTRITIS

In most cases, acute gastritis is a self-limited inflammation of short duration. However, at times, the acute inflammation may be quite severe and may be complicated by ulceration of the mucosa with bleeding from the ulcerated areas. Patients in whom the acute gastritis is associated with mucosal ulceration often have more pronounced symptoms, and the ulcerated areas may bleed profusely.

There are many causes of acute gastritis, but most are caused by nonsteroidal anti-inflammatory drugs such as aspirin, ibuprofen, and naproxen. These drugs are widely used to treat symptoms of arthritis and related musculoskeletal pain problems. The drugs act by inhibiting an enzyme called cyclooxygenase that is required for the synthesis of prostaglandins, which are potent mediators as discussed in inflammation and repair. Prostaglandins, however, are produced by many different cells and have many different functions.

Those produced by gastric epithelial cells help protect the stomach from the damaging effects of gastric acid by promoting the secretion not only of sodium bicarbonate to counteract the acid but also of mucin to coat and protect the stomach lining. Nonsteroidal anti-inflammatory drugs reduce inflammation by inhibiting the synthesis of prostaglandin mediators of inflammation, but they also inhibit the synthesis of the prostaglandins that help protect the gastric mucosa. Consequently, the mucosa becomes more vulnerable to injury from acidic gastric juice, which may lead to acute inflammation of the mucosa and may even be followed by mucosal ulceration with bleeding.

There are actually two forms of cyclooxygenase. One form (abbreviated COX-1) promotes the synthesis of the prostaglandins that protect the gastric mucosa. The other form (abbreviated COX-2) is involved in the synthesis of the prostaglandins that function as mediators of inflammation, which are responsible for the joint and muscle inflammation in patients with musculoskeletal problems. Many nonsteroidal anti-inflammatory drugs inhibit both forms of the enzyme, which suppresses inflammation by inhibiting COX-2, but puts the gastric mucosa at risk by also inhibiting COX-1. Some nonsteroidal anti-inflammatory drugs are more selective. They are called COX-2 inhibitors because they inhibit primarily the COX-2 enzyme that promotes inflammation, but have much less effect on the COX-1 enzyme that helps protect the gastric mucosa. Unfortunately, patients treated with COX-2 inhibitors had a higher risk of heart attacks and strokes than did a comparable group treated with less selective nonsteroidal anti-inflammatory drugs. Now most physicians favor limiting the use of COX-2 inhibitors unless their benefits outweigh the possible cardiovascular risks.

Excess ingestion of alcoholic beverages is another common cause of acute gastritis because the alcohol is a gastric irritant and also stimulates gastric acid secretion.

CHRONIC GASTRITIS AND ITS COMPLICATIONS: THE ROLE OF *HELICOBACTER PYLORI*

Many cases of chronic gastritis are related to growth (colonization) of a small, curved, gram-negative organism called *Helicobacter pylori* on the surface of the gastric mucosa. This unique organism grows in the layer of mucus covering the epithelial cells lining the stomach, where it can be identified by special bacterial stains, by culture, or by other specialized tests. The organism produces an enzyme called urease that decomposes urea, a normal by-product of protein metabolism that is present in small amounts in blood and body fluids. Decomposition of urea yields ammonia, a substance that neutralizes the gastric acid and allows the organism to flourish in an acid environment that would destroy other bacteria. *Helicobacter* also produces enzymes that can break down the layer of protective mucus that covers the epithelial surface. Presumably, the chronic gastritis is caused by the ammonia and other products produced by the organism that damage the gastric mucosa of susceptible persons.

Colonization of the gastric mucosa by *Helicobacter pylori* is very common, and not all persons who harbor the organism have chronic gastritis. Moreover, many persons harbor the organism, and the frequency of bacterial colonization increases with age. About 30% of persons younger than 30 years of age are colonized by *Helicobacter pylori*. By age 50, the proportion increases to about 50% and may be as high as 65% in persons older than age 65. The organism is spread from person-to-person in households by close contacts. The spread of the organisms appears to be by mouth-to-mouth contact and also by the fecal–oral route because the organism has been cultured from both dental plaque material and from fecal material.

There are also some uncommon but important long-term harmful effects of *Helicobacter* infection. Chronic gastritis caused by this organism slightly increases the risk of two different gastric tumors: gastric carcinoma and malignant lymphoma arising from lymphocytes in the gastric mucosa (called mucosa-associated lymphoid tissue). The gastric carcinoma risk occurs because the gastritis often leads to atrophy of the gastric mucosa and causes the gastric epithelium to change into an abnormal intestinal-type epithelium (a process called intestinal metaplasia). It is these cellular changes in the gastric mucosa that predispose to gastric carcinoma. The lymphoma risk probably results because the gastritis overstimulates the mucosa-associated lymphoid tissue, which may lead to unregulated growth of lymphocytes that eventually progresses to gastric lymphoma.

Acute Gastroenteritis

An inflammation involving the intestine as well as the stomach is called a gastroenteritis, and most are acute infections. Many different infectious organisms may cause acute gastroenteritis, but most cases are caused by RNA viruses. The condition is characterized by an abrupt onset of nausea, vomiting, abdominal cramps, and profuse diarrhea, which may affect only a few persons or may occur as an epidemic affecting large numbers of persons. Usually, the illness subsides spontaneously within a few days and no specific treatment is required, although severely affected persons may require intravenous fluids to replace depleted body fluids and electrolytes resulting from the diarrhea.

Some viruses (rotaviruses, astroviruses, and enteroviruses) affect primarily infants and young children and do not spread widely in the community. In contrast, another virus called a **norovirus** is more likely to infect adults and older children and may spread as an epidemic to infect many people. Previously, the virus was called Norwalk virus because it was identified first at a school in Norwalk, Ohio, where it infected half the students in the school, and then spread to infect teachers, family members, and other adults in the community. The virus is an extremely infectious RNA virus easily spread from person-to-person by hand-to-hand transmission, or by virus-contaminated food or water. The virus is resistant to inactivation by freezing, heating, and by many disinfectants, and only a few virus particles are enough to cause an infection. Although norovirus infections may occur sporadically and spread only to family members, epidemics may occur when large groups of persons are in close contact, as in schools, military bases, summer camps, cruise ships, nursing homes, hospitals, and restaurants. It is estimated that about 90% of cases of acute gastroenteritis are caused by the norovirus. There are many strains of norovirus, and a recent infection may provide some temporary immunity against the strain that caused the infection, but does not protect against other strains of the virus.

Norovirus
An extremely infectious RNA virus easily spread from person to person and by contaminated food or water

Peptic Ulcer

Peptic ulcer is a chronic ulcer that usually involves the distal stomach or proximal duodenum (FIGURE 8). The ulcer results from digestion of the mucosa by acid gastric juice. Persons who secrete large volumes of acidic gastric juice are prone to ulcers.

The initial event is probably a small, superficial erosion of the gastric or duodenal mucosa. Gastric acid and pepsin begin to digest the deeper tissues, which have

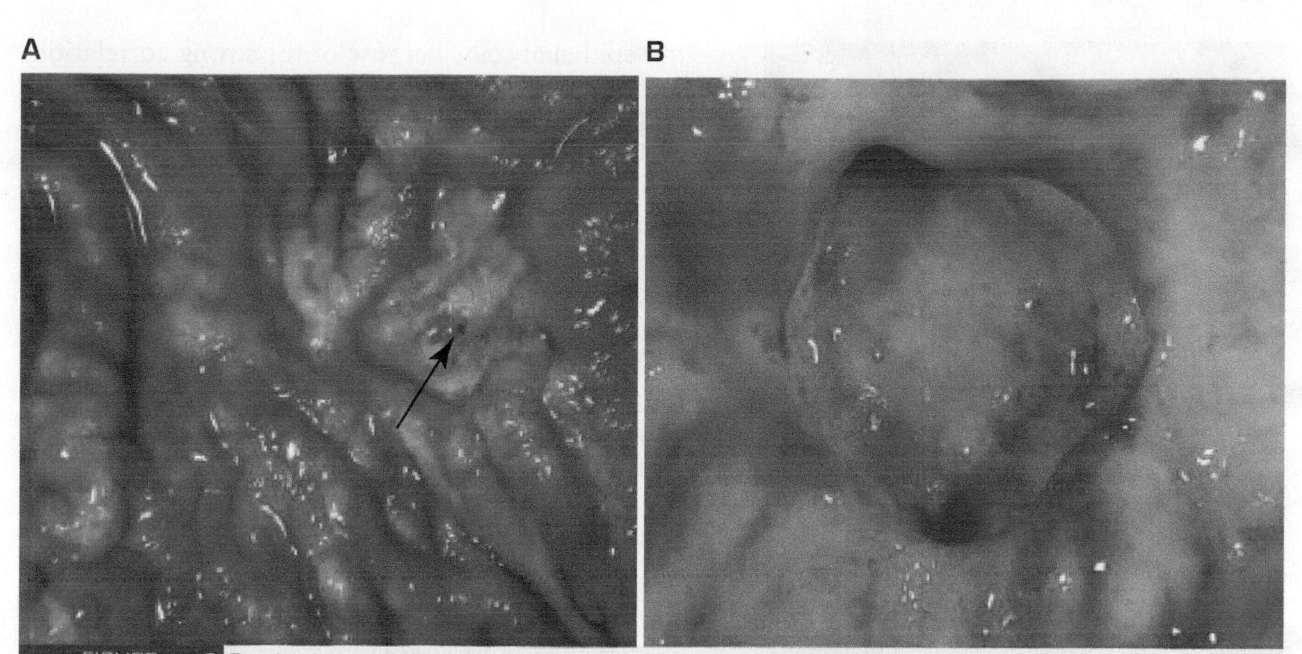

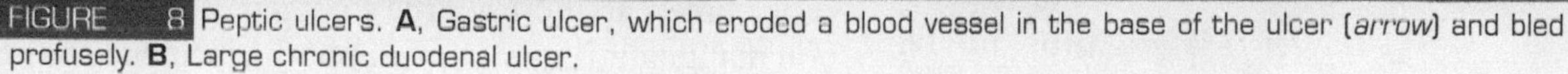

FIGURE 8 Peptic ulcers. **A**, Gastric ulcer, which eroded a blood vessel in the base of the ulcer (*arrow*) and bled profusely. **B**, Large chronic duodenal ulcer.

been denuded of covering epithelium. Attempts at healing in the presence of continuing digestion eventually lead to considerable scarring at the base of the ulcer. Clinically, ulcers produce pain that is usually relieved by ingestion of food or antacids that neutralize the gastric acid.

Helicobacter pylori, the same organism that is associated with chronic gastritis, also plays an important role in the pathogenesis of both gastric and duodenal ulcers. Presumably, the organism injures the mucosa and initiates the mucosal erosion that eventually develops into a chronic ulcer. The role of *Helicobacter* in causing a gastric ulcer is understandable because this is the same organism that causes the mucosal damage leading to chronic gastritis. Its role in causing duodenal ulcers is more difficult to explain because the organism characteristically colonizes gastric mucosa, not duodenal mucosa. Some investigators have speculated that there are small areas of gastric epithelial cells in the duodenum where the organism can grow and damage the duodenal mucosa, making it more susceptible to ulceration. An alternative explanation postulates that the organism does not damage the duodenal mucosa directly, but does so indirectly because the *Helicobacter*-induced gastritis causes the gastric mucosa to secrete excess acid, and it is the hyperacidity that causes the duodenal ulcers. According to this concept, the mucosal damage caused by the gastritis disturbs various functions of gastric mucosal cells that regulate gastric acid secretion and causes the mucosa to secrete excess acid which leads to the duodenal ulceration.

Peptic ulcer has complications: hemorrhage (bleeding), perforation, and obstruction. An ulcer that erodes into a large blood vessel may cause severe hemorrhage. An ulcer may also erode completely through the wall of the stomach or duodenum, causing a perforation of the wall through which gastric and duodenal contents leak into the peritoneal cavity, resulting in a generalized inflammation of the peritoneum, the membrane that lines the abdominal cavity and covers the exterior of the abdominal organs. The inflammation is called peritonitis. Sometimes the scarring that follows healing of a gastric ulcer may be so severe as to cause obstruction of the outlet of the stomach, called the pylorus, preventing the stomach from emptying properly.

Peptic ulcer is generally treated by antacids, which neutralize the excess gastric acid and promote healing of the ulcer, or by drugs that block the secretion of acid by the

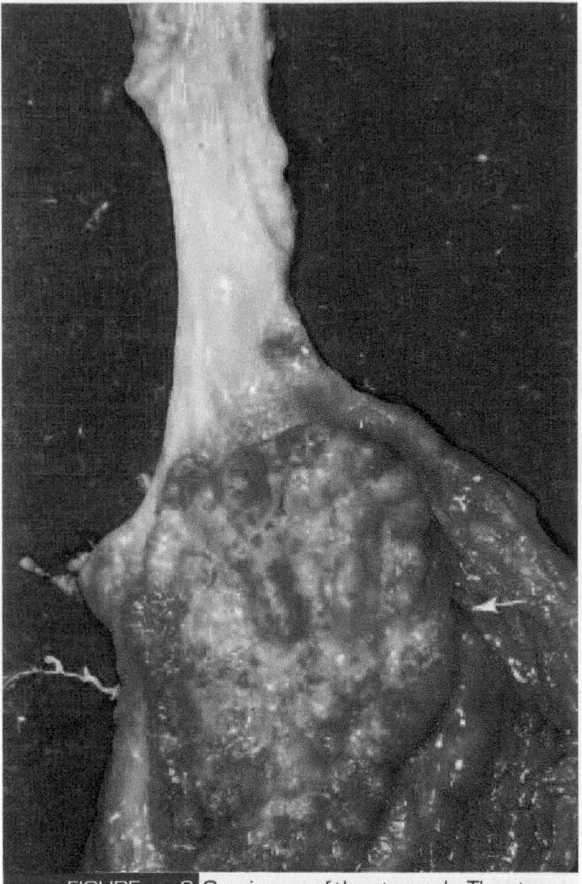
FIGURE 9 Carcinoma of the stomach. The stomach has been opened revealing a large ulcerated neoplasm arising from gastric mucosa (*arrow*) and extending upward to gastroesophageal junction. Esophagus is seen in upper part of photograph.

gastric epithelial cells. Because of the strong correlation between *Helicobacter pylori* and peptic ulcers, patients with ulcers who are colonized by this organism are often treated not only with drugs to neutralize gastric acid or suppress its secretion, but also with antibiotics and other medications to eradicate *Helicobacter pylori.* A large number of laboratory tests are available to identify the presence of *Helicobacter* in the gastric mucosa. Combined antacid and antimicrobial therapy in patients who are colonized by *Helicobacter* leads to faster healing of the ulcers and fewer recurrences than antacid treatment alone.

Surgical treatment is sometimes required if medical therapy fails to heal the ulcer or if complications develop.

Carcinoma of the Stomach

At one time, carcinoma of the stomach was the most common malignant tumor in men, but the incidence has been decreasing. The initial symptom may be only vague upper abdominal discomfort. Sometimes the first manifestation is an iron deficiency anemia, the result of chronic blood loss from the ulcerated surface of the tumor. Gastric carcinoma is treated by resection of a large part of the stomach together with the surrounding tissues and draining lymph nodes (FIGURE 9). Unfortunately, a gastric carcinoma is often far advanced by the time it causes symptoms; consequently, long-term survival of patients with stomach carcinoma is relatively poor. Sometimes, gastric carcinoma may produce symptoms similar to those of a benign peptic ulcer. At times, it may be difficult for the physician to determine whether a patient has a benign peptic ulcer of the stomach or an ulcerated gastric carcinoma. The distinction can usually be made by gastroscopy, an examination in which a flexible gastroscope is passed into the stomach so that the physician can visualize the lesion and take biopsy specimens from various areas.

Inflammatory Disease of the Intestine

Enteritis
(en-ter-ī′tis)
Inflammation of the intestine.

Colitis
(kō-lī′tis)
Inflammation of the colon, such as chronic ulcerative colitis.

The intestine may be the site of both acute and chronic inflammation. The term **enteritis** (*enteron* = bowel) is used to describe inflammation of any part of the intestinal tract. The term **colitis** denotes inflammation restricted to the colon, and the general term bowel inflammation refers to any part of the intestinal tract, either small intestine, colon, or both.

ACUTE ENTERITIS

Acute intestinal infections are usually caused by known pathogens or their toxins, as described in the discussions on pathogenic micro-organisms and animal parasites. They are generally of short duration and may subside without specific treatment, or may respond to appropriate antibiotics or other agents. Clinical manifestations include nausea, vomiting, abdominal discomfort, and passage of many loose stools. In severe infections, the bowel mucosa may be ulcerated, and the diarrheal stools may be bloody.

CHRONIC ENTERITIS

Chronic enteritis is less common and more difficult to treat. The two important types of chronic enteritis are Crohn disease and chronic ulcerative colitis. Often, the two diseases are grouped together under the general term chronic inflammatory bowel disease. Both diseases tend to be chronic, with periodic flare-ups manifested by cramplike abdominal pain and diarrhea, followed by periods when the disease is inactive. During periods of activity, the affected persons may also have systemic manifestations, including joint inflammation, eye inflammation, and various types of skin nodules and skin infections. Although the diseases have many similarities, there are also significant differences between them.

These two diseases appear to be autoimmune diseases as described in the discussion on immunity, hypersensetivity, allergy, and autoimmune diseases, and recent studies have provided further insight into their pathogenesis. Several factors working together appear to trigger the autoimmune response that leads to these diseases:

1. The ability of the immune system to regulate the immune response, which is genetically determined, is impaired in affected persons.
2. In contrast to normal bowel epithelium, which prevents the normal bacterial flora in the bowel from invading the bowel wall, the intestinal epithelium of persons with chronic enteritis is less able to resist invasion by intestinal bacteria, which is called defective epithelial barrier function.
3. Because barrier function is defective, intestinal bacteria can penetrate the epithelium and extend into the deeper tissues. The bacteria are recognized as foreign antigens by the immune system, which generates an intense cell-mediated immune response to destroy the bacteria.
4. The activated T lymphocytes and their destructive cytokines are responsible for the intestinal inflammation and necrosis in persons with chronic enteritis. However, we do not know whether the inflammatory reaction that damages the bowel is directed against intestinal bacteria that get into the intestinal wall periodically because epithelial barrier function is defective, or is an autoimmune response directed against the patient's own cells because they contain some of the same antigenic determinants (cross-reacting antigens) as those possessed by the intestinal bacteria to which the immune system has responsed.

Crohn Disease

Crohn disease is a chronic inflammation and ulceration of the bowel mucosa with marked thickening and scarring of the bowel wall (FIGURE 10). The distal ileum is a frequently involved site. The inflammation often affects scattered areas of the small bowel, leaving normal intervening segments of bowel (called "skip areas") between the areas of severe disease. Occasionally, affected persons have such severe thickening and scarring of an involved segment of bowel that the lumen becomes greatly narrowed or even completely blocked, which impedes passage of bowel contents. Crohn disease was originally called regional ileitis because the inflammatory process is often localized to the distal ileum, but now we know that the disease is not restricted to the ileum. Other parts of the small intestine may also be involved, and the disease may involve the colon as well.

Chronic Ulcerative Colitis

In contrast to Crohn disease, chronic ulcerative colitis targets the colon, not the small intestine. The inflammation is limited to the mucosa, and the bowel wall is not thickened as in Crohn disease. Frequently, the disease begins in the rectal mucosa

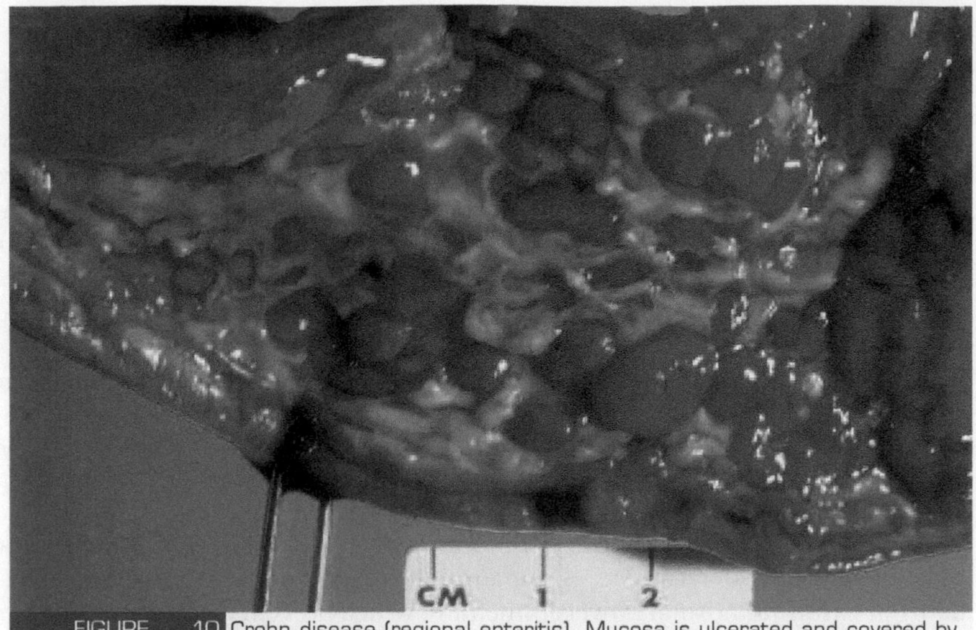

FIGURE 10 Crohn disease (regional enteritis). Mucosa is ulcerated and covered by inflammatory exudate.

but may spread progressively until eventually the entire colon is involved. In severe cases, the ulcerated mucosa may bleed profusely, leading to bloody diarrhea, and at times the inflammatory process becomes so extensive that it leads to a perforation of the colon with escape of bowel contents into the peritoneal cavity. Affected persons with long-standing disease also may develop carcinoma arising in the diseased regions of the colon or rectum.

Treament of Chronic Enteritis

Treatment of inflammatory bowel disease involves symptomatic and supportive measures, including antibiotics and corticosteroid hormones to control disease symptoms during flare-ups, and immunosuppressive drugs. Eventually, surgical resection of severely diseased bowel segments may be required in many patients. Persons with severe and extensive chronic ulcerative colitis may require total removal of the entire colon and rectum, both to control the disease and also to eliminate the risk of colon carcinoma, which is prone to occur in patients with long-standing chronic disease.

ANTIBIOTIC-ASSOCIATED COLITIS

Some persons taking broad-spectrum antibiotics develop mild diarrhea. Others, unfortunately, develop severe bloody diarrhea with abdominal pain, fever, and other systemic manifestations, which may be life threatening. In the mild cases, the intestinal mucosa is slightly inflamed. In the more severely affected persons, there are multiple ulcerations of the colonic mucosa, and the ulcerated areas are covered by masses of fibrin and inflammatory cells.

The broad-spectrum antibiotics cause the colitis by changing the intestinal bacterial flora. Most of the normal flora is destroyed by the broad-spectrum antibiotic. This allows overgrowth of an anaerobic spore-forming intestinal bacterium called *Clostridium difficile* (pronounced dif-fís-sill) that is not inhibited by the antibiotic. The organism produces two toxins that cause the intestinal inflammation and necrosis.

The diagnosis of antibiotic-associated colitis is established by detection of the bacterial toxin in the stool and by identification of the organism in stool cultures. Treatment consists of stopping the antibiotic, and in severe cases, giving a drug that inhibits anaerobic bacteria (metronidazole) or an antibiotic (vancomycin), which inhibits growth of the organism. Treatment should not include drugs that reduce the diarrhea by inhibiting intestinal motility. Such drugs prolong the illness by allowing the injurious clostridial toxins to remain in the intestine instead of being eliminated rapidly in the diarrheal stools.

Unfortunately, *C. difficile* has acquired increased virulence. Previously useful antibiotics have become less effective, and the infection may recur within 60 days after apparently successful treatment. Consequently, the incidence of the infection has more than doubled since the original cases were reported, which makes the infection the most common cause of bacterial diarrhea in the United States. Some patients have multiple recurrences of infection over several months or years, which can spread to infect other hospitalized patients. Current treatment is directed to restoring the normal bacterial population in the colon in order to discourage growth of *C. difficile* and to treat recurrences with an antibiotic that is least likely to be followed by a recurrent infection. One promising method to supplement antibiotics and reduce recurrences consists of administration of a single infusion of antibodies directed against toxins A and B, which reduces recurrences. Other studies are underway to find new antibiotics and other methods of treatment that may be able to achieve a more permanent cure of the infection.

APPENDICITIS

Appendicitis is the most common inflammatory lesion of the bowel. In many animals, the portion of the bowel represented in humans by the appendix is a large, wide-caliber intestinal segment, similar in appearance to the remainder of the colon. In humans, this segment of bowel is reduced in both size and caliber to the extent that it is a vestigial structure.

The high incidence of acute appendicitis is due primarily to the narrow caliber of the appendix, the base of which often becomes plugged by firm bits of fecal material. Because of the obstruction, the secretions normally produced by the epithelial cells lining the appendix drain poorly from the area distal to the blockage. The accumulated secretions create pressure within the appendiceal lumen. This compresses the blood vessels in the mucosa, impairing its viability (FIGURE 11). Bacteria normally present in the appendix and colon invade the devitalized wall, causing an acute inflammation.

Clinically, appendicitis is characterized by generalized abdominal pain that soon becomes localized to the right lower part (quadrant) of the abdomen. Examination of the abdomen reveals localized tenderness over the appendix when pressure is applied

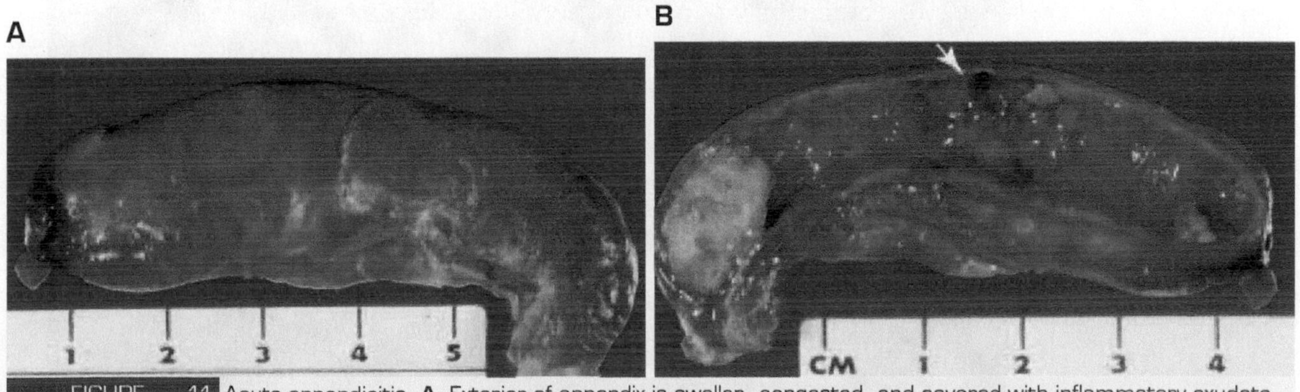

FIGURE 11 Acute appendicitis. **A**, Exterior of appendix is swollen, congested, and covered with inflammatory exudate. **B**, Appendix bisected to reveal interior. Pus within lumen has been removed. Mucosa is congested and ulcerated (*arrow*). The base of the appendix (*left side* of photograph) is plugged by a firm mass of fecal material.

to the abdomen by the fingers of the examiner. Often, the patient also experiences pain when the pressure is released suddenly (rebound tenderness). In addition, there is usually reflex contraction of the abdominal muscles (abdominal rigidity) in response to the underlying inflammation. Laboratory tests reveal that the number of polymorphonuclear leukocytes in the blood also is increased as a result of the infection. Sometimes it may be difficult to distinguish appendicitis from other conditions with similar manifestations, such as acute gastroenteritis or a gynecologic problem in a young woman such as a fallopian tube infection (salpingitis) or ruptured ovarian cyst. When the diagnosis is uncertain, other diagnostic studies such as ultrasound or CT examination, or even a laparoscopy, may help establish the correct diagnosis and lead to appropriate treatment.

Mild cases of appendicitis may heal spontaneously. More severe inflammation may lead to rupture of the appendix and peritonitis. For this reason, it is essential to identify appendicitis and remove the appendix in any patient in whom appendicitis is suspected.

MECKEL DIVERTICULUM

During embryonic development, the small intestine is connected for a time to the yolk sac of the embryo by means of a narrow tubular channel called the vitelline duct (*vitellus* = yolk). Normally, the duct disappears along with the yolk sac, and no trace persists in the adult. In about 2% of persons, however, a remnant of the vitelline duct persists as a small tubular outpouching from the distal ileum about 12–18 in proximal to the cecum. This structure is called a Meckel diverticulum (FIGURE 12). Normally, a Meckel diverticulum has the same type of epithelial lining as that lining the small intestine, but sometimes part of the epithelial lining consists of acid-secreting gastric mucosa. Most Meckel diverticula are asymptomatic, but sometimes the diverticulum becomes infected, causing the same symptoms and complications as an acute appendicitis. If a Meckel diverticulum contains misplaced (ectopic) gastric mucosa, the acidic "gastric juice" secreted by the diverticulum may cause a peptic ulcer of the diverticulum, which may be complicated by bleeding or perforation, as may occur with peptic ulcers in the stomach or duodenum. Whenever an operation is performed for a suspected appendicitis or other gastrointestinal problem, the surgeon

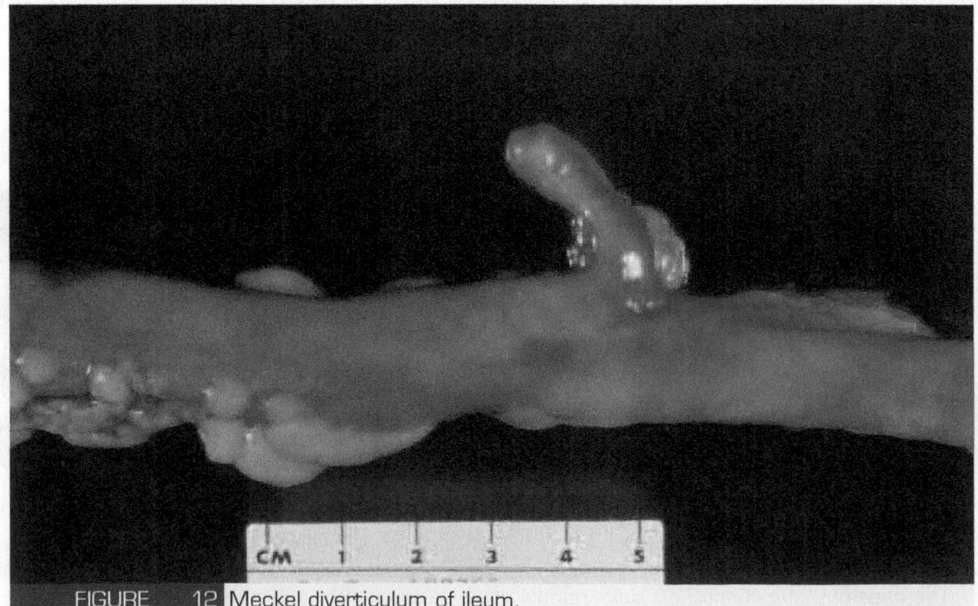

FIGURE 12 Meckel diverticulum of ileum.

always checks to see whether the patient's symptoms are caused by an inflammation or other problem in an unsuspected Meckel diverticulum.

Foreign Bodies

Accidentally swallowed foreign objects that are small and have a relatively uniform shape without sharp edges that can penetrate the bowel mucosa, such as a detached dental tooth crown, a coin, or a closed safety pin can pass through the colon without complication and can be recovered in the feces to confirm that the object has traveled safely through the bowel. However, an object with a sharp point, such as the accidentally swallowed canapé toothpick from a club sandwich, may become stuck by its tip in the intestinal mucosa and penetrate the bowel, as described in Case 1. A larger rigid object may be able to get through the small bowel but may be unable to pass through the ileocecal valve into the colon and may injure the bowel, as described in Case 2.

CASE 1

A late middle-aged man consulted a physician because of abdominal discomfort and cramps for several days. Examination of the abdomen revealed a localized area of tenderness but no evidence of peritonitis. An x-ray examination of the colon revealed a narrow irregular area in the colon of uncertain nature, and an exploratory operation was performed to determine its cause. The abnormality was caused by a large canapé toothpick that had perforated the colon with some associated inflammation in the colon surrounding the perforation site but no significant leakage of bowel contents into the peritoneal cavity (FIGURE 13). The toothpick was removed, and the site of the perforation was closed. The patient made an uneventful recovery.

Toothpick perforations of the bowel may occur when the person eating a canapé sandwich has dentures, which may interfere with oral sensation, or the subject has been drinking alcoholic beverages and is not paying attention to the food being consumed. Usually, the end of the toothpick projecting from the three-layer canapé sandwich has some identifying cellophane attached to the end of the toothpick, which designates its location. Toothpicks should be removed before starting to eat the sandwich.

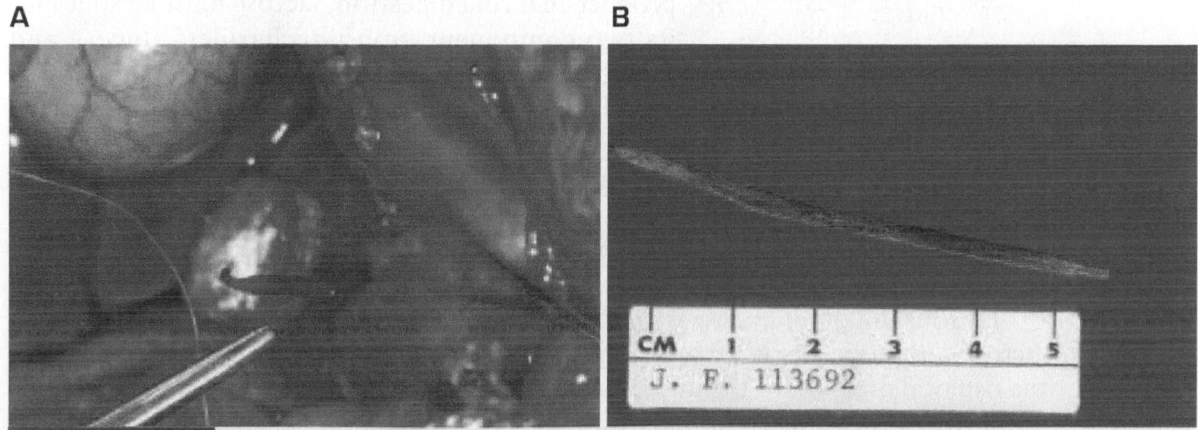

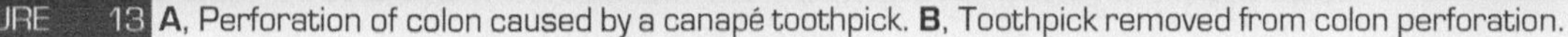

FIGURE 13 **A**, Perforation of colon caused by a canapé toothpick. **B**, Toothpick removed from colon perforation.

CASE 2

A 68-year-old diabetic nursing home resident was accustomed to leaving the nursing home on passes. When she was away from the nursing home, she was allowed to take her medications with her. One was a 25-mg tablet of thioridazine (Mellaril) provided in a unit dose package composed of a rigid foil-covered cardboard base fixed to a plastic cover with a central elevation (blister) that contains the pill. The blister pack is opened to obtain the pill by pulling the base away from the plastic cover. In the nursing home, the medications are dispensed by a nurse but opened by the patient when away from the nursing home.

A few days after she returned from the home pass, she began to experience abdominal pain and her abdomen became distended. She was hospitalized, and an operation was performed. Instead of opening the unit dose blister pack to obtain the pill, she had apparently become confused and ingested the entire unit dose package containing the pill, which had traveled through the upper gastrointestinal tract but was too big to pass through the ileocecal valve into the colon despite vigorous small bowel peristalsis. There were two parallel perforations of her ileum caused by the rigid edges of the unit dose package with an edge protruding through one of the perforations (FIGURE 14). The involved segment of ileum was excised, and the bowel segments were reconnected.

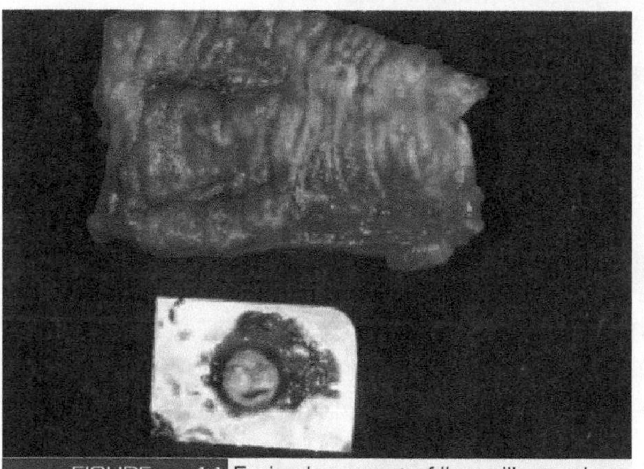

FIGURE 14 Excised segment of ileum illustrating two linear ulcerations and the pill contained in the intact unit dose package.

Disturbances of Bowel Function

FOOD INTOLERANCE

Some patients manifest crampy abdominal pain, abdominal distention, flatulence (excessive gas in the intestinal tract), and frequent loose stools as a result of food intolerance. The two most common types are

1. Lactose intolerance
2. Intolerance to the wheat protein gluten

Lactose Intolerance

Lactose is a disaccharide found in milk and dairy products. During digestion, lactose must be split into its two component monosaccharides, glucose and galactose, before it can be absorbed. This process is accomplished by an enzyme called lactase, which is present on the mucosal surface of the epithelial cells in the small intestine. The enzyme is abundant in infants and young children. In many populations, however, the concentration of lactase gradually declines to very low levels during adolescence and early adult life. The enzyme is deficient in about 20% of adult whites, 70% of American blacks, 90% of American Indians, and almost all Asians.

Persons in whom lactase is deficient are unable to digest lactose. Consequently, lactose cannot be absorbed and remains within the intestinal lumen, where it raises the osmotic pressure of the intestinal contents. Because of the high intraluminal osmotic pressure, fluid is retained within the intestinal tract instead of being absorbed normally, leading to abdominal discomfort, cramps, and diarrhea. Some of the unabsorbed lactose is fermented by bacteria in the colon, yielding lactic acid and other organic acids that further raise the intraluminal osmotic pressure and contribute to the person's discomfort. The symptoms are related to ingestion of dairy products and abate promptly when intake of dairy products is reduced or discontinued.

Gluten Intolerance

Gluten is a general term, which refers to a group of similar proteins found in wheat, rye, oats, and barley; it is the gluten in wheat flour that is responsible for imparting the elasticity to bread dough. Some persons have a hereditary predisposition to become sensitive to the protein in gluten called gliadin, and they form antigliadin antibodies and activated gliadin-sensitized T cells, which causes atrophy of the intestinal villi in the duodenum and proximal jejunum (FIGURE 15). As a result, digestion and absorption of fats and other nutrients is impaired. Several different names have been applied to this condition. The most descriptive term is **gluten enteropathy**, but the condition is also known as celiac disease or celiac sprue. Clinically, the condition is characterized by passage of frequent large, bulky stools containing much unabsorbed fat, associated with weight loss and vitamin deficiencies as a result of the impaired intestinal absorption.

Gluten enteropathy *Damage to intestinal villi caused by ingesting gluten-containing foods by persons sensitive to a protein in gluten; characterized by passage of large bulky stools containing a large amount of poorly absorbed fat.*

Diagnosis is made on the basis of the clinical features and is confirmed if biopsy of the small intestinal mucosa reveals atrophy of the intestinal villi. The specimen for biopsy is obtained by a flexible biopsy device with a small capsule on the end that is swallowed by the patient. The device is positioned in the upper jejunum and is manipulated so that a small bit of intestinal mucosa enters the capsule. Then the capsule is closed, cutting off and retaining a piece of mucosa.

Treatment by a gluten-free diet promptly cures the condition, and the intestinal villi return to normal in about 3–4 months.

IRRITABLE BOWEL SYNDROME

Some patients exhibit episodes of crampy abdominal discomfort, loud gurgling bowel sounds, and disturbed bowel function. Frequent loose stools sometimes alternate

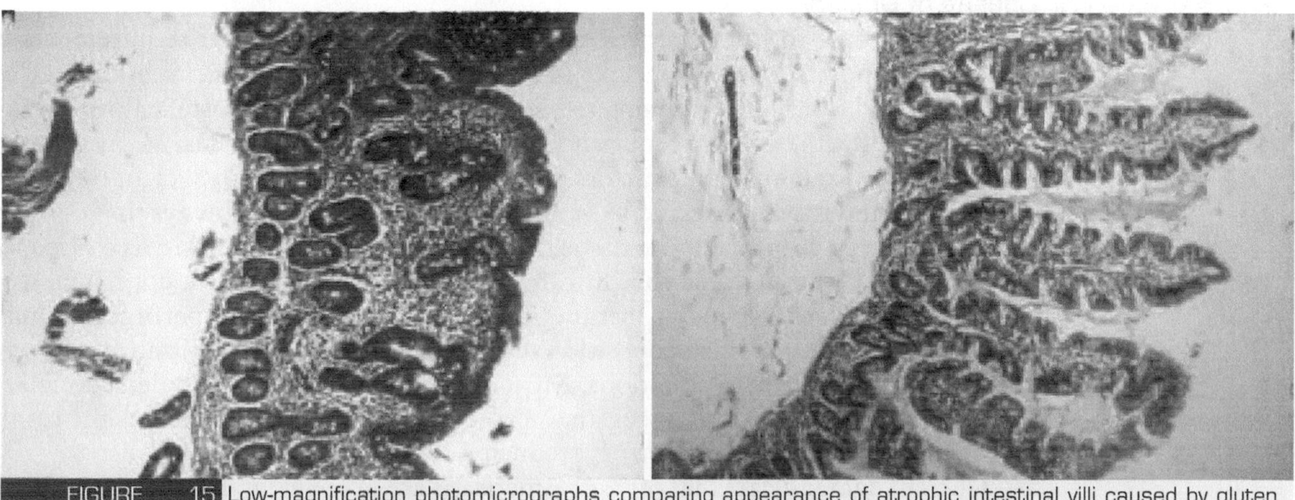

FIGURE 15 Low-magnification photomicrographs comparing appearance of atrophic intestinal villi caused by gluten sensitivity (**A**) with normal appearing villi after excluding gluten from the diet for several months (**B**).

with periods of constipation, and excessive amounts of mucus are secreted by the colonic mucosal glands. These manifestations are frequently quite distressing to the affected individual, but no structural or biochemical abnormalities can be identified to account for the functional disturbances. This condition is often called the irritable bowel syndrome. Other terms for this very common condition are spastic colitis and mucous colitis.

The diagnosis of irritable bowel syndrome is one of exclusion. The physician must rule out infections as a result of pathogenic bacteria and intestinal parasites, food intolerance, and various types of chronic enteritis such as Crohn disease and chronic ulcerative colitis.

Treatment consists of measures that reduce emotional tension and improve intestinal motility. Sometimes, substances that increase the bulk of the stool provide relief of symptoms.

INTESTINAL INFECTIONS IN HOMOSEXUAL MEN

Some homosexual men suffer from intestinal complaints that are caused by various combinations of pathogenic micro-organisms, such as *Shigella* and *Salmonella* and intestinal animal parasites such as *Entamoeba histolytica* and *Giardia*. Spread of the enteric infection is by anal–oral sexual practices that transfer the intestinal pathogens from the infected individual to his sexual partner. In some cases, the intestinal complaints may be misinterpreted as an irritable bowel syndrome if adequate diagnostic studies are not undertaken. Specific methods of treatment are available to cure these infections.

Eating Disorders

Eating disorders are conditions in which food intake is inappropriate and harmful because it leads to serious health consequences. Excessive food intake leading to obesity, which has many harmful effects on health, is the most prevalent disorder. However, abnormal eating habits associated with anorexia nervosa, bulimia nervosa, and binge eating disorders also pose serious health problems for the affected persons.

OBESITY

Causes of Obesity

Fat is the storage form of energy. Any caloric intake that exceeds requirements is stored as adipose tissue and weight is gained. Each excess pound of body weight represents the storage of approximately 3,500 calories. Weight is lost if caloric intake is reduced below the amount required for normal metabolic processes. Many genetic, environmental, and hormonal factors play a role in regulating body weight by affecting appetite and food intake and by influencing the metabolic pathways that convert food into energy or into adipose tissue. It is sometimes said that obesity is caused by an endocrine gland malfunction. In rare instances, hypothyroidism contributes to obesity by reducing the body's metabolic rate. Adrenal cortical hyperfunction may be associated with increased deposition of fat and an abnormal distribution of body fat. These are uncommon situations. Most obese individuals have no detectable endocrine or metabolic disturbances. In the vast majority of cases, obesity is the result of overeating and can be "cured" by reducing food intake.

Current data indicate that 60% of Americans are overweight. Half of the persons in this overweight group are classified as obese, which is defined as 20% or more over ideal body weight, or a body mass index of 30 or more. (Body mass index is a calculated value based on weight in kilograms divided by the square of height in meters.) Moreover, the prevalence of obesity has increased about 8% in the last decade. About 6% of women and 3% of men are more than 100% over their ideal body weight, which is called morbid obesity.

Health Consequences of Obesity

Overweight persons have a higher incidence of diabetes, hypertension, cardiovascular disease, and several other diseases than do persons of normal weight. Therefore, being significantly overweight is undesirable, and extreme obesity is a major health hazard. Obese persons have a mortality rate almost twice that of normal individuals. The excess fat is harmful to the cardiovascular system in three ways:

1. Blood volume and cardiac output must increase to nourish the excess adipose tissue, which overworks the heart.
2. Obese persons are prone to develop high blood pressure, which places a further strain on the heart and blood vessels.
3. Blood lipids are often elevated, which predisposes to arteriosclerosis of the coronary arteries.

Other systems also are adversely affected. Large masses of adipose tissue may impair normal pulmonary ventilation, producing various types of respiratory difficulty and increased susceptibility to pulmonary infection. An otherwise relatively minor respiratory illness may, in an obese person, be a catastrophe because of the increased demands placed upon already overtaxed cardiovascular and respiratory systems.

The high incidence of diabetes in obese persons is the result of an impaired ability to utilize insulin efficiently, as described in the discussion on pancreas and diabetes mellitus. Musculoskeletal disabilities are frequent because the excess weight places undue stress on the bones, joints, and ligaments. Finally, the obese individual is at a serious disadvantage if an operation is required. The operative procedure carries a higher risk, and postoperative complications are more frequent. Any surgical procedure is technically much more difficult in an obese person, and wound healing is delayed. The adipose tissue, which has a relatively poor blood supply, heals poorly and is also quite vulnerable to infection, resulting in an increased incidence of postoperative wound infections.

Another ominous effect of obesity also has been well documented. In obese persons, the death rate from cancer is 52% higher in men and 62% higher in women than are comparable death rates in men and women of normal weight. It has been estimated that 90,000 deaths from cancer could be prevented each year in the United States if men and women could maintain normal weight. The reasons for the higher mortality rate caused by obesity are probably related to higher levels of steroid hormones, insulin, and tumor-promoting growth factors in obese persons compared to persons of normal weight.

Treatment of Obesity

Most overweight persons are too heavy because they are eating too much and are not active enough. Obesity virtually always results from overeating and can be abolished by reducing food intake and becoming more active. Even small weight losses can bring significant health benefits. However, the results of treatment of obesity by dieting have been surprisingly poor because obese individuals are either unable or unwilling to reduce their caloric intake.

Because of the limited success of treating obesity by diet, various other measures have been proposed. Drugs that suppress appetite have been used, but many of these drugs have undesirable side effects.

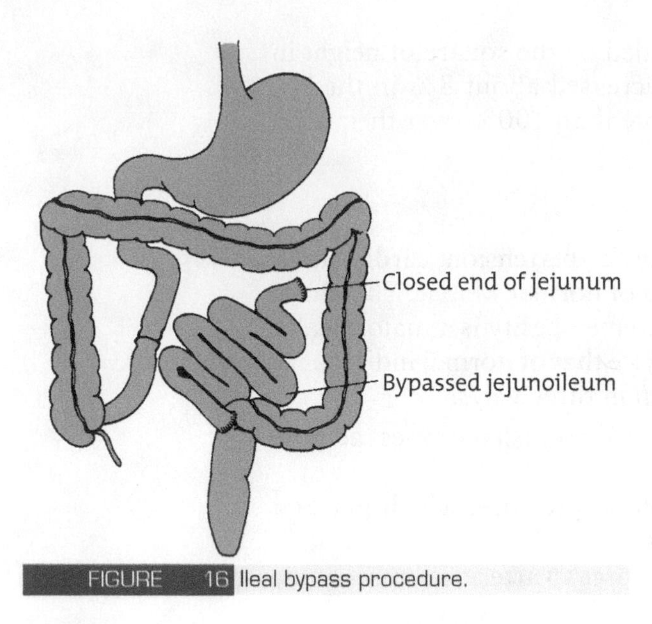

FIGURE 16 Ileal bypass procedure.

As a last resort, massive obesity is sometimes treated by various surgical operations. One of the first weight-reduction operations was called an **ileal bypass.** In this procedure, the ileum was divided about 18 cm proximal to the ileocecal valve, and the jejunum was divided about 30 cm distal to the duodenojejunal junction. Then the proximal jejunum and distal ileum were sutured together, bypassing the remaining part of the small intestine. The proximal (jejunal) end of the bypassed segment was closed. The distal end was connected to an opening made in the sigmoid colon, which permitted intestinal secretions to drain from the bypassed segment into the colon (FIGURE 16). Weight was lost because absorption of nutrients from the greatly shortened small intestine was very poor, which had the same effect as restricting food intake. Unfortunately, this drastic procedure was associated with so many late complications resulting from inadequate absorption of nutrients that it had to be abandoned. Other similar procedures were developed in which weight loss was achieved primarily by preventing absorption of nutrients, but also reduced the capacity of the stomach. Rapid weight loss was achieved but gave rise to the same problems related to impaired absorption of nutrients as the procedure it replaced, and its use is limited to special situations.

Ileal bypass
A surgical procedure performed on the small intestine to promote weight loss.

The current surgical procedures produce weight loss primarily by restricting the capacity of the stomach without resorting to drastic restriction of nutrient absorption in the small intestine. They can be performed using standard surgical incisions or by laparoscopy using small abdominal incisions (described in the general concepts of disease) and are often grouped together under the general term of "stomach stapling operations." The best known and most widely used of these procedures is called the Roux-en-Y gastric bypass, named after the man who devised it (Roux) and the Y-shaped connection made between the small bowel loops in the procedure.

Gastric bypass
An operation to treat massive obesity in which the capacity of the stomach is reduced.

In a **gastric bypass**, a line of staples is placed across the upper part of the stomach. This divides the stomach into two compartments, a very small upper compartment having a volume of only about 15 ml, and a much larger lower compartment that is continuous with the duodenum. Then the jejunum is divided. The distal cut end is anastomosed (connected) to the gastric pouch, and the proximal cut end is connected by means of a second anastomosis to the jejunum distal to the anastomosis between the jejunum and gastric pouch (FIGURE 17). When the procedure is completed, food from the gastric pouch empties directly into the jejunum. The main part of the stomach no longer receives food. Gastric secretions can drain into the duodenum normally, but the secretions enter the jejunum distal ("downstream") to the segment of jejunum receiving the contents from the gastric pouch.

Gastric bypass induces weight loss because the upper compartment of the stomach is so small that it soon becomes overdistended with food when the individual starts to eat. The subject feels "stuffed" and has to stop eating. Weight is lost by enforced reduction of food intake, but absorption of nutrients is also impeded to some extent because gastric contents are shunted into the distal jejunum, bypassing absorption from the proximal part of the small intestine. Unfortunately, gastric bypass procedures may lead to late complications in many patients: anemia caused by poor absorption of iron and vitamin B_{12} and weakening of bones (osteoporosis) as a result of inadequate calcium intake and absorption.

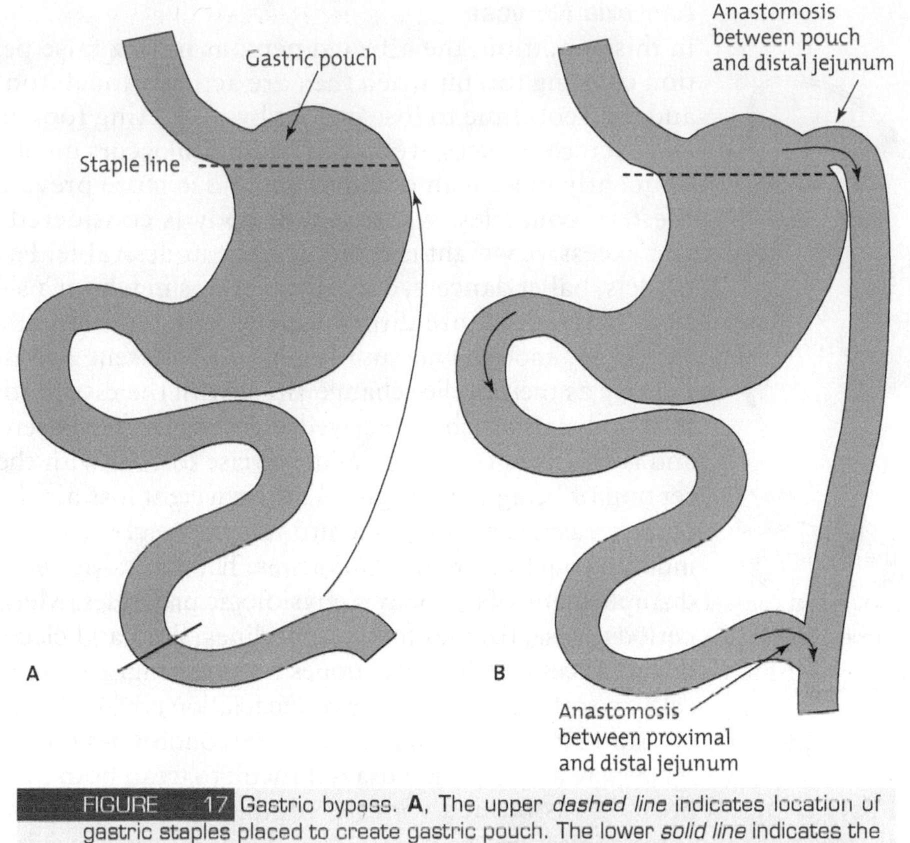

FIGURE 17 Gastric bypass. **A**, The upper *dashed line* indicates location of gastric staples placed to create gastric pouch. The lower *solid line* indicates the site where the jejunum is divided. The *arrow* indicates how the distal segment of jejunum is moved for anastomosis with gastric pouch. **B**, Completed bypass illustrating proximal and distal anastomoses. The *arrows* indicate the direction of movement of gastrointestinal contents, as described in text.

Adjustable gastric banding is another laparoscopic procedure to control food intake by placing an inflatable saline-filled adjustable gastric band around the upper part of the stomach. The band compresses the stomach to form a small upper gastric pouch that is almost completely separated from the rest of the stomach except for a very small channel that allows food in the upper gastric pouch to empty slowly into the lower part of the stomach. The amount of compression applied to the inflatable band, which controls the rate of gastric emptying, can be adjusted by adding or removing saline through a port placed under the skin of the abdomen. The procedure has the advantage of not requiring a "major redesign" of the gastrointestinal tract, but banding does not lead to as much weight loss as a gastric bypass (FIGURE 18).

Adjustable gastric banding
A method for treating obesity by applying an adjustable gastric band to the stomach in order to reduce its capacity, thereby promoting weight loss.

ANOREXIA NERVOSA AND BULIMIA NERVOSA

These two conditions are characterized by profound eating disturbances. Although they are characterized as separate disorders, there is considerable overlap between the two conditions. A more recently recognized condition called binge eating disorder, which occurs in older overweight and obese persons, is probably best considered as a variation of bulimia. Any of these conditions can lead to extreme malnutrition caused by inadequate nutrients, along with associated vitamin and mineral deficiencies. These conditions can lead to serious health consequences, which can be fatal if not adequately treated.

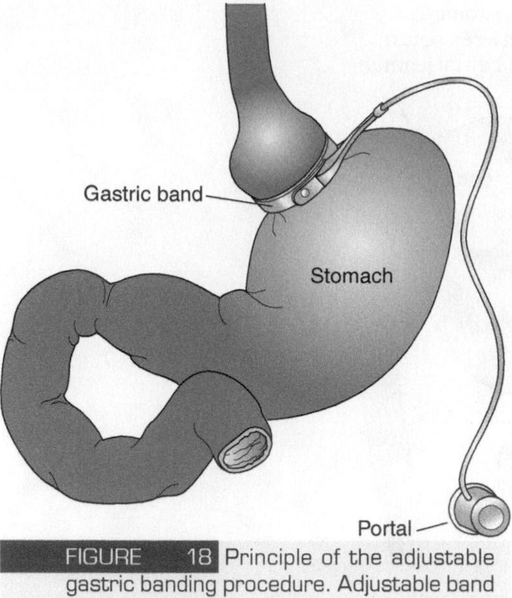

FIGURE 18 Principle of the adjustable gastric banding procedure. Adjustable band filled with saline limits capacity of stomach by constricting outflow from stomach above the band. Rate of gastric emptying can be regulated by adding or removing saline from the band.

Anorexia Nervosa

In this condition, the affected persons have a false perception of being too fat when they are actually much too thin, and they continue to lose weight by restricting food intake and exercising excessively. The condition occurs much more frequently in women than in men and is more prevalent in Western countries, where a slim body is considered ideal and excessive weight is thought to be undesirable. Fashion models, ballet dancers, and other groups in whom a slender body is required, are disproportionately represented.

Often, anorexia nervosa begins in adolescent girls during puberty as their bodies change along with the distribution of their body fat, which is perceived as getting fat from overeating and is followed by dieting and exercise to deal with the perception of being overweight. As their weight loss accelerates, other measures may be taken to reduce weight, such as self-induced vomiting or taking laxatives. The excessive weight loss disrupts many of the body's physiologic processes. Menstrual periods cease, thyroid function declines, fluid and electrolyte disturbances develop, and bones become fragile from loss of calcium (osteoporosis). Extreme emaciation is a life threatening condition that may lead to death if the condition is not treated.

Severe anorexia nervosa is difficult to treat; both the medical and psychological problems associated with the condition must be dealt with. Medical treatment requires correcting the physiologic disturbances caused by the fasting, which may require intravenous fluids and whatever other methods are needed to restore health. Psychologic treatment requires the assistance of a psychiatrist or clinical psychologist experienced in dealing with eating disorders. The affected person needs to acquire a more realistic perception of her (or his) own body, needs to understand what may have led to the eating problem, and needs to learn how to adjust eating habits to prevent a recurrence of the condition.

Bulimia Nervosa

This condition is another method of weight control that is characterized by repeated episodes of binge eating (rapidly eating an excessively large amount of food) followed by purging (self-induced vomiting) to counteract the effects of the bingeing and is followed by guilt and remorse at the inability to control the binge–purge behavior. The purging may be supplemented by taking laxatives to decrease food absorption by promoting rapid passage of digested food through the small intestine. The condition occurs most often in young women. Their body weight may fluctuate in relation to their binge–purge behavior but they do not become emaciated. Their friends and relatives usually are not aware of their problem because they look normal and carefully conceal their binge–purge behavior.

Bulimia nervosa carries with it some serious health problems. Repeated self-induced vomiting leads to dental problems caused by the corrosive effect of the gastric acid on the tooth enamel. The repeated loss of excess gastric juice may lead to metabolic alkalosis and electrolyte disturbances, as discussed in water, electrolyte, and acid–base balance. One of the most serious effects of self-induced vomiting is a tear in the mucosa of the stomach near the gastroesophageal junction, which can bleed profusely and may be fatal, as illustrated in FIGURE 7.

Treatment involves the same medical and psychological approaches used to deal with anorexia nervosa.

BINGE-EATING DISORDER

The condition called a binge eating disorder is characterized by binge eating without compensatory purging to restrict the excess calories contributed by the binge eating, and leads to weight gain. The condition occurs in overweight and obese older adults, with both genders represented in roughly equal proportions. The binge eating complicates the problems of the obese person who is trying to lose weight, and it is estimated that up 20% of persons in weight loss programs may have a binge eating problem. The same approach used to motivate a person to lose weight also applies when dealing with the additional problem posed by the binge eating.

Chronic Malnutrition: Its Causes and Effects

CAUSES OF MALNUTRITION

Malnutrition results when the intake of nutrients is insufficient to supply the body's needs either because there is insufficient food available or the food is not being used efficiently. In developing countries, inadequate food to supply the population may result from crop failure, a natural disaster such as a flood or a drought, poor food distribution, an unstable government, or other causes that impact on food production or delivery. Often, infants and children are disproportionately affected because they have a greater need for nutrients to sustain their rapid growth rate during infancy and childhood.

In modern industrialized countries, many cases of chronic malnutrition are caused by diseases that impair food intake, digestion, or absorption or by conditions that increase nutrient and protein requirements, such as an acute illness, a severe burn, or a major surgical procedure. Other persons at risk are persons living in poverty, the elderly, persons who consume alcohol in excess, drug abusers, persons with AIDS or advanced cancer, and persons with the eating disorders. Treatment consists of supplying adequate nutrients together with vitamins and minerals before the malnutrition-induced organ damage has progressed to such a degree that response to treatment is unlikely to be successful.

IDENTIFYING PERSONS AT RISK

Malnutrition in children may be a manifestation of parental neglect, which should be investigated. Malnutrition in adults should be suspected when an adult has lost weight and whose food intake or absorption have decreased for any reason or whose nutrient requirements have increased significantly as a result of disease. Prevention and early detection of malnutrition in high-risk patients facilitates early treatment. More advanced and severe malnutrition takes longer to correct.

EVALUATION AND TREATMENT

Nutritional deficiencies often involve not only inadequate food nutrients but also multiple vitamin and mineral deficiencies. Weight loss of 5–10% of normal body weight usually can be tolerated but as weight loss increases, so do the manifestations of inadequate nutrition and protein deficiency. Extreme emaciation is a life threatening condition, and loss of over 30% of body weight may be fatal.

When evaluating a malnourished subject, the initial clinical evaluation should be supplemented by laboratory tests to assess the extent of organ and tissue damage, including determination of serum albumin as an index of protein deficiency. Medical treatment requires correcting any fluid and electrolyte disturbances and other physiologic disturbances caused by the deficiencies, followed by slowly increasing calorie and protein intake, preferably by oral feeding. Appropriate vitamin and mineral supplements are also provided, along with whatever additional measures are necessary to restore health.

ALCOHOL: ITS ROLE IN MALNUTRITION

Drinking modest amounts of alcoholic beverages is considered acceptable in many cultures and even provides some health benefits by favorably influencing blood lipids. Although not classified as a nutrient, alcohol provides 7 calories per gram, which is almost as many calories as in fat. So alcohol can be categorized as a "high-calorie nonnutrient." Excess alcohol intake can cause serious problems. Rapidly drinking large amounts of alcohol in a short period can be lethal, as documented by many reports of fatal alcohol intoxication, resulting from binge drinking among high school and college students. Chronic alcohol use has its own set of potential problems. It may lead to dependence on alcohol, which can progress to alcohol addiction in susceptible individuals. Alcoholism is a common cause of malnutrition because the alcohol is substituting nonnutritive "empty calories" from alcohol for calories from food, which supply the nutrients, vitamins, and minerals that the body needs. Many of the harmful results of chronic alcoholism are related not only to the organ damage caused by excess alcohol, such as alcoholic liver disease and its complications described in the discussion on the liver and biliary system, but also from the associated vitamin deficiencies that accompany an inadequate diet.

Diverticulosis and Diverticulitis of the Colon

Outpouchings of the mucosa of the colon often project through weak areas in the muscular wall of the large intestine. These outpouchings are called diverticula (singular, **diverticulum**), and the condition is called **diverticulosis** (FIGURES 19, 20, AND 21). This is an acquired condition, in contrast to a Meckel diverticulum, which

Diverticulum
(dī-vur-tik′u-lum)
An outpouching from an organ, as from the mucosa of the colon, which projects through the muscular wall.

Diverticulosis
(dī-vur-tik-u-lō′sis)
A condition characterized by an outpouching of the colonic mucosa through weak areas in the muscular wall.

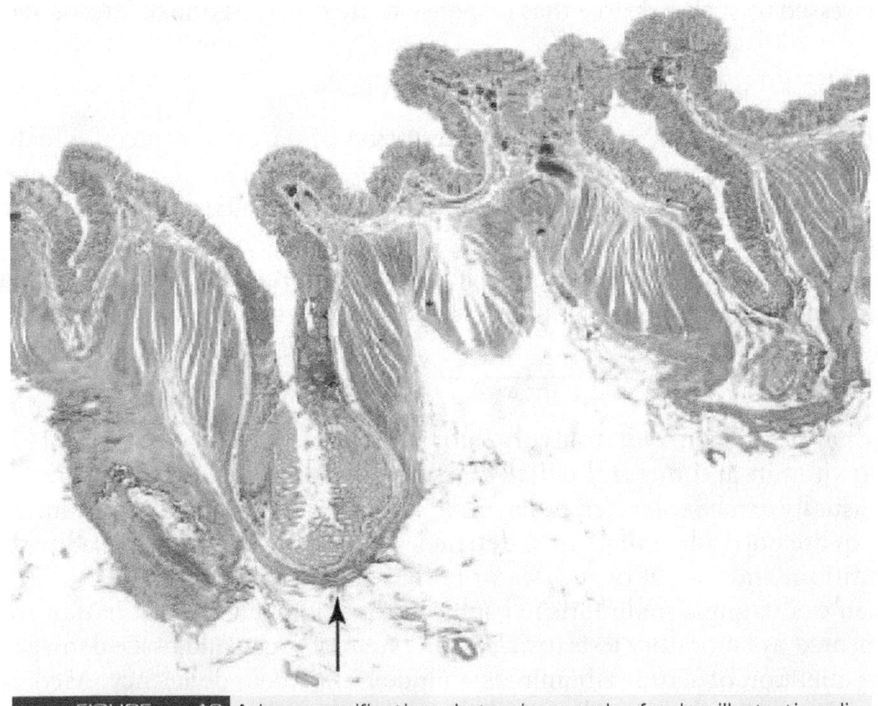

FIGURE 19 A low-magnification photomicrograph of colon illustrating diverticula. Mucosa of the colon (*upper part* of photograph) protrudes through muscular wall (*arrow*) into the serosa of colon (original magnification × 10).

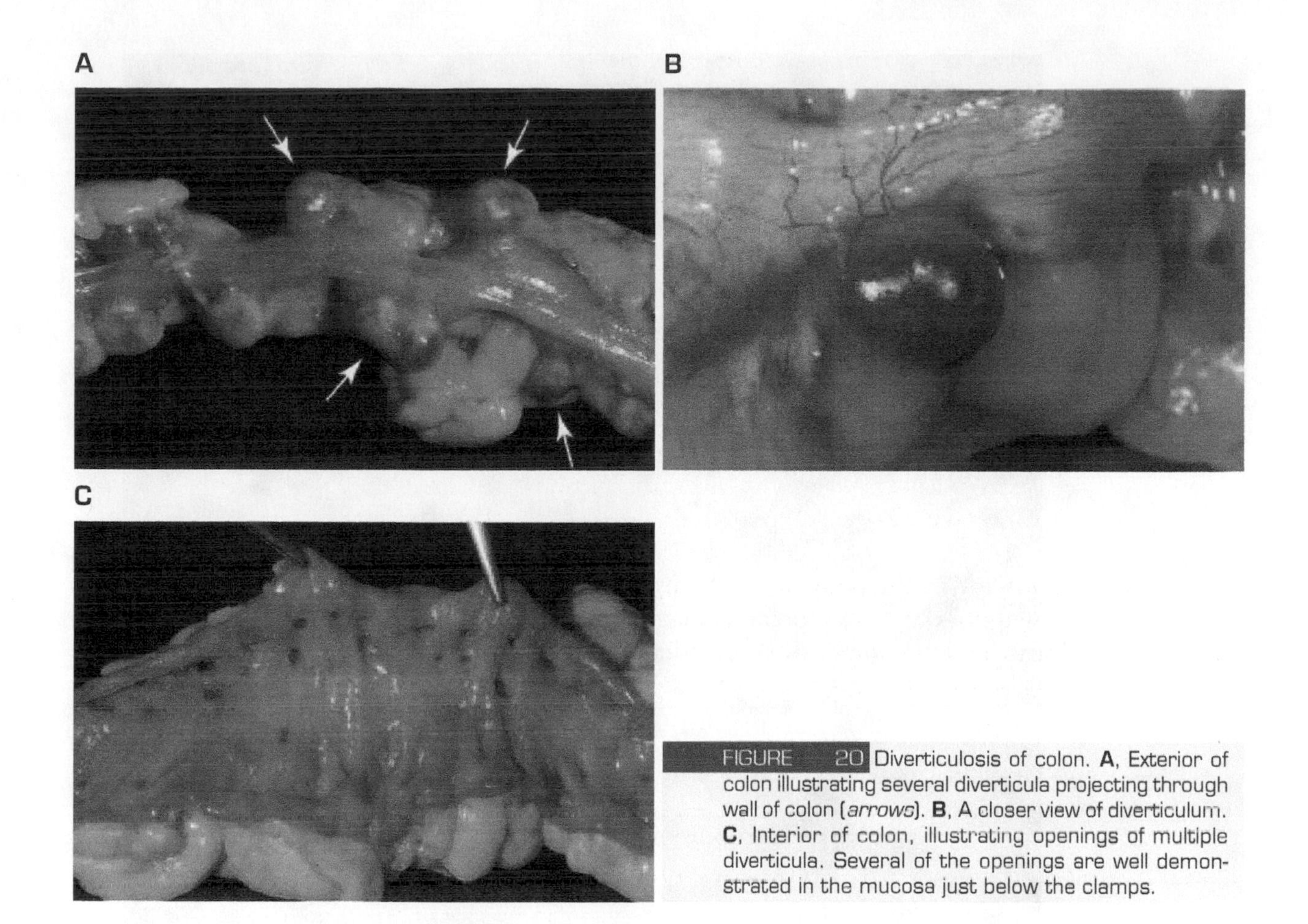

FIGURE 20 Diverticulosis of colon. **A**, Exterior of colon illustrating several diverticula projecting through wall of colon (*arrows*). **B**, A closer view of diverticulum. **C**, Interior of colon, illustrating openings of multiple diverticula. Several of the openings are well demonstrated in the mucosa just below the clamps.

is a congenital abnormality (see FIGURE 12). Diverticula, which usually occur in the distal colon, are encountered with increasing frequency in older patients. Highly refined, low-residue diets predispose to diverticula because stools are small and hard, and high intraluminal pressure must be generated by peristalsis to propel the stool through the colon. This high intracolonic pressure forces the mucosa through weak areas in the muscular wall. In contrast, people who subsist on high-residue diets have large, bulky stools that can be propelled through the colon easily at low intraluminal pressures, and diverticula occur infrequently among them.

Most diverticula are asymptomatic, but occasionally problems arise. Bits of fecal material may become trapped within these pouches and incite an inflammatory reaction called **diverticulitis**. The inflammation may be followed by considerable scarring. Occasionally, perforation of a diverticulum may occur, leading to an abscess in the pelvis. Sometimes blood vessels in the mucosa of the diverticulum may become ulcerated by abrasion from the fecal material, resulting in bleeding. Diverticula attended by such complications as infections, perforation, or bleeding are often treated by surgical resection of the affected segment of bowel.

Diverticulitis
(dī-vur-tik-u-lī′tis)
An inflammation of a diverticulum.

Intestinal Obstruction

If the normal passage of intestinal contents through the bowel is blocked, the patient is said to have an intestinal obstruction. The site of the blockage may be either the small intestine (high intestinal obstruction) or the colon (low intestinal obstruction). Bowel obstruction is always serious. The severity of the symptoms depends on the location of the obstruction, its completeness, and whether there is interference with the blood supply to the blocked segment of bowel.

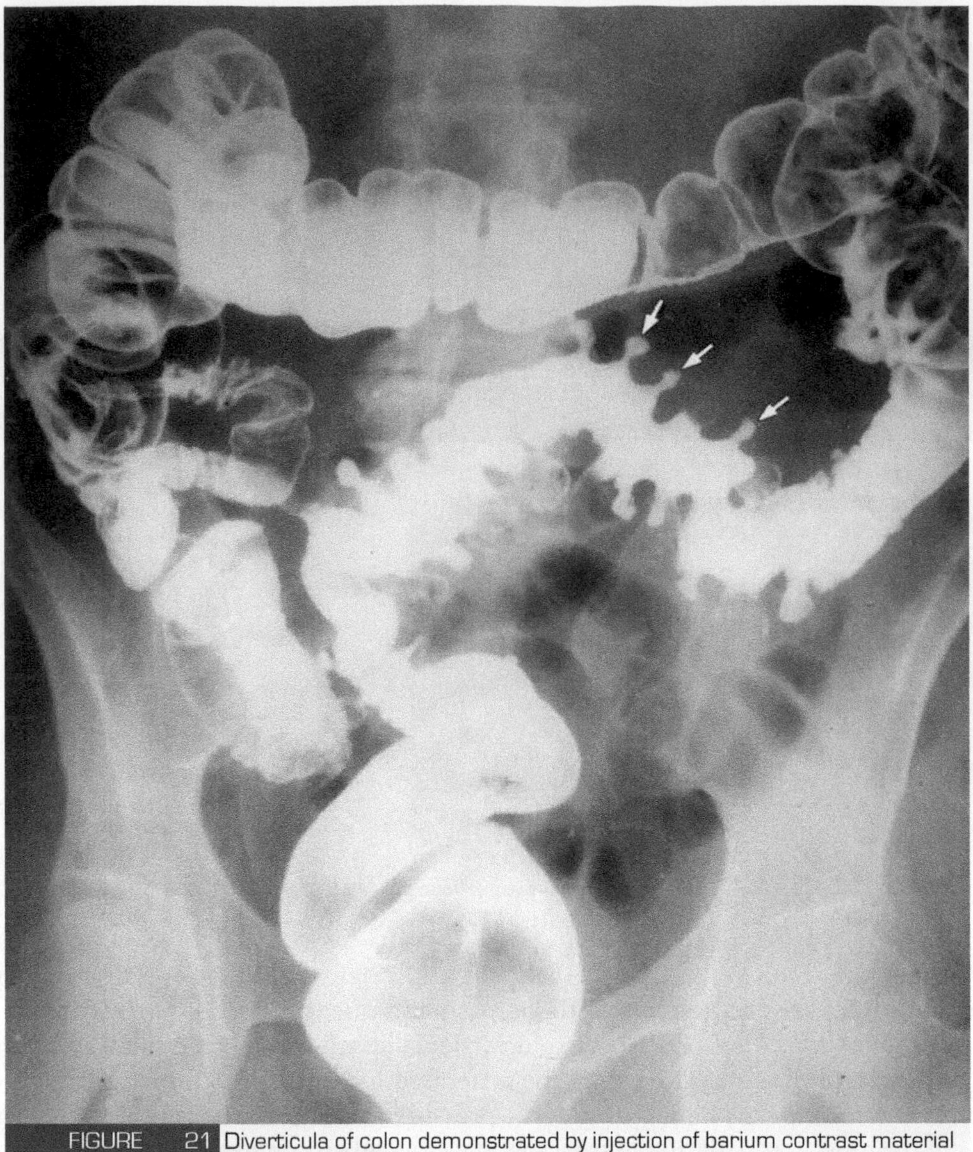

FIGURE 21 Diverticula of colon demonstrated by injection of barium contrast material into colon (barium enema). Diverticula filled with contrast material appear as projections from the mucosa (*arrows*).

Obstruction of the small intestine causes severe, crampy pain as a result of vigorous peristalsis, reflecting the attempt of the intestine to force bowel contents past the site of obstruction. This is associated with vomiting of copious amounts of gastric and upper intestinal secretions, resulting in loss of large quantities of water and electrolytes. As a consequence, the patient becomes dehydrated and develops pronounced fluid and electrolyte disturbances.

Symptoms are much less acute when the distal colon is obstructed. There may be mild, crampy abdominal pain and moderate distention of the abdomen. However, vomiting with associated loss of fluid and electrolytes is not as serious a problem as in high intestinal obstruction. Disturbances of fluid and electrolytes do not develop as rapidly.

The common causes of intestinal obstruction are as follows:

1. Intestinal adhesions
2. Hernia
3. Tumor
4. Volvulus
5. Intussusception

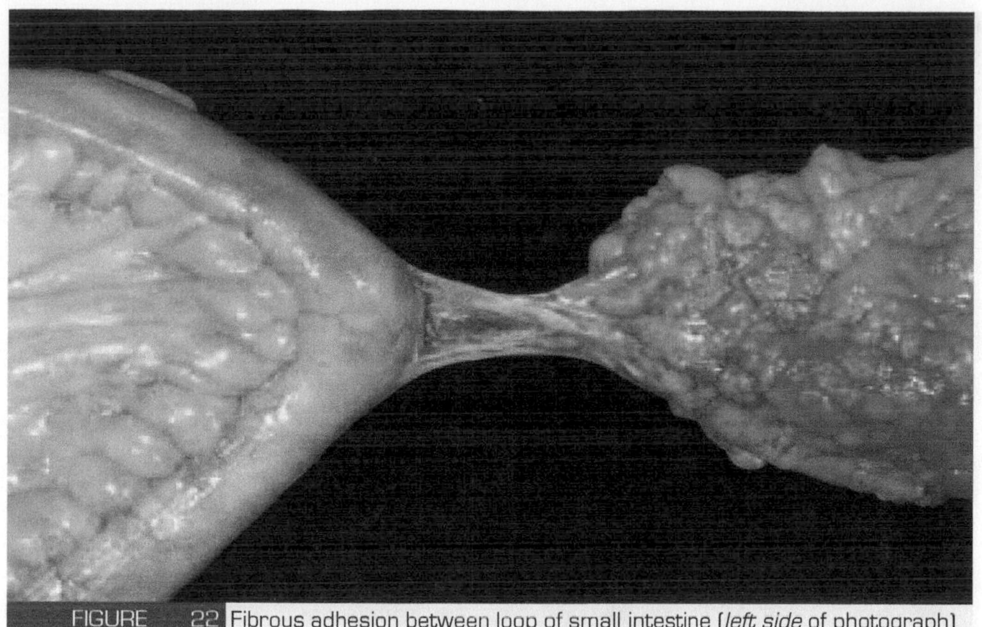

FIGURE 22 Fibrous adhesion between loop of small intestine (*left side* of photograph) and omentum.

Adhesions
(ad-hē′shuns)
Bands of fibrous tissue that form subsequent to an inflammation, and bind adjacent tissues together.

Hernia
(her′nē-yuh)
A protrusion of a loop of bowel through a narrow opening, usually in the abdominal wall.

ADHESIONS

Adhesive bands of connective tissue (**adhesions**) may form within the abdominal cavity after surgery (FIGURE 22). Sometimes a loop of bowel becomes kinked, compressed, or twisted by an adhesive band, causing obstruction proximal to the site of the adhesion.

HERNIA

A **hernia** is a protrusion of a loop of bowel through a small opening, usually in the abdominal wall. The herniated loop pushes the peritoneum ahead of it, forming the hernia sac. Inguinal hernia is quite common in men (FIGURE 23). A loop of small bowel protrudes through a weak area in the inguinal ring and may descend downward into the scrotum. Umbilical and femoral hernias occur in both sexes. In an umbilical hernia, the loop of bowel protrudes into the umbilicus through a defect in the abdominal wall (FIGURE 24). In a femoral hernia, a loop of intestine extends under the inguinal ligament along the course of the femoral vessels into the groin. If a herniated loop of bowel can be pushed back into the abdominal cavity, the hernia is said to be reducible. Occasionally, a herniated loop becomes stuck and cannot be reduced. This is called an incarcerated hernia. Sometimes the loop of bowel is so tightly constricted by the margins of the defect that allowed the herniation that the blood supply to the herniated bowel is obstructed, causing necrosis of the protruding segment of bowel. This is called a strangulated hernia and requires prompt surgical intervention.

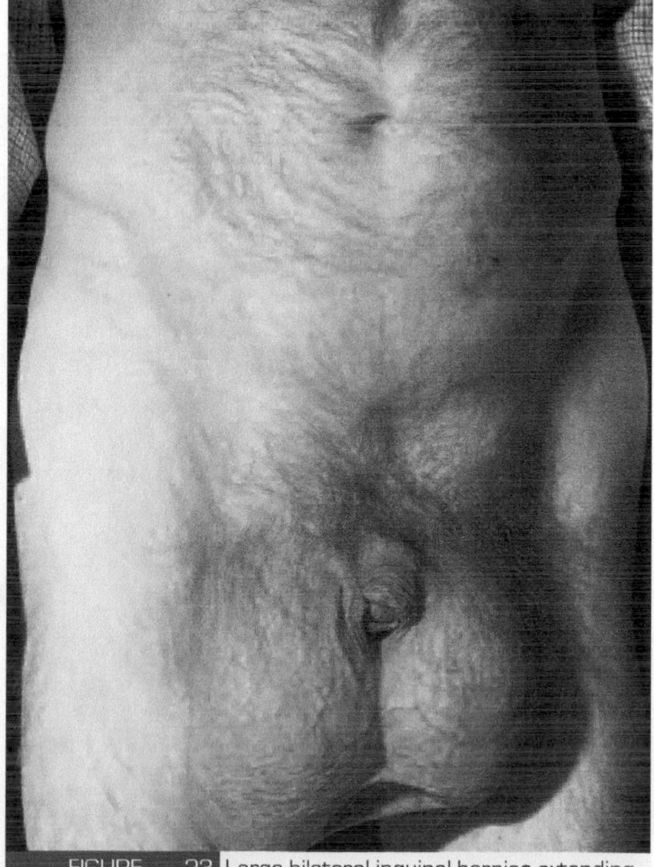

FIGURE 23 Large bilateral inguinal hernias extending into the scrotum.

Volvulus
(vol′vū-lus)
A rotary twisting of the intestine on its mesentery, with obstruction of the blood supply to the twisted segment.

Intussusception
(in′tus-us-cep′shun)
A telescoping of one segment of bowel into an adjacent segment.

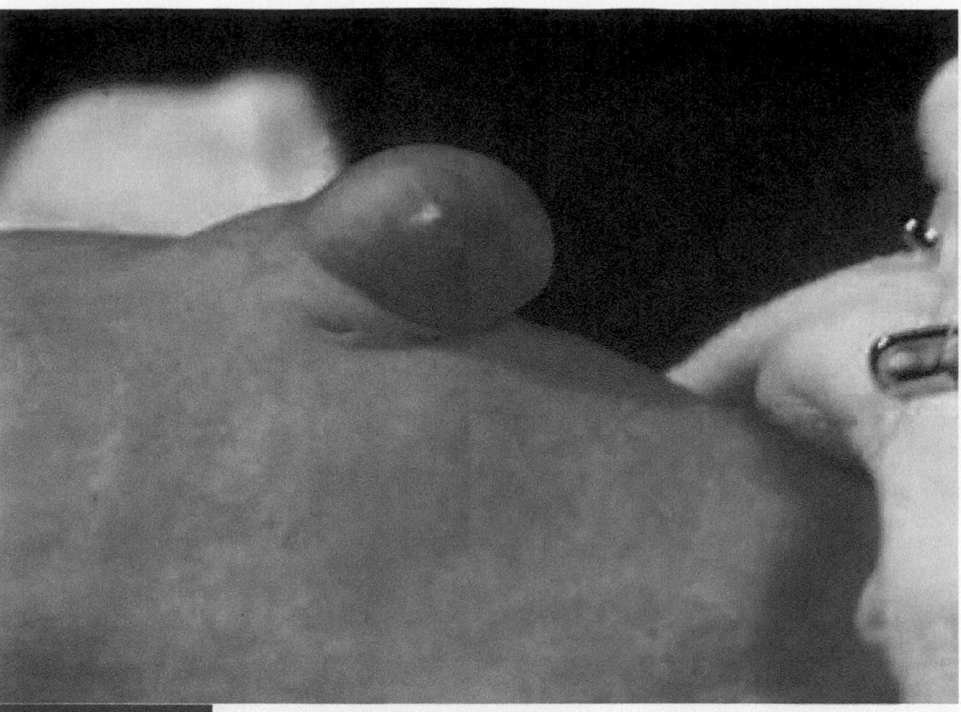

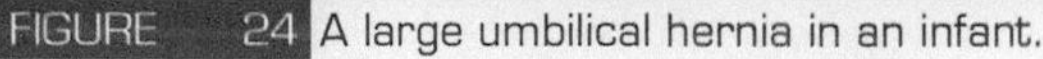
FIGURE 24 A large umbilical hernia in an infant.

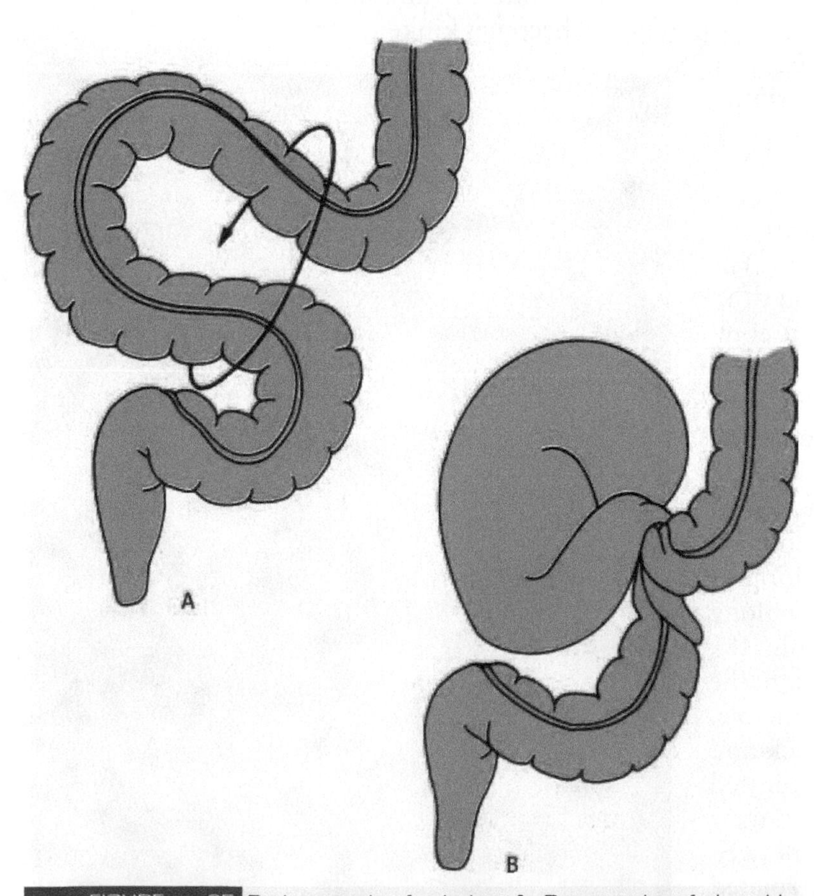

FIGURE 25 Pathogenesis of volvulus. **A**, Rotary twist of sigmoid colon on its mesentery. **B**, Obstruction of colon and interruption of its blood supply caused by volvulus.

VOLVULUS AND INTUSSUSCEPTION

A **volvulus** is a rotary twisting of the bowel on the fold of peritoneum that suspends the bowel from the posterior wall of the abdomen, which is called the mesentery of the bowel. The blood supply to the twisted segment also is impaired because the blood vessels supplying the bowel travel in the mesentery, and they are compressed when the bowel and mesentery become twisted. The sigmoid colon is the usual site (FIGURE 25).

An **intussusception** is a telescoping of one segment of bowel into an adjacent segment. This is a common cause of intestinal obstruction in children and usually results from vigorous peristalsis that telescopes the terminal ileum into the proximal colon through the ileocecal valve (FIGURE 26). In adults, the condition is usually secondary to a benign tumor of the bowel that is supported by a narrow stalk. A tumor of this type is often called a pedunculated tumor, the name being derived from the stalk (pedicle) that supports it (*pediculus* = little foot). As the tumor is propelled by a peristaltic wave, the base of the tumor exerts traction on the bowel wall at its site of attachment, causing the proximal segment of bowel to be pulled into the distal segment (FIGURES 27 AND 28).

Carcinoma of the colon may obstruct the distal colon and is a common cause of low intestinal obstruction.

Mesenteric Thrombosis

The blood supply to the gastrointestinal tract is derived from several large arteries arising from the aorta. The blood supply to most of the bowel is provided by the superior mesenteric artery. This vessel supplies blood to the entire small intestine and the proximal half of the colon. The arteries supplying the gastrointestinal tract may develop arteriosclerotic changes and become occluded by thrombosis in the same way as may other arteries. Thrombosis of the superior mesenteric artery leads to an extensive infarction of most of the bowel.

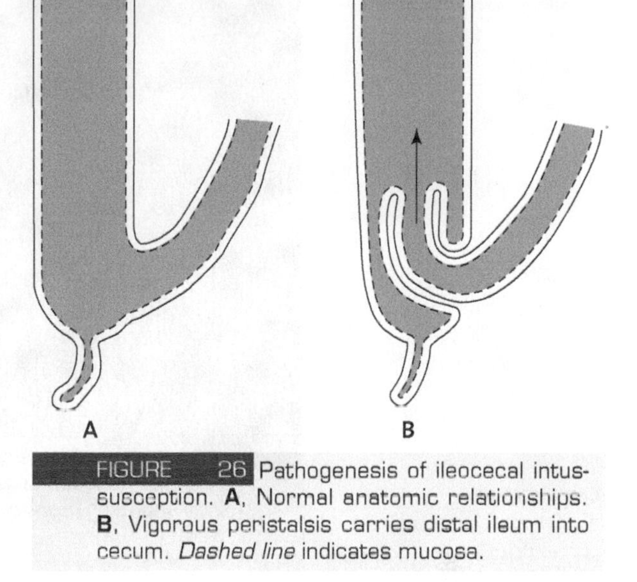

FIGURE 26 Pathogenesis of ileocecal intussusception. **A**, Normal anatomic relationships. **B**, Vigorous peristalsis carries distal ileum into cecum. *Dashed line* indicates mucosa.

Tumors of the Bowel

Tumors of the small intestine are uncommon, whereas benign pedunculated polyps of the colon occur quite frequently. Usually they do not cause symptoms, but occasionally the tip of the polyp may become eroded and cause bleeding. Often, a polyp can be removed by inserting a flexible instrument called a colonoscope into the bowel through the rectum and cutting the narrow stalk.

Imperforate anus
(im-per′for-āt)
Congenital absence of anal opening, often associated with absence of distal rectum as well.

Carcinoma of the colon is a common tumor that may arise anywhere in the large intestine or rectum. Carcinoma arising in the cecum and right half of the colon generally does not cause obstruction of the bowel because the caliber of this portion of the colon is large and the bowel contents are relatively soft. However, the tumor often becomes ulcerated and bleeds, leading to chronic iron deficiency anemia. The patient with a carcinoma of the right half of the colon may consult a physician because of weakness and fatigue caused by the anemia, without experiencing any symptoms referable to the intestinal tract.

Carcinoma of the distal portion of the colon, which has a much smaller caliber than the proximal colon, often causes partial obstruction of the bowel and leads to symptoms of lower intestinal obstruction (FIGURES 29 AND 30).

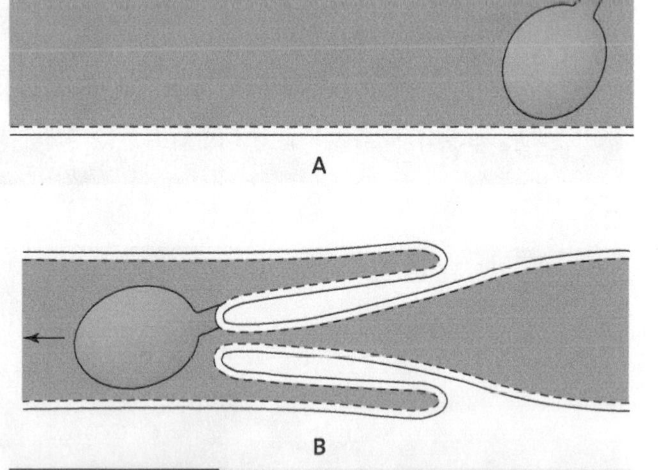

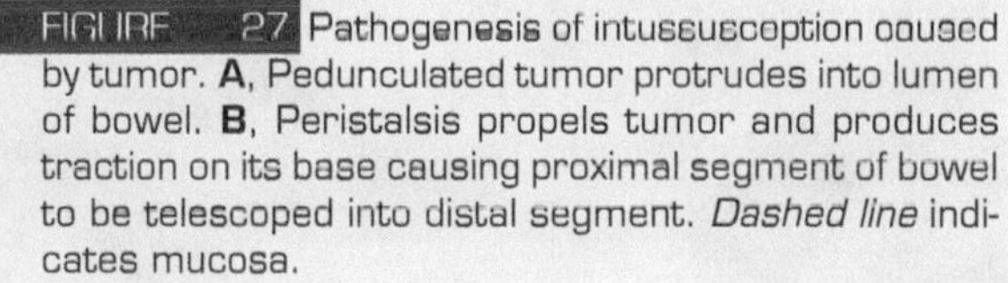

FIGURE 27 Pathogenesis of intussusception caused by tumor. **A**, Pedunculated tumor protrudes into lumen of bowel. **B**, Peristalsis propels tumor and produces traction on its base causing proximal segment of bowel to be telescoped into distal segment. *Dashed line* indicates mucosa.

Imperforate Anus

Imperforate anus is an uncommon congenital abnormality in which the colon fails to acquire a normal anal opening (FIGURE 31). There are two major types. In one type, the rectum and anus are normally formed and extend to the level of the skin, but no anal orifice is present. Often, a small tract (fistula) extends

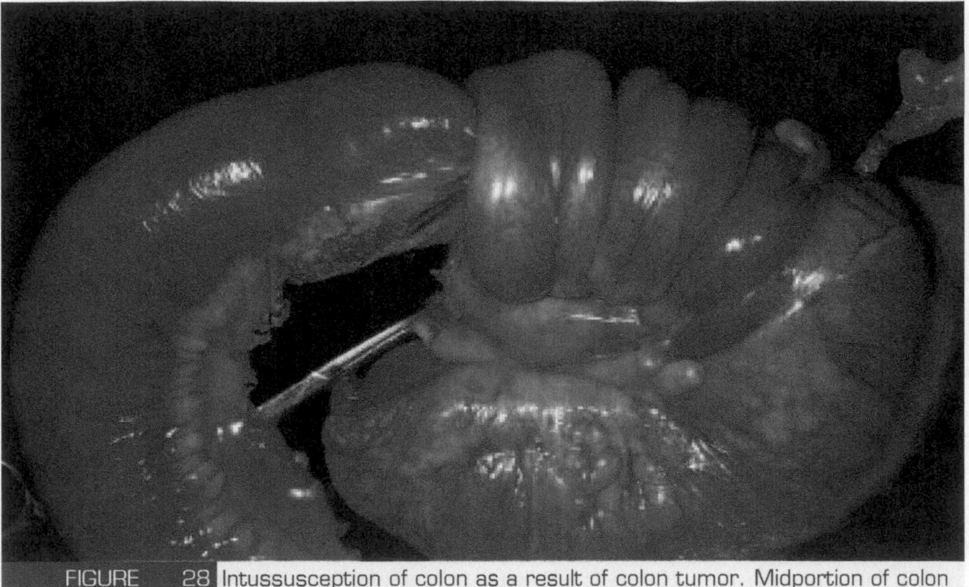

FIGURE 28 Intussusception of colon as a result of colon tumor. Midportion of colon is swollen because of telescoping of the proximal segment (*left side* of photograph) into distal segment (*right side* of photograph).

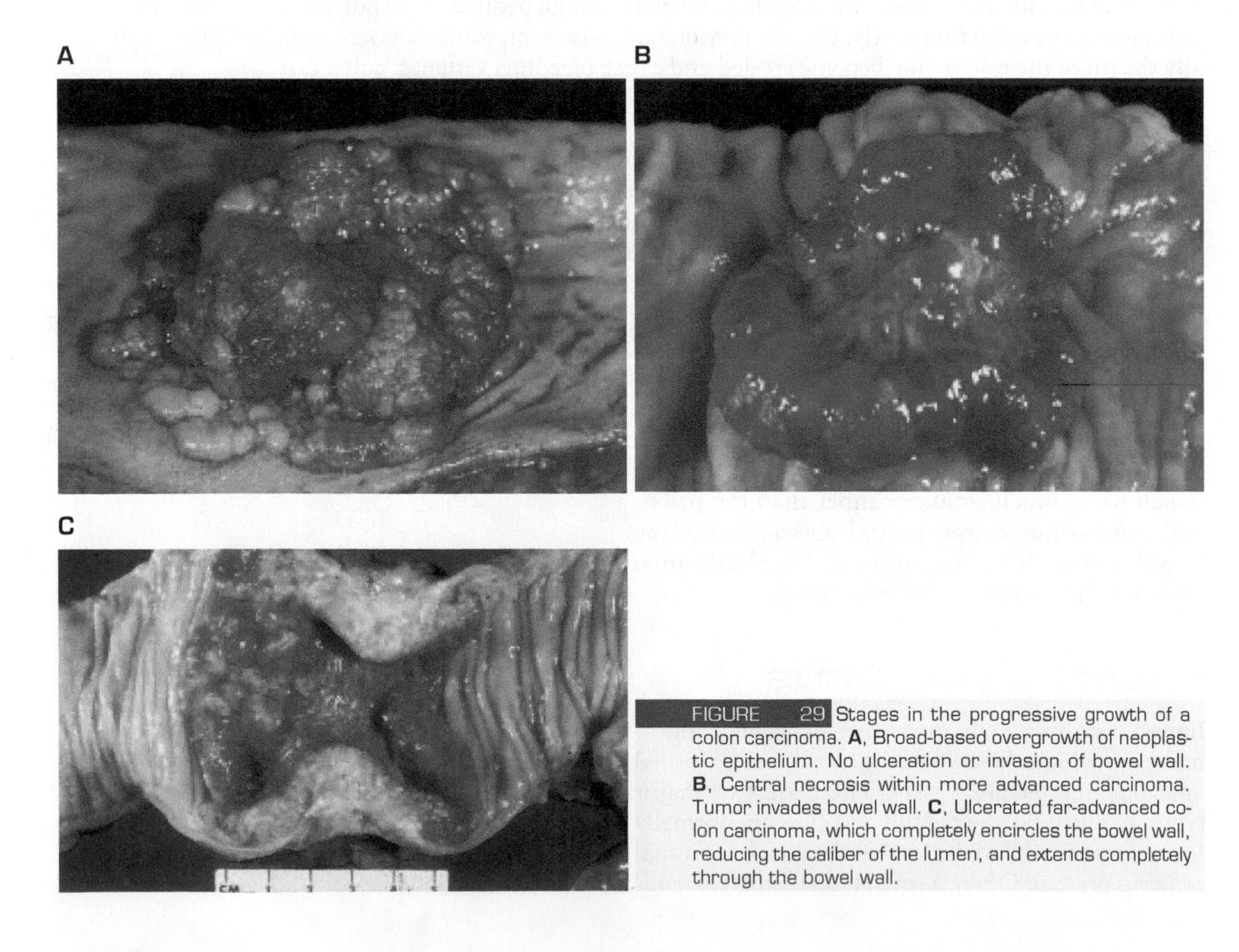

FIGURE 29 Stages in the progressive growth of a colon carcinoma. **A**, Broad-based overgrowth of neoplastic epithelium. No ulceration or invasion of bowel wall. **B**, Central necrosis within more advanced carcinoma. Tumor invades bowel wall. **C**, Ulcerated far-advanced colon carcinoma, which completely encircles the bowel wall, reducing the caliber of the lumen, and extends completely through the bowel wall.

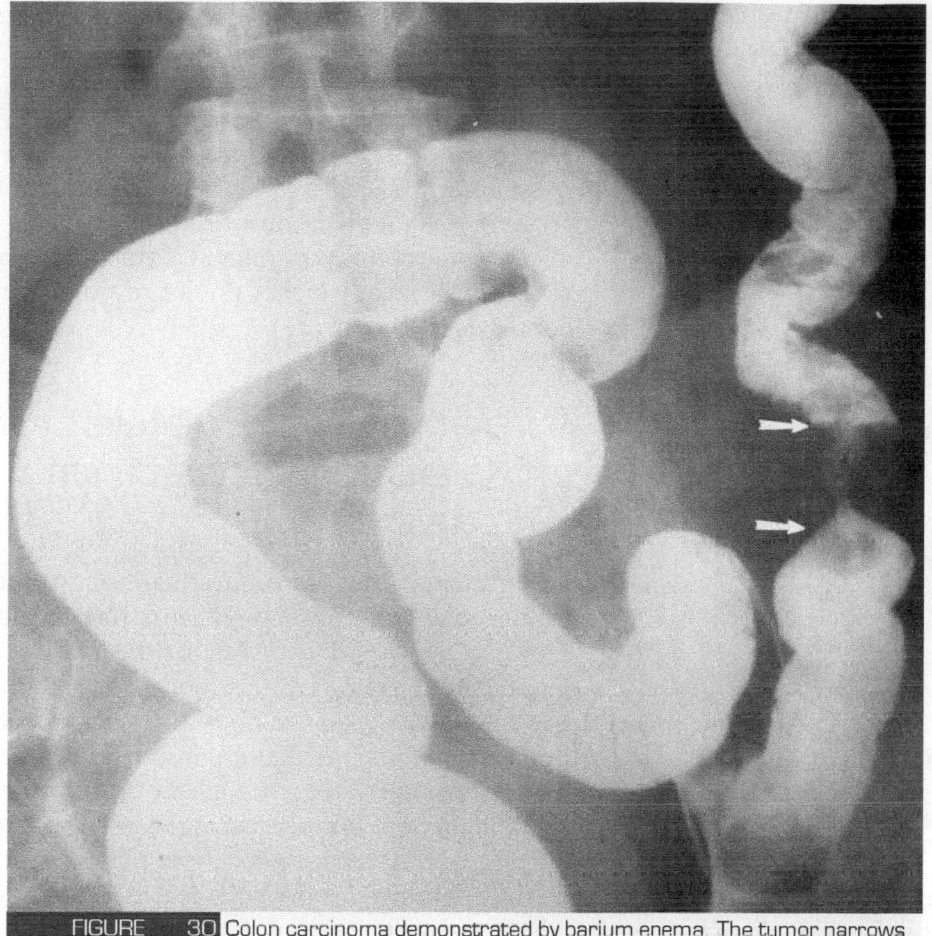

FIGURE 30 Colon carcinoma demonstrated by barium enema. The tumor narrows the lumen of the colon, which appears as a filling defect in the column of barium (*arrows*).

Hemorrhoids
(hem'or-oyds)
Varicosities of anal and rectal veins.

from the blind end of the anal canal to terminate in the urethra, in the vagina, or on the surface of the skin. Usually, this type of imperforate anus can be easily treated by excising the tissue covering the anal opening. In the second type of imperforate anus, the entire distal rectum fails to develop, and often there are associated abnormalities of the urogenital tract and skeletal system. Surgical repair of this type of abnormality is much more difficult, and results are less satisfactory.

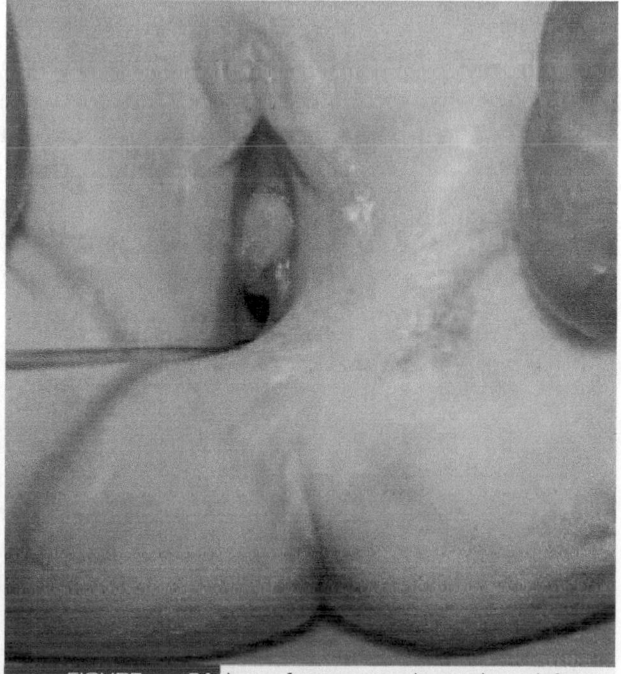

FIGURE 31 Imperforate anus in newborn infant. Metal probe has been placed in vagina.

Hemorrhoids

Hemorrhoids are varicosities of the venous plexus that drains the rectum and anus (FIGURE 32). Constipation and increased straining during bowel movements predispose to their development. Internal hemorrhoids, which involve the veins of the lower rectum, may become eroded and bleed, may become thrombosed, or may prolapse through the anus. External hemorrhoids involve the veins of the anal canal and perianal skin. They sometimes become

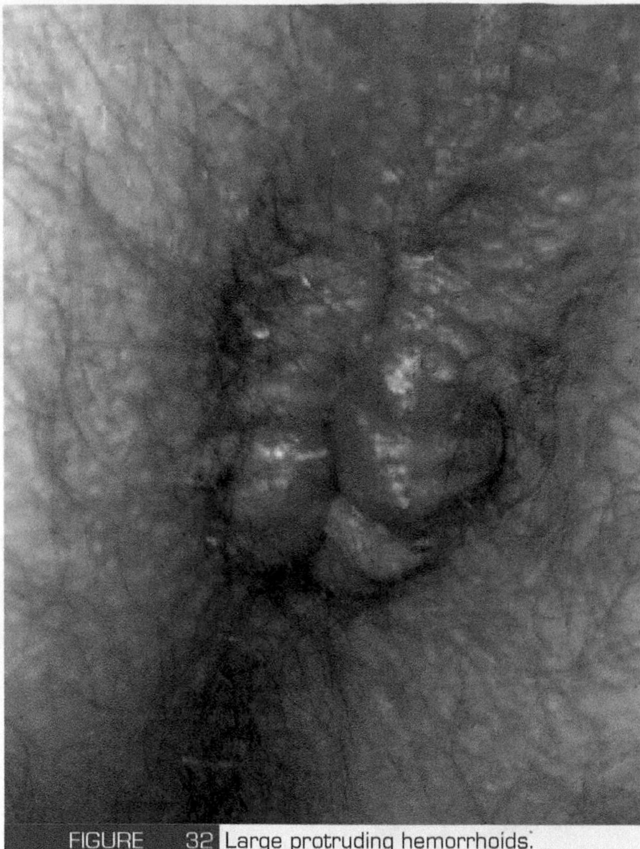

FIGURE 32 Large protruding hemorrhoids.

thrombosed, which causes considerable anorectal discomfort.

Symptoms of hemorrhoids can often be relieved by a high-fiber diet rich in fruits and vegetables, which promotes large, bulky stools that can be passed without excessive straining. Stool softeners and local application of rectal ointments may also provide temporary relief. Hemorrhoids can be removed surgically if they do not respond to more conservative therapy.

Diagnostic Evaluation of Gastrointestinal Disease

Unfortunately, the gastrointestinal tract cannot be examined as easily as many other parts of the body. However, it is possible to visualize the interior of the esophagus, the stomach, the duodenum, and the entire colon by endoscopic procedures using specially designed instruments that are inserted into the gastrointestinal tract either through the oral cavity or the anus. Endoscopy is described in the general concepts of disease in the section on diagnostic procedures.

Endoscopic procedures are generally employed if the patient experiences symptoms suggesting disease of the esophagus, stomach, or colon. Abnormal areas in the mucosa can be visualized, biopsied, and examined histologically.

Areas that cannot be visualized directly can be studied by radiologic examination. Examination of the upper gastrointestinal tract is accomplished by having the patient ingest a radiopaque material (contrast medium), allowing the clinician to visualize the transport of the material through the intestinal tract by x-ray studies. Any areas where the motility of the bowel appears abnormal, indicating disease, can be seen on the film. This technique also allows the clinician to visualize the contours of the gastrointestinal mucosa and thereby to identify the location and extent of disease affecting the bowel mucosa, such as ulcer, stricture, tumor, or an area of chronic inflammation. The colon can be studied in a similar manner by instilling radiopaque material into the bowel through the anus in order to outline the contours of the large intestine. This type of study is called a barium enema (see FIGURES 19 AND 30).

QUESTIONS FOR REVIEW

1. What is a cleft palate? What is its usual mode of inheritance? How is it treated?
2. What factors affect the development of dental caries? What complications may result from dental caries? What are the causes and possible effects of periodontal disease?
3. What are some of the major causes of esophageal obstruction? What symptoms does esophageal obstruction produce?
4. What is peptic ulcer? In what parts of the gastrointestinal tract are peptic ulcers encountered? What factors contribute to the development of peptic ulcers? What are the complications of a peptic ulcer?

5. What is the difference between Crohn disease and chronic ulcerative colitis? Diverticulosis and diverticulitis?
6. What is a Meckel diverticulum? Where is it located? What clinical manifestations can it produce?
7. What is intestinal obstruction? What symptoms does it produce? What are some of the common causes of intestinal obstruction?
8. What is the pathogenesis of acute appendicitis?
9. What symptoms and physical findings are likely to be encountered in a patient with a carcinoma of the colon? Why?
10. What is an intussusception? How is it caused? What is the difference between volvulus and intussusception?

SUPPLEMENTARY READINGS

Allen, J. J. 1995. Molecular biology of colorectal cancer: A clinician's view. *Perspectives in Colon and Rectal Surgery* 8:181–202.

- An excellent review article on genes related to cancer development, the "multiple hit" concept of cell deregulation, and the hereditary types of colon cancer.

Blaser, M. J. 1999. Where does *Helicobacter pylori* come from and why is it going away? *Journal of the American Medical Association* 282:2260–2.

- *H. pylori* infects only primates, and there is no reservoir in nature. The organism can be identified in dental plaque and in stool specimens. Very large numbers of organisms are present in the vomit of infected persons and in the air in the vicinity of the vomitus. Fewer persons are colonized by the organism as a result of better sanitation and less close family contacts, which reduces the person-to-person spread of the organism.

Brolin, R. E. 2002. Bariatric surgery and long-term control of morbid obesity. *Journal of the American Medical Association* 288:2793–6.

- Describes the magnitude of the "obesity epidemic" and the applications and limitations of various surgical procedures used to treat morbid obesity. Includes description of gastric banding and another procedure somewhat similar to the ileal bypass procedure.

Calle, E., Rodriguez, C., Walker-Thurmond, K., and Thun, M. J. 2003. Overweight, obesity, and mortality from cancer in a prospectively studied cohort of U.S. adults. *The New England Journal of Medicine* 348:1625–38.

- In a 16-year prospective study of more than 900,000 U.S. adults, increased body weight is associated with increased death rates for all cancers combined and for cancers at multiple specific sites.

Christakis, N. A., and Fowler, J. H. 2007. The spread of obesity in a large social network over 32 years. *The New England Journal of Medicine* 357:370–9.

- Evaluation of a densely connected social network of 12,067 people assessed repeatedly from 1971 to 2003 as part of the Framingham Heart Study revealed that obesity spreads within social groups, especially among close friends, siblings, and spouses, strongly suggesting that the spread of obesity among spouses, brothers and sisters, close friends, and associates may be influenced by developing shared ideas and concepts about the acceptability of overeating, weight gain, and obesity. For example, a person's chance of becoming obese increased by 57% if he or she had a close friend who was obese. Among brothers and sisters, if one became obese, the other had a 42% chance of a similar fate, and if one spouse became obese, the other spouse had a 37% chance of also becoming obese.

Crowley, L. V., Sean, J., and Wullin, G. 1984. Late effects of gastric bypass for obesity. *American Journal of Gastroenterology* 79:850–60.

- Many patients developed iron and vitamin B_{12} deficiencies and osteoporosis as late complications of gastric bypass. Hematopoietic complications usually can be prevented and are relatively easy to treat, but musculoskeletal complications are more difficult to prevent and treat.

Cummings, D. E., and Flum, D. R. 2008. Gastrointestinal surgery as a treatment for diabetes. *Journal of the American Medical Association* 299:341–3.

- Obese patients with diabetes who had laparoscopic adjustable gastric banding procedures to treat their diabetes lost weight, and 73% had remission of their diabetes. Patients who had a Roux-en-Y gastric bypass procedure sustained a greater response than gastric banding patients. It appears likely that the gastric bypass increases insulin sensitivity but also improves beta cell function.

DeMaria, E. J. 2007. Bariatric surgery for morbid obesity. *The New England Journal of Medicine* 356:2176–83.

- A discussion of the applications and limitations of the various types of surgical procedures available to reduce food intake by reducing the size of the stomach and/or impairing absorption of nutrients from the small intestine. Some of the newer laparoscopic procedures are described.

Dolin, R. 2007. Noroviruses—challenges to control. *The New England Journal of Medicine* 351: 1072–3.

- Noroviruses are the most common cause of nonbacterial gastroenteritis. Transmission is mainly by fecal–oral route. Infections may occur sporadically but may affect large groups of persons in close contact, as in cruise ships, schools, recreational areas, military facilities, and so forth. The viruses are highly infectious and resistant to inactivation. As little as 10 virus particles may cause an infection. No specific treatment is available.

DuPont, H. L. 2011. The search for effective treatment of *Clostridium difficile* infection. *The New England Journal of Medicine* 364:473–5.

- A review of the current treatment problems and need for better therapy.

Eckel, R. 2008. Clinical practice. Nonsurgical management of obesity in adults. *The New England Journal of Medicine* 358:1941–50.

- Nonsurgical treatment is described for obese patients whose body mass index is not high enough to be considered for bariatric surgery. Patients should be encouraged to set realistic goals, record food intake, and record their weight at least weekly. Applications and limitations of weight loss drugs are considered.

Fontaine, K. R., Redden, D. T., Wang, C., et al. 2003. Years of life lost due to obesity. *Journal of the American Medical Association* 289:187–93.

- Obesity greatly shortens life expectancy, especially among younger adults.

Glass, R. I., Parashar, U. D., and Estes, M. K. 2009. Norovirus gastroenteritis. *The New England Journal of Medicine* 361:1776–85.

- Noroviruses are the leading cause of gastroenteritis epidemics and also an important cause of sporadic gastroenteritis in children as well as adults. The virus is usually spread by the fecal–oral route, but may also be transmitted by person-to-person contact, as well as by particles of clothing, towels, and other fomites. Exposure to only a small number of virus particles is sufficient to cause an infection, and the infected person may begin to shed virus capable of infecting other persons when the infected subject is still asymptomatic. Moreover, the infected person, such as a food handler or restaurant employee, may continue to shed virus long after recovery from the norovirus infection, which may expose many other people. The virus can survive a wide range of temperatures from freezing to 60°C and can persist on the surfaces of household items, as well as in water and on foods. Repeated infections may occur because there are so many strains of norovirus that recovery from one infection provides very little cross protection against infection by another strain of the virus. There are no agents effective against the virus. Only symptomatic and supportive treatment of infected persons is available.

Hossain, P., Kawar, B., and El Nahas, M. E. 2007. Obesity and diabetes in the developing world—a growing challenge. *The New England Journal of Medicine* 356:213–5.

- The rates of obesity have tripled in developing countries that have adopted a Western lifestyle characterized by decreased physical activity and overconsumption of cheap high-calorie foods, and affects children as well as adults. Type 2 diabetes, cardiovascular disease, and some cancers have followed the obesity epidemic. These problems are severe in middle-income countries of Eastern Europe, Latin America, and Asia, but are rare in developing countries that continue to observe their traditional lifestyle. The obesity, diabetes, hypertension triad also targets the kidneys, leading to development of diabetic nephropathy in one-third of persons with diabetes, and its incidence has increased greatly in Asia, where diabetic nephropathy is the most common cause of end-stage renal disease in 9 of 10 Asian countries.

Kenchaiah, S., Evans, J. C., Levy, D., et al. 2002. Obesity and the risk of heart failure. *The New England Journal of Medicine* 347:305–13.

- Approximately 11% of cases of heart failure among men and 14% among women can be attributed to obesity. Efforts to promote optimal body weight may reduce the risk of heart failure.

The Longitudinal Assessment of Bariatric Surgery (LABS) consortium. 2009. Perioperative safety in the longitudinal assessment of bariatric surgery. *The New England Journal of Medicine* 361:445–54.

- Bariatric surgery is recommended as a weight control procedure in obese subjects with a body mass index (BMI) of 40 or more who do not have major coexisting obesity-related medical conditions and is also appropriate for obese subjects with a BMI of at least 35 when there are obesity-related coexisting medical problems. In this study, weight loss procedures were performed on 4,776 subjects by experienced bariatric surgeons in bariatric surgery centers. More than half of the group had coexisting medical conditions. A Roux-en-Y gastric bypass was performed on 3,412 subjects, with 87.2% performed as a laparoscopic procedure. Mortality in this group was 0.3%. Complications were considered to be death, deep vein thrombosis, pulmonary embolism, need for a subsequent operation for complications related to the initial surgery, or failure to be discharged by 30 days after surgery. The complication rate was 4.1% in the laparoscopy treatment group and 7.8% in the group treated by an open surgical procedure. Adjustable gastric banding was performed on 1,198 patients, and the complication rate was 1.0%; 166 patients underwent other rarely performed procedures that were not included in the analysis.
- In most patients, the Roux-en-Y procedure lowers blood glucose before any weight loss occurs; this effect apparently is caused by release of peptides from the intestinal mucosa that lower blood glucose and may also enhance weight loss. Obesity is a major cause of illness and death, and bariatric surgery is the only approach that consistently results in significant sustained weight loss. The short-term risks of surgery should be considered in relation to the long-term health benefits of the weight loss.

McColl, K. E. 2010. Clinical practice. *Helicobacter pylori* infection. *The New England Journal of Medicine* 362:1597–604.

► *Helicobacter pylori* lead to the development of both gastric and duodenal ulcers. The gastric ulcers begin with chronic gastritis caused by the organism, which is associated with stimulation of the gastric-secreting mucosal cells leading to increased secretion of acid gastric juice. Duodenal ulcers result from the excessive gastric acid secretion.

Nishioka, N. S., and Lauwers, G. 2006. Case records of the Massachusetts General Hospital. Case 10-2006. A 66-year-old woman with Barrett's esophagus with high-grade dysplasia. *The New England Journal of Medicine* 354:1403–9.

► Partial resection of the esophagus has many complications and less aggressive treatment is preferred. Affected area of dysplasia can be replaced by normal squamous epithelium by various methods, which are described and discussed.

O'Brien, P. E., Sawyer, S. M., Laurie, C., et al. 2010. Laparoscopic adjustable gastric banding in severely obese adolescents: A randomized trial. *Journal of the American Medical Association* 303:519–26.

► Fifty adolescents aged 15–18 having a body mass index (BMI) over 35 and obesity-related medical complications were randomly divided into two groups. Half were assigned to a program of diet, exercise, and lifestyle modification; the other half had a laparoscopic adjustable gastric banding procedure; and both groups were followed for 2 years. The goal was to achieve at least a 50% reduction of the excess weight. The lifestyle modification group achieved a 13.2% loss of excess weight, compared with a 78.8% reduction of excess weight in the gastric banding group, and also achieved greater improvement in obesity-related complications. However, long-term follow-up by trained health professionals is required to sustain the improvement obtained by the procedure.

Paulson, E. K., Kalady, M. F., and Pappas, T. N. 2003. Clinical practice. Suspected appendicitis. *The New England Journal of Medicine* 348:236–42.

► The three signs most predictive of appendicitis are right lower quadrant pain, abdominal rigidity, and migration of pain from the epigastrium to the right lower quadrant. Diagnosis in women is more difficult because of other conditions related to ovarian or tubal disease. Abdominal CT or ultrasound study is helpful for evaluating confusing cases.

Pratt, J. S., Cummings, S., Vineberg, D. A., et al. 2004. Case records of the Massachusetts General Hospital. Weekly clinicopathological exercises. Case 25-2004. A 49-year-old woman with severe obesity, diabetes, and hypertension. *The New England Journal of Medicine* 351:696–705.

► This article describes the evaluation and management of a typical patient with severe obesity being considered for bariatric (weight loss) surgery. Medical, nutritional, psychological, and surgical evaluations are described, and various surgical procedures are considered. The major obesity-related complications resolve as normal weight is restored. Diabetes improves as weight is lost and may resolve completely if the obesity-related type 2 diabetes has been present for less than 5 years. Gastric bypass patients require supplementary vitamin B_{12}, iron, calcium, and vitamin D, as absorption of these substances is impaired as a result of the bypass.

Service, G. J., Thompson, G. B., Service, J., et al. 2005. Hyperinsulinemic hypoglycemia with nesidioblastosis after gastric-bypass surgery. *The New England Journal of Medicine* 353:249–54.

► Gastric bypass ameliorates obesity-related complications, and diabetes improves rapidly even before there has been significant weight loss, apparently because the bypass of nutrients into the distal jejunum induces the release of intestinal hormones that stimulate pancreatic islets to increase insulin secretion. In some bypass patients, the prolonged islet stimulation causes hyperplasia of islets (called nesidioblastosis) and excessive insulin secretion, which leads to hypoglycemia (see also the editorial by Cummings in the same issue, pages 300–301).

Sharma, P. 2009. Clinical practice. Barrett's esophagus. *The New England Journal of Medicine* 361:2548–56.

- This condition is prone to occur in persons with gastroesophageal reflux and often leads to epithelial dysplasia that may progress to esophageal carcinoma. Various methods are available to eradicate the abnormal epithelium without resorting to a radical esophageal resection.

Suerbaum, S., and Michetti, P. 2002. *Helicobacter pylori* infection. *The New England Journal of Medicine* 347:1175–86.

- A current review article with an extensive bibliography.

Uemura, N., Okamota, S., Yamamoto, S., et al. 2001. *Helicobacter pylori* infection and the development of gastric cancer. *The New England Journal of Medicine* 345:784–9.

- Gastric cancer develops in persons with *Helicobacter pylori* infection but not in uninfected persons. Persons with gastritis associated with marked gastric atrophy and intestinal metaplasia are at risk.

OUTLINE SUMMARY

Face and Oral Cavity

CLEFT LIP AND PALATE

Face and palate formed by coalescence of cell masses.
Maldevelopment leads to defects in lip, jaw, and palate.
Multifactorial inheritance pattern.
Treatment by surgical correction of defect.

ABNORMALITIES OF TOOTH DEVELOPMENT

Missing teeth common. Multifactorial inheritance pattern.
Tetracycline stains enamel of developing teeth and may cause abnormal tooth development.
Do not give to pregnant women.
Do not give to children younger than 8 years of age.

DENTAL CARIES (TOOTH DECAY) AND ITS COMPLICATIONS

Organic acids produced by bacterial fermentation of retained food particles erode enamel.
Combined acid and bacterial action destroy tooth structure, forming cavity.
Spread of bacteria to pulp cavity causes pulp infection and toothache.
Infection may affect apex of tooth and bone in which tooth embedded.
Treatment:
Cavities treated by removing decay and filling the defect.
Pulp infection and infection in bone at apex of tooth may require antibiotics, root canal treatment, or occasionally tooth extraction.

PERIODONTAL DISEASE

An infection between roots of teeth and gums.
Spread of infection into tooth sockets may cause teeth to loosen and eventually fall out.
Various local dental treatments may control or arrest condition.

Inflammation of the Oral Cavity

STOMATITIS

Caused by various irritants.

Tumors of the Oral Cavity

CARCINOMA

Arises from squamous epithelium of oral cavity.
Treated by resection or radiation.

Diseases of the Esophagus

CARDIAC SPHINCTER DYSFUNCTION

Cardiospasm: sphincter fails to open and obstructs food transport.
Incompetent sphincter.
Reflux of acid gastric juice causes inflammation, ulceration, scarring (reflux esophagitis).
Glandular metaplasia of squamous epithelium (Barrett esophagus) carries increased risk of esophageal cancer.

MUCOSAL TEARS

Retching and vomiting lacerates mucosa, which may bleed profusely.

CARCINOMA OF ESOPHAGUS

Squamous cell carcinoma gradually narrows lumen.
May invade trachea and cause fistula.

FOOD IMPACTION

Poorly chewed meat may block esophagus.
Occurs in persons unable to chew properly.

STRICTURE

Esophagus narrowed by scar.
Ingestion of corrosive chemicals causes inflammation that heals by scarring.

Gastritis and Gastroenteritis

ACUTE

Often caused by nonsteroidal anti-inflammatory drugs or alcohol.
Acute gastroenteritis usually caused by norovirus.

CHRONIC

Often associated with *Helicobacter pylori* colonization of mucosa.

Peptic Ulcer

PATHOGENESIS

Increased acid secretions and digestive enzymes erode gastric mucosa.
Helicobacter pylori plays role in pathogenesis.

COMPLICATIONS

Bleeding.
Perforation.
Pyloric obstruction by scarring.

TREATMENT

Administer drugs to block acid secretion or neutralize acid.
Antibiotic therapy if ulcer associated with *H. pylori*.
Surgery may be required for ulcer complications.

Carcinoma of Stomach

MANIFESTATIONS AND TREATMENT

Upper abdominal discomfort.
Iron deficiency anemia from chronic blood loss.
Diagnosis established by biopsy of tumor by means of gastroscopy.
Treated by gastric resection.

Inflammatory Disease of the Intestine

ACUTE ENTERITIS

Common and self-limited.
Caused by many different organisms and bacterial toxins.

CHRONIC ENTERITIS

Crohn disease (regional enteritis).
Chronic inflammation with scarring affects distal ileum.
Treatment by resection.
Chronic ulcerative colitis.
Recurrent chronic inflammation of colon and rectum.
Various forms of medical treatment.
Often requires resection of colon.

COMPLICATIONS OF CHRONIC ENTERITIS

Nutritional disturbances from chronic diarrhea.
Bleeding.
Obstruction by scarring.
Perforation.

ANTIBIOTIC-ASSOCIATED COLITIS

Broad-spectrum antibiotics eliminate normal intestinal bacterial flora. Anaerobic *Clostridium difficile* not inhibited by broad-spectrum antibiotic.
Organism no longer held in check by normal intestinal flora.
Organism proliferates and produces toxins that injure colonic mucosa.
Severe cases treated with antibiotics directed against *Clostridium difficile*.

Appendicitis

PATHOGENESIS AND TREATMENT

Narrow caliber of appendix favors obstruction at base.
Accumulation of secretions raises intraluminal pressure, impairing viability of wall.
Intestinal bacteria invade wall.
Inflamed appendix may perforate and cause peritonitis.
Appendectomy performed in all suspected cases.

Meckel Diverticulum

PATHOGENESIS

Embryonic remnant of vitelline duct.
Appears as tubular outpouching from distal ileum.

MANIFESTATIONS AND TREATMENT

Usually asymptomatic.
Inflammation of diverticulum causes symptoms similar to appendicitis.

Foreign Bodies

Most objects with smooth edges pass through bowel without difficulty.
Objects with sharp edges may perforate bowel.
Bowel injury may result.

Disturbances of Bowel Function Caused by Food Intolerance

LACTOSE INTOLERANCE

Many adults unable to digest lactose caused by lactase deficiency.
Unabsorbed lactose raises osmotic pressure of bowel contents, leading to retention of fluid in intestinal lumen associated with cramps and diarrhea.
Symptoms abate when dairy products discontinued.

GLUTEN INTOLERANCE

Hypersensitivity to wheat protein leads to impaired intestinal absorption and atrophy of intestinal villi.
Diagnosis established by small bowel biopsy.

Treatment by gluten-free diet relieves symptoms and villi return to normal.

Irritable Bowel Syndrome

PATHOGENESIS AND MANIFESTATIONS

Disturbed bowel function without structural or biochemical abnormalities.

A diagnosis of exclusion.

Symptomatic treatment relieves symptoms.

Symptomatic treatment may also improve intestinal motility.

Intestinal Infections in Homosexual Men

PATHOGENESIS AND MANIFESTATIONS

Intestinal complaints among homosexual men caused by bacterial–parasitic infections spread by sexual practices.

May be misinterpreted as irritable bowel syndrome.

Specific treatment given after diagnostic studies completed.

Eating Disorders

OBESITY

Calorie intake exceeds requirement.

Major health consequences.

- *Cardiovascular disease.*
- *Musculoskeletal problems.*
- *Impaired pulmonary function.*
- *Operation carries high risk.*
- *Higher death rate from cancer.*

Treatment.

- *Medical management often ineffective.*
- *Surgical treatment: gastric bypass or adjustable gastric banding.*

ANOREXIA NERVOSA AND BULIMIA NERVOSA

Anorexia nervosa.

- *False perception of being fat despite marked weight loss.*
- *Food intake restricted to lose weight.*
- *Self-induced vomiting and laxatives may be used to promote weight loss.*
- *Organ system abnormalities occur related to food restriction.*
- *Requires psychiatric–medical treatment by persons experienced in dealing with eating disorders.*

Bulimia nervosa.

- *Binge eating followed by self-induced vomiting.*
- *Usually weight maintained. Family and friends may not be aware of behavior.*
- *Risk of gastric mucosa tears from retching and vomiting.*
- *Dental problems and metabolic alkalosis from vomiting-induced loss of gastric acid.*
- *Treatment similar to treatment of anorexia nervosa.*

BINGE EATING DISORDERS

Characterized by binge eating without self-induced vomiting leading to weight gain.

Affects older adults and complicates problems of person trying to lose weight.

Treatment requires patient motivation, as when dealing with overeating problems.

CHRONIC MALNUTRITION

In developing countries caused by inadequate food or poor distribution.

In industrialized countries usually caused by diseases that impair food utilization.

Identify and treat persons at risk.

Diverticulosis and Diverticulitis of Colon

PATHOGENESIS

Outpouching of colonic mucosa through weak areas in wall.

Chronic constipation and low-residue diet predisposes.

COMPLICATIONS

Inflammation.

Bleeding.

TREATMENT

Asymptomatic diverticula do not require treatment.

Surgical resection of affected bowel if complications occur.

Intestinal Obstruction

HIGH INTESTINAL OBSTRUCTION

Crampy pain and vomiting.

Severe water and electrolyte disturbances develop rapidly.

LOW INTESTINAL OBSTRUCTION

Mild crampy pain and distention.

Water and electrolyte disturbances not a major problem.

CAUSES

Adhesions: from previous surgery.

Hernia: protrusion of bowel through weak area in abdominal wall.

Volvulus: rotary twisting of sigmoid colon on its mesentery.

Intussusception: telescoping of one segment of bowel into adjacent segment.

- *As a result of vigorous peristalsis.*
- *Caused by pedunculated tumor.*

Mesenteric Thrombosis

PATHOGENESIS

Superior mesenteric artery supplies small bowel and proximal half of colon.

Artery may become blocked by thrombus, embolus, or atheroma.

Obstruction of artery causes extensive bowel infarction.

Tumors of Bowel

SMALL INTESTINE

Small-bowel tumors are uncommon.

COLON

Benign polyps.

Carcinoma.

Left half of colon: tumors often obstruct colon.

Right half of colon: usually causes chronic blood loss but does not obstruct.

Imperforate Anus

MANIFESTATIONS AND TREATMENT

Congenitally absent anal opening, sometimes with absent distal rectum as well.

Can be corrected surgically.

Hemorrhoids

PATHOGENESIS

Varicose veins of hemorrhoidal venous plexus.

Constipation predisposes.

CLASSIFICATION

Internal hemorrhoids: may bleed or prolapse or become thrombosed.

External hemorrhoids: may become thrombosed.

TREATMENT

Conservative treatment preferred.

Can be treated surgically if not responsive to conservative therapy.

Diagnostic Evaluation of Gastrointestinal Tract Disease

DIAGNOSTIC METHODS

Endoscopy: tube inserted to visualize interior of gastrointestinal tract. Biopsies performed if indicated.

X-ray studies.

http://health.jbpub.com/humandisease/9e

Human Disease Online is a great source for supplementary human disease information for both students and instructors. Visit this website to find a variety of useful tools for learning, thinking, and teaching.

The Nervous System

LEARNING OBJECTIVES

1. Describe the normal structure and basic functions of the brain, meninges, and cerebrospinal fluid as they relate to neurologic disease.
2. Define muscle tone and voluntary motor activity, and relate these concepts to the two forms of muscle paralysis.
3. Explain the pathogenesis and clinical manifestations of closure defect of the central nervous system. Name the techniques used for prenatal diagnosis.
4. Describe the pathogenesis and manifestations of hydrocephalus, and relate them to treatment measures.
5. Name the causes, manifestations, and treatment of transient ischemic attacks.
6. Differentiate between the two principal types of stroke in regard to pathogenesis, prognosis, and treatment.
7. Describe the pathogenesis, manifestations, and treatment of congenital cerebral aneurysms.
8. Name the types of tumors that affect the central nervous system, and explain their origin, pathogenesis, clinical manifestations, and treatment.
9. Explain the pathogenesis, major clinical manifestations, and general principles of treatment of Parkinson disease, meningitis, and multiple sclerosis.

Structure and Function

The central nervous system (CNS) consists of the brain and spinal cord, surrounded by several membranes called **meninges**. The firm, fibrous outer membrane is called the **dura**. The thin inner membrane, which adheres to the surface of the brain and spinal cord, is called the **pia**. The middle membrane, interposed between the pia and the dura, is called the **arachnoid**. The space between the arachnoid and the underlying pia is called the **subarachnoid space**. It contains cerebrospinal fluid (CSF) together with fine strands of arachnoidal connective tissue that extend through the space and attach to the tips of the gyri.

meninges (men-in′jēz) The membranes covering the brain and spinal cord.

dura (dū′rä) The outer covering of the brain and spinal cord.

pia (pē′yuh) The innermost of the three membranes covering the brain and spinal cord.

arachnoid (ar-ak′noyd) The middle of the three meninges that cover the brain and spinal cord.

subarachnoid space (sub-är-ak′noyd) The space between the arachnoid and the pia, containing large blood vessels supplying the brain.

oligodendroglia (ol′ig-ō-den-drog′li-ah) One type of neuroglia that surrounds nerve fibers within the central nervous system.

The *brain* is divided into the *cerebrum, brain stem,* and *cerebellum.* The brain is hollow, containing four interconnected cavities called ventricles. Arterial blood is supplied to the brain by large blood vessels entering the base of the skull. These arteries join to form a circle of vessels (*the circle of Willis*) at the base of the brain. Branches from the circle extend outward to supply all parts of the brain. Venous blood is returned from the brain into large venous sinuses in the dura, which eventually drain into the jugular veins.

The brain and spinal cord are surrounded by cerebrospinal fluid and are encased within protective bony structures: the *cranium* and the *vertebral column*. The bony case protects the soft and rather fragile nervous tissue, and the cerebrospinal fluid acts as a hydrostatic cushion to insulate the brain from shocks and blows.

The nerve tissue of the brain and spinal cord is composed of nerve cells called neurons and supporting cells called neuroglia. Each individual neuron has a central body and one or more long processes extending from the cell body to transmit the impulses. Processes carrying impulses into the nerve cell are called dendrites, and those carrying impulses out of the nerve cell are called axons. Sometimes the general term *nerve fiber* is used when referring to either type. Neurons are frequently arranged in chains; the neurons interconnect with other neurons to transmit impulses, but they are not in direct contact with one another. They are separated by minute gaps called *synapses*. The transmission of a nerve impulse across a synapse is by means of a chemical called a *neurotransmitter* that is released from the end of an axon and activates receptors on the dendrite or cell body of the adjacent neuron. There are several types of neurotransmitters, and each type of neuron has its own specific type. When a nerve fiber leaves the central nervous system, it becomes invested by cells called *Schwann cells* that wrap around the fiber. These cells produce the myelin that insulates the fiber. The myelin surrounding nerve fibers within the central nervous system is produced by glial cells called **oligodendroglia**.

A nerve that transmits impulses into the nervous system is called a *sensory nerve* or *afferent nerve* (*ad* = to + *ferre* = carry). A *motor nerve* or *efferent nerve* (*e* = away) conducts impulses from brain or spinal cord to muscle. The gray matter of the brain and cord is composed primarily of nerve cells and their processes. The *white matter* consists mostly of bundles of nerve fibers covered by fatty myelin sheaths.

The nervous system may be regarded as a giant switchboard, receiving sensory impulses and relaying this information to brain and spinal cord centers concerned with perception of sensation and with motor activity. The cerebral cortex receives sensory input and initiates voluntary motor activity. In the depths of each cerebral hemisphere are masses of gray matter: the thalami and the basal ganglia (basal nuclei). The paired thalami function as relay stations that receive sensory impulses from lower levels and transmit them to the cortex. The basal ganglia in each hemisphere are part of a complex neuron system that is concerned with control of automatic functions that do not require constant attention, such as walking. The brain stem also contains neurons that are involved in multiple functions not under direct cortical control, and also carries the bundles of nerve fibers that pass to higher and lower levels within the CNS. The cerebellum regulates muscle tone, coordination, posture, and balance.

The spinal cord is the continuation of the brain stem. Its central gray matter receives sensory input from spinal nerves entering the cord, and motor neurons exit from the cord to innervate muscles. Spinal sensory and motor neurons are involved in many reflex functions not under cortical control, and are also activated by motor impulses originating from cortical neurons. The spinal motor neurons in turn discharge impulses to the skeletal muscles that they supply, causing them to contract.

The fiber tracts conveying sensory impulses to the cortex and those conveying motor impulses from the cortex cross within the brain stem to the opposite side as they transmit impulses to their destination. Consequently, the right hemisphere registers sensation from the left half of the body and innervates the muscles on the left side. Conversely, the left hemisphere receives sensation from the right side of the body and activates muscles on the right side.

Development of the Nervous System

In the embryo, the CNS first appears as a thickened band of surface cells (ectoderm) called the neural plate. Its lateral margins become elevated to form neural folds, and the two folds then fuse to form a hollow tube called the neural tube. Fusion begins in the middle of the developing tube and progresses toward both ends until a completely closed tube is formed by the end of the fourth week of embryonic development. Three expansions, called the forebrain, midbrain, and hindbrain, develop from one end of the neural tube (Figure 1). The other end remains narrow and becomes the spinal cord.

The *cerebral hemispheres* develop as lateral outgrowths from the forebrain and soon overgrow the remaining parts of the brain. The remainder of the forebrain becomes the *diencephalon*, which is located between the cerebral hemispheres (*dia* = between + *encephalon* = brain). The *midbrain* persists as a small area connecting the forebrain and the hindbrain. The hindbrain gives rise to parts of the brain called the *pons*, *medulla*, and *cerebellum*. The diencephalon, midbrain, pons, and medulla together form the *brain stem*. The central cavity within the neural tube develops into the *ventricular system* of the adult brain. The embryonic cells (mesoderm) surrounding the developing neural tube give rise to the cranial cavity, vertebral bodies, and adjacent tissues.

Muscle Tone and Voluntary Muscle Contraction

A skeletal muscle contracts in response to impulses discharged from motor neurons in the spinal cord or from corresponding neurons of the cranial nerves in the brain stem. Voluntary motor activity is controlled by two separate motor systems. One system, called the *pyramidal system*, controls voluntary motor functions, and the other system, called the *extrapyramidal system*, regulates muscle groups concerned primarily with balance, posture, and coordination.

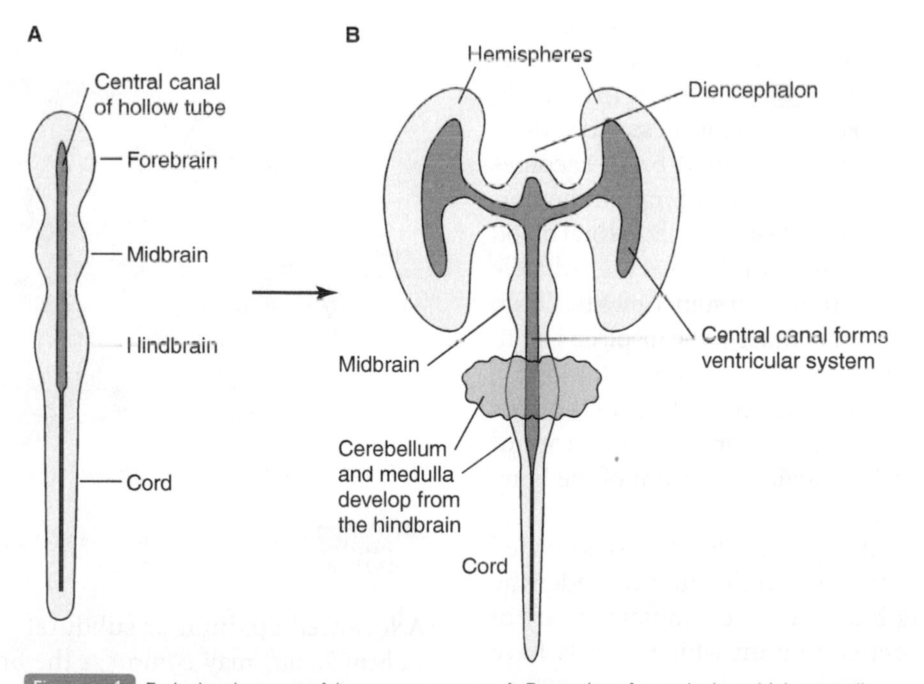

Figure 1 Early development of the nervous system. **A**, Formation of neural tube, which normally closes at both ends. Central canal in tube is the precursor of the ventricular system. **B**, Cerebral hemispheres grow from the forebrain and the central region becomes the diencephalon. The hindbrain forms the medulla and cerebellum. The tube becomes the ventricular system. The two lateral ventricles follow the contours of the developing hemispheres, which communicate with the third ventricle in the diencephalon by channels called interventricular foramina. The channel in the midbrain becomes the cerebral aqueduct, which expands into the fourth ventricle in the medulla. Each ventricle develops a choroid plexus to make the cerebrospinal fluid that flows through the ventricular system, exits through openings in the fourth ventricle, and circulates around the brain and spinal cord.

The pyramidal system and the extrapyramidal system function together as a single system under cortical control to produce the smooth integrated functions of muscle groups involved in voluntary motor activity. Malfunction of the extrapyramidal system leads to loss of coordinated motor functions. The muscles do not function smoothly, and the malfunction also gives rise to abnormal uncontrollable muscular movements.

Muscle Paralysis

A muscle that is no longer subject to voluntary control is said to be paralyzed. There are two different types of paralysis:

1. *Flaccid paralysis* results when the spinal motor neurons are destroyed by disease, as in poliomyelitis.
2. *Spastic paralysis* results from disease affecting the cortical motor neurons or their fibers, as occurs when a person has a stroke.

Spastic paralysis occurs more frequently than flaccid paralysis because cortical neurons are more often damaged by disease than are spinal motor neurons.

Cerebral Injury

The brain is well protected from moderate trauma. However, a severe blow may injure the brain, and sometimes the skull also is fractured (Figure 2). Injury to the brain may be manifested by loss of consciousness and various neurologic disturbances. The injured brain becomes swollen and often shows evidence of pinpoint hemorrhages caused by disruption of small intracerebral blood vessels. Usually the brain injury is located immediately adjacent to the site of the blow, but sometimes the brain injury is caused by violent contact of the displaced brain against the cranial cavity on the side opposite the injury. For example, the force of a blow to the back of the head may displace the brain forward, injuring the front of the brain where it strikes against the front of the bony cranial cavity (Figure 3).

Sometimes a head injury tears blood vessels located between the cranial bones and the dura or under the dura. The escaping blood may accumulate in any of several locations, depending on which vessels have been damaged:

1. Between the outer layer of dura and the cranial bones (*epidural hemorrhage*)
2. Between the dura and the arachnoid (*subdural hemorrhage*)
3. Between the arachnoid and the pia (*subarachnoid hemorrhage*)

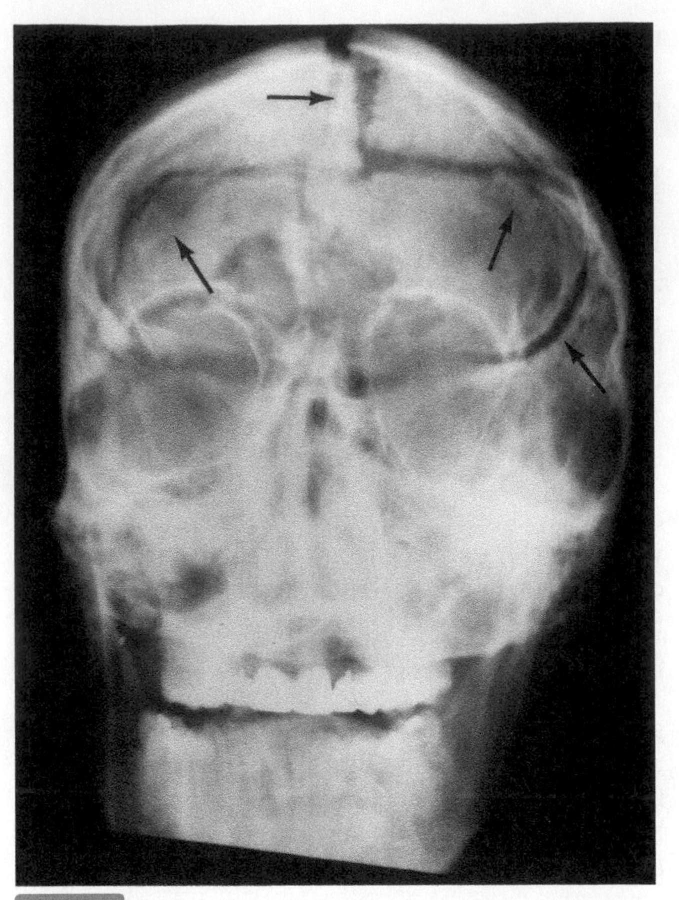

Figure 2 Skull x-ray illustrating large skull fracture (*arrows*) associated with extensive injury to underlying brain.

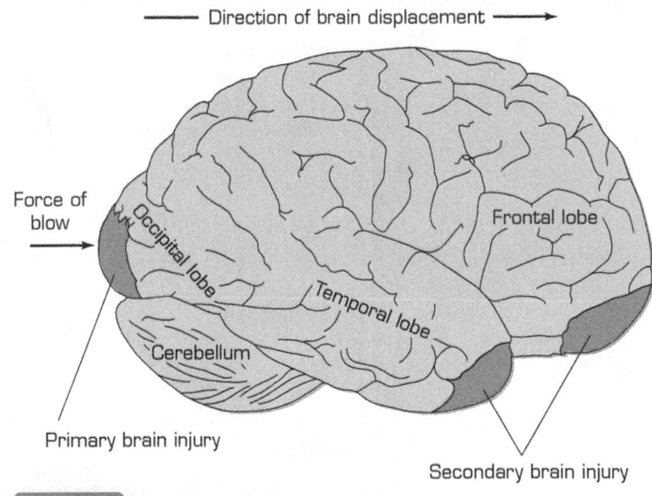

Figure 3 Mechanism of injury to frontal and temporal poles of brain caused by a blow to the back of the head.

A localized epidural or subdural collection of blood (a *hematoma*) may compress the brain and impair its function. In a subarachnoid hemorrhage, the blood often mixes with the cerebrospinal fluid and spreads diffusely through the subarachnoid space.

Unfortunately, the rigid cranial cavity, which normally serves a protective function, is a disadvantage if the brain is seriously injured. The brain often swells at the site of injury, and the unyielding cranial cavity restricts the swelling and compresses the swollen brain, leading to high intracranial pressure. The elevated pressure adversely affects cerebral function and may also interfere with the blood supply to the brain by compressing cerebral blood vessels.

Neural Tube Defects

Failure of either end of the neural tube to close properly leads to serious congenital malformations called *neural tube defects*, which involve not only the nervous system but the surrounding tissues as well. A closure defect involving the end of the tube destined to form the cerebral hemispheres (called the *cephalic end*) leads to a condition called **anencephaly** (*ana* = without + *encephalon* = brain). **Spina bifida** results if the opposite end of the tube (the *caudal* end) fails to close normally. These are the two most common congenital malformations of the nervous system. The combined incidence of these malformations is about 2 per 1,000 births in the United States and even higher in some other countries. The malformations follow a multifactorial pattern of inheritance and tend to recur in subsequent pregnancies. If parents have already given birth to an offspring with a neural tube defect, the risk of recurrence in a subsequent pregnancy is approximately 1 in 20. The risk is 1 in 10 when the parents have had two affected infants.

A deficiency of folic acid during the early part of pregnancy when the neural tube is forming plays an important role in causing neural tube defects. Intake of 0.4–0.8 mg of folic acid daily beginning one month before conception and during the early part of pregnancy (first trimester) can reduce by one-half the frequency of neural tube defects. However, these defects follow a multifactorial inheritance pattern, and the folic acid deficiency functions along with genetic factors to cause the neural tube defect.

Anencephaly

Anencephaly occurs most commonly in female infants and is incompatible with postnatal life. Because the cephalic end of the neural tube fails to close, the exposed neural tissue undergoes secondary degenerative changes that convert it into a mass of vascular connective tissue intermixed with masses of degenerated brain and choroid plexus. The anencephalic infant has a striking appearance (Figure 4). The brain is absent, as are the soft tissues of the scalp and the bones making up the vertex of the skull. The exposed base of the skull is covered only by a vascular membrane. The base of the cranial cavity is abnormally formed,

anencephaly (an-en-seff′uh-lē) A congenital malformation: absence of brain, cranial vault, and scalp as a result of defective closure of the neural tube.

spina bifida (spī′-nuh bif′fid-duh) Incomplete closure of vertebral arches over the spinal cord, sometimes associated with protrusion of meninges and neural tissue through the defect (*cystic spina bifida*).

A

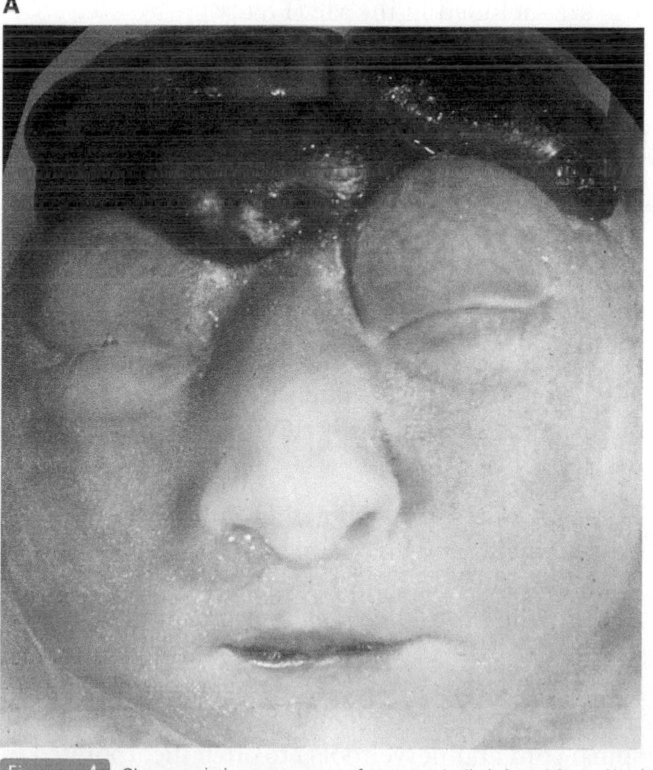

B

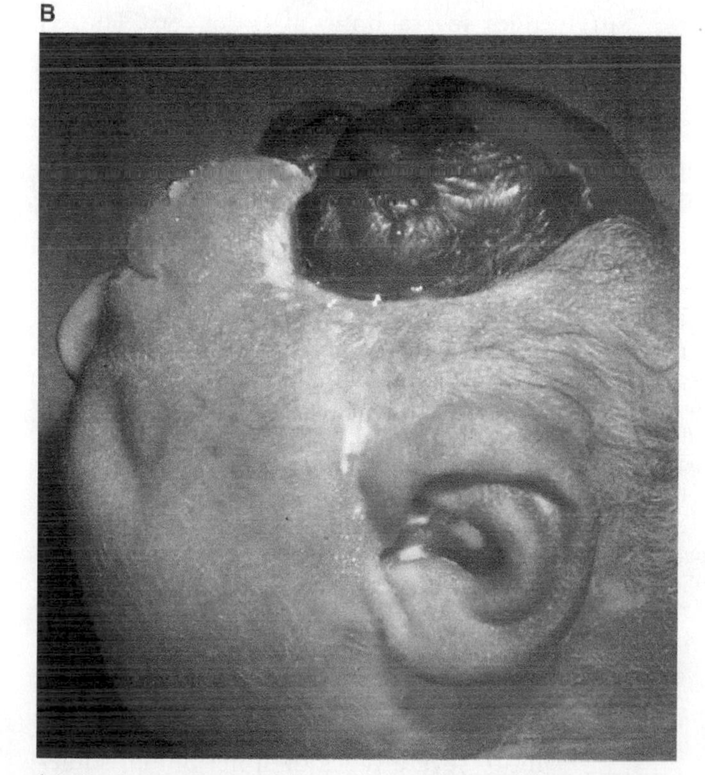

Figure 4 Characteristic appearance of anencephalic infant. Most of brain, top of skull, and scalp are absent. Maldevelopment of skull causes protrusion of eyes. **A**, Frontal view. **B**, Lateral view.

and the orbits are shallow, causing the eyes to bulge outward. The trunk is short, the shoulders are broad, and the neck is not normal; the head arises directly from the trunk and cannot be flexed.

The following case illustrates some of the obstetric problems associated with anencephaly.

Case Study 1

A female anencephalic infant was born to a 28-year-old woman who was pregnant for the first time. The fetal heartbeat could be heard by the obstetrician throughout the last part of the pregnancy. When the patient's abdomen was examined near term, the obstetrician became concerned about the possibility of anencephaly because of the inability to feel the fetal head. An x-ray film taken of the patient's abdomen confirmed the clinical impression because only the base of the fetal skull could be seen in the x-ray film. The bones of the cranial vault were absent. The rest of the fetal skeleton appeared normally formed. The patient was delivered at term with some difficulty because the anencephalic head was unable to flex normally as it passed through the mother's pelvis, and the infant was delivered face first. The infant survived for several hours after delivery. The autopsy revealed complete absence of the cerebral hemispheres, the cerebellum, and most of the brain stem.

Spina Bifida

meningocele (men-in′go-sēl) A protrusion of meninges through a defect in the spinal vertebral arches.

meningomyelocele (men-ing-gō-mī′el-ō-sēl) A type of spina bifida characterized by protrusion of meninges and cord through the defect in the vertebral arches.

Malformations of the opposite (caudal) end of the neural tube and related vertebral arches are generally considered together under the term *spina bifida*. This term means literally *split spine* and refers to the characteristic failure of fusion of the vertebral arches common to all types of spina bifida (Figure 5). Failure of fusion of vertebral arches in the lower lumbar region occurring as an isolated abnormality is called *occult spina bifida* (Figure 5A); this type produces no clinical symptoms. The more severe types of spina bifida, sometimes called collectively *cystic spina bifida*, are

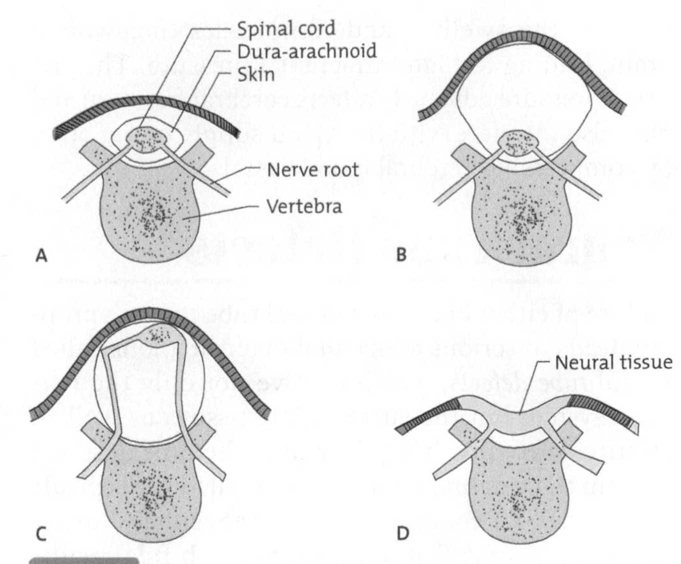

Figure 5 Various types of spina bifida. **A,** Occult spina bifida. Failure of formation of vertebral arches. No protrusion of meninges. **B,** Meningocele. Meninges protrude through defect in the vertebral arches. Cord and nerve trunks are not present in the sac. **C,** Meningomyelocele. Protrusion of both meninges and nerve tissue. The spinal cord and nerve trunks are frequently incorporated into the wall of the sac. **D,** Failure of the neural tube to form and separate from the surface ectoderm. The neural tissue is continuous with the adjacent skin.

characterized by a saclike protrusion of meninges or meninges and nerve tissue through the defect in the vertebral arches. The malformation is called a **meningocele** if the protrusion consists only of meninges (Figure 5B) and is called a **meningomyelocele** (*myelo* = cord) if parts of the spinal cord or nerve roots also are included in the sac (Figure 5C).

In meningomyelocele, there is often a severe neurologic deficit below the level of the sac because the nerve tissue is actually incorporated into the wall of the sac and is disorganized so that the conduction of nerve impulses is impaired or completely interrupted. In the most severe (and fortunately rare) form of spina bifida, the caudal end of the neural tube completely fails to close. The distal end of the spinal cord is represented by a flattened mass of nerve tissue that is continuous with the adjacent skin (Figure 5D). The larger meningomyelocele sacs often are covered not by skin but merely by a thin, easily ruptured membrane composed only of meninges (Figure 6).

Treatment of Spina Bifida Occult spina bifida is asymptomatic, and no treatment is required. A meningocele usually can be repaired without difficulty by excising the sac and closing the spinal dura, and the results are usually very satisfactory. Unfortunately, a large meningomyelocele is much more difficult to treat, and results are much less satisfactory. Because spinal cord and nerve roots are often incorporated in the sac, there is frequently some loss of sensation and

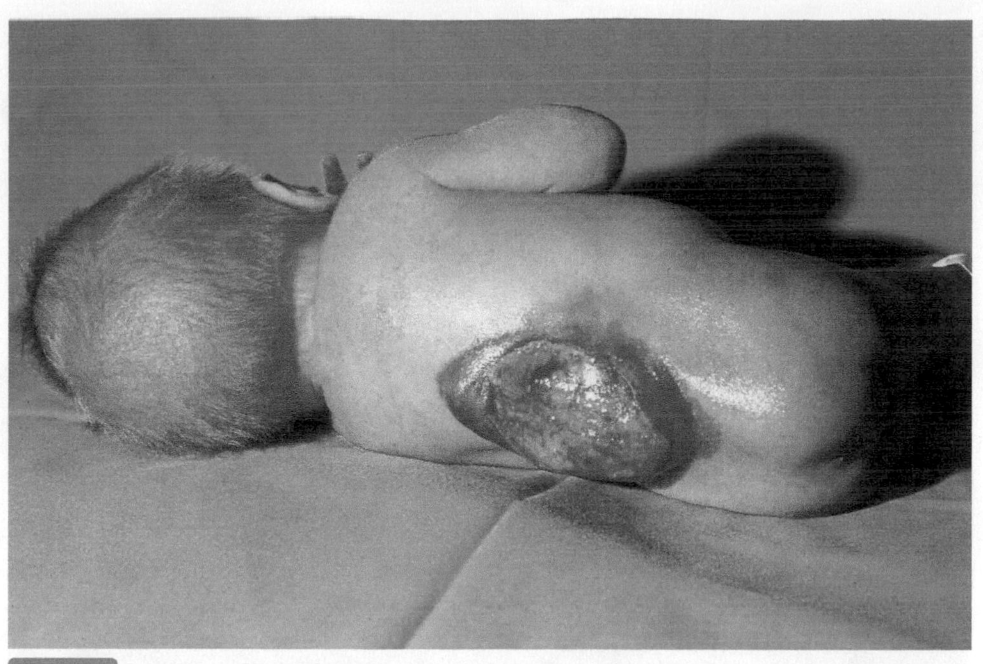

Figure 6 Large thoracic meningomyelocele covered only by a thin membrane. This condition is associated with neurologic disturbances resulting from incorporation of neural tissue into the wall of the sac.

motor power in the lower extremities. Bowel and bladder function also may be impaired, leading to stasis of urine in the bladder and predisposing to urinary tract infections. These individuals are managed best by a team of specialists in a medical center specializing in the care of patients with severe disabilities of this type. Many patients can be treated successfully and are able to lead happy and productive lives despite their disability.

Prenatal Detection of Neural Tube Defects

It is usually possible to identify a fetus with a neural tube defect prior to birth. An elevated concentration of **alpha fetoprotein (AFP)** detected on a routine screening test of maternal blood may suggest the possibility of a neural tube defect, and the defect can be confirmed by an ultrasound examination of the fetus performed at about 16-weeks' gestation.

Alpha fetoprotein is produced in the fetal liver beginning early in pregnancy and can be readily detected in the fetal blood. The concentration in fetal blood is highest at about 13 weeks and then gradually declines. A small amount of AFP normally diffuses from the fetal blood into the amnionic fluid and also into the mother's blood. High amnionic fluid AFP levels are encountered when the fetus is anencephalic or has a cystic spina bifida in which the defect is covered only by a thin membrane. Consequently, AFP can more easily diffuse from the fetal blood and cerebrospinal fluid into the amnionic fluid, and AFP levels are much higher than in a normal pregnancy.

Hydrocephalus

Cerebrospinal fluid serves as a protective cushion around the brain and spinal cord. The fluid is secreted by the choroid plexuses of the ventricles. It flows from the lateral ventricles into the third ventricle, through the cerebral aqueduct (*aqueduct of Sylvius*) into the fourth ventricle and then out into the subarachnoid space through three small openings in the roof and lateral walls of the fourth ventricle. The fluid circulates around the cord and over the convexity of the brain and is resorbed into the large venous sinuses in the dura. Secretion of cerebrospinal fluid continues even if the flow of fluid through the ventricular system is blocked. Obstruction to the normal circulation of spinal fluid distends the ventricles proximal to the site of obstruction, with associated compression atrophy of brain tissue around the dilated ventricles. This condition, which is called **hydrocephalus**, may be either congenital or acquired (Figure 7).

alpha fetoprotein (AFP) (al'fuh fē'tō-prō'tēn) Protein produced by fetal liver early in gestation. Sometimes produced by tumor cells. Level is elevated in amnionic fluid when fetus has neural tube defect.

hydrocephalus Dilatation of the ventricular system caused by pressure arising from accumulation of cerebrospinal fluid within the ventricles.

Congenital Hydrocephalus *Congenital hydrocephalus* is usually caused by a congenital abnormality in the ventricular system, either a congenital obstruction or abnormal formation of the cerebral aqueduct, a narrow channel connecting the third and fourth ventricles, or failure of the openings in

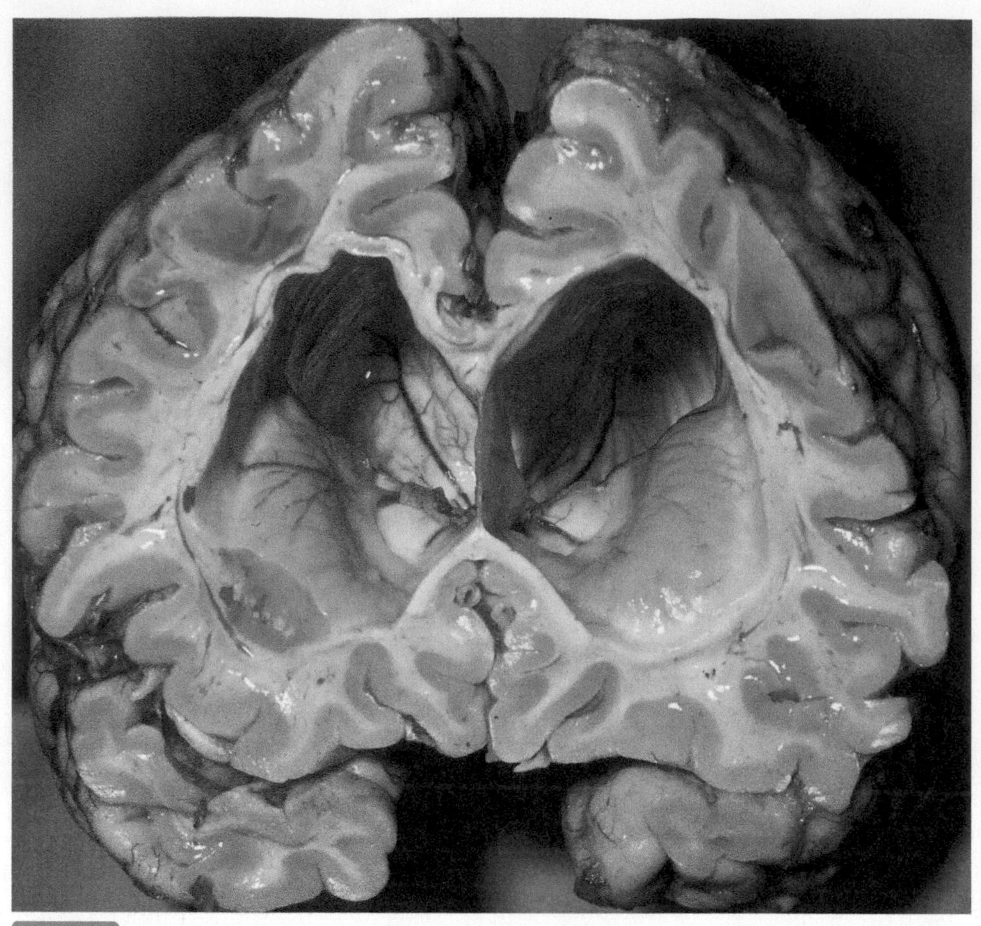

Figure 7 Coronal section of brain revealing marked dilatation of ventricles in patient with congenital hydrocephalus.

the roof and lateral walls of the fourth ventricle to form normally, which blocks escape of cerebrospinal fluid into the subarachnoid space. An aqueduct obstruction leads to distention of the lateral and third ventricles. An obstruction of the outlet channels in the fourth ventricle leads to distention of all four ventricles. Because the distention develops before the skull bones have fused, the head enlarges greatly and the brain undergoes pronounced atrophy secondary to compression by the dilated ventricles. Hydrocephalus may occur in the fetus prior to birth, and the head may become so large that it is unable to enter the maternal pelvis during labor. More often, the hydrocephalus develops insidiously after birth.

Acquired Hydrocephalus *Acquired hydrocephalus* is most commonly caused by obstruction of the circulation of the cerebrospinal fluid in the region of the fourth ventricle by fibrous adhesions, which sometimes form after a bacterial infection of the meninges (meningitis) and block the outflow of fluid from the fourth ventricle, or by blockage of the ventricular system secondary to a brain tumor. Acquired hydrocephalus develops after the skull bones fuse, and the skull cannot enlarge as in the congenital form of hydrocephalus.

Treatment of Hydrocephalus Hydrocephalus can often be treated successfully by inserting a plastic tube into one of the dilated ventricles and rerouting (*shunting*) the fluid into another part of the body where it can be absorbed. The fluid can be shunted into the right atrium (*ventriculoatrial shunt*) or into the peritoneal cavity (*ventriculoperitoneal shunt*). A small opening is made in the skull to allow insertion of a plastic drainage tube through cerebral hemisphere into one of the dilated lateral ventricles. The other end of the tube is passed through the subcutaneous tissues behind the ear. In a ventriculoatrial shunt, the tube is inserted into the jugular vein and threaded down the vein so that the tip is positioned in the right atrium. In the more commonly used ventriculoperitoneal shunt the tube is passed through the subcutaneous tissues of the neck, chest, and upper abdomen and introduced into the abdominal cavity through a small incision in the peritoneum. Whatever type of shunt is used, a one-way valve is incorporated in the tube to prevent any reflux of blood or peritoneal fluid into the ventricles (Figure 8).

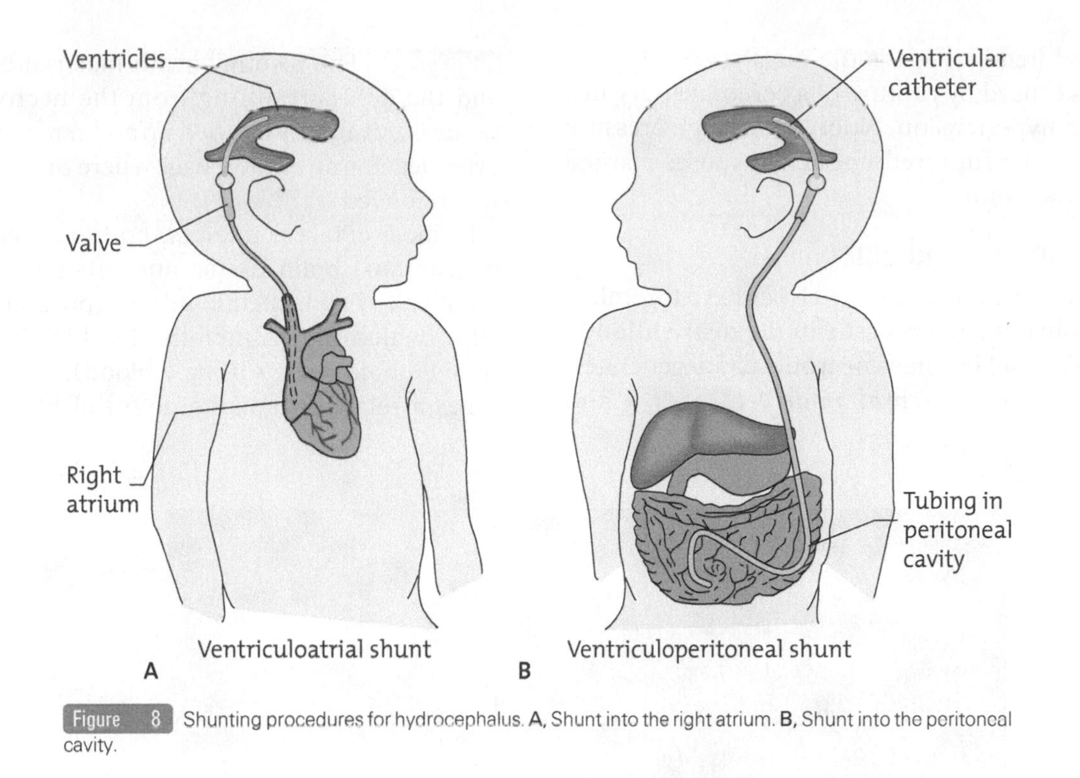

Figure 8 Shunting procedures for hydrocephalus. **A**, Shunt into the right atrium. **B**, Shunt into the peritoneal cavity.

Case 2 illustrates some of the obstetric and pediatric problems encountered when hydrocephalus occurs in the fetus before delivery.

Case Study 2

A 24-year-old woman who was pregnant for the first time noted marked enlargement of her abdomen during the last part of pregnancy. X-ray examination of the abdomen revealed a hydrocephalic infant having a head diameter that was larger than the diameter of the mother's pelvis, indicating that delivery could not be accomplished vaginally. At term, an elective cesarean section was performed, and the infant was evaluated soon after delivery by a neurosurgeon. A shunt was performed in order to control the progressing hydrocephalus. The shunt prevented further enlargement of the head, and the infant did reasonably well after this operation.

Stroke

The term **stroke**, also called a **cerebrovascular accident** or simply **CVA**, is used to designate any injury to brain tissue resulting from disturbance of blood supply to the brain and encompasses three conditions: (1) cerebral thrombosis, (2) cerebral embolism, and (3) cerebral hemorrhage.

A **cerebral thrombosis**, as indicated by the name, results from thrombosis of a cerebral artery narrowed by arteriosclerosis and is the cause of most strokes.

A **cerebral embolus**, which occurs less frequently than a cerebral thrombosis, is caused by blockage of a cerebral artery by a fragment of a blood clot dislodged from the surface of an ulcerated arteriosclerotic plaque in the carotid artery and carried to the brain, or from a blood clot that formed within the heart. Three cardiac conditions predispose to cerebral emboli:

1. A mural thrombus that formed on the wall of the left ventricle adjacent to a healing myocardial infarct.
2. A thrombus that formed on the rough surface of a diseased mitral or aortic valve.
3. A small thrombus in the left atrial appendage (auricle) of a person with atrial fibrillation. Atrial thrombi tend to develop because the atria are not contracting normally. Consequently, the blood pools in the atrial appendages instead of being ejected normally, which predisposes to formation of blood clots in the stagnant atrial appendage blood.

stroke Any injury to the brain caused by disturbance of its blood supply.

cerebrovascular accident (CVA) An injury to the brain resulting in a disturbance of cerebral blood flow caused by a cerebral thrombosis, cerebral embolism, or cerebral hemorrhage.

cerebral thrombosis A stroke caused by thrombosis of an arteriosclerotic cerebral artery.

cerebral embolus A stroke caused by blockage of a cerebral artery by a blood clot that had formed elsewhere in the circulatory system and was transported in the bloodstream to the brain.

A **cerebral hemorrhage** is the most serious type of stroke. It is caused by rupture of a cerebral artery in a person with hypertension. Blood under high pressure escapes from the ruptured vessel and causes marked damage to the brain.

Cerebral Thrombi and Emboli

When a cerebral artery is blocked by either a thrombus on an embolus, the brain tissue in the distribution of the blocked vessel becomes necrotic and degenerates, which is called a *cerebral infarct* (Figure 9 and Figure 10). The myelin sheath material breaks down and the debris resulting from the necrosis of brain tissue is eventually cleaned up and removed by phagocytes, leaving an empty space where the necrotic tissue was removed (Figure 11).

In most cerebral infarcts, no blood leaks into the degenerated brain tissue, and this type of infarct is often called an ischemic infarct (pronounced *is-key-mik*), which means literally that blood is held back (*ischo* = hold back + *heme* = blood). However, sometimes a relatively small amount of blood leaks into

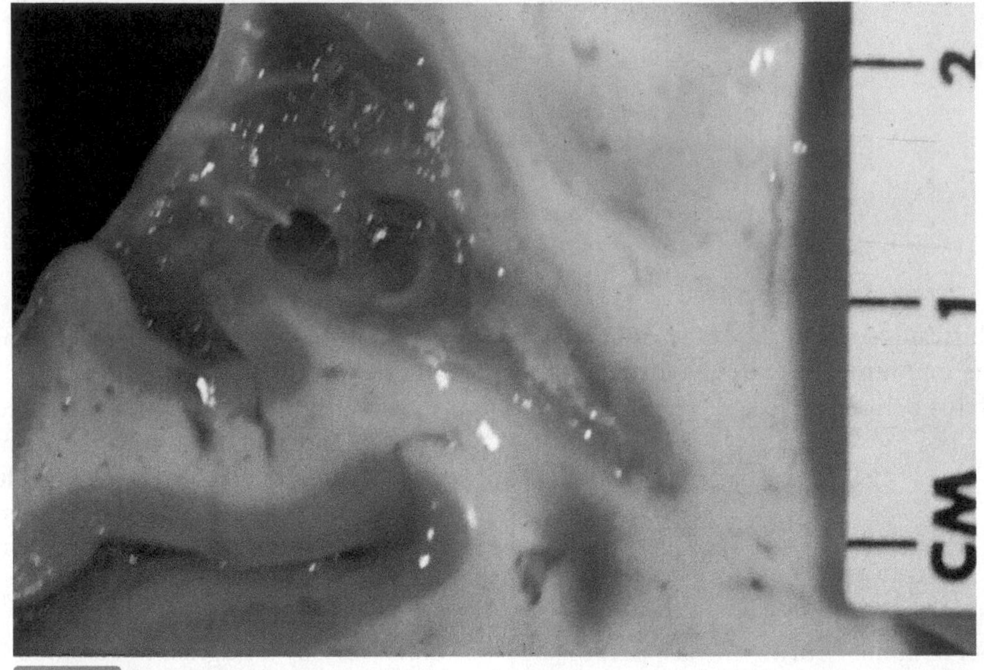

Figure 9 A small, older infarct of the cerebral cortex that is undergoing cystic breakdown (encephalomalacia).

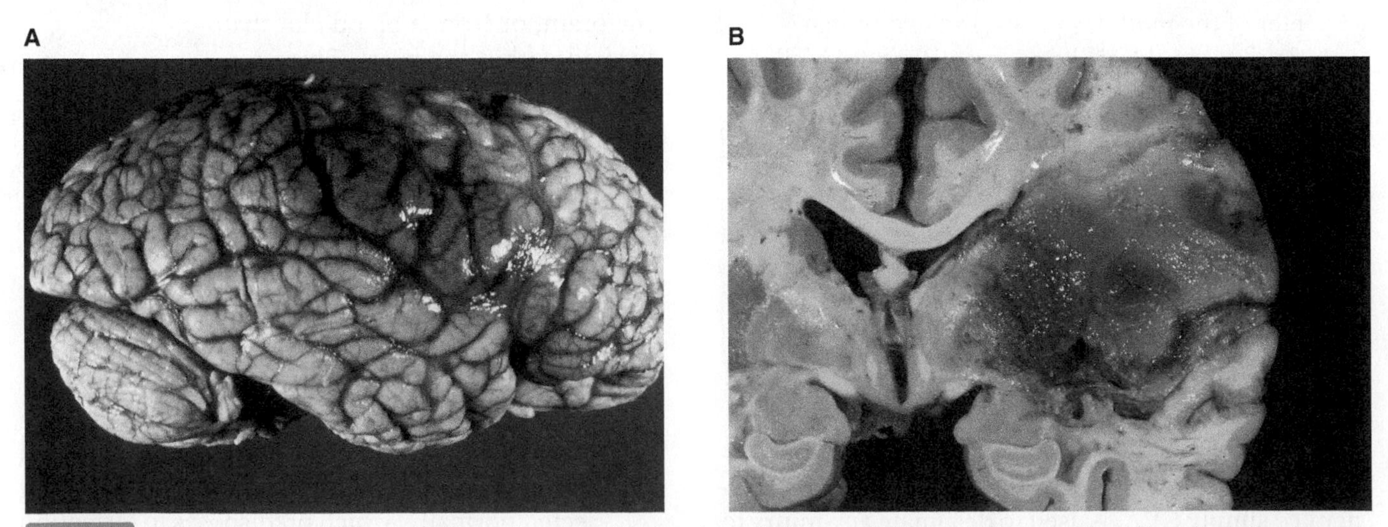

Figure 10 Large recent infarct of right cerebral hemisphere caused by thrombosis of middle cerebral artery. **A**, External surface of brain illustrating the swollen, dark, infarcted area in the right hemisphere. **B**, Coronal section through hemispheres at level of basal ganglia. Cerebral tissue is necrotic and discolored and involves a large part of the hemisphere.

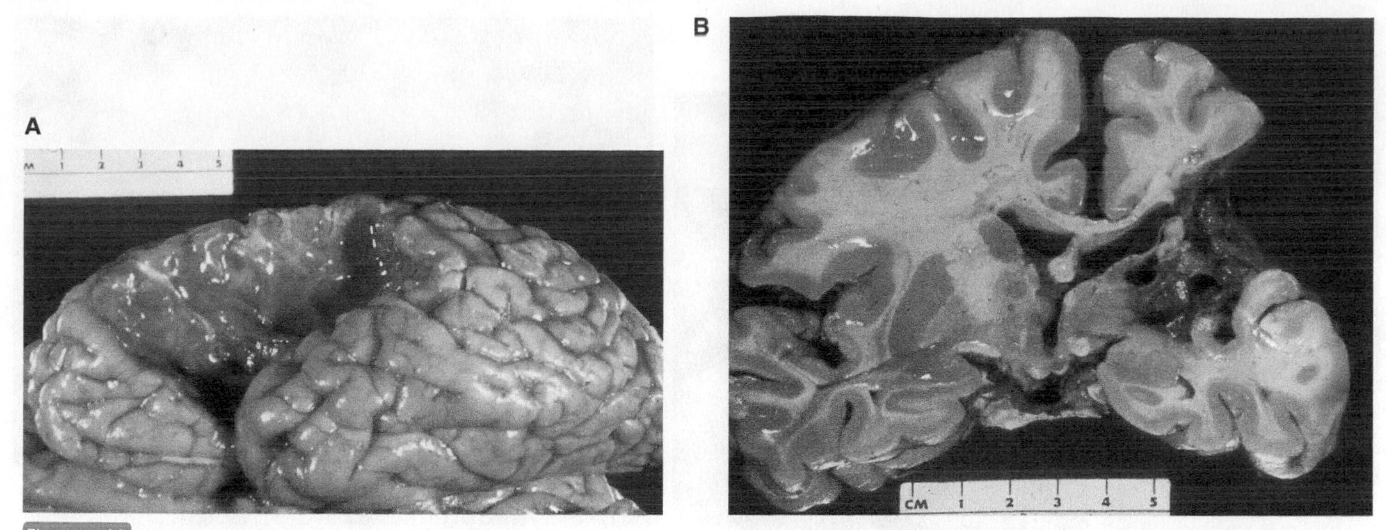

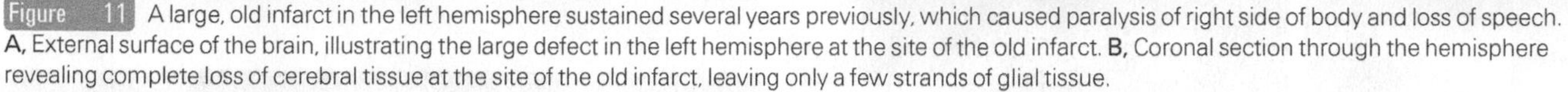

Figure 11 A large, old infarct in the left hemisphere sustained several years previously, which caused paralysis of right side of body and loss of speech. **A**, External surface of the brain, illustrating the large defect in the left hemisphere at the site of the old infarct. **B**, Coronal section through the hemisphere revealing complete loss of cerebral tissue at the site of the old infarct, leaving only a few strands of glial tissue.

the degenerated brain tissue from adjacent damaged cerebral blood vessels, as illustrated in Figure 10.

Some patients who have had a stroke caused by thrombosis of a cerebral artery may benefit from the same type of thrombolytic drugs used to dissolve blood clots in coronary arteries. Unfortunately, there is very little time available to restore flow through a blocked cerebral artery before permanent brain damage occurs, and sometimes the thrombolytic drug treatment may be complicated by hemorrhage within the damaged brain tissue.

Stroke Caused by Arteriosclerosis of Extracranial Arteries

A stroke may also be caused by atherosclerosis of one of the major arteries arising from the aorta to supply the brain, before the vessel enters the cranial cavity. A commonly affected site is at the origin of the internal carotid artery in the neck, where atheromatous plaques may narrow the lumen and reduce cerebral blood flow. The plaques may also become ulcerated, and thrombi may form on the roughened surfaces. Bits of arteriosclerotic debris or thrombus material may break loose from the plaque and be carried into the blood vessels in the brain, where they may block small cerebral arteries. Rarely, the internal carotid artery may become completely blocked by a thrombus that has formed on the roughened surface of the artery, leading to a large cerebral infarction. Figure 12 illustrates the possible effects of arteriosclerosis of the internal carotid artery in the neck.

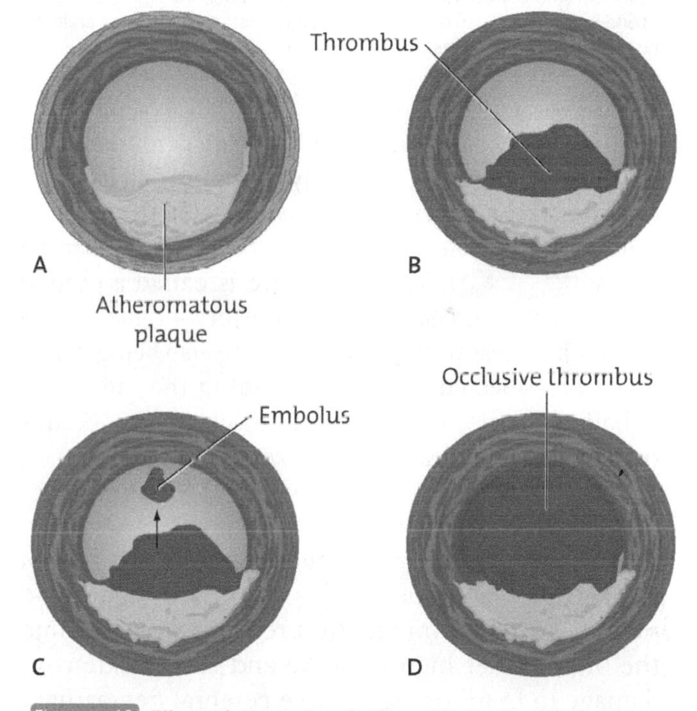

Figure 12 Effects of atherosclerosis of carotid artery in neck. **A**, Atherosclerotic plaque narrows vessel lumen, and surface frequently becomes ulcerated. **B**, Formation of thrombus on ulcerated surface of plaque, further narrowing vessel lumen. **C**, Thrombus material dislodged from plaque to form an embolus, which is carried to the brain. **D**, Complete occlusion of artery by thrombus.

Diagnosis of Extracranial Vascular Disease

Cerebral blood flow can be studied by injecting a radiopaque dye into the carotid and vertebral arteries that arise from the arch of the aorta to supply the brain. In this procedure, called a *cerebral angiogram*, the course of the dye is followed by serial x-ray studies, using methods similar to those used to visualize the coronary arteries. Arteriosclerotic plaques that

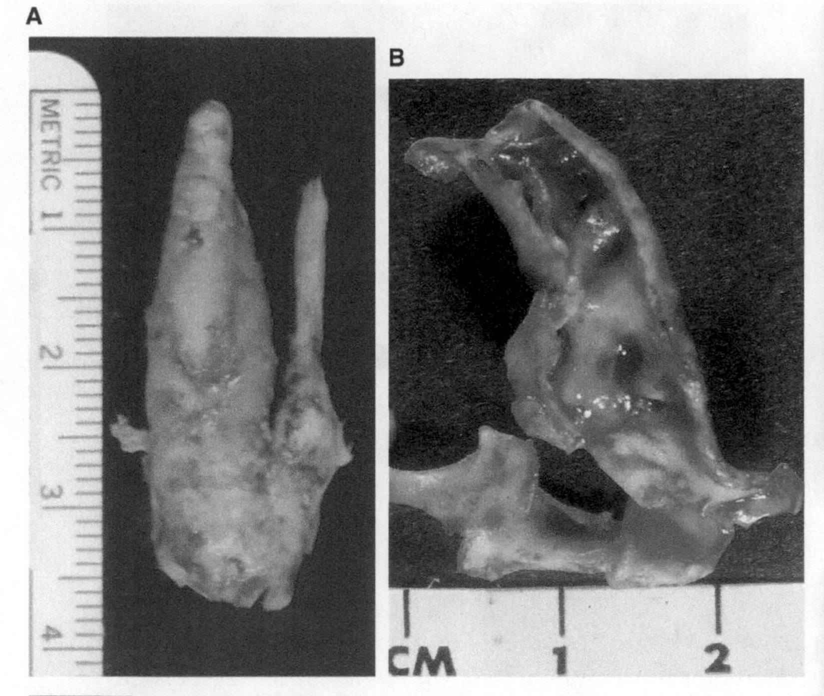

Figure 13 Carotid endarterectomy. **A,** Resected atherosclerotic plaque material has the contour of the common carotid artery and its two major branches, where it formed. **B,** An opened endarterectomy specimen revealing rough internal surface with areas of ulceration and hemorrhage in the atheromatous plaque.

occlude the carotid artery and impede cerebral blood flow can be removed surgically by making an incision in the carotid artery and dissecting out the arteriosclerotic lining and plaque, thereby opening up the artery (Figure 13). The procedure is called a *carotid endarterectomy* (*endo* = within + artery + *tome* = incision). Other less invasive methods are also being investigated in selected patients, including the same type of balloon angioplasty and stent insertion procedures that are used to treat coronary artery plaques.

Cerebral Hemorrhage

A *cerebral hemorrhage* is a much more serious type of stroke that occurs in persons who have high blood pressure. Blood from the ruptured vessel escapes into the brain under high pressure and causes extensive damage to brain tissue. A large cerebral hemorrhage is frequently fatal (Figure 14).

It is possible to distinguish a cerebral infarct from a cerebral hemorrhage by a specialized x-ray study called a computed tomographic (CT) scan. A CT scan can localize abnormal areas in the brain and determine their density. A cerebral hemorrhage appears as a dense area within the brain because blood is denser than normal brain tissue (Figure 15). In contrast, an infarct is often swollen by edema and appears less dense than normal brain tissue. Magnetic resonance imaging (MRI) provides similar information and is equally effective.

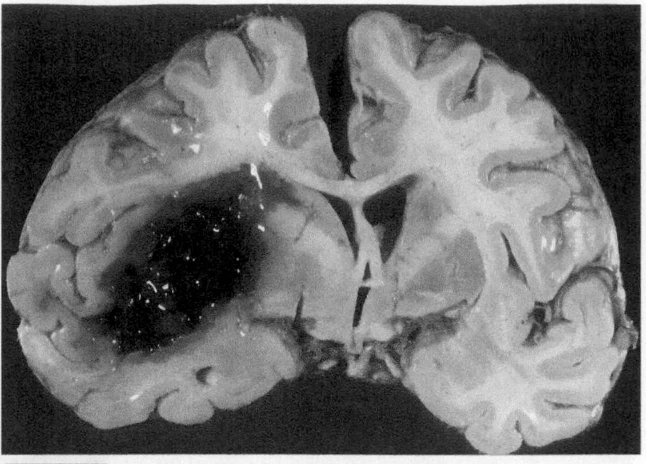

Figure 14 Coronal section of brain illustrating large cerebral hemorrhage that has compressed and displaced the cerebral ventricles.

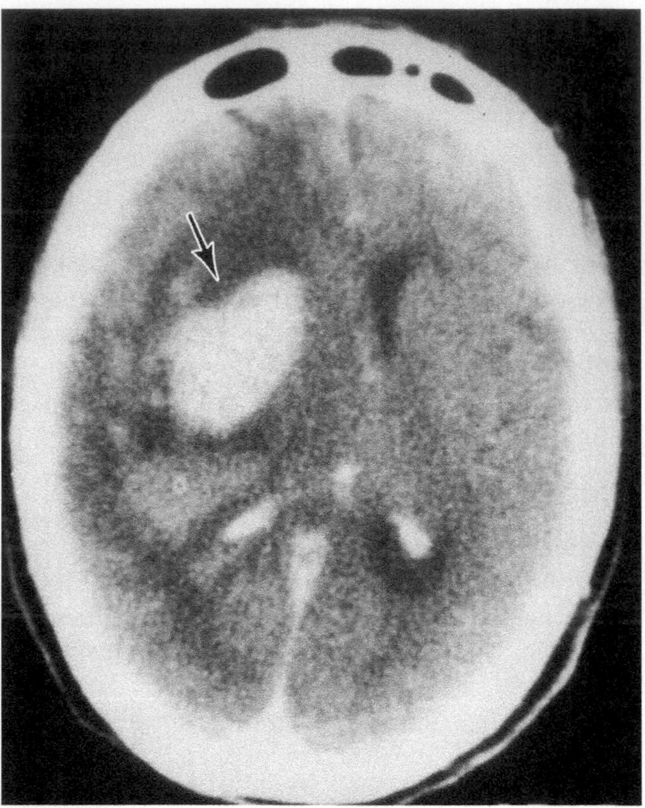

Figure 15 A computed tomographic (CT) scan of a patient with cerebral hemorrhage (*arrow*), which appears white because blood is denser than brain tissue.

Manifestations of Stroke

The clinical effects of a stroke depend on the location of the brain damage and the amount of brain tissue injured. Small infarcts may cause little functional disturbance and are usually followed by prompt recovery with little or no residual disability. Unfortunately, many strokes result from occlusions of the middle cerebral artery or one of its major branches or from a hemorrhage in a part of the brain supplied by the artery. Frequently the injury is extensive and causes partial paralysis by disrupting the nerve fibers that carry impulses to the spinal motor neurons and motor neurons of the cranial nerves. Nerve fibers carrying sensory impulses to the cortex are often damaged as well, leading to various sensory disturbances.

As mentioned earlier, sensory and motor fiber tracts cross in the brain stem as they ascend or descend; so the motor neurons from the right cerebral hemisphere supply the left side of the body, and sensory impulses received by this hemisphere come from the left side of the body. Conversely, the left hemisphere controls the right half of the body and receives sensory input from the right side. Consequently, a stroke involving one cerebral hemisphere often leads to weakness or paralysis on the opposite side, called **hemiplegia** (*hemi* = half + *plege* = stroke) or *hemiparesis* (*paresis* = weakness) and often to some sensory impairment on the paralyzed side as well. Speech also may be affected, but usually the affected individual does not lose consciousness.

Rehabilitation of the Stroke Patient

Many patients who suffer a major stroke are partially paralyzed, and some may have speech impairment as well. Rehabilitation, which is begun as soon as possible, helps the patient achieve several goals:

1. To regain the ability to walk
2. To relearn self-care activities, such as washing, combing the hair, and eating, which may have been impaired by the stroke
3. To prevent stiffness and limitation of motion in the joints of the paralyzed limbs
4. To make an emotional adjustment to the disability

These goals are achieved primarily by a program of exercises and relearning. If speech is impaired, speech therapy also is started. Many patients can learn to walk again, although in some cases a leg brace and cane may be required. It is more difficult to regain useful function in a paralyzed upper limb.

Transient Ischemic Attack

The term **transient ischemic attack**, often abbreviated **TIA**, refers to brief episodes of neurologic dysfunction such as temporary paralysis of an arm or leg, loss of speech, or disturbances of vision. The episodes, which tend to occur in older persons, last from a few minutes to a few hours and clear completely. They are usually caused by bits of thrombus or arteriosclerotic debris that break loose from an ulcerated plaque in the internal carotid artery and obstruct a small cerebral artery. The episodes are brief because the obstructing debris or small clot becomes fragmented and dissolved, and the circulation through the blocked vessel is restored before permanent damage to brain tissue occurs.

About one-third of patients with transient ischemic attacks eventually suffer a major stroke, but most have no further difficulties. Treatment consists either of surgical resection of the ulcerated plaque in the carotid artery by means of a *carotid endarterectomy* or administration of drugs that decrease the likelihood that thrombi will form on the ulcerated plaques. A narrowing of the carotid artery is significant if the lumen of the artery is reduced by 50 percent. This degree of narrowing corresponds to a 75 percent reduction in the cross-section area of the lumen and is associated with a large reduction in flow rate through the artery.

hemiplegia (hem-ē-plē´-jē-uh) Paralysis of one side of the body.

transient ischemic attack (TIA) (isskē´mik) Temporary cerebral dysfunction as a result of transient obstruction of a cerebral vessel by a bit of atheromatous debris or blood clot usually embolized from an arteriosclerotic plaque in the carotid artery.

Cerebral Aneurysm

Occasionally, aneurysms occur in the large cerebral arteries at the base of the brain. The most common type, a *congenital cerebral aneurysm*, results from a congenital defect in the elastic and muscular tissue of the vessel wall, usually at the point where the artery branches. Because of the congenital weakness, the lining of the arterial wall (*intima*) eventually protrudes through the defect at the point of branching, leading to the formation of a saclike outpouching (Figure 16).

Although the weakness of the vessel wall is congenital, the actual aneurysm does not develop until young

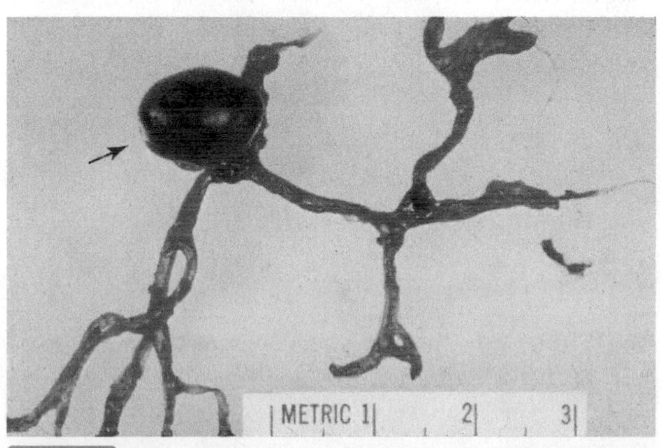

Figure 16 Dissection of vessels from the brain of a person with large congenital cerebral aneurysm (*arrow*).

adulthood or middle age. Persons with congenital polycystic kidney disease are prone to develop aneurysms of this type. Congenital aneurysms are hazardous because they may rupture, producing severe and sometimes fatal subarachnoid hemorrhage within the cranial cavity (Figure 17). Persons with high blood pressure are especially prone to this complication. The initial symptoms of a ruptured aneurysm are severe headache and a stiff neck. The headache results from the increased intracranial pressure caused by the sudden escape of blood into the subarachnoid space. The stiff neck occurs because the escaping blood irritates the meninges, setting off reflex contraction of the neck muscles.

The location of the aneurysm can be determined by a *cerebral angiogram*. Radiopaque material (contrast medium) is injected into the arteries supplying the brain and fills the aneurysm sac, defining both its size and position (Figure 18). Treatment usually consists of occluding (closing off) the aneurysm. Often this can be accomplished by applying a small metal clip to the narrow neck of the sac at its attachment to the arterial wall, but other procedures may be used depending on the size and location of the aneurysm.

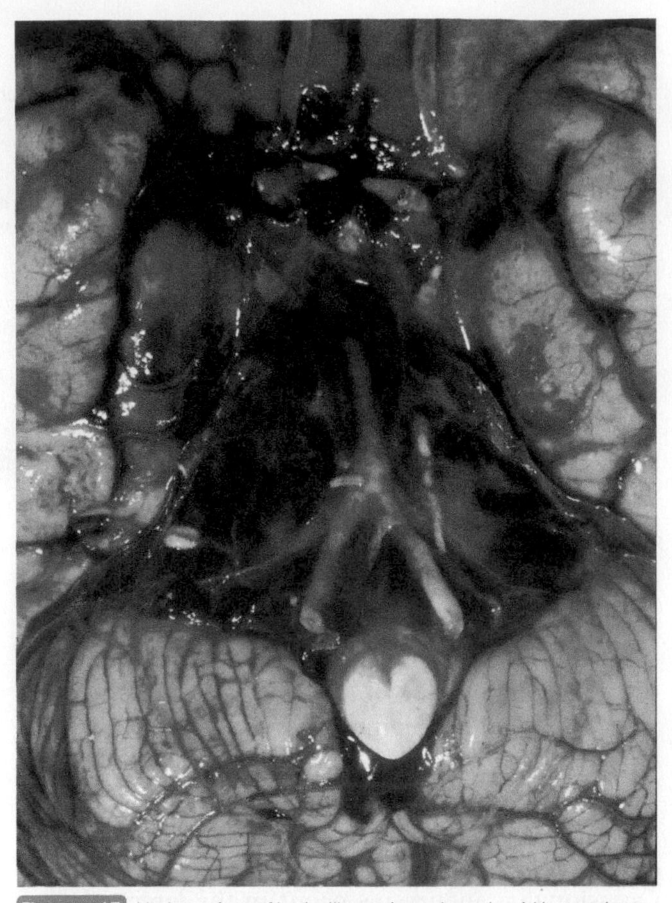

Figure 17 Undersurface of brain, illustrating subarachnoid hemorrhage secondary to ruptured cerebral aneurysm.

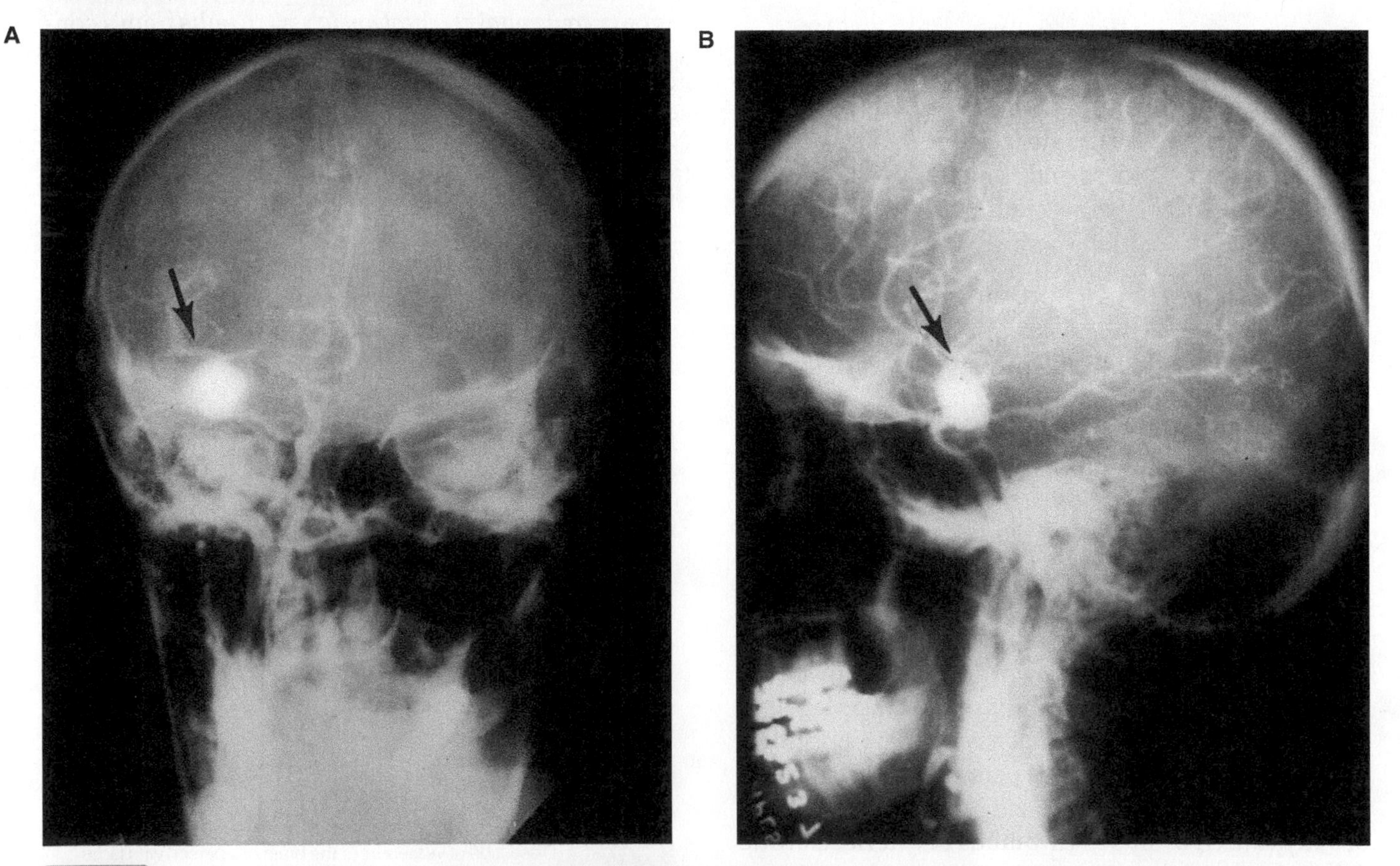

Figure 18 A cerebral aneurysm (*arrow*) demonstrated by an angiogram. **A**, Front view. **B**, Side view.

Infections of the Nervous System

Many different organisms can infect the nervous system, including bacteria, viruses, and fungi. An infection that predominantly affects the meninges surrounding the brain and spinal cord is called a **meningitis**. An infection of the brain tissue is called an **encephalitis**. If both brain and meninges are affected, the term *meningoencephalitis* is often used. An infection of the spinal cord is called a **myelitis**.

The manifestations of an infection of the CNS are those of any systemic infection: elevated temperature and other nonspecific symptoms. In addition, there are manifestations of meningeal irritation, consisting of a headache and a stiff neck. Involvement of brain tissue is associated with alteration of consciousness and neurologic symptoms resulting from dysfunction of localized areas within the brain.

Diagnosis of a CNS infection is established by examination of the spinal fluid, which contains a large number of leukocytes and an elevated protein concentration if infection is present. In bacterial infections, the leukocytes are primarily neutrophils, whereas lymphocytes predominate in viral infections. In bacterial and fungus infections, the organism responsible for the infection can often be identified in stained smears prepared from the spinal fluid and by culture of the spinal fluid.

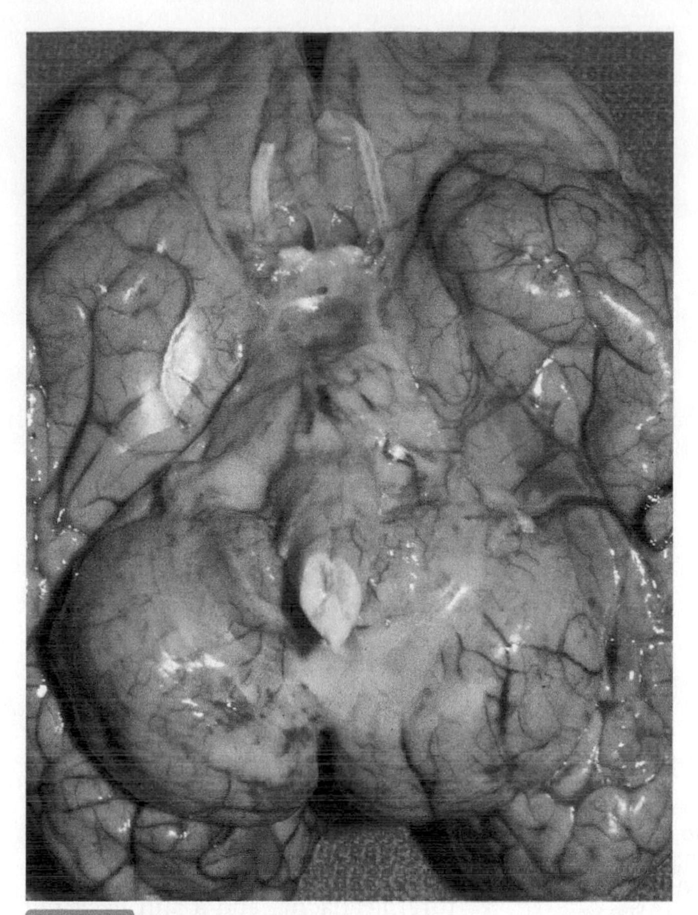

Figure 19 Bacterial meningitis, illustrating purulent exudate in the meninges. Exudate is most noticeable over the pons (*middle* of photograph) and cerebellum.

Meningitis Caused by Bacteria and Fungi

Two organisms are responsible for most cases of bacterial meningitis: the meningococcus (*Neisseria meningitides*) and the pneumococcus (*Streptococcus pneumoniae*) as illustrated in Figure 19. Until recently, a third organism, *Hemophilus influenzae*, was a common cause of meningitis in children. Now infants and children are routinely immunized against this organism, and *Hemophilus influenzae* meningitis, as well as other infections caused by this organism, occurs much less frequently than in the past.

Meningococcal infections occur primarily in young adults and often become epidemic where people live in close quarters, such as college dormitories and army camps. If an individual develops meningococcal meningitis, persons who have had close contact with the infected individual are treated with prophylactic antibiotics. If several cases occur in a community, college dormitory, or army camp, mass immunizations are undertaken to prevent an epidemic of meningococcal meningitis. In contrast, pneumococcal meningitis occurs sporadically in older adults, but it is not transmitted from person to person as is meningococcal meningitis. Consequently, persons who have had contact with an individual who develops pneumococcal meningitis do not require antibiotic prophylaxis, and communitywide immunizations are not required. Other bacteria may occasionally cause meningitis, especially in persons whose immunologic defenses have been weakened by disease or immunosuppressive therapy, or under conditions in which bacteria are introduced directly into the nervous system.

meningitis (men-in-jī'tis) Inflammation of the meninges.

encephalitis (en-sef-äl-ī'tis) An inflammation of the brain.

myelitis (mī-el-ī'tis) An inflammation of the spinal cord.

Bacterial meningitis is often preceded by a mild upper-respiratory infection, during which small numbers of bacteria gain access to the bloodstream. The bacteria are carried to the meninges, where they localize and initiate an acute infection. Occasionally, the pathogens may spread directly to the meninges from a sinus or middle-ear infection, or they may be introduced into the nervous system directly from a serious head injury such as a gunshot wound or other severe injury in which the scalp is lacerated and the skull is fractured.

Meningitis caused by the tubercle bacillus or a pathogenic fungus is uncommon and tends to be chronic rather than acute. *Tuberculous meningitis* results from spread of bacteria from a primary infection in the lung. *Fungus meningitis* also is usually secondary to a fungal infection of the lung, and many of the cases develop in immunocompromised persons. Bacterial and fungal infections are treated with appropriate antibiotics.

Viral Infections

Many viruses can infect the nervous system, including the measles and mumps viruses, various intestinal and respiratory viruses, the herpes simplex virus, cytomegalovirus, poliomyelitis virus, and an important group of viruses called *arboviruses*.

Manifestations of Nervous System Virus Infection

A viral infection may affect either the meninges (meningitis) or the brain tissue (encephalitis). A viral infection restricted to the meninges is often called *aseptic meningitis* to distinguish it from *suppurative* (pus-producing) *meningitis* caused by pathogenic bacteria. The affected individual has an elevated temperature, headache, and a stiff neck but does not usually appear seriously ill and recovers completely. *Viral encephalitis* is a much more serious infection. Affected patients are often very sick and exhibit various neurologic disturbances, such as confusion, disorientation, coma, cranial nerve dysfunction, weakness, and paralysis. Some cases are fatal, and patients who recover may be left with some permanent neurologic disability. Unfortunately, there is no specific treatment for most cases of viral encephalitis. However, some antiviral drugs may be effective if administered early in the course of the disease.

poliomyelitis
(pō´lē-yo-mī-e-lī´tis) An inflammation of the gray matter of the spinal cord, caused by a virus.

Arbovirus Infections

This important group of viruses is responsible for many cases of meningitis and encephalitis. The viruses infect birds and animals as well as humans and are transmitted by mosquitoes. The term *arbovirus* is a contraction of the term *arthropod–borne-virus*. Several different types of arboviral encephalitis are recognized. In the United States, *western equine encephalitis* occurs primarily in the West, and *eastern equine encephalitis* in the eastern part of the country. Two other types of encephalitis, called *St. Louis encephalitis* and *California encephalitis*, are not limited to the area implied by their names but are quite widely distributed.

West Nile Virus Infections The West Nile virus was first identified in 1937 in an infected woman living in the West Nile province of Uganda in Africa. From there the virus soon spread to Europe, where it became established and eventually spread to the United States in 1999, where the first case was identified in a person living in the New York City area.

Soon afterwards the virus spread rapidly through the United States, as well as into Canada and Mexico, where it caused the largest outbreak of arbovirus infections ever recorded in the Western Hemisphere. The West Nile virus infects many species of wild birds, horses, and other animals, as well as people, and many species of mosquitoes can transmit the virus. The virus can also be transmitted across the placenta from a pregnant virus-infected mother to her infant and in breast milk from an infected mother to a nursing infant.

Most persons infected with West Nile virus have no symptoms of infection, but about 20 percent of infected persons develop a fever and neurologic manifestations that can vary from mild aseptic meningitis to severe and sometimes fatal encephalitis. Some affected persons have developed a poliomyelitislike flaccid paralysis. No vaccine is available to immunize against the virus, and no antiviral therapy is available to treat the disease.

Poliomyelitis **Poliomyelitis** was formerly a very important and serious disease that caused much disability and many deaths. The virus enters the body through the gastrointestinal tract, localizing in the gray matter of the spinal cord and sometimes also in the cell bodies of cranial nerves in the brain stem. Destruction of motor neurons leads to paralysis of the muscles supplied by the affected neurons. The name of the disease refers to the affinity of the virus for the gray matter of the spinal cord (*polios* = gray). Fortunately, widespread immunization has eliminated this disease in the developed countries of the world, and an extensive immunization effort directed toward persons at risk in third world countries may soon lead to worldwide elimination of poliomyelitis. Hopefully, poliomyelitis will soon join smallpox as another disease that has been completely eradicated by an effective immunization program.

The Postpolio Syndrome About half the persons who survived paralytic poliomyelitis have begun to experience slowly progressive muscular atrophy, weakness, and muscle fatigue, and the onset of these manifestations began many years after the original episode of acute poliomyelitis from which they had recovered. The weakness usually involves muscles or muscle groups that had been affected during the original bout of poliomyelitis and from which the individual had made a partial or apparent complete recovery. This late-onset muscle weakness and muscle atrophy have been called the *postpolio syndrome*.

The exact cause of the postpolio syndrome is unknown. One likely explanation is that the surviving spinal motor neurons that were not damaged by poliomyelitis took over the function of the spinal neurons destroyed by poliomyelitis. These neurons established new axon connections with the muscle fibers that had lost their nerve supply, thereby reestablishing function in the previously paralyzed muscles. Overuse of the muscles with their reestablished nerve supply eventually caused the overworked neurons to fail many years later, which led to weakness and atrophy of the involved muscles as they gradually lost their nerve supply. Unfortunately, there is no specific treatment that can restore function to the muscles that have become weak and atrophic.

Creutzfeldt–Jakob Disease

Named after the physicians who described it, Creutzfeldt–Jakob (CJ) disease is a very unusual disease caused by a very unusual infectious agent. The disease occurs sporadically but can also be transmitted like an infectious disease, from contact with the infected tissues of a person with the disease.

The infectious agent is unusually resistant to inactivation by heat, by many disinfectants, and by ultraviolet light, but it can be destroyed by autoclaving or by household bleach. CJ is caused by an abnormal form of a specific protein called a **prion**, which is a contracted term for *proteinaceous infectious particle.* The normal form of the protein (the "good prion") is found in the cell membranes of neurons and in some other tissues. The abnormal form of the protein (the "bad prion") is identical except for the way the protein is folded, which causes the protein to have a different configuration (conformation) when viewed in three dimensions. The abnormal prion is able to function as an infectious agent because of its ability to convert normal prions into abnormal forms. As progressively more prion proteins are converted into abnormal forms, a self-perpetuating chain reaction follows as the newly formed abnormal prions convert more normal prions. As the abnormal prion proteins continue to accumulate, they disrupt the functions of the brain cells, which leads to the characteristic clinical and histologic manifestations of CJ disease.

The sporadic cases of CJ disease, which occur in older adults (as does Alzheimer disease described in a following section), are caused by a spontaneous mutation of a normal gene, and the mutated gene codes for the abnormal prion protein responsible for CJ disease.

Clinically, CJ disease is characterized by rapidly progressive mental deterioration (*dementia*) associated with neurologic disturbances. The disease is usually fatal within 6 months after the onset of symptoms. Histologically, the brains of affected persons contain a large number of vacuoles within the neurons, which causes the affected brain tissue to have a spongy appearance. The affected neurons degenerate, and astrocytes proliferate in response to the neuron loss; however, there is no inflammatory reaction (Figure 20). Unfortunately, no treatment is available for this devastating disease.

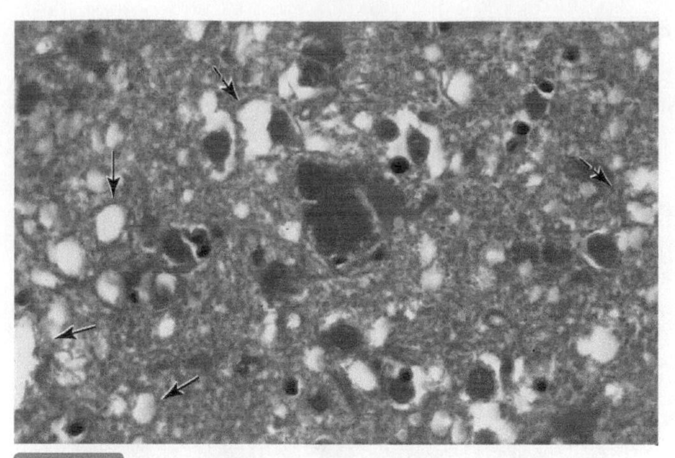

Figure 20 A photomicrograph of cerebral tissue from patient with Creutzfeldt–Jakob disease, illustrating multiple small vacuoles throughout the cortex (*arrows*) with loss of neurons and proliferation of astrocytes but no inflammatory reaction. The clump of eosinophilic material in the center of the photomicrograph is an aggregate of abnormal prion protein (original magnification × 400).

The cases of CJ disease caused by contact with infected tissues have been traced to biologic products or tissue contaminated with abnormal prions, such as cornea and organ transplants obtained from persons with unsuspected CJ disease.

prion (prī′-on) A protein infectious particle responsible for Creutzfeldt-Jakob disease and some other degenerative diseases of the nervous system.

Mad Cow Disease

Somewhat similar prion diseases occur in animals, which can be transmitted between animals of the same or different species by feeding animal tissues from infected animals to healthy animals. One such prion-related disease occurs in cattle and has raised concerns that it may cause CJ disease in humans. The cattle disease was recognized in 1985 when several dairy cows in the United Kingdom developed bovine spongiform encephalopathy, a prion disease that is usually called by the more familiar term *mad cow disease* because of the bizarre behavior of infected animals. During subsequent years, the number of infected cows increased to over 170,000. This epidemic was traced to cattle feed that had been mixed with protein-rich tissues obtained from sheep that had been infected with a similar prion

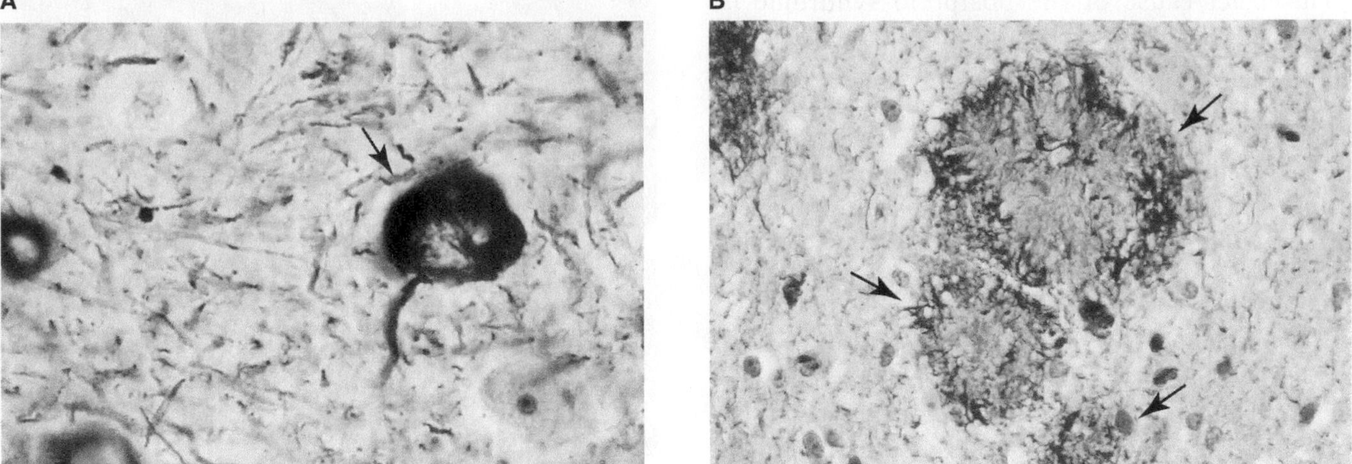

Figure 21 Alzheimer disease. **A**, Thickened neurofilaments encircle and obscure nucleus of nerve cells (*arrow*) forming neurofibrillary tangle (silver stain, original magnification × 400). **B**, Three neuritic plaques (*arrows*), composed of broken masses of thickened neurofilaments (silver stain, original magnification × 100).

disease. This feeding practice was discontinued, and the frequency of the cattle disease declined. Now use of animal tissues in animal feed is banned in both Britain and the United States.

The disease in cattle was followed several years later by cases of CJ disease, which had clinical features that were somewhat different from the usual manifestations of CJ disease, and has been called *new variant Creutzfeldt–Jakob disease*. This variant disease was contracted from eating meat from infected cows, and many people were concerned that more cases would occur since there was a lag time between consumption of infected beef and onset of clinical manifestations, but a great increase in new cases has not materialized.

Alzheimer Disease

Alzheimer disease (ahls′-hīm-er) A degenerative disease of the nervous system with characteristic structural abnormalities within neurons.

multiple sclerosis Chronic disease characterized by focal areas of demyelination in the central nervous system, followed by glial scarring.

astrocyte A large stellate cell having highly branched processes. Forms the structural framework of the nervous system. One of the neuroglial cells.

Alzheimer disease is a chronic progressive disease that affects primarily middle-aged and older persons. The disease is characterized by progressive failure of recent memory and difficulties in thinking, reasoning, and judgment; it is often associated with emotional disturbances such as depression, anxiety, and irritability.

The brains of affected patients exhibit progressive loss of neurons with atrophy of cerebral cortex and two rather characteristic histologic changes: *neurofibrillary tangles* and *neuritic plaques*. Neurofibrillary tangles result from degenerative changes affecting the thin, delicate, wirelike neurofilaments, which are located within the cytoplasm of the neurons. They become converted into thick, tangled, ropy masses encircling or displacing the nuclei of nerve cells and are demonstrated by special stains containing silver compounds (Figure 21A). Neuritic plaques are masses of broken, thickened nerve filaments that stain intensely with silver-containing stains and that surround a core of acellular protein material, called *amyloid protein*, with distinct staining properties (Figure 21B). In general, there is a correlation between the degree of intellectual deterioration and the severity of the histopathologic changes. The brains of patients with advanced Alzheimer disease contain large numbers of neuritic plaques and neurofibrillary tangles, whereas those with mild disease have less-striking changes.

The diagnosis of Alzheimer disease is made by excluding other conditions that can impair brain function, such as chronic infections of the nervous system or multiple strokes. Unfortunately, there is no specific treatment that can arrest the relentless progression of the disease, although some drugs may be useful to improve cerebral function temporarily.

Multiple Sclerosis

Multiple sclerosis is a chronic disease characterized by focal randomly distributed degeneration of the myelin sheaths covering groups of nerve fibers in the brain and spinal cord. The areas of demyelination disrupt the conduction of nerve impulses, and the damaged areas eventually heal by proliferation of fibers made by neuroglial cells called **astrocytes** (Figure 22). The disease is named from the multiple areas of demyelination, and the term sclerosis refers to the proliferation of fibers made by astrocytes, although the fiber proliferation is not the same as a fibrous tissue scar

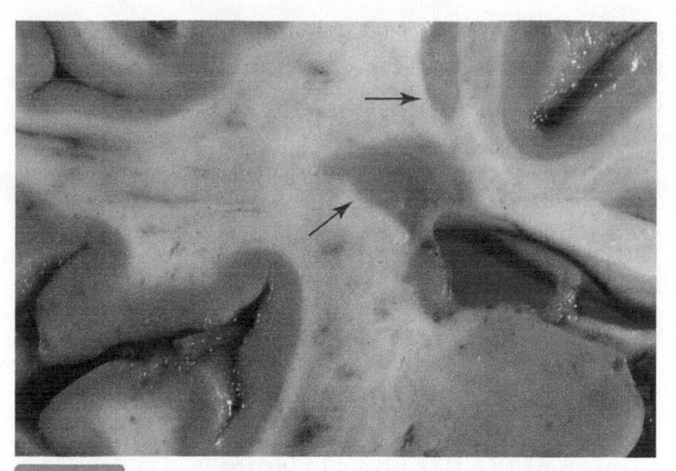

Figure 22 Coronal section of brain illustrating areas of glial scarring (*arrows*) adjacent to ventricle in multiple sclerosis. The demyelinated areas appear much darker than the adjacent normal white matter because of loss of myelin.

made by connective tissue cells. The discrete areas of myelin loss with glial scarring are called multiple sclerosis plaques. They are readily demonstrated within the nervous systems of affected persons by means of magnetic resonance imaging (MRI). This diagnostic procedure is extremely useful for evaluating patients with neurologic disease in whom multiple sclerosis is suspected (Figure 23).

Multiple sclerosis is a disease of young adults. The onset of symptoms before the age of 15 or after the age of 40 is rare. Clinically, the disease is characterized by periodic episodes of acute neurologic disturbances, the nature depending on the location of the demyelination. Each episode is followed by a period of recovery and remission. The course of the disease is prolonged and quite unpredictable, with repeated acute episodes followed by remissions extending over many years. Eventually, the neurologic disabilities become permanent as a consequence of multiple areas of glial scarring, which impair conduction of nerve impulses in the brain and spinal cord. There is no specific treatment that can arrest the progression of the disease. A number of measures, however, are available to relieve symptoms, shorten the recovery from an acute episode, and minimize the neurologic disabilities. Much evidence indicates that multiple sclerosis is an autoimmune disease, possibly initiated by a viral infection in a genetically predisposed person that stimulates an abnormal immune response manifested by focal demyelination of nerve tissue.

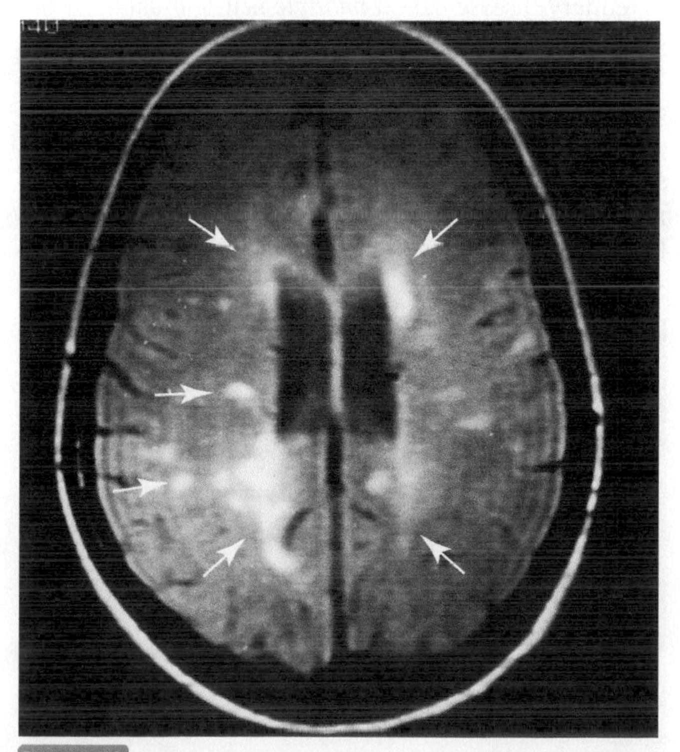

Figure 23 Multiple sclerosis demonstrated by MRI. The ventricular system is well demonstrated in the *center* of the photograph. Dense white areas adjacent to posterior horns of the ventricles and scattered throughout the brain lateral to the ventricles (*arrows*) are multiple sclerosis plaques.

Parkinson Disease

Parkinson disease is a chronic disabling disease characterized by rigidity of voluntary muscles and tremor of fingers and extremities. The disease results from a progressive loss of neurons in a part of the midbrain called the substantia nigra. The axons of these neurons synapse with neurons in the basal ganglia, where they release the neurotransmitter dopamine, and this is one of the important connections of the extrapyramidal motor system. As a result of the progressive neuron loss in the substantia nigra, fewer fibers are available to release dopamine in the basal ganglia, and the concentration of dopamine in the basal ganglia falls. The muscular rigidity, increased muscle tone, and abnormal repetitive involuntary movements, which are common manifestations of the disease, result from the deranged function of the extrapyramidal system.

Parkinson disease A chronic disease of the central nervous system characterized by rigidity and tremor, caused by decreased concentration of dopamine in the central nervous system.

The manifestations of the disease can be relieved by a drug called L-*dopa*, which is converted within the brain into dopamine. The drug therapy alleviates symptoms because it raises the concentration of dopamine in the basal ganglia, thereby supplying the neurotransmitter that is deficient. Various other drugs also have been used successfully to control the manifestations of Parkinson disease. Treatment, however, does not arrest the progressive neuron loss in the substantia nigra, nor does it stop the progression of the disease.

Huntington Disease

This is an uncommon but relatively well-known hereditary autosomal dominant disease that is characterized by progressive mental deterioration associated with abnormal jerky and writhing movements. The first manifestations in affected persons occur between ages 30 to 50 years. The disease progresses slowly and is usually fatal within about 15 to 20 years. Huntington disease causes progressive atrophy of groups of neurons called basal ganglia that are located deep within the cerebral hemispheres. These structures are part of the extrapyramidal motor system, which regulates smooth and coordinated muscle movements, and damage to the system gives rise to the abnormal movements characteristic of the disease. The cerebral cortex is also affected, which eventually leads to dementia as the disease progresses. CT scans of affected subjects demonstrate the cortical and basal ganglia atrophy characteristic of the disease.

Unfortunately, there is no way to arrest the progression of the disease, but drugs are available to help control some of its manifestations. Children of persons with Huntington disease should be offered genetic counseling and should be advised that they can be tested to determine whether they carry the abnormal gene. However, not all of the children of affected persons want this information. Some prefer living with an uncertain future rather than being tested and possibly learning that they carry the abnormal gene and are destined to acquire the disease.

Degenerative Diseases of Motor Neurons

A group of diseases of unknown cause affecting middle-aged and older adults is characterized by degeneration of motor neurons in the cortex, of cranial nerve neurons in the brain stem, and of spinal motor neurons. Most cases occur sporadically, and no hereditary background can be identified. Many of these diseases receive specific names, depending on which neuron groups are affected most severely, and the clinical manifestations of the neuron degeneration depend on which part of the nervous system suffers the greatest degenerative changes. In general, the symptoms are rapidly progressive muscular weakness leading to severe incapacitation and breathing difficulties resulting from weakness or paralysis of respiratory muscles. Death usually results from respiratory failure, often complicated by superimposed pulmonary infections. Unfortunately, there is no way to arrest the relentless progression of these devastating diseases. One of the best known of these neuronal degenerative diseases is called *amyotrophic lateral sclerosis*, better known as Lou Gehrig disease.

Tumors of the Nervous System

Tumors of the nervous system may arise from three sites:

1. The peripheral nerves
2. The meninges
3. Cells within the brain or spinal cord

Tumors of the Peripheral Nerves

Tumors of peripheral nerves arise from the Schwann cells that surround the nerve fibers. Such tumors may be solitary or multiple, benign or malignant.

Most solitary Schwann cell tumors are benign. They form discrete, well-circumscribed nodules attached to larger nerve trunks and usually can be dissected easily from the adjacent nerve. This type of tumor is often called a *neuroma*, although the terms *schwannoma* or *neurofibroma* also are used. Sometimes a neuroma arises from one of the cranial nerves at the base of the brain or from one of the spinal nerves within the spinal canal. A tumor in either of these locations is much more difficult to remove.

Multiple tumors of the peripheral nerves occur in a hereditary disease called *multiple neurofibromatosis* or *von Recklinghausen* disease, an uncommon condition transmitted as a Mendelian dominant trait. In this condition, the skin is disfigured by multiple tumors that grow from the cutaneous nerves and appear as variously sized nodules covering the entire body (Figure 24). The nodules are usually associated with localized light-brown patches of hyperpigmented skin. Multiple tumors

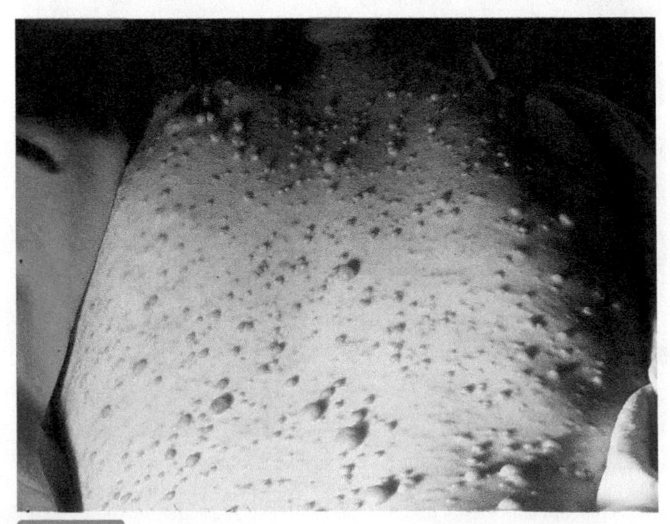

Figure 24 Multiple skin tumors in a patient with multiple neurofibromatosis.

also arise from the more deeply placed nerves supplying the internal organs. There is no specific treatment for this disease. Large tumors that encroach on vital organs or are cosmetically disfiguring can be removed surgically.

Tumors of the Brain

Malignant tumors arising in the breast, colon, lung, or other sites frequently metastasize to the brain. *Primary brain tumors* are less common than metastatic tumors. They may arise from the meninges, from the glial-supporting tissues of the brain, from the cells lining the ventricular system, or rarely from other tissues such as the blood vessels within the brain. Neuromas may also arise from the cranial nerves, as described in the foregoing section. Tumors do not develop from neurons because adult nerve cells are no longer capable of cell division.

A tumor of meninges is called a **meningioma**. This is a well-circumscribed benign tumor arising from arachnoid cells and is firmly adherent to the dura. The tumor causes symptoms as a result of compression of the underlying brain and can be removed successfully if it is located in an accessible location.

Any tumor of neuroglial origin is called a **glioma**. These tumors are further classified according to the type of glial-supporting cell from which the neoplasm arises. The most common type arises from astrocytes and is called an *astrocytoma*. A special name, *glioblastoma multiforme*, is applied to a highly undifferentiated, rapidly growing astrocytoma. The name describes the primitive appearance of the neoplastic astrocytes (*blast* = primitive cell) and their great variability in shape and appearance (*multiform* = having many shapes). Gliomas arise less frequently from other supporting cells. Lymphomas also may arise within the CNS and they are relatively common tumors in patients with AIDS.

Primary CNS tumors do not normally spread outside the nervous system, but many carry a poor prognosis because they often lie deep within the brain. Treatment consists of surgical resection of as much of the tumor as possible. In selected cases, surgery is followed by radiation and sometimes by anticancer chemotherapy as well. Primary lymphomas respond poorly to treatment, although radiotherapy may control the tumor for a time.

The symptoms of a brain tumor depend on the size and location of the neoplasm. Headache is a common initial manifestation because the increased volume within the cranial cavity caused by the tumor raises the intracranial pressure. Growth of the tumor also disrupts nerve cells and fiber tracts within the brain, leading to various neurologic disturbances.

Tumors of the Spinal Cord

The types of tumors that affect the brain may also occur in the spinal cord. In addition, metastatic tumors within the vertebral bodies or **multiple myeloma**, a tumor of plasma cells within the bone marrow, may extend from the vertebrae to compress or invade the adjacent spinal cord. If this occurs, sensation and motor function below the level of cord injury may be partially or completely lost.

Peripheral Nerve Disorders

Peripheral nerves and nerve roots may undergo demyelination and varying degrees of axon degeneration, and the condition is usually called peripheral neuritis. Clinical manifestations depend on the degree of nerve degeneration and on which nerves are affected. Involvement of a single nerve is usually secondary to injury or external compression. A frequently compressed nerve is the median nerve as it travels into the hand accompanied by the flexor tendons that attach to the thumb and fingers. These structures all travel through a narrow channel called the carpal tunnel that is interposed between the carpal bones posteriorly and a dense fibrous tissue ligament anteriorly. The nerve compression causes pain and **paresthesia** (abnormal sensations such as burning, numbness, and tingling) in the index and middle fingers, together with decreased sensation in the part of the hand supplied by the nerve. The small muscles of the hand at the base of the thumb, which are supplied by the nerve, may also undergo atrophy. Sometimes symptoms can be relieved by conservative measures such as injecting a corticosteroid mixed with a local anesthetic into the confined space (called the *carpal tunnel*) in which the nerve is compressed. In many cases, however, it may be necessary to cut the ligament that forms the anterior boundary of the carpal tunnel, thereby enlarging the tunnel to relieve the median nerve compression.

meningioma (men-in-jē-ō′muh) A benign tumor arising from the meninges.

glioma (glē-ō′muh) Any brain tumor arising from glial (supporting) cells of the brain.

multiple myeloma (my-el-ō′muh) A malignant neoplasm of plasma cells.

paresthesia (par-es-thē′ze-ah) An abnormal sensation, such as burning, prickling, or numbness.

polyneuritis (päl-ē-nū-rī′tis) An inflammation of multiple nerves.

Polyneuritis (Peripheral Neuritis)

Polyneuritis, also called *peripheral neuritis*, is characterized by progressive muscular weakness, numbness and tingling, tenderness, and pain in the parts of the body supplied by the peripheral nerves (called the *distribution* of the nerves). Often the muscles supplied by the involved nerves also exhibit some degree of atrophy. Usually the weakness and sensory disturbances affect the distal parts of the limbs, whereas strength and sensation remain relatively normal in the proximal parts of the extremities. This "glove-and-stocking" pattern of sensory and motor dysfunction is quite characteristic of polyneuritis. Most cases result from systemic diseases such as long-standing diabetes or various autoimmune diseases, or from occupational exposure to toxic drugs, heavy metals, or industrial compounds. Alcoholism is another common cause of peripheral neuritis, which is probably related to a coexisting vitamin B deficiency. Treatment of the alcoholism and its associated vitamin and nutrient deficiencies may improve the peripheral neuritis.

Neurologic Manifestations of Human Immunodeficiency Virus Infections

The nervous system is often involved in persons infected with the human immunodeficiency virus (AIDS virus). Neurologic manifestations of AIDS virus infections fall into three large categories:

1. Infections of the nervous system directly caused by the AIDS virus
2. Infections of the nervous system caused by opportunistic pathogens
3. AIDS-related tumors of the nervous system

HIV Infections of the Nervous System

Although HIV causes its major damage by infecting and destroying helper T lymphocytes, the virus also infects monocytes that can transport the virus into the brain, where it can injure the nervous system. In some patients, the infection may be manifested as acute viral meningitis occurring soon after the initial infection with the virus. In others, the infection causes a more chronic progressive degeneration of the brain with symptoms similar to those of Alzheimer disease, which is called *AIDS-related dementia* or *AIDS encephalopathy* (*encephalon* = brain + *pathy* = disease).

Opportunistic Infections of the Nervous System

Many of the opportunistic viruses, bacteria, fungi, and parasites that afflict AIDS patients can cause a primary infection of the nervous system. The clinical manifestations depend on the location of the infection within the nervous system and the amount of neurologic damage caused by the pathogen. Some of the more common opportunistic infections of the nervous system are those caused by the herpesvirus, cytomegalovirus, the fungus *Cryptococcus neoformans* and the protozoan parasite *Toxoplasma gondii*. Some of these infections respond to appropriate antibiotics and chemotherapeutic agents.

AIDS-Related Tumors

Persons with AIDS are at risk of various malignant tumors, especially Kaposi sarcoma and lymphoma, and these tumors may metastasize to the nervous system as well as to other sites within the body. AIDS patients may also develop primary lymphomas of the nervous system. These tumors carry a very poor prognosis and do not respond well to treatment.

CHAPTER REVIEW

Summary

This chapter begins with an overview of the structure and function of the nervous system, which can be regarded as a giant switchboard receiving nerve impulses and relaying them to their proper destination. The pyramidal and extrapyramidal motor systems function together to facilitate both voluntary motor activity and motor functions concerned with maintaining posture, balance, and coordination of activities such as walking, running, or swimming. Muscle paralysis results when its connection with the nervous system is lost. Flaccid paralysis results when spinal motor neurons are destroyed by disease, such as poliomyelitis, and the affected muscles become atrophic. Spastic paralysis results from damage to cortical neurons or their axons that connect with spinal neurons, as after a stroke. Control of the affected muscles is lost but the muscles do not become atrophic.

The brain is well protected within the cranial cavity but may be damaged by a severe blow, and the skull may fracture. Intracerebral bleeding may follow. If the neural tube does not form normally, the brain or spinal cord may be affected. Anencephaly is incompatible with postnatal life. Spina bifida may vary from only defective formation of the bony arch overlying the spinal cord to a profound developmental disturbance called a meningomyelocele. Results of treatment depend on the severity of the malformation. Hydrocephalus is a distention of the ventricular system caused by an obstruction of cerebrospinal fluid (CSF) movement through the ventricular system. In infants the head enlarges because the cranial bones have not fused, which does not occur in an affected adult. Treatment involves shunting the fluid through a tube extending from the dilated ventricular system into the peritoneal cavity, where the CSF is reabsorbed into the circulation by blood vessels within the peritoneal cavity.

A stroke, also called a cerebrovascular accident or CVA, may result from a thrombosis of a cerebral blood vessel, an embolus from a thrombus within the heart or overlying an atheromatous plaque in the internal carotid artery, or from rupture of an intracerebral blood vessel in a person with severe hypertension; a cerebral hemorrhage follows, which is a life-threatening catastrophe. A transient ischemic attack, often called a TIA, is a brief episode of neurologic dysfunction that subsides in a short time, and is usually caused by short-duration blockage of a cerebral artery by atheromatous plaque material or a bit of thrombus material extruded from a plaque within the internal carotid artery. A cerebral aneurysm results from a congenital defect in the muscle or elastic tissue in the wall of an artery at the base of the brain; the protrusion usually occurs where the artery branches. The lining of the artery (intima) projects as a saclike extension from the artery, which may rupture and cause a subarachnoid hemorrhage. Various methods are available to prevent rupture of a known aneurysm, or to deal with the results of a ruptured aneurysm.

Infections of the nervous system may be caused by bacteria, such as the meningococcus or pneumococcus, or by viruses such as the West Nile virus. Less commonly the mycobacterium causing tuberculosis may infect the meninges, and various fungi may infect immunocompromised persons. Appropriate antibiotics are available to treat many of these infections. An entirely different problem results from an infection caused by the abnormal prion that causes sporadic Creutzfeldt–Jakob (CJ) disease, and the new variant CJ disease caused by ingestion of meat from cows infected with mad cow disease (bovine spongiform encephalopathy).

A number of other diseases affect the nervous system and impair CNS function including (1) Alzheimer disease, caused by progressive neuron loss and neuritic plaques; (2) Parkinson disease, caused by degeneration of dopamine-producing cells in the midbrain; (3) multiple sclerosis, an autoimmune disease affecting the white matter of the nervous system; and (4) Huntington disease, a progressive hereditary disease affecting the basal ganglia that disrupts the functions of the extrapyramidal system.

There are also several degenerative diseases of unknown cause affecting middle-aged and older adults. The diseases are characterized by progressive nerve cell degeneration, leading to progressive muscular weakness, eventually affecting respiratory muscles and leading to death from respiratory failure. The best known of these is a condition called amyotrophic lateral sclerosis, better known as Lou Gehrig disease.

Various primary tumors also affect the nervous system, arising from peripheral nerves (neuromas and neurofibromas), and from neuroglial cells (various gliomas including astrocytomas and the highly malignant glioblastoma multiforme). One relatively common hereditary disease is characterized by the formation of multiple neurofibromas in the skin and deeper tissues, which is called multiple neurofibromatosis. Metastatic tumors may also involve the nervous system.

Peripheral nerve degeneration is called peripheral neuritis, and many cases are caused by harmful drugs or other agents, or as a result of nutritional deficiencies in persons with chronic alcoholism. Isolated nerve degeneration may also follow nerve compression, as in the carpal tunnel syndrome where the nerve is compressed within the carpal tunnel as it passes through the wrist. Some cases of polyneuritis appear to be a manifestation of an autoimmune disease. An HIV infection may also affect the nervous system, presenting as a meningitislike syndrome during the initial infection, as an infection by various opportunist pathogens in persons with AIDS, or occasionally as a malignant lymphoma related to failure of the immune defense system in an AIDS patient.

Questions for Review

1. Briefly describe the organization of the central nervous system. Describe the function and circulation of cerebrospinal fluid.
2. What are some of the possible effects of a severe blow to the head?
3. What is a stroke? What are the common causes of a stroke? What is a congenital aneurysm of the circle of Willis?
4. What are the common causes of hydrocephalus? How does a brain tumor cause hydrocephalus?
5. What is a neural tube defect? How can it be recognized before birth?
6. What is meant by the following terms: *arachnoid*, *subdural hemorrhage*, *anencephaly*, and *meningioma*?
7. What is a transient ischemic attack? How is it treated?
8. Describe the common tumors of the nervous system. What are their clinical manifestations?
9. What is the difference between a polyneuritis (peripheral neuritis) and an isolated nerve compression, as in the carpal tunnel syndrome?
10. Compare Creutzfeldt–Jakob disease and Alzheimer disease.
11. Describe the role of magnetic resonance imaging in the diagnosis of multiple sclerosis.
12. Describe the effects of human immunodeficiency virus infections on the nervous system.

Supplementary Reading

Brown, P. 1997. The risk of spongiform encephalopathy ("mad cow disease") to human health. *Journal of the American Medical Association* 278:1008–11.

A review of the variant form of Creutzfeldt–Jakob disease transmitted from infected cattle to humans.

Caplan, L. R. 1998. Stroke treatment: Promising but still struggling [Editorial]. *Journal of the American Medical Association* 279:1304–6.

Many technical advances have improved the management of affected patients. Thrombolytic therapy may be helpful in selected cases, but carries a risk of causing a brain hemorrhage and must be used within a few hours after the onset of stroke symptoms.

Centers for Disease Control and Prevention. 1993. Recommendations for use of folic acid to reduce the number of spina bifida cases and other neural tube defects. *Journal of the American Medical Association* 269:1233–38.

All women of childbearing age should consume 0.4 mg of folic acid per day to reduce their risk of having a pregnancy affected with a neural tube defect.

DeAngelis, L. M. 2001. Brain tumors. *New England Journal of Medicine* 344:114–23.

A comprehensive review article dealing with the clinical features, classification, diagnosis, prognosis, and management of the various types of glial and meningeal tumors.

Hollander, H., Schaefer, P. W., and Hedley-Whyte, E. T. 2005. Case 22-2005: An 81-year-old man with cough, fever, and altered mental status. *New England Journal of Medicine* 353:287–95.

A clinical and pathological case study of an older man with the fatal West Nile virus infection. Autopsy revealed encephalomyelitis with the most marked damage in spinal cord anterior horn cells and in motor nuclei of the brain stem, changes similar to those encountered in poliomyelitis. Less marked changes were also detected in the thalamus, cerebellum, and cerebral cortex.

JAMA Patient Page. 1998. How do you know when someone is having a stroke? *Journal of the American Medical Association* 279:1324.

A review for the lay person of risk factors, manifestations, and what to do when someone is having a stroke.

Johnson, R. T., and Gibbs, C. J., Jr., 1998. Creutzfeldt–Jakob disease and related transmissible spongiform encephalopathies. *New England Journal of Medicine* 339:1994–2004.

This review article discusses the relationship of mad cow disease to Creutzfeldt–Jakob disease.

Jubelt, B., and Agre, J. C. 2000. Characteristics and management of postpolio syndrome. *Journal of the American Medical Association* 284:412–14.

A discussion of clinical manifestations and management of postpolio syndrome, which affects about half the persons who developed paralytic poliomyelitis many years previously.

Noseworthy, J. H., Lucchinetti, C., Rodriguez, M., and Weinshenker, B. G. 2000. Multiple sclerosis. *New England Journal of Medicine* 343:938–52.

A comprehensive review of clinical manifestations, epidemiologic features, genetic factors, and treatment.

Ojemann, R. G. 1981. Management of unruptured intracranial aneurysm [Editorial]. *New England Journal of Medicine* 304:725–26.

From approximately 3 to 4 percent of patients each year with an asymptomatic aneurysm will experience cerebral hemorrhage as the result of rupture. The larger the aneurysm, the greater the likelihood of rupture. Aneurysm larger than 7 mm should be treated surgically.

Sacco, R. L. 2001. Extracranial carotid stenosis. *New England Journal of Medicine* 345:1113–18.

A review of methods of treatment, risk of strokes and other complications under various conditions, and guidelines for treatment. Patients with symptoms who have severe carotid artery stenosis should be treated surgically.

Tyler, K. L. 2003. Creutzfeldt–Jakob disease [Perspective]. *New England Journal of Medicine* 348:681–82.

Current status of new variant Creutzfeldt–Jakob disease and tests available for diagnosis. The number of new cases in the United Kingdom is decreasing.

Interactive Activities

Matching

Match the disease or condition in the left column with its characteristic features or manifestations in the right column.

Disease or Condition	Features or Manifestations
1. Alzheimer disease	A. Demyelinating disease
2. Glioblastoma	B. Brain degeneration caused by abnormal prions
3. Transient ischemic attack	C. Neuritic plaques and neurofibrillary change in cerebral neurons
4. Neurofibroma	D. Nerve compression
5. Mad cow disease	E. Progressive nerve cell degeneration in older adult
6. Lou Gehrig disease	F. Malignant brain tumor
7. Carpal tunnel syndrome	G. Protrusion of meninges through defect in spine
8. Multiple sclerosis	H. Enlarged ventricles
9. Cystic spina bifida	I. Benign tumor of nerve
10. Hydrocephalus	J. Short episode of neurologic dysfunction.

True or False

Mark the answer true (T) or false (F) in the space provided.

1. Lou Gehrig disease is caused by abnormal prions that destroy brain tissue. _____
2. Multiple neurofibromatosis is a hereditary disease resulting in formation of multiple benign tumors in skin and deeper tissues. _____
3. Anencephaly results from failure of the neural tube to close normally. ____
4. A saclike protrusion of the lining of a cerebral artery through a defect in the arterial wall is called a cystic spina bifida. ____
5. The frequency of neural tube defects can be reduced significantly by ingestion of folic acid before conception and during pregnancy. ____
6. Most glioblastomas in older adults respond well to treatment and have a good prognosis. ____
7. Persons who had poliomyelitis many years ago with muscle paralysis who have recovered muscle function may have a recurrence of their paralysis many years later. ____

8. Mad cow disease is a type of rabies that causes the cows to become aggressive and hostile. ____
9. New variant Creutzfeldt–Jakob disease is acquired from eating meat from cows infected with abnormal prions. ____
10. The West Nile virus usually causes a measleslike skin rash. _____

Critical Thinking

1. Jane Anderson said that her 62-year-old father was drinking coffee in a restaurant and he had a brief episode when he lost the strength in his hand and dropped the cup, spilling his coffee. The hand weakness persisted for about 30 minutes and then his muscle strength returned. She asks you what this means and should she be concerned about it. What would you tell her?
2. Susan Smith is a 25-year-old computer operator who has begun to experience pain in the right wrist and hand especially after she has been working at the computer for a long period of time. She also has developed some weakness on some of her thumb muscles. She asks you what to do about this. What would you tell her?

Answers

Matching: 1C; 3J; 5B; 7D; 9G

True or False: 1F; 3T; 5T; 7T; 9T

Critical Thinking:

1. Jane's dad had a transient ischemic attack (TIA) probably caused by temporary plugging of an artery in the brain by arteriosclerotic plaque material or a bit of thrombus material on the surface of a plaque in his carotid artery that soon was removed by the body's protective mechanisms, and blood flow returned. The TIA is a manifestation of vascular disease and he should have a further investigation to evaluate his cardiovascular system and see whether the carotid artery is the source.

The Musculoskeletal System

LEARNING OBJECTIVES

1. Name the common congenital abnormalities of the skeletal system.
2. List the three major types of arthritis. Describe their pathogenesis and clinical manifestations, and explain the methods of treatment.
3. Describe the causes and effects of osteoporosis, and name the methods of treatment.
4. Describe the structure of the intervertebral disks, and explain their function. Describe the clinical manifestations of a herniated disk.
5. Compare the pathogenesis and clinical manifestations of muscular atrophy and muscular dystrophy. Name and describe the common types of each.
6. Describe the pathogenesis, manifestations, and treatment of myasthenia gravis.
7. Describe the manifestations, complications, and treatment of scoliosis.

Structure and Function of the Skeletal System

The skeleton is the rigid supporting structure of the body. All bones have the same basic structure. They are composed of an outer layer of *compact bone*, the cortex, and an inner, spongy layer in which the bone is arranged in a loose meshed latticework of thin strands called *bone trabeculae*. The spaces between the trabeculae contain the bone marrow, which consists of fat and blood-forming tissue.

Individual bones vary in size and appearance. They may be long, short, flat, or irregular in shape. The typical long bone, such as is found in the upper and lower limbs, has a tubular shape with expanded ends. The *shaft* is the long cylindrical part, and the expanded ends of the shaft are called the *epiphyses*. The center of the shaft is hollowed out to form the marrow cavity, which is filled with fat and bone marrow. This type of construction provides considerable strength without excessive weight.

Bone is a specialized type of connective tissue. It is composed of a dense connective-tissue framework (called osteoid before it is calcified) which soon becomes impregnated with calcium phosphate salts along with smaller amounts of calcium carbonate and other minerals. Three different types of cells are found in bone: osteoblasts, osteocytes, and osteoclasts. *Osteoblasts* are the active bone-forming cells that produce the collagenous bone matrix. They secrete an enzyme, *alkaline phosphatase*, that promotes deposition of calcium phosphate salts in the bone matrix to calcify the bone. As the bone matrix is formed and calcified, the osteoblasts become incorporated within the bone and become transformed into relatively inactive mature bone cells called *osteocytes*. Osteoclasts are multinucleated cells concerned with bone resorption. They remove the bone matrix by phagocytosis, dissolve the bone salts, and release the calcium and phosphate ions into the circulation. Bone is not a static structure. It is continually being broken down and reformed, and calcium salts in bone and calcium ions in the blood and body fluid are continuously interchanged.

In general, the strength and thickness of the bones depend on the activities of the individual. A person accustomed to strenuous physical labor has thicker, heavier bones than one who is normally engaged in light, sedentary activities. If an extremity is immobilized and is not allowed to bear weight, as after a fracture, the immobilized bone undergoes significant thinning and decalcification, called disuse atrophy.

The bones of the skeleton are connected by *joints*. There are three types: fibrous joints, cartilaginous joints, and synovial joints. In a *fibrous joint*, such as occurs between the bones of the skull, the bones are firmly joined by fibrous tissue to form a firm union called a *suture line*. In a *cartilaginous joint*, such as occurs between adjacent vertebral bodies in the spine and between the pubic bones of the pelvis (symphysis pubis), the ends of the bones are joined by fibrocartilage. Joints of this type have very little mobility. A *synovial joint* is a movable joint. The ends of the bones that move against one another are covered by smooth hyaline cartilage, which is called the *articular cartilage* (*articulare* = to connect). The ends of the bones are held together by dense fibrous bands (ligaments). The joint capsule is lined by a thin synovial membrane (the *synovium*), which secretes a small amount of mucinous fluid to lubricate the joint.

intramembranous bone formation Direct formation of bone by osteoblasts without prior formation of a cartilage model.

endochondral bone formation (en-dō-kon′drul) Formation of bone as, first, a cartilage model that is then reabsorbed and converted into bone.

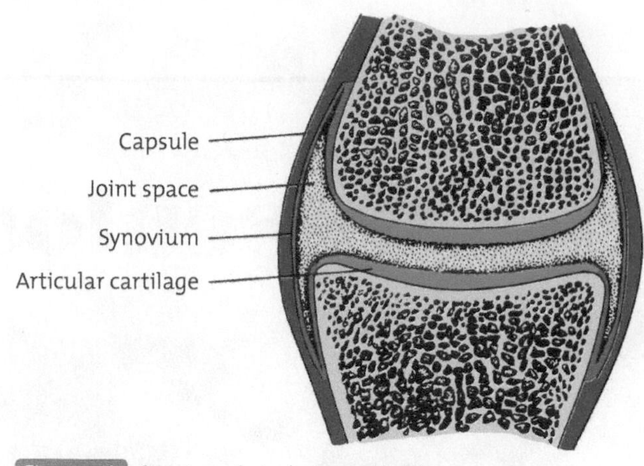

Figure 1 Structure of a typical movable joint.

Figure 1 illustrates the structure of a typical movable joint. Figure 2 illustrates the histologic appearance of the articular cartilage and underlying bone, and the appearance of a normal synovium. In joint disease, the structures are altered by inflammation and degeneration, leading to derangement in the functions of the joints.

Bone Formation

There are two types of bone formation, and they are fundamentally similar. In one type, called **intramembranous bone formation**, the embryonic connective-tissue cells (mesodermal cells) are transformed directly into bone-forming cells (osteoblasts). The osteoblasts secrete a collagenous material called *osteoid*, which then becomes calcified to form bone. The bones of the vertex of the skull, the facial bones, and a few other bones are formed in this manner. Most of the skeletal system, however, is formed by a process called **endochondral bone formation** (*endo* = within + *chondral* = cartilage). In endochondral bone formation, the mesodermal cells differentiate first into cartilage cells, and the bones are formed initially as cartilage models. The cartilage is then absorbed and replaced by bone. Conversion of cartilage into bone is accomplished by vascular bone-forming mesoderm, which invades the cartilage. The areas of active bone formation are termed *centers of ossification*.

Bones that have been preformed in cartilage undergo ossification at specific times throughout fetal and postnatal life. The time of appearance of the various centers of ossification is characteristic for each bone. In the long bones, ossification begins first in the shaft; later, centers of ossification form at the ends (epiphyses) of the bone. The actively growing zone of cartilage between the shaft and the epiphysis of a long bone is called the epiphyseal plate.

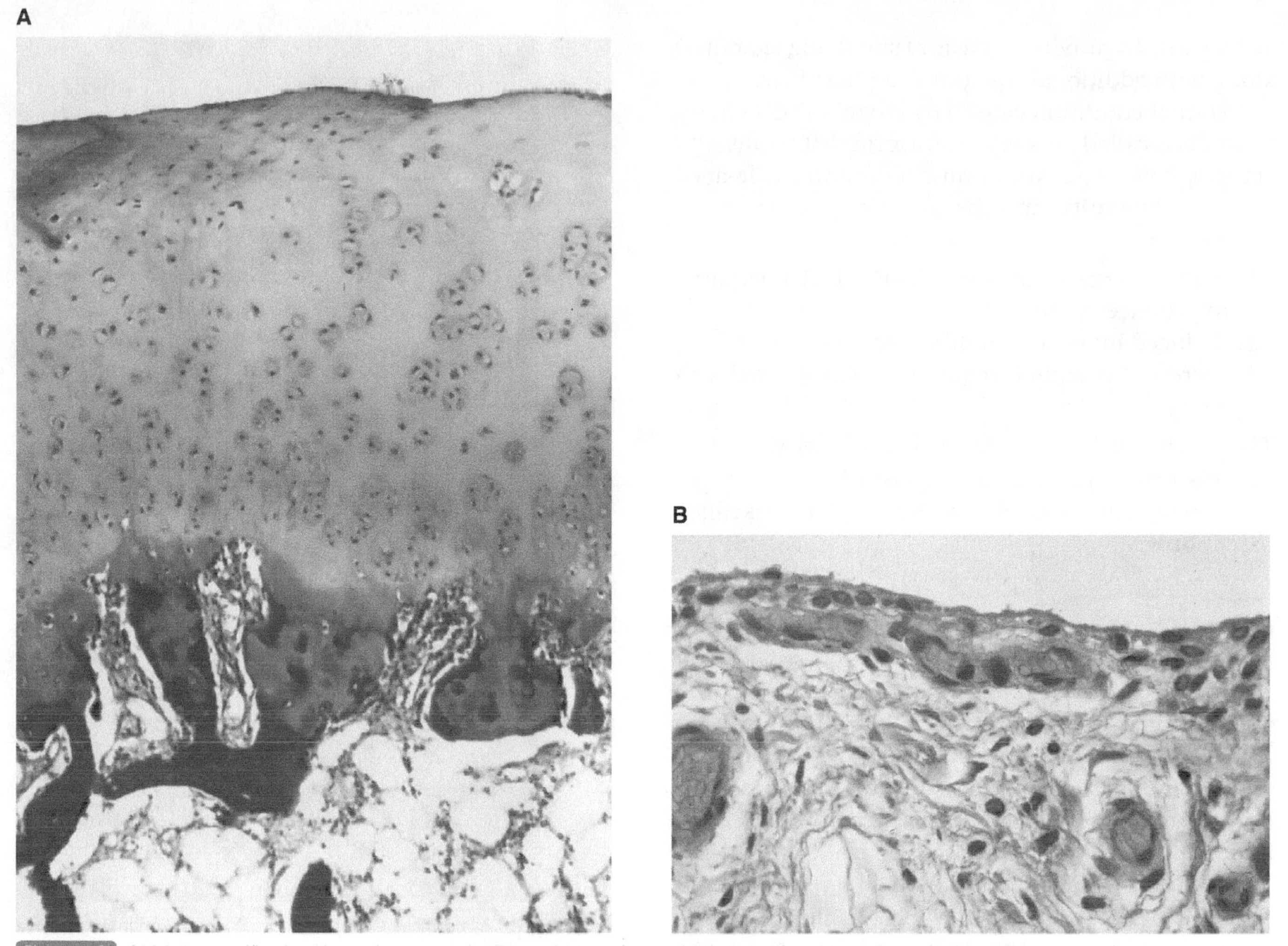

Figure 2 **A**, A low-magnification photomicrograph of cellular structure of normal articular surface, illustrating articular cartilage at *top* of photograph, junction of bone and cartilage in *middle* of photograph, and normal bone with fatty bone marrow at *bottom* of photograph (original magnification × 40). **B**, Normal synovium composed of synovial cells (*top* of photograph) covering loose connective tissue.

Bone Growth

Bone grows in both length and thickness and is continually remodeled as it grows by absorption of bone in some areas and formation of new bone in others. Bone grows thicker by adding to its external surface newly formed bone that is produced by the periosteum, a layer of specialized connective-tissue cells surrounding the bone. The periosteal cells differentiate into osteoblasts, which in turn produce bone. Growth in the length of bone is the result of proliferation of cartilage at the epiphyseal plate, which is converted into bone. Growth in bone length continues into adolescence. Eventually, epiphyseal growth ceases, and the cartilagenous epiphyseal plate becomes converted into bone—called closure of the epiphyses. Thereafter, no further growth in length of bone is possible.

Normal bone growth and maturation require a normal amount of vitamin D, which can be obtained by exposure of the skin to sunlight, or obtained from the diet in vitamin D-fortified milk and other foods. Normal amounts of calcium and phosphate are also needed to calcify the bone as it is formed, and the parathyroid glands, which regulate the level of blood calcium, must function normally.

Bone Growth Disturbances Caused by Vitamin D Deficiency Children lacking adequate vitamin D develop rickets, which is an uncommon disease because most children receive vitamin D supplements. However, if vitamin D is insufficient, calcium is not absorbed normally from the intestinal tract and the blood calcium tends to fall. The parathyroid glands respond to the low calcium by increasing the secretion of parathyroid hormone, which raises blood calcium but also causes the level of phosphate in the blood to fall. As a result, the deposition of calcium phosphate in the bone matrix is impaired because there is not enough phosphate available to combine with calcium, and the bone matrix is not adequately calcified. Osteoid is formed in excess at the epiphyseal ends of the growing bones, but it lacks strength because it is so poorly calcified. Consequently, the weakened bones tend to become bowed when weight bearing is attempted. Treatment consists of supplying vitamin D along with additional calcium and phosphate.

A similar condition caused by vitamin D deficiency in adults is called *osteomalacia*, a term that means *softening of bone*. The condition occurs in middle-aged and elderly adults, and the deficiency is caused by several factors:

1. Inadequate exposure to sunlight, which is required to produce vitamin D
2. Reduced intake of vitamin D-fortified foods
3. Increased vitamin D requirements associated with aging

The poorly calcified bone formed in persons with osteomalacia may contribute to the loss of bone strength and bone density associated with aging, which is called **osteoporosis**.

Congenital Malformations

Abnormal Bone Formation

The two most important genetically determined diseases of the skeletal system that result from abnormal bone formation are achondroplasia and osteogenesis imperfecta.

In **achondroplasia**, endochondral bone formation is faulty. The abnormality, which is transmitted as a Mendelian dominant trait, is characterized by disturbed endochondral bone formation at the epiphyseal plates (growth centers) of the long bones. The disturbance impairs growth of the extremities, causing a type of dwarfism in which the limbs are disproportionately short in relation to the trunk (*achondroplastic dwarfism*). The head is also abnormally formed because of disturbed endochondral ossification of the bones forming the base of the skull, and there is usually also an exaggerated curvature (lordosis) of the lumbar spine (Figure 3).

osteoporosis (ä′stē-ō-por-ō′sis) Generalized thinning and demineralization of bone that tends to occur in postmenopausal women.

achondroplasia (a-kon-dro-pla′zi-yuh) A congenital disturbance of endochondral bone formation that causes a type of dwarfism.

osteogenesis imperfecta A congenital disturbance of bone formation characterized by excessively thin and delicate bones that are easily broken.

clubfoot Congenital malposition of foot. In most common type, foot is turned inward at ankle and heel is elevated.

Osteogenesis imperfecta (meaning literally "imperfect bone formation") is characterized by the formation of very thin and delicate bones that are easily broken under very minimal stress. In the most severe cases, the infant is born with multiple fractures. Some fractures occur before birth, having been sustained as a result of the very minor stresses resulting from the movements of the fetus within the uterus; other fractures occur during delivery. The intrauterine fractures of the extremities usually heal in poor alignment, causing the limbs to appear bent and disproportionately short (Figure 4). In milder forms of the disease, the abnormal fragility of the bone may not become apparent until childhood or adolescence.

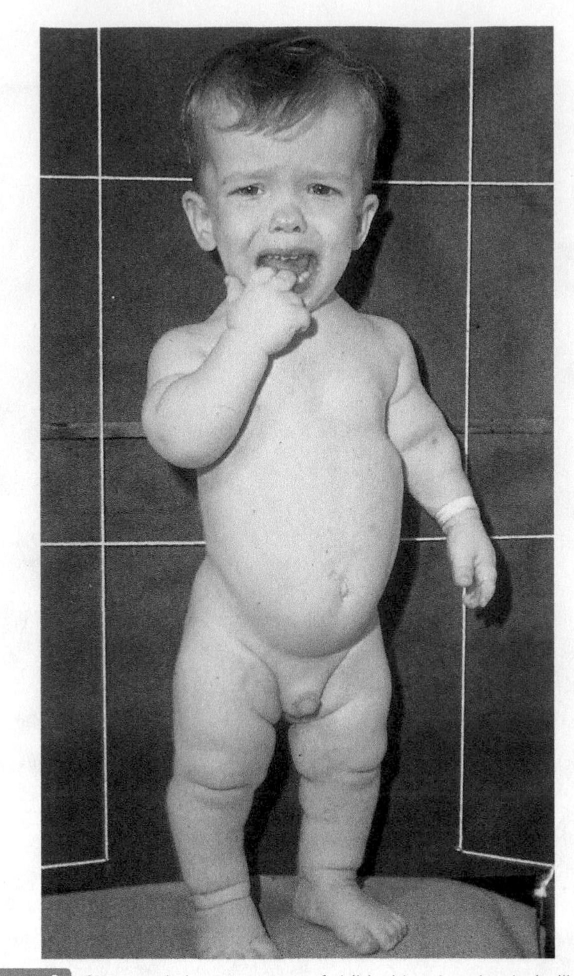

Figure 3 Characteristic appearance of child with achondroplasia, illustrating the relatively large head and disproportionate shortening of the extremities.

Congenital Clubfoot (Talipes)

Clubfoot is a relatively common congenital abnormality, having an incidence of about 1 in 1000 infants. The malformation is characterized by an abnormal position of the foot that prevents normal weight-bearing, and the affected individual tends to walk on the ankle rather than on the sole of the foot (*talus* = ankle + *pes* = foot). Figure 5 illustrates the most common type of clubfoot deformity called *talipes equinovarus*, in which the foot is turned inward at the ankle (varus position) and fixed in tiptoe (equinus) position. Often the malposition can be corrected by application of casts or splints. Surgical correction may be required if more conservative treatment is not successful.

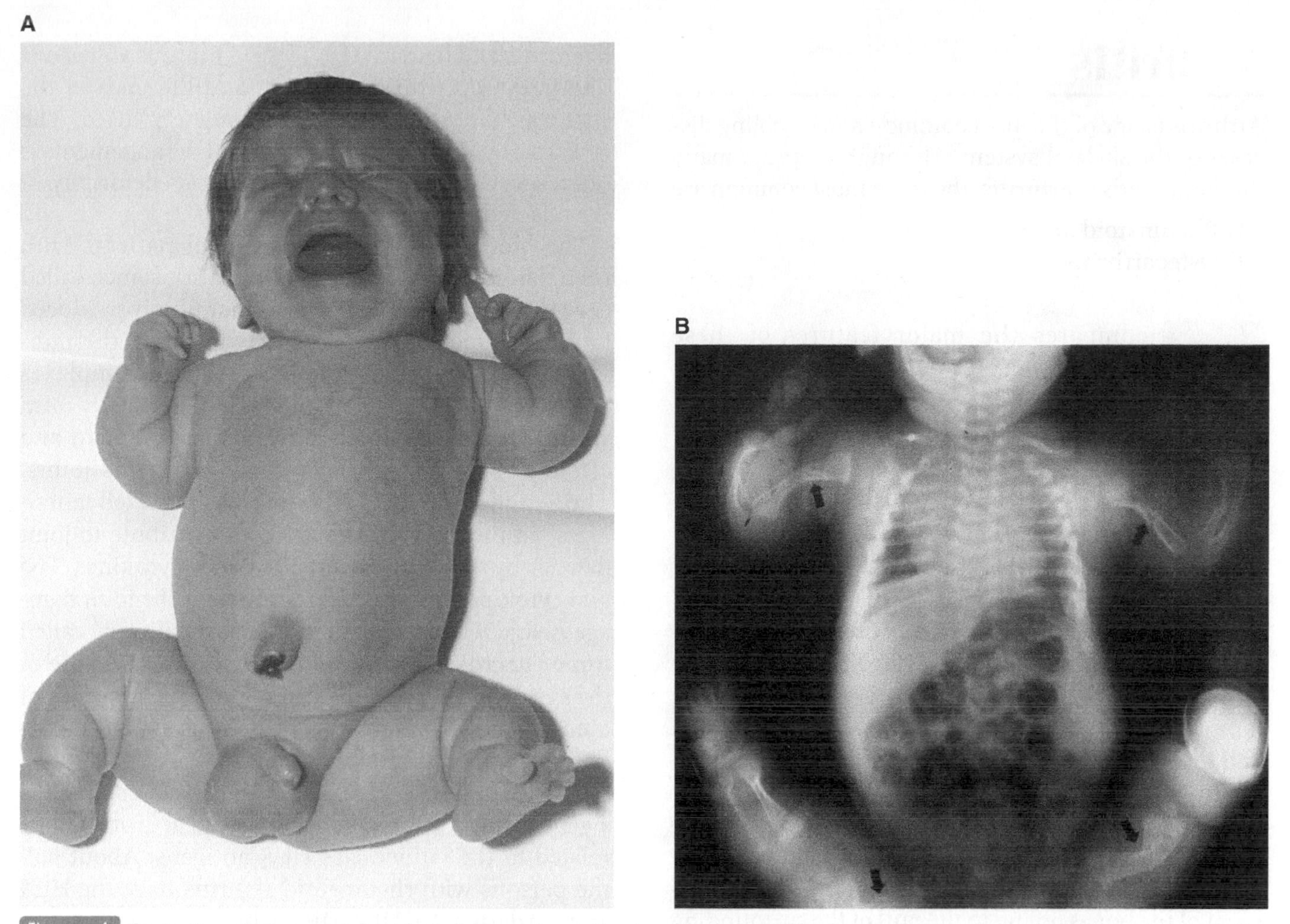

Figure 4 Severe form of osteogenesis imperfecta. **A,** Shortening and bowing of the limbs resulting from multiple intrauterine fractures that have healed in poor alignment. **B,** X-ray film showing multiple fractures of ribs and limb bones, some showing poor alignment and evidence of healing. *Arrows* indicate the location of four fractures.

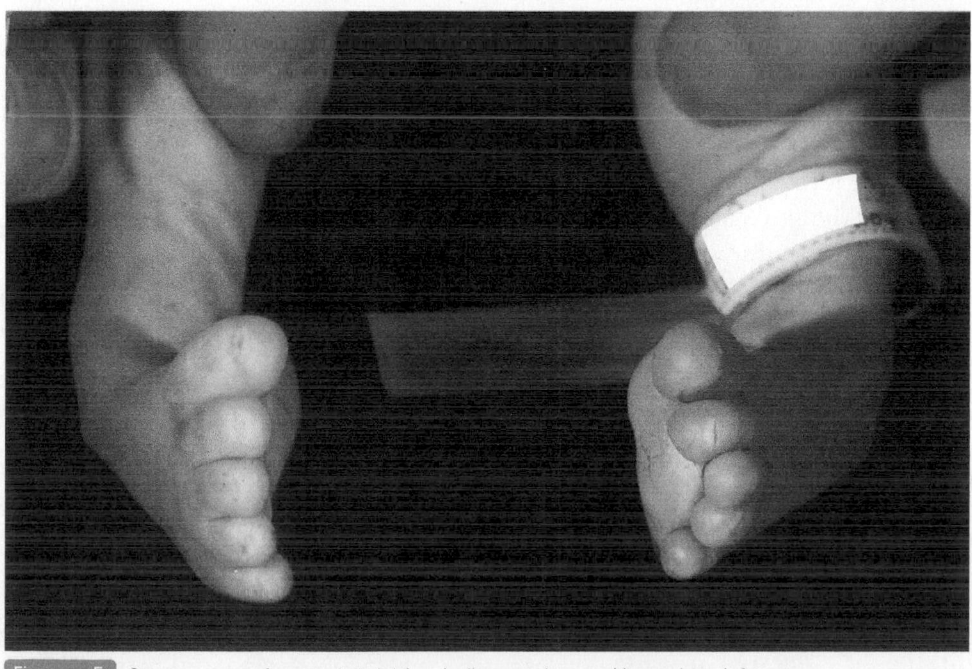

Figure 5 Common type of congenital clubfoot (*talipes equinovarus*) in newborn infant.

Arthritis

Arthritis is one of the most common and disabling diseases of the skeletal system. Although there are many different kinds of arthritis, the three most common are

1. Rheumatoid arthritis
2. Osteoarthritis
3. Gout

Table 1 compares the major features of these conditions.

Rheumatoid Arthritis

Rheumatoid arthritis is a systemic disease affecting the connective tissues throughout the body, but the most pronounced clinical manifestations are in the joints. Clinically, the disease is seen as a chronic, disabling, and often deforming arthritis affecting several joints. Rheumatoid arthritis is encountered most frequently in young and middle-aged women; it usually affects the small joints of the hands and feet. In the joints, the arthritis produces a chronic inflammation and thickening of the synovial membrane. The inflammatory tissue extends over the surface of the articular cartilage, destroying the cartilage (Figure 6). The severe damage to the articular surfaces makes the joint unstable; this in turn leads to deviation or displacement of the bones owing to the pull of the surrounding ligaments and tendons (Figure 7). Fibrous adhesions often develop within the joint, and the ends of the adjacent bones may become completely fused. The end result of these various structural derangements is often severe disability and conspicuous deformity of the affected joints (Figure 8).

The blood and synovial tissues of patients with rheumatoid arthritis often contain a substance called *rheumatoid factor*, which is an autoantibody produced by B lymphocytes that is directed against the individual's own gamma globulin. Immune complexes composed of gamma globulin and autoantibody form within the joints, which activates complement and attracts inflammatory cells that damage the joints. The lymphocytes and macrophages (activated monocytes) in the synovial tissues also contribute to joint damage by secreting various injurious cytokines. The two cytokines responsible for much of the joint damage characteristic of rheumatoid arthritis are called **tumor necrosis factor** and **interleukin-1**. Because of the systemic nature of the disease and the presence of autoantibodies, rheumatoid arthritis is usually classified as one of the autoimmune diseases.

As with some other autoimmune diseases, there is a genetic susceptibility to rheumatoid arthritis that is related to the individual's HLA antigens. About half the persons with rheumatoid arthritis have the HLA antigen designated HLA-DR4, which is present in only

Table 1 Comparison of Major Features of Common Types of Arthritis

	Rheumatoid Arthritis	Osteoarthritis	Gout
Age and sex of usual patient	Young and middle-aged, female	Adult, older persons, both sexes	Middle-aged, male
Major characteristic	Systemic disease with major effects in joints; causes chronic synovitis	"Wear-and-tear" degeneration of articular cartilage	Disturbance of purine metabolism; acute episodes caused by crystals of uric acid in joints
Secondary effects of disease	Ingrowth of inflammatory tissue over cartilage destroys cartilage, leads to destruction of joint space; deformities common	Overgrowth of bone; thickening of periarticular soft tissues	Deposits of uric acid in joints with damage to joints (gouty arthritis); soft tissue tophi
Joints usually affected	Small joints of hands and feet	Major weight-bearing joints	Small joints; joint at base of great toe often affected
Special features	Autoantibody against gamma globulin (rheumatoid factor)	No systemic symptoms or biochemical abnormalities	High blood level of uri

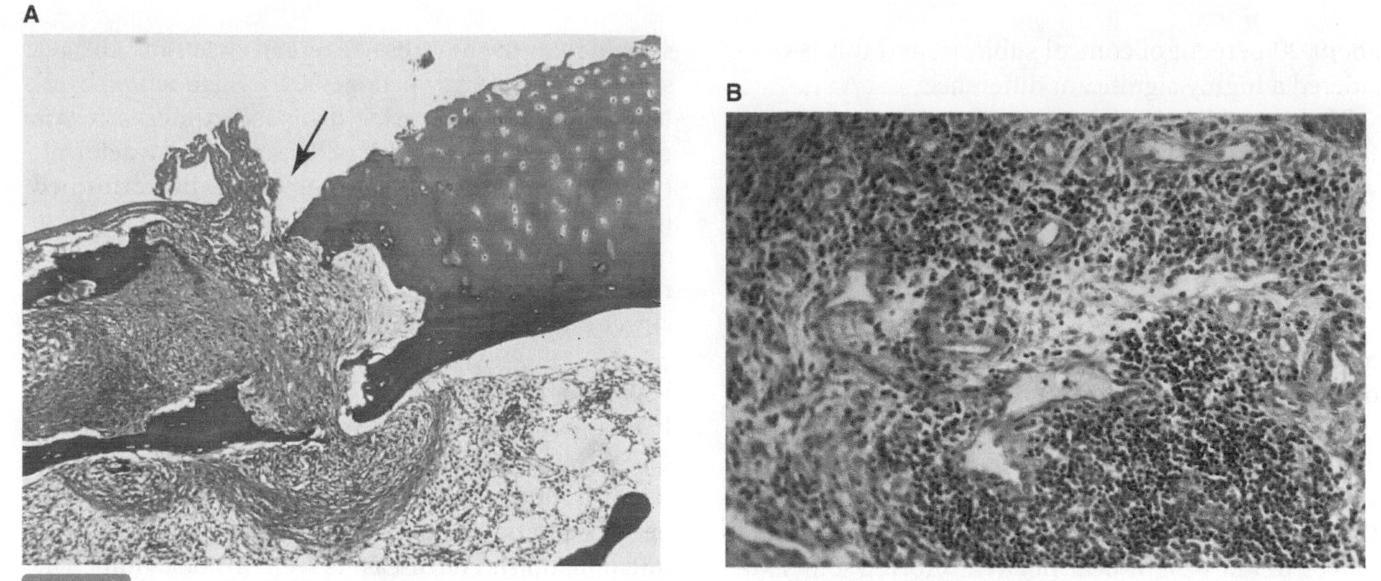

Figure 6 Rheumatoid arthritis. **A**, Low-magnification photomicrograph illustrating destruction of articular cartilage by inflammatory reaction (*arrow*) extending from synovial surface (original magnification × 25). **B**, Photomicrograph of chronic inflammatory reaction in synovium (original magnification × 100).

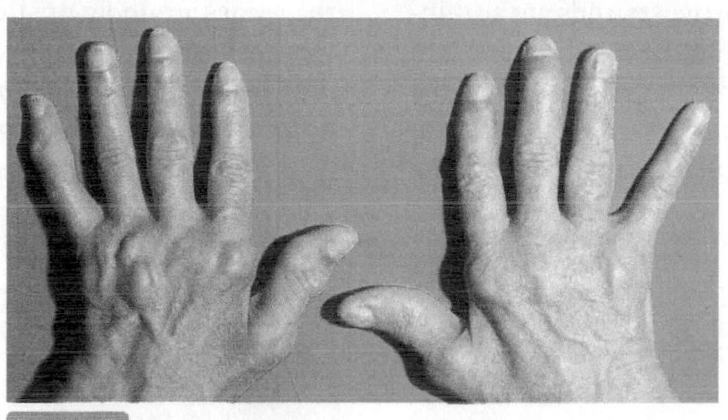

Figure 7 Rheumatoid arthritis. Early manifestations, illustrating swelling of knuckle joints (metacarpophalangeal joints) as a result of inflammation.

rheumatoid arthritis (rōōm′uh-toyd) A systemic disease primarily affecting the synovium with major manifestations in the small joints.

tumor necrosis factor A cytokine that can destroy foreign or abnormal cells.

interleukin-1 (in-ter-loo′-kin) A cvytokine that promotes lymphocyte proliferation and maturation and also produces mediators of inflammation that causes inflammation, which may lead to tissue damage.

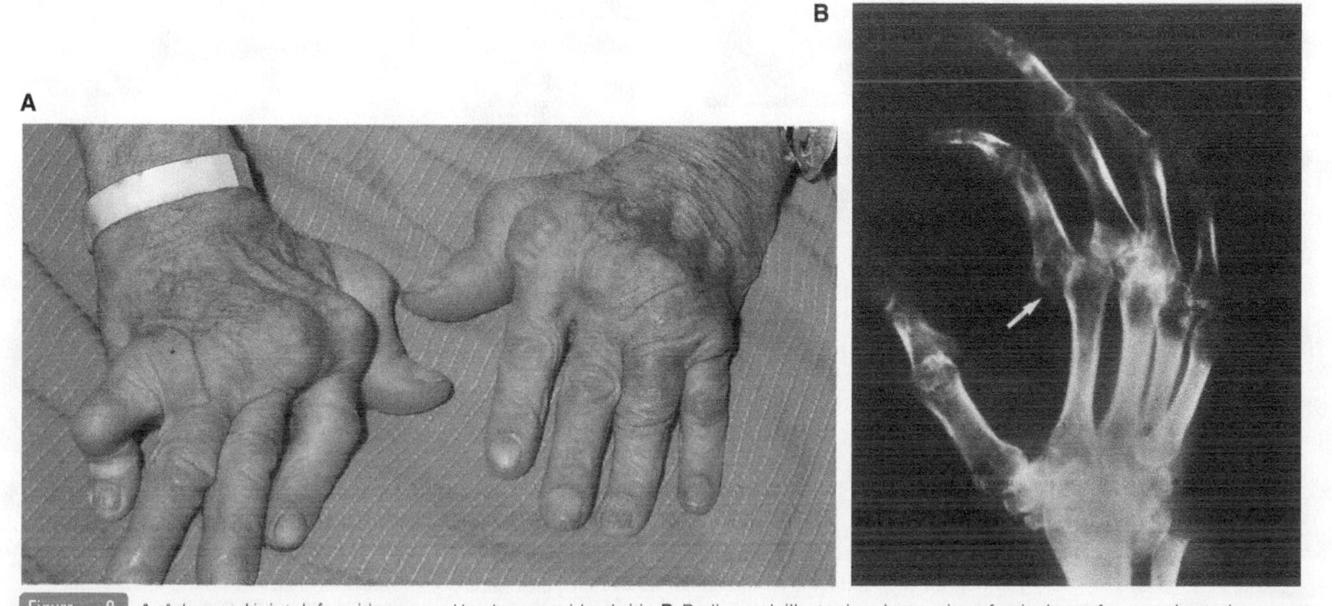

Figure 8 **A**, Advanced joint deformities caused by rheumatoid arthritis. **B**, Radiograph illustrating destruction of articular surfaces and anterior dislocation of base of index finger (*arrow*) as a result of joint instability.

about 20 percent of control subjects, and this is considered a highly significant difference.

Rheumatoid arthritis tends to fluctuate in severity. Periods in which the disease is active may alternate with periods in which it is inactive. Although there is no cure for rheumatoid arthritis, a number of measures can be used to control the disease and minimize its attending disability and deformity.

The primary objectives of treatment are reduction of joint inflammation and pain, maximal preservation of joint function, and prevention of joint deformity if possible. Treatment consists of rest periods for several hours every day while the disease is active, use of splints to support inflamed joints and reduce deformities caused by muscle spasm, and use of crutches and braces to aid weight-bearing. The affected joints are exercised gently in order to preserve joint mobility and muscle strength. Anti-inflammatory drugs such as aspirin are prescribed to reduce inflammation within the joints. In selected cases, corticosteroids are administered orally or injected into the affected joints. Often other measures are used to slow the progression of the disease, which are grouped under the general term of *disease-modifying anti-rheumatic drugs*. Many take several weeks or months to exert an effect, and all have some toxicity. Many patients are treated with a cytotoxic immunosuppressive drug called methotrexate combined with other drugs. If severe joint deformities develop, surgical procedures can be performed to improve joint function. These measures include excision of thickened inflamed synovium, surgical correction of joint dislocations, or even complete reconstruction of damaged joints.

Osteoarthritis

In contrast to rheumatoid arthritis, which is a systemic disease, **osteoarthritis** is a result of "wear-and-tear" degeneration of one or more of the major weight-bearing joints (*osteo* = bone + *arthro* = joint + *itis* = inflammation). The disease is seen in older adults. The primary change in osteoarthritis is degeneration of the articular cartilage, leading to roughening of the articular surfaces of the bones (Figure 9). As a consequence, the bones grate against one another when the joint moves, instead of gliding smoothly. Degeneration of the cartilage sometimes leaves large areas of underlying bone exposed. Secondary overgrowth of bone frequently occurs in response to the trauma of

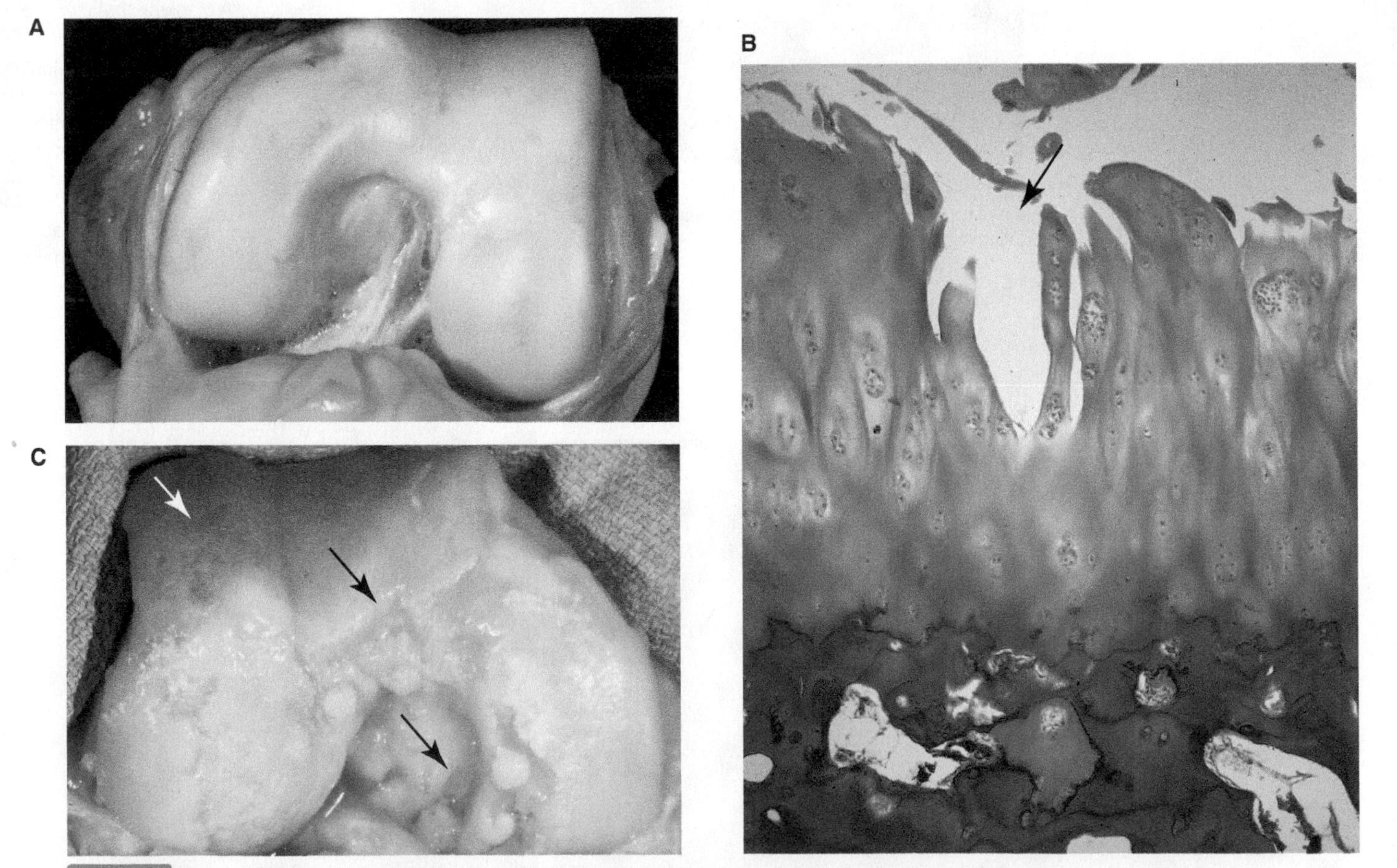

Figure 9 A, Knee joint, illustrating smooth articular surface of femoral condyles. B, Early histologic changes of osteoarthritis, illustrating splitting and fragmentation of articular cartilage (*arrow*) (original magnification × 160). Compare with normal articular cartilage in Figure 2A. C, Advanced osteoarthritis, illustrating loss of articular cartilage (*left arrow*) and nodular overgrowth of bone (*right arrows*).

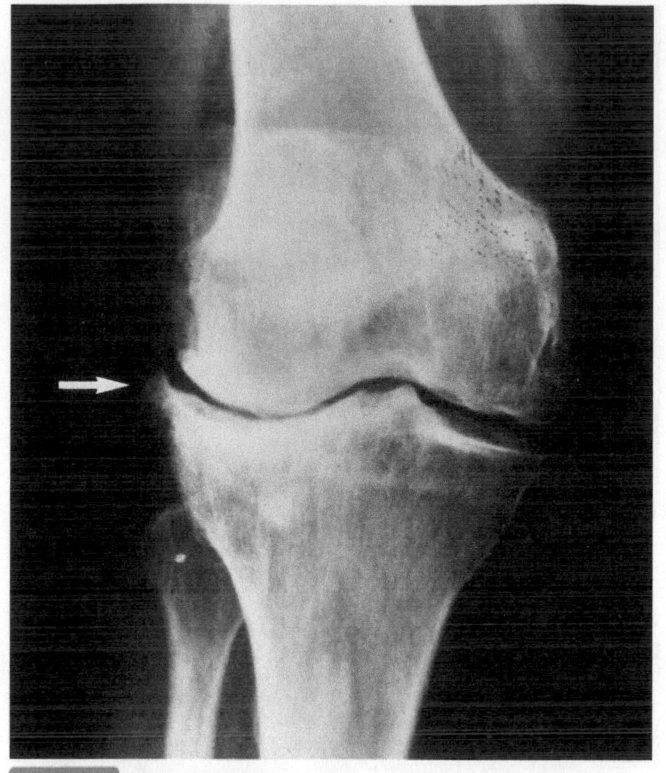

Figure 10 Osteoarthritis. Radiograph illustrates increased bone density of femoral condyle (*left side* of photograph) and adjacent tibia, with overgrowth of bone at margin of tibia (*arrow*).

weight-bearing (Figure 10), and some thickening of the synovium and adjacent soft tissues is also common.

Clinically, persons with osteoarthritis experience stiffness, creaking, and some pain on motion of the joints, but disability is usually not severe, and the joints are not destroyed. However, occasional patients may experience considerable pain and disability from advanced arthritis affecting one or both hip joints. In such cases, it is possible to remove the affected femoral head and articular surface of the hip bone surgically and to replace them with an artificial hip joint. Similar types of joint replacement procedures have been performed on the knee joint and some other joints as well. Joint replacement operations can provide excellent pain relief and greatly improved joint function in many patients.

Gout

Gout is a clinical syndrome associated with an elevated level of uric acid in the blood and body fluids (hyperuricemia), leading to precipitation of uric acid as sodium urate crystals in joints and other tissues. In most patients, the condition is caused by a metabolic disorder of purine metabolism, which leads to an overproduction of uric acid, an inadequate excretion of uric acid, or a combination of both. This condition is called **primary gout** to distinguish it from the much less common **secondary gout** in which the elevated uric acid is secondary to some other disease or condition.

Primary Gout Purines are double-ring nitrogen compounds that are used to form the nucleotides adenine and guanine. Along with the pyrimidine nucleotides, they make up the large DNA molecules within the nuclei of our cells. Although our body can produce purines from nonpurine precursor substances, most of the purines that we use to make nucleoproteins for new cells are salvaged (recycled) from our own worn-out cells when the cells are broken down. The purines that are not salvaged and recycled are converted into the end-product uric acid, which is excreted in the urine. Because uric acid is not very soluble in body fluids, any significant elevation may lead to precipitation of the uric acid in joints and other tissues.

Clinically, the person afflicted with gout experiences periodic episodes of extremely painful acute arthritis usually involving initially only a single joint, often the joint at the base of the great toe (Figure 11A). The acute episodes are caused by crystallization of uric acid within the joint, which incites an intense inflammatory reaction. Gradually the symptoms of an acute attack subside, and joint function returns to normal until the next attack. If the disease is not treated, however, the attacks last longer, occur more frequently, and may involve several joints. Eventually, lumpy masses called gouty tophi are deposited in the soft tissues around the joints (Figure 11B) and in other locations. The tophi consist of large masses of urate surrounded by macrophages, multinucleated giant cells, and fibrous tissue. When viewed under polarized light, the needle-like urate crystals have a characteristic appearance diagnostic of gout (Figure 12). In untreated patients, masses of urate crystals deposited in and around the articular surfaces of the joints damage the joint surfaces and adjacent bone; this is called *gouty arthritis* (Figure 13).

In many persons with gout, the disease also targets the kidneys and urinary tract. Many develop uric acid kidney stones. The uric acid also may precipitate from the tubular filtrate within the kidney tubules, which blocks the tubules, damages the

osteoarthritis (ä′stē-ō) A "wear and tear" degeneration of the major weight-bearing joints.

gout A disorder of nucleoprotein metabolism characterized by elevated uric acid and deposition of uric acid in and around joints.

primary gout A metabolic disease caused by overproduction of uric acid, reduced excretion of uric acid, or a combination of both factors. Clinical manifestations are related to precipitation of uric acid in joints, kidneys, and other sites.

secondary gout Elevated uric acid and clinical manifestations of gout not caused by the metabolic disease, primary gout, but instead caused by some other disease that raises the blood uric acid excessively, such as kidney failure or excessive breakdown of white blood cells in patients with leukemia.

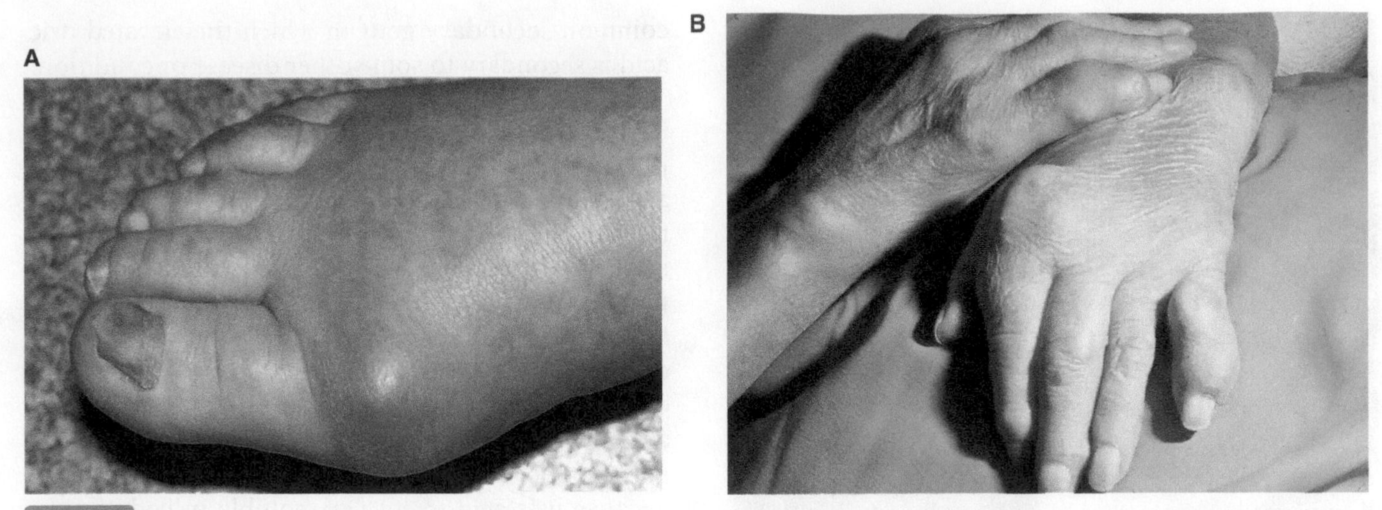

Figure 11 A, Acute gout affecting right great toe (© Dr. Allan Harris/Phototake). B, Deformities of hands caused by accumulation of uric acid crystals (tophi) in and around finger joints.

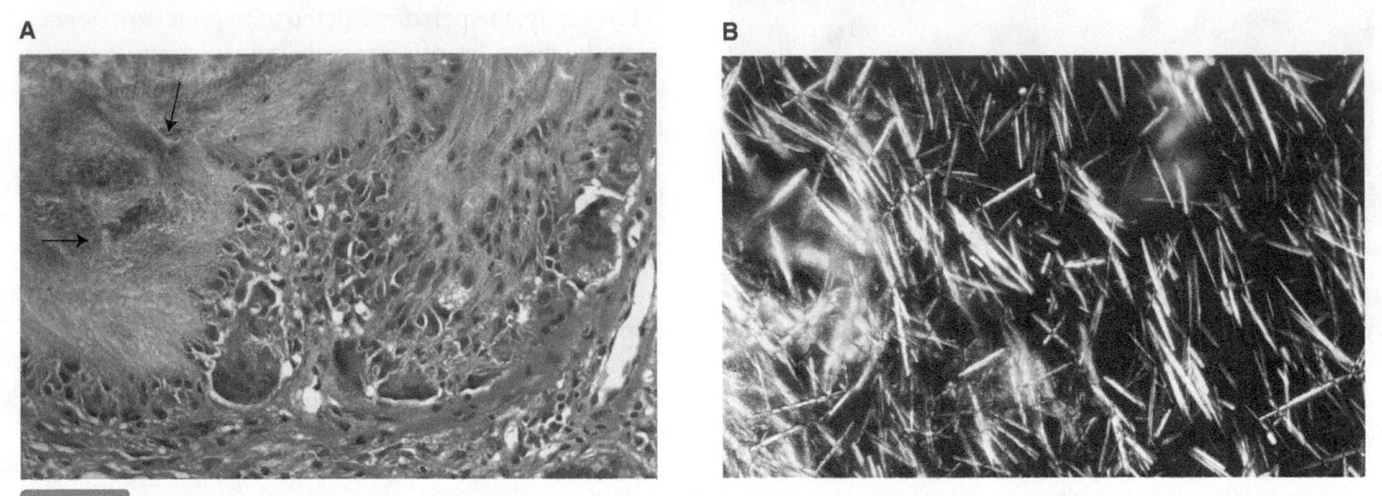

Figure 12 A, Margin of tophus illustrating mass of urate crystals (*arrows*) and adjacent zone of macrophages, multinucleated giant cells, and fibrous tissue formed in response to crystal deposits (original magnification × 250). B, Characteristic histologic appearance of needlelike sodium urate crystals from tophus viewed under polarized light (original magnification × 400).

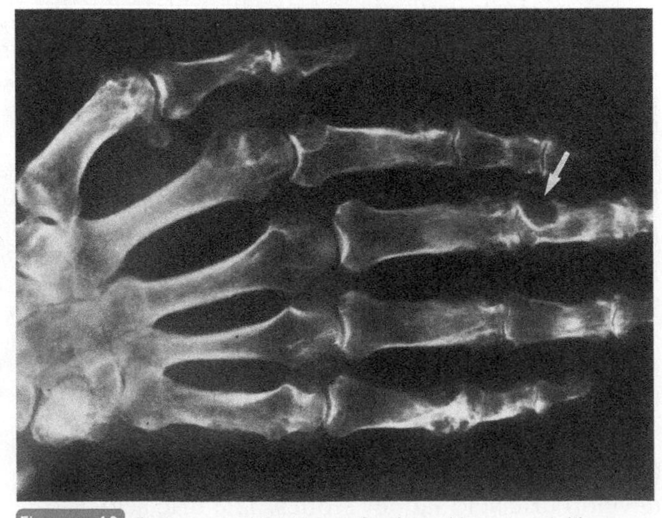

Figure 13 Radiograph of right hand of patient with gouty arthritis illustrating area of bone destruction (*arrow*) caused by masses of uric acid crystals.

kidneys, and impairs renal function. This condition is called *urate nephropathy*.

Gout is treated by administering drugs that reduce the concentration of uric acid in the blood by interfering with the formation of uric acid within the body, or by promoting the excretion of uric acid by the kidneys.

Secondary Gout Other conditions may also raise blood uric acid, caused either by inadequate excretion of uric acid or excessive breakdown of nucleoprotein. Sometimes the uric acid level may be so high that the uric acid precipitates from the blood and produces the same manifestations as gout caused by the metabolic disorder of purine metabolism. This condition is often called *secondary gout* because the elevated uric acid is secondary to some other disease, either a kidney-related problem in which uric acid excretion is impaired or a blood disease characterized by a marked overproduction of white blood cells. For example, patients with kidney failure may have high blood uric acid because the diseased kidneys are unable to excrete the uric acid efficiently, and some diuretics also may impair renal uric acid excretion. Hyperuricemia may be a problem in patients with leukemia who have a greatly increased number of white blood cells, especially after treatment with drugs that destroy the leukemic cells and release large amounts of nucleoprotein from the disrupted cells. The breakdown of the nucleoprotein yields a large amount of uric acid derived from the purine-containing nucleotides in the nucleoprotein. In these conditions, there is no underlying metabolic defect of purine metabolism.

Fracture

A **fracture** is a break in bone. In a *simple fracture*, the bone is broken into only two pieces. The term *comminuted fracture* is used when the bone is shattered into several pieces. A *compound fracture* is one in which the overlying skin has been broken. A compound fracture is more serious than the other types because of the possibility that bacteria may invade the fracture site and cause secondary infection of bone (*osteomyelitis*).

After a fracture, the ends of the broken bone may remain aligned, or they may be displaced out of position. The term *reduction of a fracture* refers to realigning the ends of the broken bone so that the bone will heal in its normal anatomic position. Sometimes a bone may become so weakened by disease such as metastatic tumor that it breaks after minimal stress (for example, coughing or sneezing). A fracture of this type through a diseased area in bone is called a *pathologic fracture*.

Osteomyelitis

Osteomyelitis is an infection of bone and adjacent marrow cavity (*osteo* = bone + *myelos* = marrow + *itis* = inflammation) that is usually the result of staphylococci or various gram-negative bacteria. The infecting organisms gain access to bone in two ways:

1. They may be transported to bone from a distant site by way of the bloodstream, which is called *hematogenous osteomyelitis*.
2. Bacteria may be implanted directly in the bone from various causes.

Hematogenous Osteomyelitis

Hematogenous osteomyelitis is more common in children than in adults. The bacteria are usually carried to the bone from a skin infection, such as a boil, from a kidney infection, or from some other distant site. In children, the organisms tend to lodge in the growing end of the bone on the diaphyseal (shaft) side of the epiphyseal plate, where they proliferate and incite an acute inflammation. Local injury to bone near its very vascular growing end seems to favor localization of bacteria in the bone, probably because a small hemorrhage forms secondary to the injury, and the collection of blood provides conditions favorable for the growth of bacteria.

fracture (frak-tūr) A broken bone.

Hematogenous osteomyelitis sometimes occurs in adults. Although hematogenous osteomyelitis may affect any bone, the infection frequently localizes in the vertebral bodies rather than in the long bones. Probably the stresses and trauma associated with weight-bearing predispose to localization in the spine.

Osteomyelitis as a Result of Direct Implantation of Bacteria

Various conditions may expose bone to direct infection, including compound fractures, gunshot wounds, or other severe injuries affecting bone. Various surgical procedures performed on bone, such as open reduction and internal fixation of fractures or total joint replacement, may also be complicated by osteomyelitis. Chronic ulcers of the feet, which sometimes develop in diabetic patients, may expose the small bones of the feet to chronic infection.

Clinical Manifestations and Treatment

Usually, osteomyelitis is manifested as an acute febrile illness associated with localized pain, tenderness, and swelling over the affected bone.

Osteomyelitis is treated by a prolonged course of antibiotic therapy. In some patients, the infection may become chronic and may recur periodically. Chronic osteomyelitis is much more difficult to treat. In addition to intensive antibiotic treatment, surgical procedures may be required to remove infected degenerated bone and drain collections of pus in the bone.

Pathogenic fungi, tubercle bacilli, and various unusual opportunistic organisms may at times cause osteomyelitis, especially in immunocompromised adults. The infections are treated by appropriate antibiotics supplemented by various surgical procedures, if needed.

Tumors of Bone

Bone is often affected by metastatic tumors. Carcinoma of breast or prostate, as well as many other tumors, frequently metastasize to bone (Figure 14). Occasionally, the skeletal system may be so heavily infiltrated

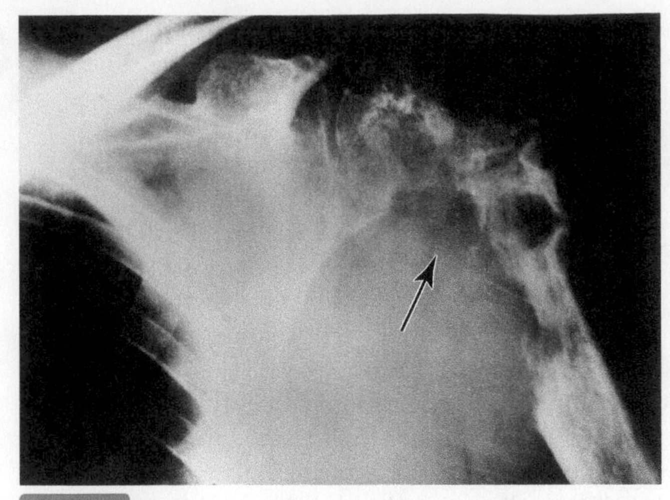

Figure 14 Metastatic carcinoma in the humerus. The primary tumor was in the kidney. Bone destruction by metastatic carcinoma is indicated by marked irregularity in the contour of the head and neck of the humerus (*arrow*).

by tumor that hematopoietic cells within the marrow are crowded out, leading to anemia, leukopenia, and thrombocytopenia. Nodular deposits of neoplastic plasma cells are frequently present throughout the skeletal system in multiple myeloma. Benign cysts and benign tumors of bone are encountered occasionally, but primary malignant tumors of bone are unusual. A malignant tumor of cartilage is called a *chondrosarcoma*. One arising from bone-forming cells is called an *osteosarcoma*.

Osteoporosis

Osteoporosis, literally meaning "porous bones," is a generalized thinning and demineralization of the entire skeletal system. Most cases are found in postmenopausal women, beginning in their 50s, and a significant degree of osteoporosis is said to be present in approximately one-fourth of all women in their 60s. Osteoporosis develops whenever bone resorption exceeds bone production. The incidence is high in postmenopausal women because the loss of ovarian function results in estrogen deficiency. Estrogen inhibits bone resorption, and loss of estrogen accelerates the rate of bone resorption, which results in slowly progressive thinning of the bones. Osteoporosis also develops in older men, but it occurs at a much later age and is usually less severe than in women.

The osteoporotic bones are quite fragile and susceptible to fracture. Fractures of vertebral bodies are frequent, either from the stress of weight-bearing or after minor exertion (Figure 15). Such fractures produce back pain and tenderness and are often characterized by collapse of the anterior portions of the vertebral bodies (*compression fractures*). Collapse of vertebral bodies may compress the spinal nerve roots passing through the intervertebral foramina, causing pain to radiate along the course of the compressed nerve.

Maximum bone density is attained in young adults, and then it slowly but steadily declines as they get

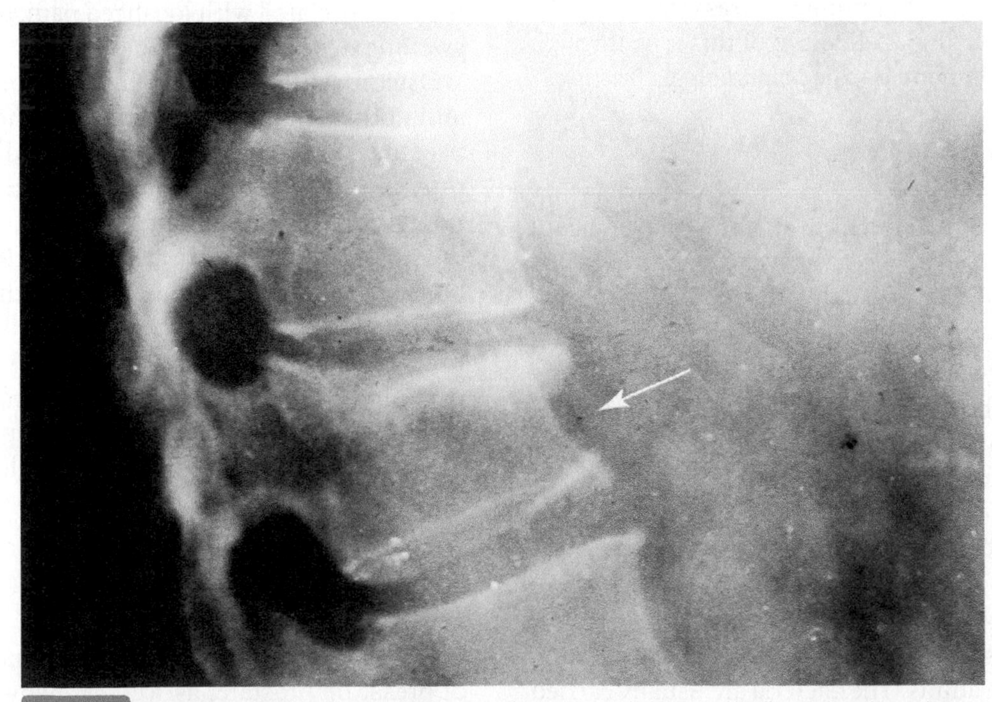

Figure 15 Osteoporosis with a compression fracture of vertebral body. Vertebral bodies are less dense than normal, and the front of one vertebral body has collapsed (*arrow*). Compare the compression fracture in this vertebral body with the vertebra above in which the anterior and posterior surfaces are the same height.

older. The greater the bone density one has as a young adult, the longer it will take before there is enough bone loss to increase the risk of fractures. To use an analogy, bone density is like a savings account at a bank where money is deposited for retirement. The more money one has accumulated, the longer it takes before the savings account is depleted.

Bone loss can be retarded by regular weight-bearing exercises, which help maintain bone density, by a high-calcium diet and calcium supplements if necessary to ensure an adequate calcium intake, and by an adequate intake of vitamin D, which is required to promote calcium absorption from the intestine and incorporation into bone. Estrogens are no longer recommended to retard bone loss in postmenopausal women because of the long-term risks associated with estrogen use.

Once marked osteoporosis has developed and fractures occur, it is difficult to restore bone density. A number of drugs are available that may be helpful. Each has advantages and disadvantages.

Significant loss of bone density may also occur in women athletes who engage in prolonged, intense physical activity, such as runners and gymnasts. The high level of physical activity triggers the hypothalamus and pituitary gland to increase adrenal corticosteroid output as an adaptation to the exercise-induced stress. This event, however, is also associated with a fall in the pituitary gonadotropic hormones that stimulate ovarian function. The ovaries, no longer adequately stimulated by pituitary gonadotropins, fail to produce adequate estrogen, which leads to cessation of menses called *exercise-induced amenorrhea*. In addition, the estrogen-deficient athlete is also at risk of the same type of estrogen-deficiency osteoporosis that develops in postmenopausal women and is subject to the same osteoporosis-related complications.

Osteoporosis related to exercise-induced amenorrhea can be prevented by reducing the level of physical activity enough to reestablish normal menstrual cycles. Alternatively, the athlete who elects to continue the same level of exercise can reduce her risk of osteoporosis by taking supplementary estrogen and progesterone hormones to replace the missing ovarian hormones and by taking calcium supplements.

X-ray and radioisotope methods are now available that make a quantitative assessment of a patient's bone density and compare the results with normal ranges established for persons of the same age and sex. Those patients whose bones are losing mineral content to a greater extent or more rapidly than normal are at high risk of fractures and other complications related to osteoporosis. They should be treated vigorously in an attempt to retard further bone demineralization.

Structure and Function of the Spine

The vertebral column forms the central axis of the body. It consists of a series of vertebrae joined by intervertebral disks and fibrous ligaments. The vertebral column has four curves. The *cervical* and *lumbar curves* arch forward. Those in the thoracic and sacral regions bend in the opposite direction (Figure 16A).

A typical vertebra has a large cylindrical *body* and a *bony arch* that encloses the spinal canal and protects the spinal cord. The parts of the arch that extend posteriorly from the body are called the *pedicles*, and the parts that roof the spinal canal are called the *laminae* (singular, *lamina*). A single midline spinous process projects posteriorly from the bony arch, and paired *transverse processes* extend laterally (Figure 16B).

When the vertebrae are viewed from the side, the superior and inferior margins of the vertebral pedicles appear concave. Small disklike articular surfaces called *articular processes* are present on the upper and lower surfaces of each vertebral arch, and the vertebral bodies articulate with each other by means of small *synovial joints*. The spaces between the concave surfaces of the pedicles of adjacent vertebrae form oval openings

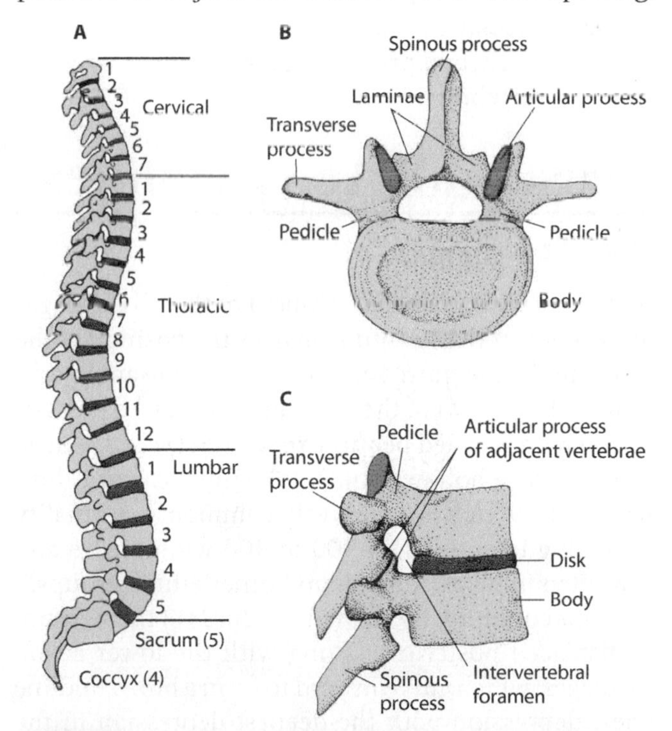

Figure 16 A, Side view of vertebral column illustrating normal curves. Vertebrae are numbered. B, Structure of typical vertebra viewed from above. The vertebral arch extends posteriorly from the vertebral body. The spinous process projects posteriorly from the arch, and the transverse processes project laterally. The articular processes of adjacent vertebrae articulate with each other by means of small synovial joints. C, Side view of two vertebrae, illustrating the intervertebral disk, articular processes, and intervertebral foramen.

called *intervertebral foramina* (singular, *foramen*), through which the spinal nerves leave the spinal canal (Figure 16C).

intervertebral disk A fibrocartilaginous joint between adjacent vertebral bodies.

annulus fibrosus (an´ū-lus) The dense peripheral ring of fibrocartilage making up the intervertebral disk.

nucleus pulposus (nū´klē-us) The soft elastic center of the intervertebral disk.

scoliosis (sko-lee-oh´-sis) An abnormal lateral curvature of the spine.

idiopathic scoliosis (id´-ē-opath´-ik skō-lē-ō´-sis) Lateral curvature of the spine. Idiopathic means cause of condition is unknown.

The **intervertebral disks**, interposed between adjacent vertebral bodies, consist of a peripheral fibrous ring, the annulus fibrosus, and a soft central *nucleus pulposus*. The **annulus fibrosus** ("fibrous ring") is structured as a ring of interlacing connective-tissue bundles firmly adherent to adjacent vertebral bodies. Longitudinal bands of connective tissue called the *anterior* and *posterior longitudinal ligaments* run the entire length of the vertebral column to reinforce the annulus. The **nucleus pulposus** ("pulpy nucleus") consists of a gelatinous material containing a carbohydrate substance called a mucopolysaccharide that contains about 80 percent water. Because of its very high water content, it is relatively incompressible.

The intervertebral disks function somewhat like shock absorbers. Pressure applied to the disks is distributed evenly around the annulus by the soft nucleus pulposus, absorbing the forces of compression to some extent, and preventing direct impact between adjacent vertebral bodies.

Chest Wall Abnormalities

Pectus Excavatum

Abnormal growth and attachment of the rib cartilages to the body of the sternum changes the position of the sternum. In the most common and important condition the lower part of the sternum is displaced posteriorly, which is called **pectus excavatum** (*pectus* = chest + *excavatum* = hollowed out), sometimes called a "funnel chest," which is a relatively common abnormality occurring in about 1 in 300 to 400 white males and less often in white females and other ethnic groups.

In this condition the lower two-thirds of the sternum is displaced posteriorly along with the lower costal cartilages, which curve inward to form a broad midline chest depression with the deepest depression in the lowest part of the sternum. The posterior displacement of the sternum appears to be caused by excessive unbalanced growth of the lower costal cartilages 3 through 5, which push the sternum posteriorly. The abnormality usually becomes apparent soon after birth, progresses during childhood, and becomes even more pronounced during the rapid skeletal growth phase associated with adolescence, but does not progress after skeletal growth ceases. About 40 percent of affected persons also have a family member with pectus excavatum.

A relatively minor posterior sternal depression may not encroach to a signficant extent on the heart or the adjacent pleural cavities, but can be a psychological problem for a teenager concerned about his or her body image. However, a marked posterior sternal depression can compromise both caridac and pulmonary function. The reduced space available to the heart between the posterior surface of the sternum and the throacic spine compresses and displaces the heart laterally, which reduces cardiac output, especially during exercise when heart rate and cardiac output increase. In addition, the laterally displaced heart projects further into the left pleural cavity, leaving less space available for full expansion of the left lung during exercise; as a result, pulmonary ventilation becomes less efficient. The impaired exercise-related cardiopulmonary function leads to reduced exercise tolerance, which becomes more marked as the person ages. Only a severe sternal depression is treated surgically, which involves moving the sternum into a more normal position to enlarge the space available for the heart located in the mediastinum between the sternum and spine.

Marfan Syndrome: Connective Tissue Disease

The two important types of connective tissue are the widely distributed collagen fibers that provide strength but lack flexibility, and elastic tissue fibers that can stretch and return to their former shape when the stretching force cesases. Elastic fibers are abundant in blood vessels when their elasticity permits the aorta and its branches to stretch and recoil in response to the blood pumped into the vessels during ventricular systole. Elastic fibers are present in many other tissues along with collagen fibers, which perform various "stretchability" functions in the skin and subcutaneous tissues, as well as in the eyes where they attach the lens to the ciliary body in the correct position required for normal vision.

Connective tissue fibers are constructed from a precursor protein called *fibrillin*, and a mutation of the gene coding for fibrillin (*FBN1*) gives rise to a group of abnormalities grouped together as a relatively common disease called **Marfan syndrome**. Its incidence is about 1 in 5,000 persons and usually this condition is transmitted as a dominant trait. Less often the disease is not transmitted from a parent, but instead results from a new, spontaneous *FBN1* gene mutation in the affected person. When the mutation is transmitted from a parent its severity may differ among affected individuals in the same family. This gene mutation leads to excessive growth in height, excessively long, thin fingers and toes with excessive joint flexibility, and various chest wall abnomalities, usually pectus excavatum. The fibers that hold the lens in correct position behind the iris may not be able to maintain the lens in proper position, which leads to visual disturbances. However, the most serious complications of Marfan syndrome involve the cardiovascular system, which is caused by defective elastic fibers in the aorta. As a result, the aorta gradually dilates because the defective elastic fibers in the aortic wall are unable to maintain the normal shape of the aorta. Excessive dilation of the aorta may lead to a dissecting aneurysm of the aorta and its complications. If the excessive dilation occurs in the ascending aorta, the cusps of the aortic valve, which are attached to the dilated aorta, are unable to fit closely together in diastole to close the aortic value, which leads to aortic value insufficiency. Mitral valve function is also compromised because the mitral valve leaflets do not fit together as well in diastole as the aorta dilates. There is no specific non-surgical treatment for the disease, although some drugs may retard the rate of the aortic dilation and reduce the risk of a dissecting aneurysm. Surgical procedures are also available to treat the complications caused by dilation of the aorta and disturbed valve functions. Annual ultrasound examinations are recommended to monitor the progression of the aortic dilation, which may require eventual surgical repair in order to reduce the risk of a dissecting aneurysm or rupture of the aorta.

Since Marfan syndrome is associated with pectus excavatum, it has been suggested that they may be related connective tissue diseases. In one series of cases one-third of the group of patients treated for pectus excavatum were later considered to have Marfan syndrome.

Scoliosis

Scoliosis is an abnormal lateral curvature of the spine and is a common abnormality that is estimated to occur in about 4 percent of people. A small percentage of cases result from a congenital abnormality of a spinal vertebra that disturbs the normal vertical alignment of the spinal vertebrae, or results from a neurologic problem that disturbs the innervation of the muscles that maintain the spinal vertebrae in proper position. The vast majority of cases, however, occur during adolescence as the teenager is growing, and we don't know why this occurs. This condition is called **idiopathic scoliosis**. (The term *idiopathic* means that we don't know why this condition develops.) Scoliosis occurs much more frequently in adolescent girls than in boys.

The spinal curvatures lead to an asymmetry of the trunk so one shoulder is higher than the other, and the pelvis is tilted so that one iliac crest is higher than its counterpart on the opposite side. Some degree of rotation of the vertebrae accompanies the curvatures, which may lead to some asymmetry of the ribs that attach to the thoracic vertebrae (Figure 17A). Posterior protrusion of the ribs on one side of the thorax may cause a noticeable humplike deformity.

If scoliosis is identified, x-rays are taken to measure the extent of the curvature. A small curvature may not require treatment, but the adolescent needs to be checked periodically because some curves may get worse as the adolescent grows. Usually a curvature doesn't progress after the teenager stops growing, but a marked curvature may continue to get worse even after growth stops. Severe degrees of scoliosis may cause significant disability. A marked thoracic curvature greatly reduces the size of the thorax, which interferes with lung function (Figure 17B).

Treatment depends on the degree of curvature. Slight curves may not require

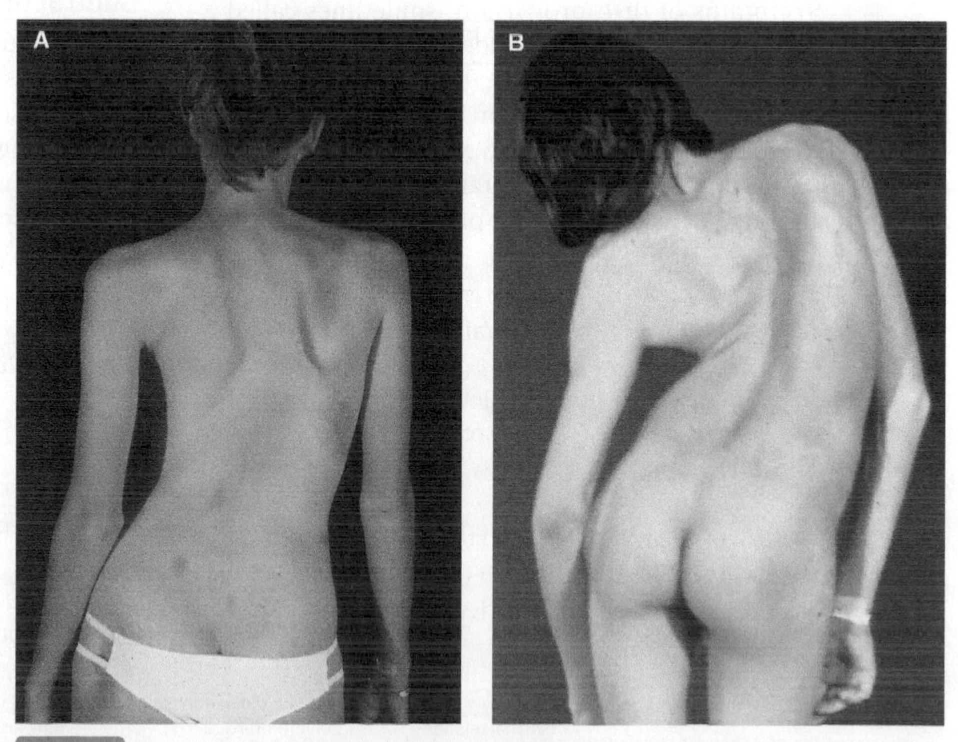

Figure 17 Scoliosis. **A**, Moderate scoliosis. **B**, Severe scoliosis that caused marked asymmetry of trunk and greatly reduced the size of the thoracic cavities, interfering with pulmonary function.

treatment but should be watched because the curve may get worse. A growing teenager with a curvature that is getting worse is treated by means of a spinal brace to help maintain the normal position of the spine and stop the progression of the curvature. A marked scoliosis may require surgical treatment, and various surgical procedures are used to stabilize the spine and correct the curvature.

Intervertebral Disk Disease

With age, the intervertebral disks undergo a progressive wear-and-tear degeneration of both the nucleus and the annulus. The nucleus becomes denser because its water content is reduced, and the annulus becomes weakened and thinned. When marked compression force is applied to the anterior part of the disk during flexion of the spine, the nucleus is forced posteriorly against the weakened annulus, and part of the nucleus may be forced into the spinal canal through a weak area or tear in the annulus (Figure 18). Generally, a disk protrusion occurs in the lumbosacral region because this is the part of the vertebral column where the disks are subject to the greatest mechanical compression during lifting. The disk usually protrudes in a posterolateral direction because the dense posterior longitudinal ligament reinforces the annulus in the midline, preventing a direct posterior protrusion.

Symptoms of disk protrusion, sometimes called a "slipped disk," consist of sudden onset of acute back pain after an episode of lifting. Frequently, the pain is also felt in the leg and thigh on the side of the protrusion. This occurs because the extruded disk material often impinges on lumbosacral nerve roots, causing pain to radiate along the course of the nerve compressed by the protruded nucleus pulposus. Treatment consists of bed rest and measures to minimize pain and disability, such as administration of aspirin or other pain-relieving medications, local application of heat, and use of muscle-relaxing drugs to relieve spasm of the back muscles that occurs after a disk protrusion and contributes to the disability. Protruded disk material may be resorbed, and the tear in the annulus may be repaired by fibrous tissue. Sometimes, however, surgical removal of the protruded disk material may be required. CT and MRI scans, noninvasive radiologic excaminations, can be used to identify a disk protrusion (Figure 19).

Structure and Function of Skeletal Muscle

Muscle cells are highly specialized contractile cells. Three different types of muscle are recognized: smooth muscle, skeletal muscle, and cardiac muscle. Smooth muscle is found in the walls of the gastrointestinal tract, biliary tract, urogenital system, respiratory tract, and blood vessels. Skeletal muscle is attached to the skeleton by tendons and ligaments; it functions in voluntary muscular activity. Cardiac muscle closely resembles skeletal muscle but has certain special features related to its function of producing rhythmic contractions of the heart. A discussion of skeletal muscle, the great bulk of muscle within the body, follows.

Contraction of Skeletal Muscle

Skeletal muscles are long, straplike fibers that measure as much as 30 centimeters in length. The cytoplasm (sarcoplasm) contains multiple nuclei located just beneath the cell membrane (sarcolemma). Filling the cytoplasm are long threadlike myofibrils composed of the contractile myofilaments actin and myosin. The

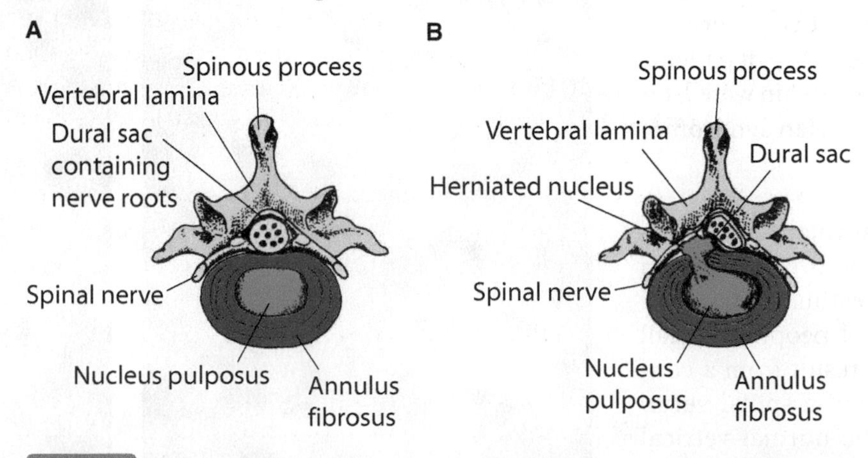

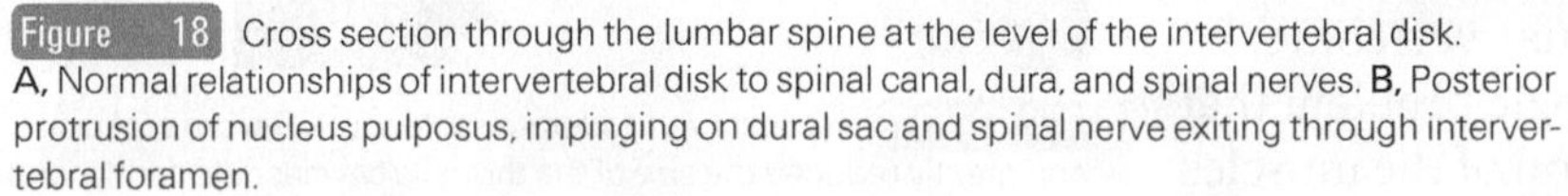
Figure 18 Cross section through the lumbar spine at the level of the intervertebral disk. **A**, Normal relationships of intervertebral disk to spinal canal, dura, and spinal nerves. **B**, Posterior protrusion of nucleus pulposus, impinging on dural sac and spinal nerve exiting through intervertebral foramen.

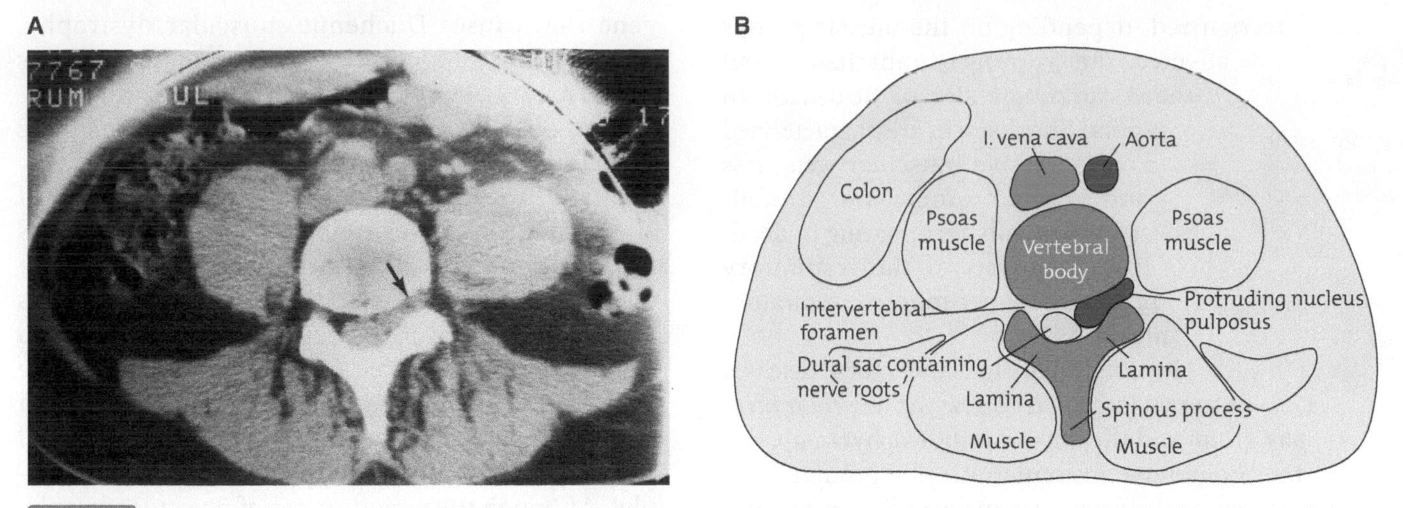

Figure 19 A, CT scan of lumbar region. Protruding nucleus pulposus (*arrow*) is located adjacent to dural sac and fills intervertebral foramen (*arrow*). Compare with appearance of normal intervertebral foramen on opposite side. B, Schematic of anatomic structures and lesion as demonstrated on CT scan.

cytoplasm also contains many energy-rich organic compounds, ions, and enzymes required for the metabolic activity of the muscle cell.

Muscle cells contract in response to motor nerve impulses conveyed to the muscle. The area of communication between the nerve endings and the muscle cell is called the *myoneural junction*. The actual stimulation of the muscle cell is the result of a chemical called **acetylcholine**, which is released from the nerve endings at the myoneural junction and interacts with acetylcholine receptors on the surface of the muscle fibers. The chemical mediator acetylcholine initiates the biochemical chain of events that causes the actin and myosin filaments to slide together, which leads to shortening of the muscle fiber. The duration of the chemical mediator is quite brief because this substance is rapidly broken down by the enzyme *cholinesterase*, which is present at the myoneural junction.

Factors Affecting Muscular Structure and Function

The normal structural and functional integrity of skeletal muscle depends on an intact nerve supply, normal transmission of impulses across the myoneural junction, and normal metabolic processes within the muscle cell.

Skeletal muscles that are not used or muscles deprived of their nerve supply undergo marked atrophy. Conversely, when additional work is required of the muscles, they undergo hypertrophy in response to the increased demands.

Diseases of skeletal muscle are uncommon. The principal disorders consist of inflammatory lesions, muscular atrophy, degeneration (dystrophy) of muscle, and disturbance of impulse conduction at the myoneural junction.

Inflammation of Muscle (Myositis)

Localized Myositis

Small areas of inflammation in skeletal muscle are encountered in many systemic diseases. Inflammation of muscle may also follow injury or muscular overexertion. The inflammation is secondary to necrosis and disruption of muscle cells and is associated with swelling and tenderness of the affected muscle. The inflammation gradually subsides as the muscle injury heals.

Generalized Myositis

Generalized inflammation of skeletal muscle (polymyositis) is an uncommon but serious systemic disease of unknown etiology, characterized by widespread degeneration and inflammation of skeletal muscle. One type of polymyositis, associated with swelling and inflammation of the skin, is called *dermatomyositis*. These disorders are often classified as autoimmune connective tissue (collagen) diseases because of the necrosis of connective tissue fibers in the affected muscles and because these diseases are presumed to have an immunologic basis.

acetylcholine
(as-et-il-kō'lēn) A chemical secreted by nerve endings that activates neurons or muscle cells.

Muscular Atrophy and Muscular Dystrophy

A group of relatively rare diseases is characterized by progressive atrophy or degeneration of skeletal muscle. Many are hereditary. Various clinical syndromes are

myasthenia gravis (mī-as-thē′nē-uh grä′vis) An autoimmune disease characterized by abnormal fatigability of muscle and caused by an autoantibody that damages the acetylcholine receptors at the myoneural junction.

recognized, depending on the muscle groups affected, the patterns of inheritance, and the rate of progression of the disease. In general, the diseases are characterized by progressive muscular weakness and gradually increasing disability, eventually terminating in death from paralysis of the respiratory muscles or superimposed respiratory infection.

It is customary to classify these diseases into two large categories: the *muscular atrophy group* and the *muscular dystrophy group.*

In the progressive muscular atrophy group of diseases, the muscular weakness and atrophy are secondary to progressive degeneration of motor nerve cells in the cerebral cortex, brain stem, and spinal cord. The clinical manifestations are related to the location of the degenerating nerve cells within the CNS and the rate at which the neuronal degeneration progresses.

In the muscular dystrophy group, the nerve supply to the muscles is unaffected. The basic disturbance is an abnormality in the muscle fibers that causes them to degenerate. The most common and severe type is called *Duchenne muscular dystrophy*, and a milder form of muscular dystrophy is called *Becker muscular dystrophy*. Both forms result from the mutation of a large gene on the X chromosome, and the disease is transmitted as an X-linked trait to male children of women who carry the defective gene. The normal gene codes for a muscle protein called *dystrophin*, which is located on the inner surface of the sarcolemma, where it plays a role in maintaining the structure and functions of the muscle fibers.

As a result of the gene mutation, dystrophin is absent in the muscle fibers of persons afflicted with Duchenne muscular dystrophy and is apparently responsible for the manifestations of the disease, which appear first during early childhood and progress rapidly, leading to death in late adolescence or early adulthood. The muscles primarily affected are those of the lower extremities, trunk, hips, and shoulder girdle. Often the extent of atrophy is masked because the muscles are infiltrated by fat and fibrous tissue as they atrophy. The fat infiltration may at times be so extreme that the affected muscles appear hypertrophied, leading to the paradox of profound muscular weakness in an individual whose muscles appear very well developed. The apparent hypertrophy is an illusion, which is why the term *pseudohypertrophic* is applied to this type of muscular dystrophy.

The less-severe Becker muscular dystrophy also is caused by a mutation of the same dystrophin-producing gene that causes Duchenne muscular dystrophy. Dystrophin is produced by the mutated gene but is either abnormal or produced in insufficient amounts. In both diseases, the muscle enzyme creatine kinase (CK) leaks from the abnormal muscle fibers, and very high enzyme levels can be detected in the blood of affected persons. (This is the same enzyme that leaks from heart muscle when the muscle is damaged.) The diagnosis of muscular dystrophy is made on the basis of the clinical features together with the very high CK blood concentration. Genetic testing reveals the gene mutation, and muscle biopsies reveal absence of dystrophin in Duchenne dystrophy and an abnormal or reduced amount of dystrophin in Becker dystrophy. Although the various types of muscular atrophy and muscular dystrophy are uncommon, they are of major concern not only to the patient, but to the family because of the hereditary nature of many of these illnesses. Unfortunately, there is no way at present to arrest the relentless progression of the disease.

Gene therapy to eventually allow insertion of replacement genes in muscle fibers to code for the synthesis of the missing or defective dystrophin is being actively investigated but has not yet been successful.

Myasthenia Gravis

Myasthenia gravis is a chronic disease characterized by abnormal fatigability of the voluntary muscles as a result of an abnormality at the myoneural junction. Fatigue develops rapidly when the muscles are used and subsides when they are rested. Often, the dysfunction is most conspicuous in the small muscles of the face and in the muscles concerned with eye movement (extraocular muscles). Myasthenia gravis appears to be an autoimmune disease. The blood of affected patients contains an autoantibody directed against acetylcholine receptors on the surface of the muscle fibers at the myoneural junction. The manifestations of the disease occur because the antibody damages and greatly reduces the number of receptors available to interact with the acetylcholine liberated from motor nerve endings.

Symptoms can be relieved by drugs that inhibit the action of the enzyme cholinesterase. This prolongs the action of the chemical mediator acetylcholine so that it can continue to stimulate the reduced numbers of receptors for a longer time. Many patients with myasthenia gravis have either a tumor or a benign hyperplasia of the thymus gland, which is probably also related to a disturbance of the immune system. Patients with hyperplasia or a tumor of the thymus gland sometimes are improved by removal of the thymus.

CHAPTER REVIEW

Summary

Our skeleton is our rigid supporting framework composed of dense connective tissue impregnated with calcium salts. Normal bone structure depends on a normal amount of calcium in our diet, normal amounts of vitamin D, and normal parathyroid gland function. Achondroplasia and osteogenesis imperfecta are genetically determined abnormalities affecting bone formation and clubfoot (talipes) results from abnormal positioning of the limb skeleton.

The three principal types of arthritis are osteoarthritis, rheumatoid arthritis, and gout. Osteoarthritis is a "wear-and-tear" degeneration of the articular cartilage of a weight-bearing joint that exposes the underlying bone, followed by reactive proliferation of the exposed bone. Rheumatoid arthritis is an autoimmune disease that targets the synovium and leads to secondary destruction of joint surfaces; joint instability follows, often association with misalignment or dislocation of affected bones, and associated disability. Treatment is directed toward controlling the autoimmune-mediated joint damage. Gout is a disorder of purine metabolism that leads to elevated uric acid (as sodium urate) in blood and body fluids. Because urate is not very soluble, it is prone to precipitate from solution in and around joints when its concentration is higher than normal, leading to episodes of acute joint pain as well as progressive joint damage resulting from the urate deposits. Urate may also precipitate from the tubular fluid within the kidney tubules, plugging the tubules and leading to kidney damage as well as joint damage caused by gout.

Bones are sturdy, but they may break, and fractures are classified based on the characteristics of the fracture. The most serious type is a compound fracture in which the overlying skin is broken, exposing the fracture site to infection. A bone may also break if it has been weakened by disease, such as by a deposit of metastatic carcinoma. Such a disease-associated fracture is called a pathologic fracture.

An infection in a bone is called osteomyelitis, which is usually caused by a pathogenic bacteria carried to the bone in the bloodstream from an infection elsewhere in the body (hematogenous spread), or introduced directly into the bone, as may occur following a compound fracture or as a complication of a surgical procedure, such as a hip replacement operation. Treatment consists of antibiotics, sometimes supplemented by surgical procedures.

Malignant tumors may involve bone. Primary bone tumors such as osteosarcoma or chondrosarcoma are uncommon. Most are metastatic tumors spreading from other sites, such as colon, breast, prostate, or lung. Myeloma, a neoplasm of plasma cells, is also relatively common, and may cause multiple areas of bone destruction.

Loss of bone density (osteoporosis) predisposes to fracture, and the condition occurs most frequently in postmenopausal women. It is easier to prevent excessive bone loss by adequate calcium intake, vitamin D, and weight-bearing exercise than it is to restore bone density after it has been lost. However, various treatments are available and are effective.

Chest wall abnormalities result from abnormal growth and attachment of the rib cartilages to the body of the sternum, which changes the position of the sternum. In the most common and important condition the lower part of the sternum is displaced posteriorly, which is called pectus excavatum (*pectus* = chest + *excavatum* = hollowed out), but this condition may also occur as part of a system connective disease called Marfan syndrome.

The spine that supports us may cause problems, such as scoliosis. Early detection and treatment prevent severe disability. Another common problem is a herniated intervertebral disk impinging on a nerve root and causing back pain radiating down the leg. Treatment may require surgical removal of the herniated disk tissue.

Myositis is an inflammation of skeletal muscle. Mild localized myositis may follow injury from overexertion. Generalized myositis is a systemic autoimmune disease and is more difficult to treat. Progressive muscular atrophy results from degeneration of nerve cells supplying the affected muscles for which there is no treatment. Muscular dystrophy is a hereditary X-linked disease affecting the muscle protein dystrophin, which leads to progressive muscle degeneration. Myasthenia gravis is an autoimmune disease in which the antibody targets acetylcholine receptors at the muscle–nerve junction, which impairs transmission of nerve impulses from nerve to muscle. Symptoms are relieved by drugs that prolong the action of acetylcholine. Some affected patients have a tumor of the thymus (thymoma) and can be improved by removing the thymic tumor.

Questions for Review

1. Describe the structure of the typical movable joint (see Figure 1).
2. What are the three most common types of arthritis? What are their distinguishing features (see Table 1)?
3. What is the difference between a simple fracture and a compound fracture? What are the complications of a compound fracture? What is a comminuted fracture? A pathologic fracture?
4. What is osteoporosis? Why does it develop? What symptoms and complications result from osteoporosis?
5. What is a "slipped disk"? Why does it occur? Why does it sometimes produce pain radiating down the leg? How is it treated?
6. What is meant by the following terms: *osteoporosis*, *multiple myeloma*, *nucleus pulposus*, *rheumatoid factor*?
7. What are the types of muscle cells?
8. What is meant by the following terms: *myoneural junction*, *acetylcholine*, and *myositis*?
9. What is the difference between muscular atrophy and muscular dystrophy? What are the most common types of atrophic disease of the muscles? Of dystrophic disease?
10. What is myasthenia gravis? What is its relationship to the immune system? How is it treated?

Supplementary Reading

Arn, P. H., Scherer, L. R., Haller, J. A. Jr., and Pyeritz, R. E. 1989. Outcome of pectus excavatum in patients with Marfan syndrome and in the general population. *Journal of Pediatrics* 115:954–8.

Records of 28 patients with Marfan syndrome were compared with 30 age-matched control patients with presumed pectus excavatum. Isolated pectus excavatum may indicate an underlying connective tissue disorder such as Marfan syndrom.

Brender, E. 2005. Vitamin D. *Journal of the American Medical Association* 394:2386.

A short, one-page article designed for patient education describing the amount of sunlight exposure required to ensure adequate vitamin D (10–15 minutes twice per week), the diseases resulting from the deficiency (rickets and osteomalacia), the persons at risk of deficiency (breastfed infants receiving less than 2 cups a day of vitamin D-fortified formula or milk, persons with dark pigmented skin, persons with very limited sun exposure, persons with fat malabsorption diseases, persons with liver or kidney disease, persons in the northern hemisphere during winter).

Cauley, J., Lui, L. Y., Ensrud, K. E., et al. 2005. Bone mineral density and the risk of incident nonspinal fracture in black and white women. *Journal of the American Medical Association* 293:2102–8.

Age, female sex, slender body configuration, and white race are well-known risk factors for osteoporosis. Although many factors affect bone mineral density (BMD), middle-aged and older black men and women have higher BMD and lower fracture rates than whites. Decreased total hip and femoral neck BMD is associated with increased fracture risk in both black and white women. At any level of BMD, fracture rates in black women were 30 to 40 percent lower than in white women. Separate race-specific databases may be appropriate to define osteoporosis and fracture risk in black and white women.

Drinkwater, B. L., Nilson, K., Ott, S., and Chesnut, C. H. 1986. Bone mineral density after resumption of menses in amenorrheic athletes. *Journal of the American Medical Association* 256:380–82.

Bone mass may not be completely restored.

Felson, D. T. 2006. Osteoarthritis of the knee. *New England Journal of Medicine* 354:841–48.

Describes risk factors, manifestations, and principle of treatment.

Holick, M. F. 2007. Vitamin D deficiency. *New England Journal of Medicine* 357:266–81.

Vitamin D deficiency is still a problem despite fortification of foods with supplements. In adults the deficiency may increase the risk of bone fractures by contributing to the development of osteoporosis, and may also cause osteomalacia. Without vitamin D only about 10–15 percent of dietary calcium and about 60 percent of phosphorous is absorbed. Most cells and tissues in the body have vitamin D receptors, and vitamin D has many effects unrelated to the skeletal system. Vitamin D inhibits cell proliferation of both normal cells and cancer cells, and promotes normal differentiation of cells. Vitamin D is required for normal immune system function, which may explain why black Americans, who are often vitamin D deficient, are more prone to tuberculosis than are whites, and tend to have more aggressive disease. People living at higher or lower latitudes (farther away from the equator where sunlight is most intense and prolonged) have a greater risk of a number of diseases than are persons living closer to the equator. Current recommendations for vitamin D supplements are too low, and many persons are vitamin D deficient.

Johnson, R. J., and Rideout, B. A. 2004. Uric acid and diet—Insights in the epidemic of cardiovascular disease. *New England Journal of Medicine* 350:1071–73.

Neither the total protein intake nor the intake of purine-rich vegetables was correlated with the development of gout. Gout is most common among persons whose diet is high in meat and low in dairy products. Genetic and other factors also modulate the uric acid levels. Many persons with chronic gout and persisting high uric acid develop urate nephropathy. Diets that contain abundant fruits, vegetables, and low-fat dairy foods not only reduce the frequency of hypertension but also the frequency of gout.

LeBoff, M. S., Kohlmeier, L., Hurwitz, S., et al. 1999. Occult vitamin D deficiency in postmenopausal U.S. women with acute hip fracture. *Journal of the American Medical Association* 281:1505–11.

Many postmenopausal women with hip fractures have occult vitamin D deficiency, which impairs absorption of calcium and mineralization of bone and also stimulates compensatory increase in parathyroid hormone secretion. These factors predispose to fractures. Older people need 600 IU of vitamin D daily, which should be increased to 800 IU in winter.

Loucks, A. B., Mortola, J. F., and Girton, S. S. C. 1990. Alterations in the hypothalamic–pituitary–ovarian and the hypothalamic–pituitary–adrenal axis in athletic women. *Journal of Clinical Endocrinology and Metabolism* 68: 402–11.

Describes pathophysiology of exercise-induced amenorrhea.

O'Dell, J. R. 2004. Therapeutic strategies for rheumatoid arthritis. *New England Journal of Medicine* 350:2591–602.

Irreversible joint damage occurs early in rheumatoid arthritis. Early diagnosis and prompt treatment with disease-modifying antirheumatic drugs (DMARD) are essential to minimize joint damage. Nonsteroidal anti-inflammatory drugs improve symptoms but do not slow the progression of the disease. Corticosteroid drugs suppress inflammation and slow disease progression but have significant side effects. DMARD vary in effectiveness and toxicity. Methotrexate is the most widely used, and many patients are treated with methotrexate combined with two other DMARD agents. Tumor necrosis factor inhibitor drugs are generally reserved for patients whose disease cannot be controlled by a combined therapy with DMARD.

Raisz, L. G. 2005. Screening for osteoporosis. *New England Journal of Medicine* 353:164–71.

Measurement of bone mineral density at the lumbar spine and proximal femur is a reliable and safe way to assess the risk of fracture. Screening should provide an estimate of fracture risk during the subsequent 5 or 20 years.

Rott, K. T., and Agudelo, C. A. 2003. Gout. *Journal of the American Medical Association* 289:2857–60.

Current concepts on pathogenesis, factors raising uric acid, clinical manifestations, drugs available for treating gout, and new treatment methods being investigated.

Shahinian, V. B., Kuo, Y. F., Freeman, J. L., and Goodwin, J. S. 2005. Risk of fracture after androgen deprivation for prostate cancer. *New England Journal of Medicine* 532:154–64.

Orchiectomy or drug-induced suppression of testicular function in men with prostate cancer significantly increases their risk of fractures by promoting more rapid decline in bone density resulting from loss of androgens.

Interactive Activities

Matching

Match the type of arthritis on the right with the disease characteristic on the left.

1. Affects primarily small bones of the hands and feet
2. Autoantibodies formed
3. Disturbed purine metabolism
4. Major weight-bearing joints involved
5. Fragmentation and degeneration of articular cartilage
6. Destructive cytokines produced by inflammatory cells
7. Uric acid deposits in and around joints
8. May lead to kidney damage

A. Osteoarthritis
B. Rheumatoid arthritis
C. Gout

True or False

Indicate whether each statement is true or false by writing T or F at the end of the statement.

1. Most patients with gout have autoantibodies directed against articular cartilage that damage the joints. _____
2. Myasthenia gravis is an autoimmune disease in which the autoantibody targets acetylcholine receptors at the myoneural junction. ____
3. Muscular dystrophy results from degeneration of motor neurons in the spinal cord. ____
4. Rheumatoid arthritis is caused by degeneration of the articular cartilage in weight-bearing joints. ____

Critical Thinking

1. Mary Jones is a college student who has heard that the risk of osteoporosis developing later in life can be minimized by measures that promote strong bones. What should she do to promote strong bones and minimize her osteoporosis risk?

2. John Cunningham is a middle-aged man who had an acute episode of pain and swelling at the base of his great toe. What conditions could account for the pain and swelling? What measures would help establish the cause of the condition?

Answers

Matching: 1B; 3C; 5A; 7C

True or False: 1F; 3F

Critical Thinking:

1. Mary should consume an adequate diet containing sufficient calcium, phosphate, and vitamin D. Moderate exercise, but not excessive, which leads to exercise-induced amenorrhea.

The Urinary System

LEARNING OBJECTIVES

1. Describe the normal structures of the kidneys and their functions.
2. Explain the pathogenesis of glomerulonephritis, nephrosis, nephrosclerosis, and glomerulosclerosis. Describe the clinical manifestations of each of these disorders.
3. Describe the clinical manifestations and complications of urinary tract infections.
4. List the causes of renal tubular injury. Describe the manifestations of tubular injury and the treatments for each disorder.
5. Explain the mechanism for formation of urinary tract calculi. Describe the complications of stone formation. Explain the manifestations of urinary tract obstruction.
6. Differentiate the major forms of cystic disease of the kidney and their prognoses. Name the more common kinds of tumors affecting the urinary tract.
7. Describe the causes, clinical manifestations, and treatment of renal failure.
8. Describe the principles and techniques of hemodialysis.

Structure and Function of the Urinary System

The urinary system (FIGURE 1A) consists of

1. The kidneys, which produce the urine
2. An excretory duct system (renal calyces, renal pelves, and ureters) that transports the urine

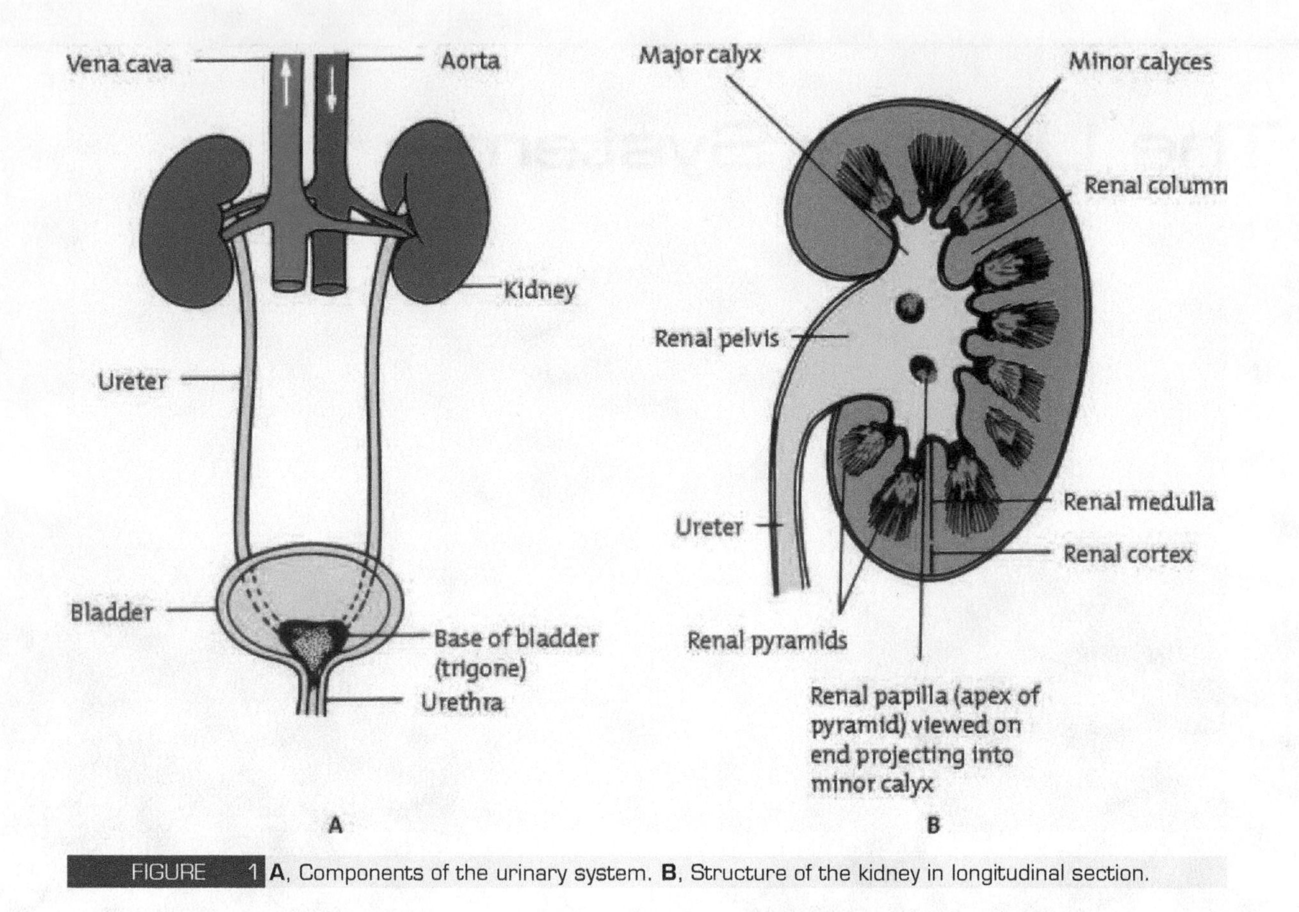

FIGURE 1 **A**, Components of the urinary system. **B**, Structure of the kidney in longitudinal section.

3. The bladder, where the urine is stored
4. The urethra, which conveys the urine from the bladder for excretion

THE KIDNEYS

The kidneys are paired, bean-shaped organs located along the back body wall below the diaphragm and adjacent to the vertebral column. Their structure is illustrated in FIGURE 1B. The region where the blood vessels enter and leave and where the ureter exits to descend to the bladder is called the hilus of the kidney. The expanded upper end of the ureter is the renal pelvis (plural, pelves). The pelvis divides into several large branches called the major calyces (singular, calyx), and these in turn subdivide to form the minor calyces. The renal substance is divided into an outer cortex and an inner medulla. The cone-shaped masses of renal tissue in the medulla that project into the minor calyces are called the renal pyramids, and the tip of each pyramid is called the renal papilla. Columns of cortical tissue that extend into the medulla between the pyramids are called the renal columns.

The calyces and pelves convey the urine into the ureters, which extend downward to enter the posterior wall of the bladder near its base, as illustrated in Figure 1A. Each ureter enters the bladder at an angle so that, when the bladder contracts, its muscular wall compresses the ureters as they run obliquely through it, somewhat like a one-way valve. This prevents backflow of urine into the ureters during voiding (urination). The ureteral openings in the bladder are also partially covered by folds of mucosa that help prevent retrograde flow of urine.

THE URETERS

The ureters are muscular tubes that propel the urine into the bladder by wavelike contractions of their muscular walls (**peristalsis**). Urine is discharged into the bladder in spurts. It does not drain by gravity.

Peristalsis
The wavelike contractions of the wall of the alimentary tract that propel contents through the bowel.

THE BLADDER AND URETHRA

The urinary bladder is the distensible reservoir for urine. It is lined by transitional epithelium continuous with that which lines the remainder of the urinary tract. The opening of the urethra is located at the base of the bladder, and the ureteral openings are located on either side and behind the urethral opening. The triangular area at the base of the bladder bounded by the two ureteral orifices posteriorly, and the urethral orifice anteriorly, is called the trigone of the bladder (*tri* = three).

Function of the Kidneys

The kidneys are important excretory organs, functioning along with the lungs in excreting the waste products of food metabolism. Carbon dioxide and water are end-products of carbohydrate and fat metabolism. Protein metabolism produces urea, as well as various acids, which only the kidneys can excrete. The kidneys also play an important role in regulating mineral and water balance by excreting minerals and water that have been ingested in excess of the body's requirements and conserving minerals and water as required. It has been said that the internal environment of the body is determined not by what a person ingests but rather by what the kidneys retain.

The kidneys serve an endocrine function as well. Specialized cells in the kidneys elaborate a hormone called **erythropoietin**, which regulates red blood cell production in the bone marrow, and another humoral substance called **renin**, which takes part in the regulation of the blood pressure.

Erythropoietin (er-ith-rō-poy′e-tin)
A humoral substance made by the kidneys that regulates hematopoiesis.

Renin (ren′in)
A humoral substance secreted by the kidneys in response to fall in blood pressure, blood volume, or sodium concentration.

Nephron (nef′rän)
The glomerulus and renal tubule.

Bowman's capsule
The cuplike expanded end of the nephron that surrounds the tuft of glomerular capillaries.

THE NEPHRON

The basic structural and functional unit of the kidney is the **nephron**, and there are about one million nephrons in each kidney. Each nephron consists of a glomerulus and a renal tubule. The glomerulus is a tuft of capillaries supplied by an afferent glomerular arteriole. The capillaries of the glomerulus then recombine into an efferent glomerular arteriole, which in turn breaks up into a network of capillaries that supplies the renal tubule. The site where the afferent arteriole enters the glomerulus and the efferent arteriole exits is called the vascular pole of the glomerulus.

The histologic structure of the glomerulus and related structures is illustrated schematically in FIGURE 2. The expanded proximal end of the tubule is called **Bowman's capsule**. The tuft of capillaries that make up the glomerulus is pushed into Bowman's capsule much as one would push a fist into a balloon. The layer of Bowman's capsule cells, which is pushed in (invaginated), becomes closely applied to the capillaries of the glomerulus and is called the visceral layer of Bowman's capsule or simply the glomerular epithelium. The cells of this layer have long, footlike cytoplasmic processes and are usually called podocytes (*podos* = foot) (Figure 2A). The outer layer of Bowman's capsule is called the parietal layer of Bowman's capsule, or simply the capsular epithelium. The space between the two layers, into which the urine filters, is called Bowman's space.

The capillary tuft is held together and supported by groups of highly specialized cells embedded in a basement membranelike material. The cells are located between the capillaries and are concentrated at the vascular pole of the glomerulus. Because of

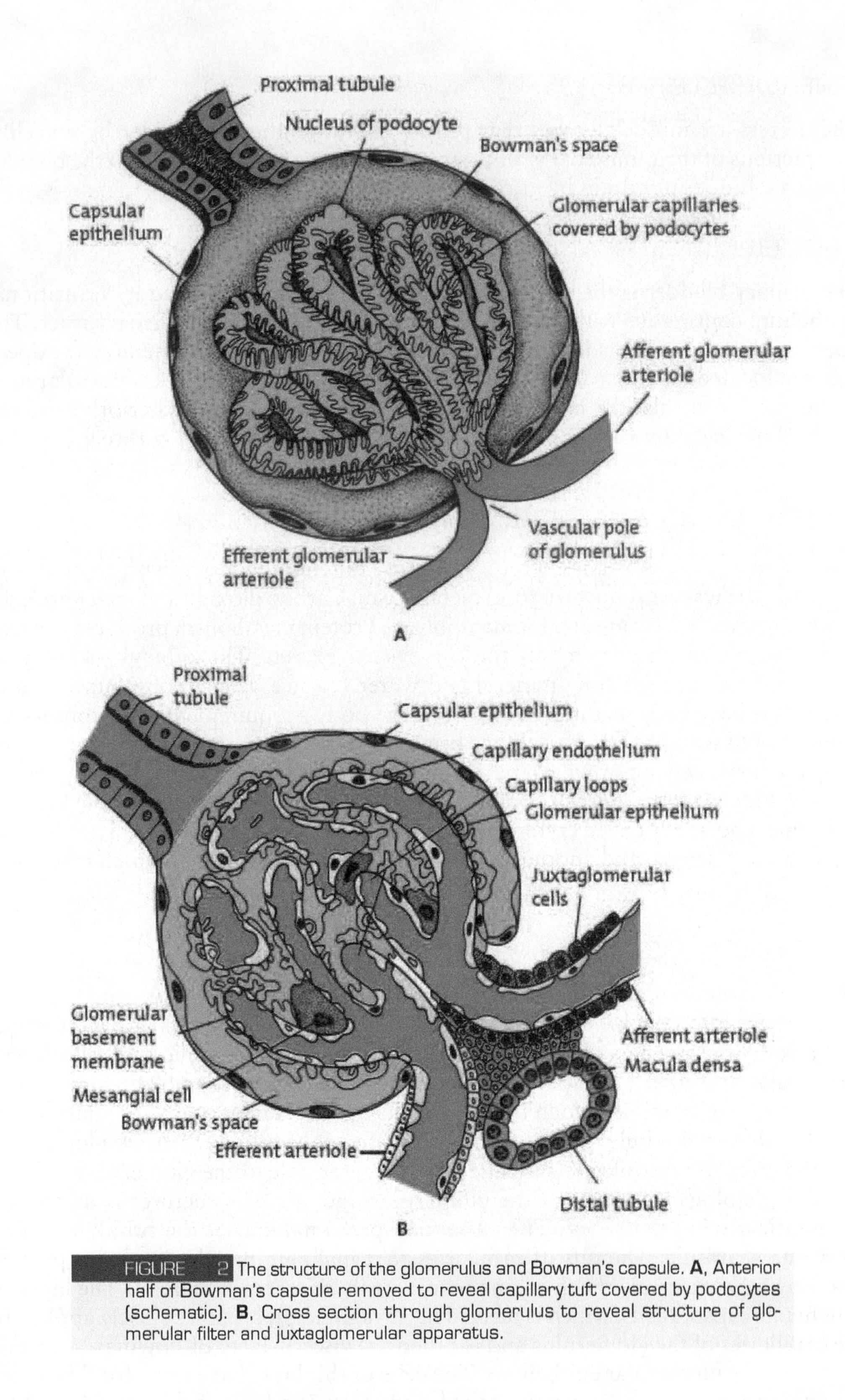

FIGURE 2 The structure of the glomerulus and Bowman's capsule. **A**, Anterior half of Bowman's capsule removed to reveal capillary tuft covered by podocytes (schematic). **B**, Cross section through glomerulus to reveal structure of glomerular filter and juxtaglomerular apparatus.

Mesangial cell
(mes-an′jē-yul)
Modified connective-tissue cells at the vascular pole of the glomerulus that hold the capillary tuft together.

Juxtaglomerular apparatus
(jux′tu-glo-mār′ū-lär)
A specialized group of cells at the vascular pole of the glomerulus that regulates blood flow through the glomerulus of the kidneys.

their location between the capillaries, they are called **mesangial cells** (*meso* = middle + *angio* = vessel). In addition to their support function, they are also contractile cells that play a role in regulating glomerular filtration by varying the caliber of the capillaries, and they are also phagocytic cells. Also located at the vascular pole is a specialized cluster of cells called the **juxtaglomerular apparatus** (*juxta* = near to), which regulates blood flow through the glomerulus. It also plays a role in regulating blood pressure by producing renin, as described in a later section. The juxtaglomerular apparatus consists of three parts:

1. The macula densa, a condensation of cells in the distal part of the renal tubule, where it is in contact with the vascular pole of the glomerulus
2. The juxtaglomerular cells, which are specialized renin-containing smooth muscle cells located in the wall of the afferent glomerular arteriole at the vascular pole of the glomerulus
3. A group of extraglomerular mesangial cells that are continuous with those within the glomerulus and interposed between the vascular pole of the glomerulus and the macula densa (Figure 2B)

Water and soluble material filter from the blood through the glomerular capillaries into Bowman's space. When visualized by electron microscopy, the membrane through which the filtrate passes can be seen to consist of three layers, as depicted in FIGURE 3. The inner layer is formed by the endothelium of the glomerular capillaries. The cytoplasm is very thin and is perforated by many small holes called fenestrations (*fenestra* = window). Most of the fenestrations are open, but some, called pseudofenestrations (*pseudo* = false), are covered by a thin membrane containing a central knob. This layer is freely permeable to water and to many large molecules. The middle layer is the porous basement membrane that supports the capillary endothelium. The outer layer is composed of the podocytes. Their highly branched cytoplasmic processes are called **foot processes,** and their terminal branches are called **pedicels** ("little feet"). The pedicels are attached to the basement membrane, and the pedicels of one cell interdigitate with others from the same cell or adjacent cells. The narrow spaces between adjacent interdigitating pedicels are called **filtration slits**. Each slit is covered by a thin membrane called a **filtration membrane** and is reinforced by a filamentous ridge. The filtration membranes are less porous than the other layers of the glomerular filter and perform much of the filtration.

Foot processes
The highly branched cytoplasmic processes of the podocytes covering the glomerular capillaries of the kidneys.

Pedicel
(ped'i-cel)
One of the small terminal processes of the podocytes that cover the glomerular capillaries.

Filtration slits
The narrow spaces between the pedicels of the podocytes that cover the glomerular capillaries of the kidneys.

Filtration membrane
The thin membrane covering the filtration slit between pedicels of the podocytes that cover the glomerular capillaries of the kidneys.

The renal tubules are long tubes that measure as much as 4 cm in length. The proximal end of the tubule is invaginated by the glomerulus, and its distal end empties into a collecting tubule. The tubule is divided into three parts (FIGURE 4):

1. The proximal convoluted tubule
2. The loop of Henle
3. The distal convoluted tubule

The proximal convoluted tubule is the greatly coiled first part of the tubule, its convolutions being located very close to the glomerulus. The loop of Henle is a U-shaped segment composed of descending and ascending limbs joined by a short segment. The descending limb and proximal half of the ascending limb are lined by flat epithelial cells, forming the thin segment of Henle's loop. The distal part of the ascending limb, called the thick segment of Henle's loop, is lined by tall columnar epithelium similar to that lining the distal tubule. The loop descends from the cortex into the medulla and then bends back sharply, returning to the cortex close to the vascular pole of its own glomerulus, where it becomes continuous with the distal convoluted tubule. The distal convoluted tubule is much shorter than the proximal tubule. It empties into a collecting tubule, which passes through the medulla to drain into one of the minor calyces at the apex of a renal pyramid (renal papilla).

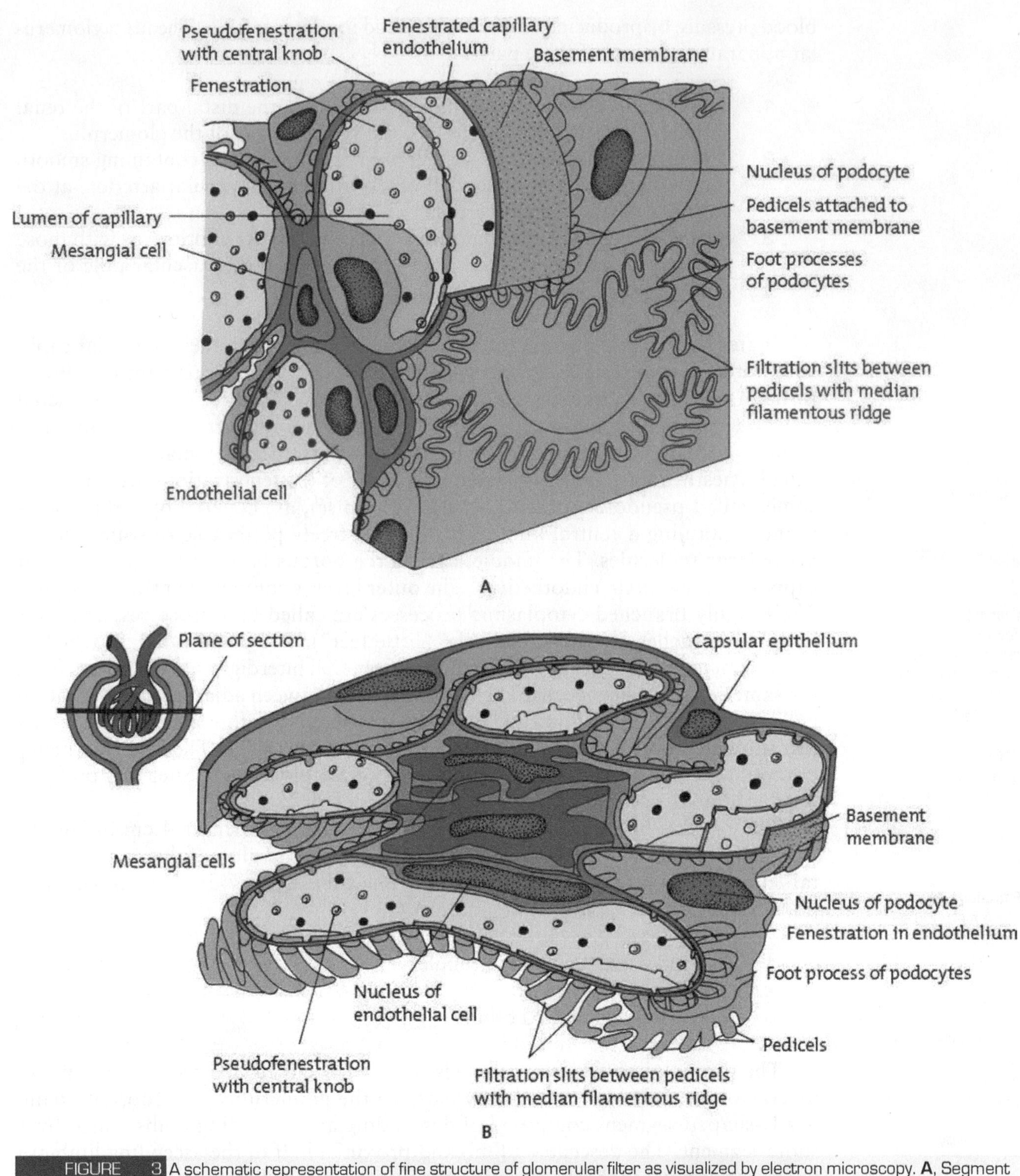

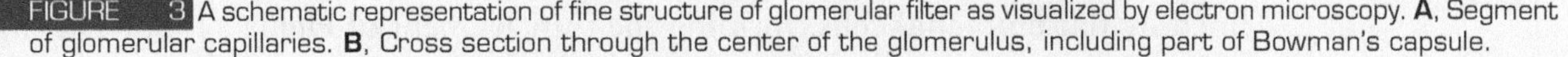
FIGURE 3 A schematic representation of fine structure of glomerular filter as visualized by electron microscopy. **A**, Segment of glomerular capillaries. **B**, Cross section through the center of the glomerulus, including part of Bowman's capsule.

The renal tubules selectively reabsorb water, minerals, and other substances that are to be conserved and excrete unwanted materials that are eliminated. Urine is the glomerular filtrate that remains after most of the water and important constituents have been reabsorbed by the renal tubules, and other substances excreted by the renal tubules have been added.

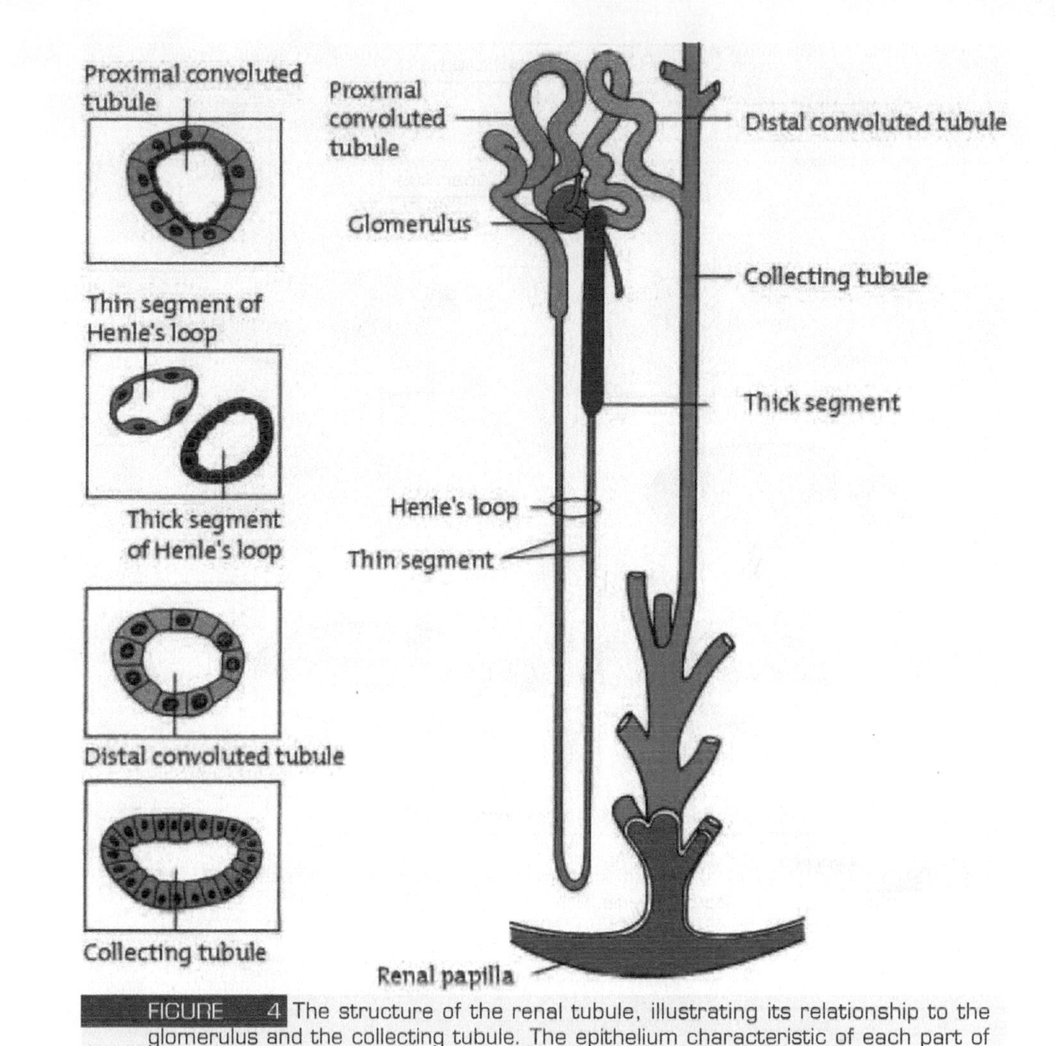

FIGURE 4 The structure of the renal tubule, illustrating its relationship to the glomerulus and the collecting tubule. The epithelium characteristic of each part of the renal tubule and the collecting tubule are also illustrated.

Renin (ren′in)
A humoral substance secreted by the kidneys in response to fall in blood pressure, blood volume, or sodium concentration.

Angiotensinogen (an-jee-o-ten-sin′-o-gen)
A blood protein converted to angiotensin I by renin secreted by the kidneys. Part of the renin-angiotensin-aldosterone system.

Angiotensin (an-jē-o-ten′sin)
A component of the renin-angiotensin-aldosterone system that raises blood pressure by constricting blood vessels and stimulating the adrenal grand to secrete aldosterone, which increases blood volume.

Angiotensin converting enzyme
An enzyme that converts angiotensin I to angiotensin II.

Aldosterone
A steroid hormone produced by the adrenal cortex that regulates the rate of sodium absorption from the renal tubules.

RENAL REGULATION OF BLOOD PRESSURE AND BLOOD VOLUME

The kidneys play a major role in regulating both the blood pressure and blood volume by secreting renin, which is released into the bloodstream from the juxtaglomerular cells in the walls of the afferent glomerular arterioles. **Renin** is an enzyme that interacts with a blood protein called **angiotensinogen** and splits off a short peptide fragment called **angiotensin I.** Then, as the blood flows through the lungs, the newly formed angiotensin I is almost immediately converted to **angiotensin II** by an enzyme called **angiotensin-converting enzyme** (abbreviated ACE) that is present in the endothelium of the pulmonary capillaries.

Angiotensin II is a powerful vasoconstrictor that raises the blood pressure by causing the peripheral arterioles to constrict. Angiotensin II also stimulates the adrenal cortex to secrete a steroid hormone called **aldosterone,** which increases reabsorption of sodium chloride and water by the kidneys. As a result, the blood volume is increased by the greater volume of salt and water entering the circulation, and the blood pressure rises because there is more fluid within the vascular system. Thus, renin regulates blood pressure both by controlling the degree of arteriolar vasoconstriction and by regulating the volume of fluid within the circulation. The system is self-regulating because renin secretion declines as blood pressure, volume, and sodium concentration are restored to normal (FIGURE 5).

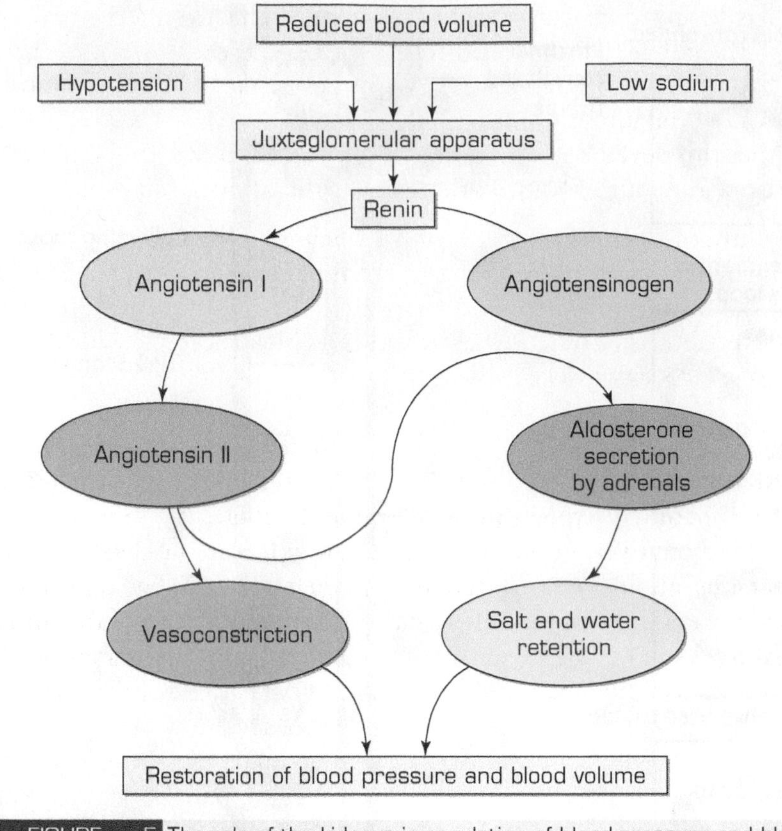

FIGURE 5 The role of the kidneys in regulation of blood pressure and blood volume, as described in the text.

REQUIREMENTS FOR NORMAL RENAL FUNCTION

The functions of the two kidneys reflect the sum of the functions of their individual nephrons. For a nephron to function normally, the following conditions must be satisfied:

1. There must be free flow of blood through the glomerular capillaries.
2. The glomerular filter must function normally. An adequate volume of filtrate must be produced, but the filter must restrict passage of blood cells and proteins.
3. The tubules must be able to selectively reabsorb important substances from the filtrate and to excrete other constituents into the filtrate.
4. The urine formed by the nephron must be able to flow freely from the kidney into the bladder and out of the urethra.

Derangement of any of these functions results in kidney disease.

Developmental Disturbances

The urinary system develops from several different components. The kidneys form from masses of primitive connective tissue (mesoderm) located along the back body wall of the embryo. The bladder develops as an offshoot of the lower end of the intestinal tract. The ureters, renal pelves, renal calyces (the urinary drainage system), and the renal collecting tubules derive from paired tubular structures called ureteric buds. Each bud grows upward from the developing bladder and connects with the kidney that is forming on the corresponding side. The kidneys begin their development within the pelvis. Later, as the embryo grows, the kidneys and their excretory ducts come to occupy a higher location, until eventually they ascend to reach their final positions in the upper lumbar region (FIGURE 6A).

Sometimes this developmental process is disturbed, and congenital malformations result. Three of the more common developmental abnormalities are:

1. Failure of one or both kidneys to develop, which is called renal agenesis
2. Formation of extra ureters and renal pelves, which are called duplications of the urinary tract
3. Malpositions of one or both kidneys, which is often associated with fusion of the two kidneys

Renal agenesis (*a* = without + *genesis* = formation) may affect one or both kidneys. Bilateral renal agenesis is uncommon. It often accompanies other congenital malformations and is incompatible with postnatal life. In contrast, unilateral renal agenesis (FIGURE 6B) is a relatively common condition that has an incidence of about one in a thousand persons, about the same frequency as cleft palate. When one kidney is absent, the other kidney enlarges and is able to carry out the functions of the missing kidney; so the affected person is usually not inconvenienced by the abnormality. The recognition of this condition, however, is of great importance to the clinician who is treating an individual with kidney disease because one can never assume that the patient has two kidneys. Before a surgeon performs a kidney operation, diagnostic studies must always be performed first in order to ascertain that the patient has two kidneys. Such precautions are essential to prevent inadvertent removal of a solitary kidney.

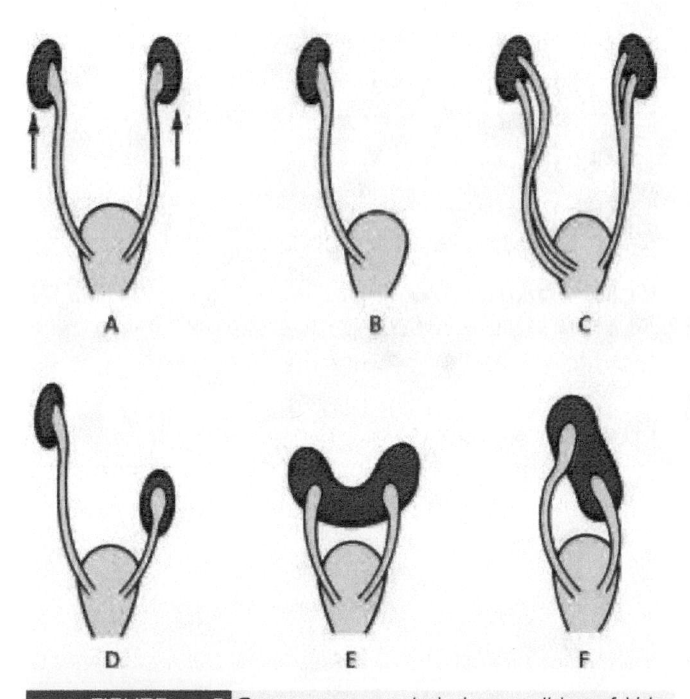

FIGURE 6 Common congenital abnormalities of kidneys and urinary tract. **A**, Normal ascent of kidneys. **B**, Unilateral renal agenesis. **C**, Various types of duplications of ureters and renal pelves resulting from formation of an extra ureteric bud (*left*) or premature splitting of a single ureteric bud (*right*). **D**, Failure of one kidney to ascend to normal position. **E**, Horseshoe kidney resulting from fusion of lower poles of kidneys. **F**, Fusion of the lower pole of one kidney to the upper pole of opposite kidney, which has failed to ascend normally.

Duplications of the urinary tract may be unilateral or bilateral. Sometimes, a kidney has an extra renal pelvis and ureter that drains separately into the bladder (complete duplication). Sometimes, double ureters draining the kidney unite to form a single ureter just before entering the bladder (partial duplication). Duplications result from abnormal prenatal development of the ureteric buds. A complete duplication results when an extra ureteric bud develops and gives rise to a separate excretory system draining the kidney on the affected side. If the ureteric bud branches after it has formed, only the upper part of the excretory system is duplicated; the lower part of the ureter is not duplicated and enters the bladder normally (FIGURE 6C).

Abnormalities of position and fusion of the kidneys may occur if both kidneys remain in the pelvis where they began their development or if they ascend only part way (FIGURE 6D). Kidneys that fail to ascend normally are in very close approximation as they develop and may become fused. One of the more common fusion abnormalities is a union of the lower poles of the two kidneys to form a U-shaped mass of renal tissue called a horseshoe kidney (FIGURE 6E). In other cases, when the kidneys ascend abnormally, the upper pole of one kidney may become fused to the lower pole of the other (FIGURE 6F).

Renal duplications, malpositions, and fusions often are of little clinical significance. At times, however, drainage of urine may be impeded by the abnormalities, causing the urine to stagnate and predisposing the patient to urinary infections. Another important developmental abnormality called congenital polycystic kidney disease is considered in the section on renal cysts.

Glomerulonephritis

Glomerulonephritis is an inflammation of the glomeruli caused by an antigen–antibody reaction within the glomerular capillaries. The interaction of antigen and antibody activates complement and liberates mediators that attract polymorphonuclear leukocytes. The actual glomerular injury is caused by destructive lysosomal enzymes that are released from the leukocytes that have accumulated within the glomeruli.

Glomerulonephritis (glo-mär′ŭ-lō-nef-rī′tis) *An inflammation of the glomeruli caused by either antigen–antibody complexes trapped in the glomeruli or by antiglomerular basement membrane antibodies.*

The antigen–antibody reaction within the glomeruli may take place in two ways. In most cases, the antigen and antibody interact within the circulation, forming small clumps called immune complexes. These are deposited in the walls of the glomerular capillaries as the blood filters through the glomeruli. Glomerulonephritis that occurs in this way is called immune-complex glomerulonephritis. Less commonly, the glomerular inflammation is caused by an autoantibody directed against the basement membranes of the glomerular capillaries. This type of glomerulonephritis is called antiglomerular basement membrane (anti-GBM) glomerulonephritis. FIGURE 7 illustrates the histologic appearance of these two types of glomerulonephritis compared with the appearance of a normal glomerulus.

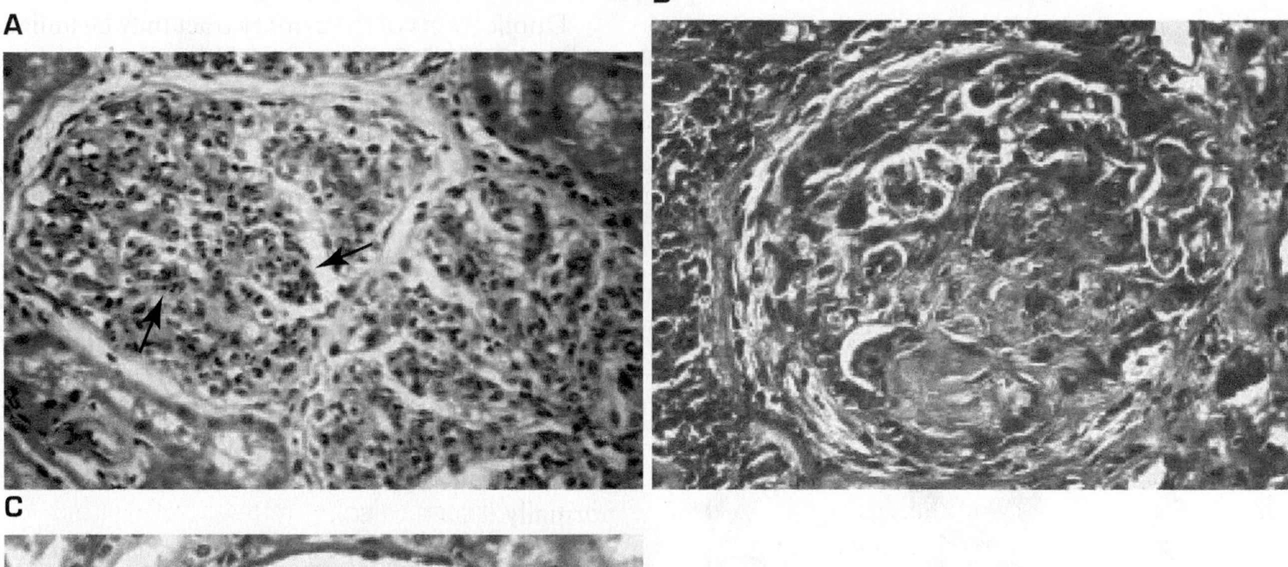

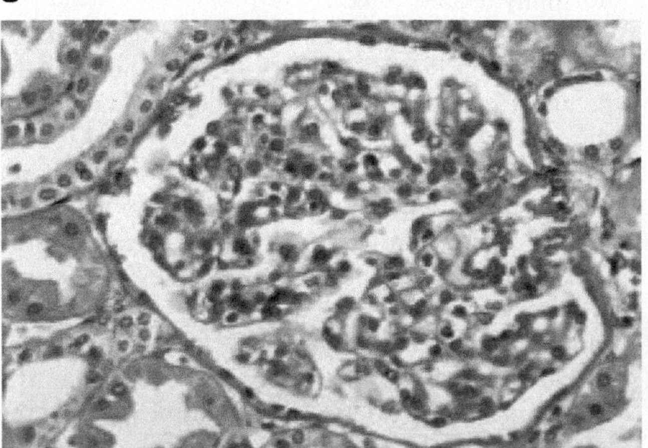

FIGURE 7 **A**, Immune complex glomerulonephritis. Two glomeruli in the photograph contain large numbers of neutrophils (*arrows*). **B**, Anti-GBM glomerulonephritis, revealing severe glomerular injury and scarring. **C**, Normal glomerulus for comparison (original magnifications × 400).

IMMUNE-COMPLEX GLOMERULONEPHRITIS

Immune-complex glomerulonephritis may develop as a complication about 2 weeks after infection by certain beta streptococci, the same type of organism that causes the familiar streptococcal sore throat. However, glomerular inflammation occurs only in a small percentage of patients with streptococcal infections. In affected subjects, the body responds to the streptococcal infection by forming antistreptococcal antibodies that interact in the bloodstream with soluble antigens from the streptococci to form immune complexes. Some of the antigen–antibody complexes are small enough to pass completely through the walls of the glomerular capillaries and be excreted in the urine. Larger complexes, however, pass through the endothelium and basement membranes of the glomerular capillaries but become trapped between the filtration slits of the glomerular epithelial cells, where they induce an inflammatory reaction.

Acute glomerulonephritis may at times follow other bacterial infections or viral infections. The mechanism of glomerular injury is similar to that of poststreptococcal glomerulonephritis. Immune complexes composed of a bacterial or viral antigen and its corresponding antibody interact in the circulation and are trapped in the glomeruli, where they produce inflammation and injury by activating complement and attracting leukocytes (Figure 7A).

The signs and symptoms of glomerulonephritis are related to the changes within the glomeruli. Many glomeruli are completely blocked by inflammation, and thus, less blood is filtered and less urine is excreted. As urinary output is reduced, waste products are retained and accumulate in the blood. Other glomeruli, damaged by lysosomal enzymes, are no longer able to function as efficient filters. Protein and red cells leak through the damaged glomerular capillary walls and are excreted in the urine. Frequently, masses of red cells and protein accumulate within the tubules and become molded to the shape of the renal tubules before finally being excreted. These structures, which are called urinary casts, are an important indication of glomerular injury.

In most cases, glomerulonephritis subsides spontaneously and the patient recovers completely without residual kidney damage. Occasionally, the disease is so severe that the patient requires dialysis treatment for renal insufficiency. In some patients, the glomerulonephritis never heals completely. The disease becomes chronic, progresses slowly, and eventually causes renal failure. Patients with chronic poststreptococcal glomerulonephritis who develop a streptococcal sore throat or other streptococcal infection may experience recurrent episodes of acute glomerulonephritis. This is analogous to the situation in rheumatic fever in which recurrent beta-streptococcal infections are sometimes followed by recurrent episodes of rheumatic fever.

Immune-complex glomerulonephritis may also occur in association with autoimmune diseases in which autoantibody-containing immune complexes become trapped in renal glomeruli, as in lupus erythematosus (discussion on immunity, hypersensitivity, allergy, and autoimmune diseases). Another relatively common type of immune-complex glomerulonephritis is associated with proliferation of mesangial cells and accumulation of immune complexes containing immunoglobulin A (IgA) within the cells. Because of the type of immunoglobulin associated with the disease, it is often called IgA nephropathy. Unfortunately, in many patients, this type of glomerulonephritis becomes chronic and slowly progressive.

ANTI-GBM GLOMERULONEPHRITIS

Glomerulonephritis caused by autoantibodies directed against glomerular basement membranes (anti-GBM glomerulonephritis) is a type of autoimmune disease. It is a relatively uncommon cause of acute glomerulonephritis. In some patients, the anti-GBM antibodies may also injure the basement membranes of the pulmonary capillaries and may cause intrapulmonary hemorrhage as well as acute glomerulonephritis.

It is possible to distinguish immune-complex glomerulonephritis from anti-GBM glomerulonephritis by special studies performed on kidney tissue obtained by renal biopsy. Immune-complex glomerulonephritis is characterized by large, irregular, lumpy deposits composed of antigen, antibody, and complement. These deposits form along the outer surface of the glomerular basement membranes, where the complexes have been trapped between the filtration slits of the glomerular epithelial cells. In contrast, anti-GBM nephritis is characterized by a relatively uniform layer of antibody and complement deposited along the inner surface of the glomerular basement membranes.

Case 1 illustrates the clinical features of glomerulonephritis that lead to renal failure and demonstrates the use of renal biopsy.

CASE 1

A 51-year-old man was admitted to the hospital because of cough, chest pain, and weight loss. Physical examination was essentially normal. The urine contained a moderate amount of protein and many red cells. Blood urea nitrogen was 87 mg/dl (normal range 10–20 mg/dl). Blood pH was reduced to 7.2 (normal range 7.35–7.45). Plasma bicarbonate was reduced to 15 meq/L (normal range 24–28 meq/L). A renal biopsy revealed an active glomerulonephritis (Figure 7B). By means of special studies, immunoglobulins and complement were identified uniformly attached to the glomerular basement membranes. The lesion was interpreted as glomerulonephritis secondary to antiglomerular basement membrane antibodies. The patient was referred to another center for dialysis and further treatment.

Nephrotic Syndrome

The term **nephrotic syndrome** refers to a group of abnormalities characterized by a severe loss of protein in the urine. Urinary excretion of protein is so great that the body is unable to manufacture protein fast enough to keep up with the losses and the concentration of protein in the blood plasma falls. This, in turn, causes significant edema owing to the low plasma osmotic pressure (discussion on circulatory disturbances). Nephrotic syndrome may be produced by a number of different types of renal diseases. The basic cause is injury to the glomerulus that allows proteins to leak through the damaged basement membrane. Because the albumin molecule is much smaller than the globulin molecule, a disproportionately large amount of albumin is lost in the urine. The osmotic pressure of the plasma falls to such an extent that excessive amounts of fluid leak from the capillaries into the interstitial tissues and body cavities. Patients with the nephrotic syndrome have marked leg edema, and often fluid collects in the abdominal cavity (called **ascites**); sometimes; fluid also accumulates in the pleural cavities (called **hydrothorax**).

Nephrotic syndrome
(nef-rä′tik sin′drōm)
A generalized edema resulting from excessive protein loss in the urine, caused by various types of renal disease.

Ascites
(a-si′tēz)
Accumulation of fluid in the abdominal cavity.

Hydrothorax
(hī-drō-thor′ax)
Accumulation of fluid in the pleural cavity.

When the nephrotic syndrome occurs in children, it is usually caused by a relatively minimal abnormality in the foot processes of the glomerular epithelial cells. Nephrotic syndrome caused by this type of glomerular abnormality responds to corticosteroid therapy, and most children recover completely, as illustrated by Case 2.

CASE 2

A 6-year-old boy complained of abdominal discomfort. His mother noted that his face, abdomen, scrotum, and legs were very edematous. His urine contained large amounts of protein and a few casts. His serum protein and serum albumin were both much lower than normal. Additional studies of serum proteins by electrophoresis were also consistent with nephrotic syndrome. The child was hospitalized, placed on a low-sodium diet, and treated with adrenal corticosteroid hormones. The edema gradually subsided, and the corticosteroids were gradually discontinued. He was discharged after a 2-week hospitalization.

In contrast to the favorable outcome in children, the nephrotic syndrome in adults is usually a manifestation of progressive, more serious renal disease in which there are marked structural changes in the glomeruli. Some cases result from chronic progressive glomerulonephritis; others result from glomerular damage resulting from long-standing diabetes, as described later, or from a connective-tissue disease affecting the kidney, such as lupus erythematosus. Some other relatively uncommon types of kidney disease involving the glomeruli may also produce nephrotic syndrome.

Nephrosclerosis
Thickening and narrowing of the afferent glomerular arterioles as a result of disease.

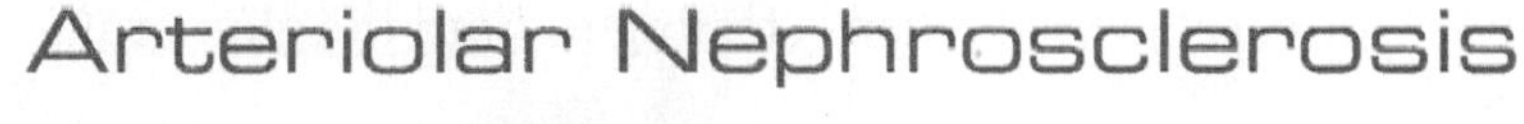

Arteriolar Nephrosclerosis

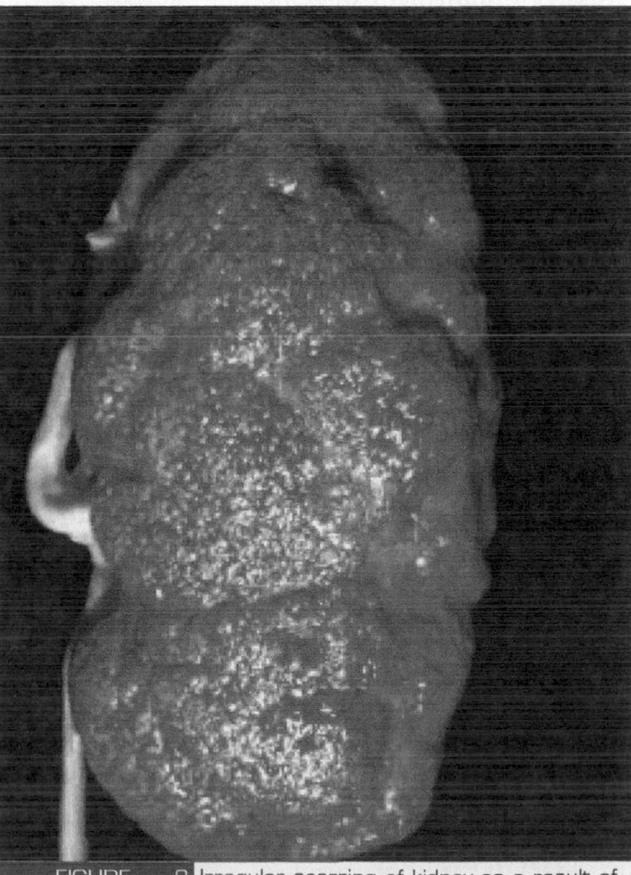

FIGURE 8 Irregular scarring of kidney as a result of nephrosclerosis.

Arteriolar nephrosclerosis (sometimes called simply **nephrosclerosis**) is a complication of severe hypertension. Because of the extreme elevation of the systemic blood pressure, the small arterioles and arteries throughout the body are called on to carry blood at a much higher pressure than normal. As a result, the blood vessels undergo severe degenerative changes characterized by thickening and narrowing of the lumens; this reduces blood flow through the narrowed arterioles. The name of the disease, which means literally "sclerosis of the arterioles of the nephrons," refers to these characteristic renal vascular changes. Glomerular filtration is reduced because the arterioles are greatly narrowed. The renal tubules, which are also supplied by the glomerular arterioles, also undergo degenerative changes. Eventually, the kidneys become shrunken and scarred as a result of reduction of their blood supply (FIGURE 8). Patients with severe nephrosclerosis may die from renal insufficiency, as well as from the effects of the severe hypertension.

Diabetic Nephropathy

Persons with long-standing diabetes mellitus often develop progressive renal damage. The glomerular

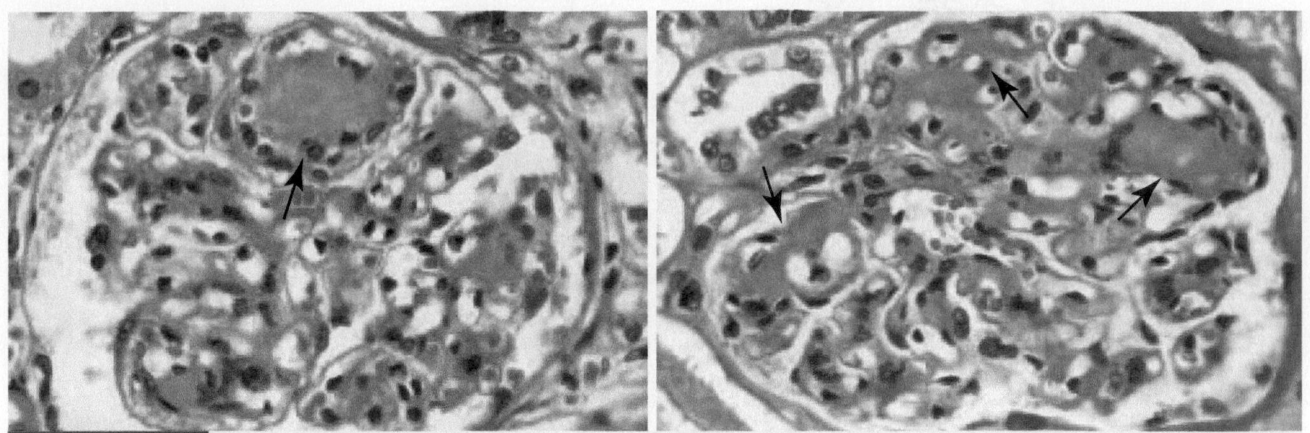

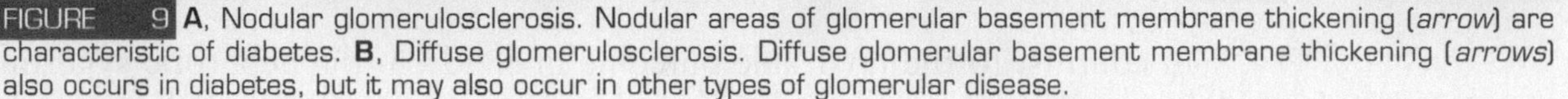

FIGURE 9 **A**, Nodular glomerulosclerosis. Nodular areas of glomerular basement membrane thickening (*arrow*) are characteristic of diabetes. **B**, Diffuse glomerulosclerosis. Diffuse glomerular basement membrane thickening (*arrows*) also occurs in diabetes, but it may also occur in other types of glomerular disease.

basement membranes exhibit characteristic nodular and diffuse thickening called **diabetic glomerulosclerosis** (FIGURE 9), which disturbs glomerular function. Usually there is also severe sclerosis of the glomerular arterioles, impairing the flow of blood to the glomeruli and tubules. Sometimes the general term **diabetic nephropathy** (*nephros* = kidney + *path* = disease) is used when referring to both the glomerular and the arteriolar lesions.

Diabetic glomerulosclerosis
(glo-mĕr′ū-lō-skler-rō′sis)
Diffuse and nodular thickening of glomerular basement membranes, a common occurrence in patients with long-standing diabetes mellitus.

Diabetic nephropathy
Kidney damage affecting primarily the kidney blood vessels (arterioles) and glomeruli caused by diabetes.

Clinically, the condition is characterized by progressive impairment of renal function that may eventually lead to renal failure. Protein leaks through the diseased glomeruli and is lost in the urine. In some patients, so much protein is lost that the nephrotic syndrome develops. There is no specific treatment that can arrest the progression of the disease. A renal transplant may be required if the patient develops renal failure. (Diabetes mellitus and its complications are considered in the pancreas and diabetes mellitus discussion.)

GOUT-ASSOCIATED NEPHROPATHY

Persons with gout, described in the discussion on the musculoskeletal system, have a higher than normal concentration of relatively insoluble uric acid in their blood and body fluids, which leads to periodic episodes of acute joint inflammation (gouty arthritis) caused by precipitation of uric acid as sodium urate crystals in their joints. Although the skeletal manifestations of gout are well known, gout also frequently affects the kidneys and urinary tract. Many patients develop kidney stones, described later in this chapter. Sodium urate crystals may also precipitate from the tubular filtrate within the Henle's loops and in the collecting tubules within the renal pyramids where the tubular filtrate is very concentrated. The precipitates obstruct and damage the renal tubules, which is followed by scarring and impaired renal function, a condition called **urate nephropathy** (FIGURE 10).

Urate nephropathy
(nĕf-rop′-uh-thē)
Kidney damage caused by precipitation of urate crystals within the kidney tubules of a person with gout.

Infections of the Urinary Tract

Urinary tract infections are common and may be either acute or chronic. An infection that affects only the bladder is called **cystitis** (*cystis* = bladder). If the upper urinary tract is infected, the term is **pyelonephritis** (*pyelo* = pelvis + *nephros* = kidney + *itis*

Cystitis
(sis-tī′tis)
Inflammation of the bladder.

Pyelonephritis
(pī′el-ō-nef-rī′tis)
A bacterial infection of the kidney and renal pelvis.

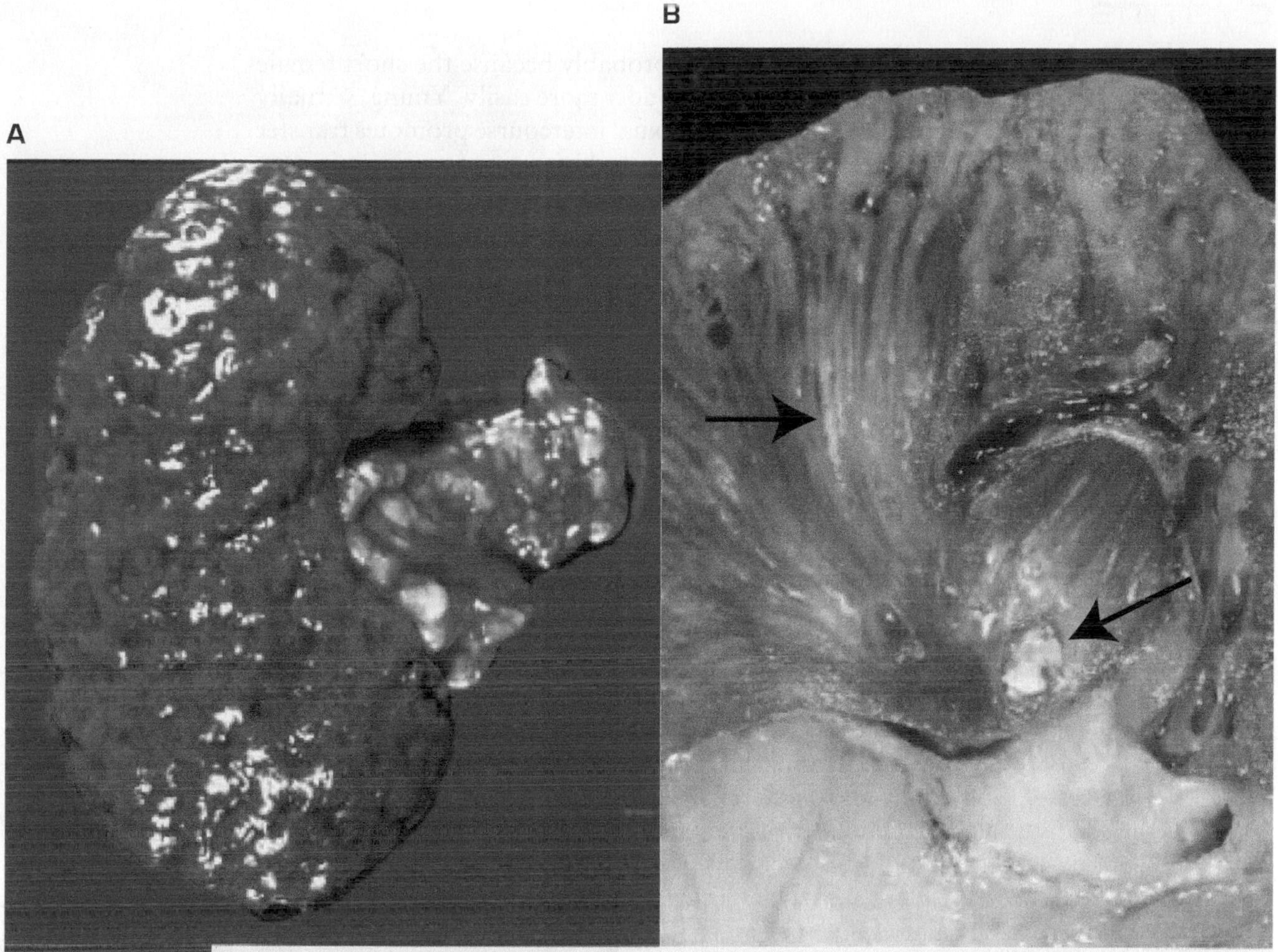

FIGURE 10 **A**, Urate nephropathy showing multiple depressed scars involving kidney cortex caused by kidney damage resulting from tubular obstruction by urate crystals. **B**, Section of kidney revealing white urate deposits within renal pyramid (*upper arrow*) and large urate deposit near tip of pyramid (*lower arrow*).

= inflammation). Most infections are caused by gram-negative intestinal bacteria. These organisms often contaminate the perianal and genital areas and gain access to the urinary tract by ascending the urethra.

Free urine flow, large urine volume, and complete emptying of the bladder protect against urinary tract infections because any bacteria that enter the bladder are soon flushed out during urination instead of being retained to multiply in the bladder urine. An acid urine is an additional defense against infection because most bacteria grow poorly in an acid environment. On the other hand, several conditions predispose to urinary tract infections:

1. Any condition that impairs free drainage of urine increases the likelihood of infection because stagnation of urine favors multiplication of any bacteria that enter the urinary tract.
2. Injury to the mucosa of the urinary tract, as by a kidney stone (calculus) or foreign body, disrupts the protective epithelium, permitting bacteria to invade the deeper tissues and set up an infection.
3. Introduction of a catheter or instrument into the bladder may carry bacteria into the urinary tract when the catheter or instrument is introduced and may also injure the bladder mucosa.

CYSTITIS

Cystitis is more common in women than in men, probably because the short female urethra allows infectious organisms to enter the bladder more easily. Young, sexually active women are especially predisposed because sexual intercourse promotes transfer of bacteria from the distal urethra into the bladder and may cause minor injury to the mucosa at the base of the bladder (trigone). Cystitis is also common in older men who cannot empty their bladders completely because of an enlarged prostate gland (discussion on the male reproductive system). The urine remaining in the bladder after voiding favors multiplication of bacteria and may lead to infection.

The manifestations of cystitis result from congestion and inflammation of the bladder (vesical) mucosa. The patient complains of burning pain on urination and a desire to urinate frequently. The urine contains many bacteria and leukocytes. Cystitis is not usually a serious problem and generally responds promptly to antibiotics. Sometimes, however, the infection may spread into the upper urinary tract to affect the renal pelvis and kidney.

PYELONEPHRITIS

Most cases of pyelonephritis are secondary to spread of infection from the bladder (ascending pyelonephritis), but occasionally, the organisms are carried to the kidneys through the bloodstream (hematogenous pyelonephritis). The symptoms of pyelonephritis are those of an acute infection, together with localized pain and tenderness over the affected kidney. Histologically, the infected portion of the kidney is infiltrated by masses of leukocytes and bacteria, and many of the renal tubules in the inflamed area are filled with leukocytes (FIGURE 11). Because cystitis and pyelonephritis are frequently associated, the patient also experiences urinary frequency and pain on urination; the urine contains many bacteria and leukocytes. Treatment is with appropriate antibiotics, together with measures directed at correcting any abnormalities in the lower urinary tract that may impede drainage of urine and predispose to infection.

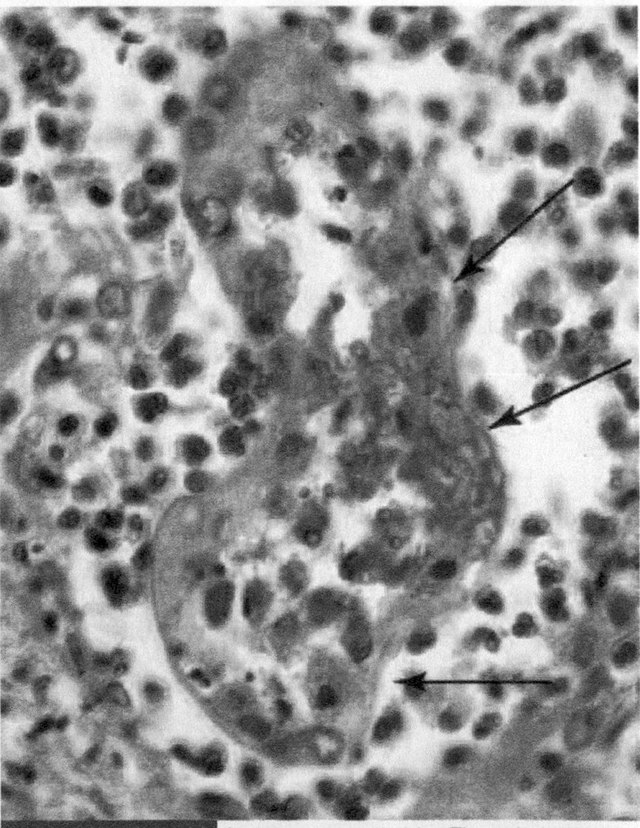

FIGURE 11 Acute pyelonephritis. The tubule in the center of field contains masses of bacteria that extend through wall of tubule (*middle arrow.*) Some tubule cells are necrotic (*upper and lower arrows*). Many neutrophils surround the tubules (original magnification × 400).

Most episodes of pyelonephritis respond promptly to treatment. If part of the kidney is severely damaged by the infection, the injured area heals by scarring. The main danger of pyelonephritis lies in the tendency of the disease to become chronic and recurrent. With each subsequent attack, more kidney tissue may be destroyed and healed by scarring. After many episodes of infection, the kidneys may become markedly scarred and shrunken, until the patient eventually exhibits manifestations of renal insufficiency.

VESICOURETERAL REFLUX AND INFECTION

Normally, effective mechanisms prevent urine from flowing upward from the bladder into the ureters during urination. Sometimes, however, these

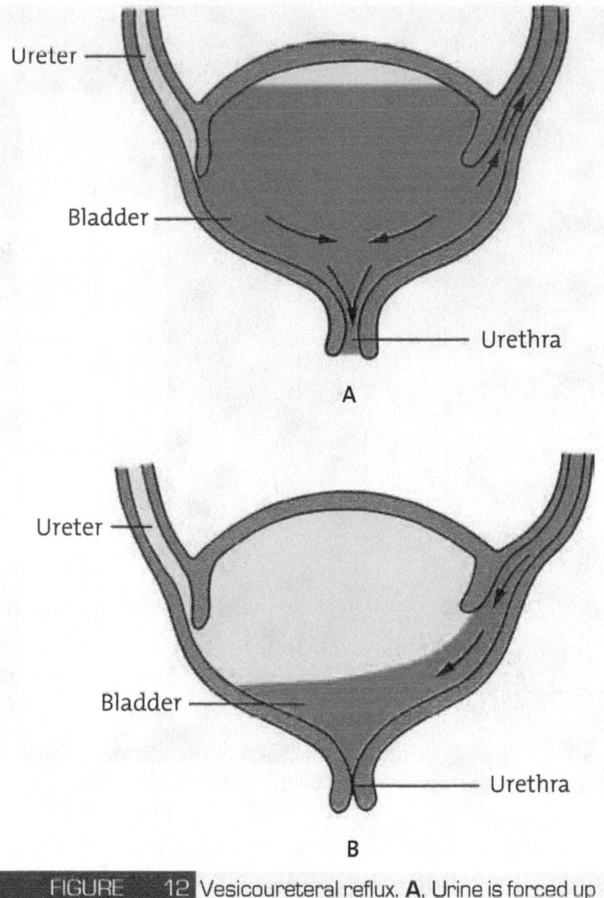

FIGURE 12 Vesicoureteral reflux. **A**, Urine is forced up one ureter during voiding (*right side* of illustration) because of defective function of the vesicoureteral valve. **B**, Urine flows back into bladder after voiding, which prevents complete emptying of bladder and predisposes to infection.

mechanisms are defective, permitting urine to flow retrograde (reflux) into one or both ureters when the bladder contracts during urination. This condition is called **vesicoureteral reflux.** It predisposes to urinary tract infection by preventing complete emptying of the bladder. The urine forced into the ureters during voiding flows back into the bladder at the completion of urination; so residual urine remains in the bladder (FIGURE 12). Bacteria also may be carried into the upper urinary tract by the reflux of urine; this predisposes to pyelonephritis.

Calculi

Stones may form anywhere in the urinary tract. They are usually called **calculi** (singular, calculus), which is a Latin word meaning "little stone" or "pebble." Most are composed either of uric acid or of a mixture of calcium salts. Three factors predispose to stone formation: increased concentration of salts in the urine, infection of the urinary tract, and urinary tract obstruction.

A greatly increased excretion of salts in the urine causes the urine to become supersaturated, and the salts may precipitate to form calculi, especially if the urine is concentrated. For example, in the disease called **gout** (discussion on the musculoskeletal system), excretion of uric acid is often greatly increased, which may cause uric acid to precipitate from the urine and form uric acid calculi. In conditions characterized by hyperfunction of the parathyroid glands, which regulate calcium metabolism (discussion on the endocrine glands), excessive calcium is excreted in the urine, often with the subsequent formation of urinary tract calculi composed of calcium salts.

Infection predisposes to calculi primarily by reducing the solubility of the salts in the urine. Clusters of bacteria also serve as sites where urinary salts may crystallize to form the stone.

Obstruction of the outflow of urine predisposes to stone formation by causing stagnation of urine, and urinary salts tend to precipitate out. Stagnation also predisposes to infection, which further increases the likelihood of stone formation.

Most calculi are small, but occasionally, they may gradually increase in size to form large branching structures that adopt the contour of the renal pelvis and calyces where they have formed. This kind of structure is called a **staghorn calculus** because it vaguely resembles the antlers of a male deer (FIGURE 13). Smaller stones sometimes pass into the ureter. The smooth muscle of the ureter contracts spasmodically to propel the stone along the ureter, causing **renal colic**—paroxysms of intense flank pain radiating into the groin. Frequently, the rough edges of the stone injure the lining of the ureter, causing red blood cells to appear in the urine. Many stones can be passed through the ureter and excreted in the urine, but some become impacted in the ureter and must be removed. A stone lodged in the distal ureter can usually be removed by inserting a cystoscope into the bladder and then passing a specially designed catheterlike instrument through the cystoscope into the

Vesicoureteral reflux
(ves′i-kō-ū r-ēt′er-al)
Retrograde flow of urine from the bladder into the ureter during voiding.

Calculus
A stone formed within the body, as in the kidney or gallbladder.

Gout
A disorder of nucleoprotein metabolism characterized by elevated uric acid and deposition of uric acid in and around joints.

Staghorn calculus
(kal′kū-lus)
A large renal calculus that has adopted the configuration of the renal pelvis and calyces where it formed.

Renal colic
Intense flank pain radiating into the groin, resulting from passage of a renal calculus into the ureter.

ureter. The instrument is constructed to snare the stone, which is then pulled through the ureter into the bladder and extracted through the cystoscope. A stone lodged in the proximal ureter is usually broken into fragments by a procedure called **shock wave lithotripsy**, a procedure that can break into small fragments a large stone that is too big to pass through the ureter so that the smaller pieces can be excreted in the urine instead of requiring a surgical procedure to remove the stone. The usual method for fragmenting a calculus involves positioning the recumbent patient on a specially designed table. Above the table is x-ray equipment capable of visualizing the location of the stone within the kidney. Below the table is a device called a lithotriptor, which can generate electrically produced shock waves capable of fragmenting the stone. When the exact location of the stone has been determined by x-ray examination, the shock wave–generating equipment is focused very precisely on the kidney stone, and shock waves directed at the stone fragment the stone into fine particles that are excreted in the urine.

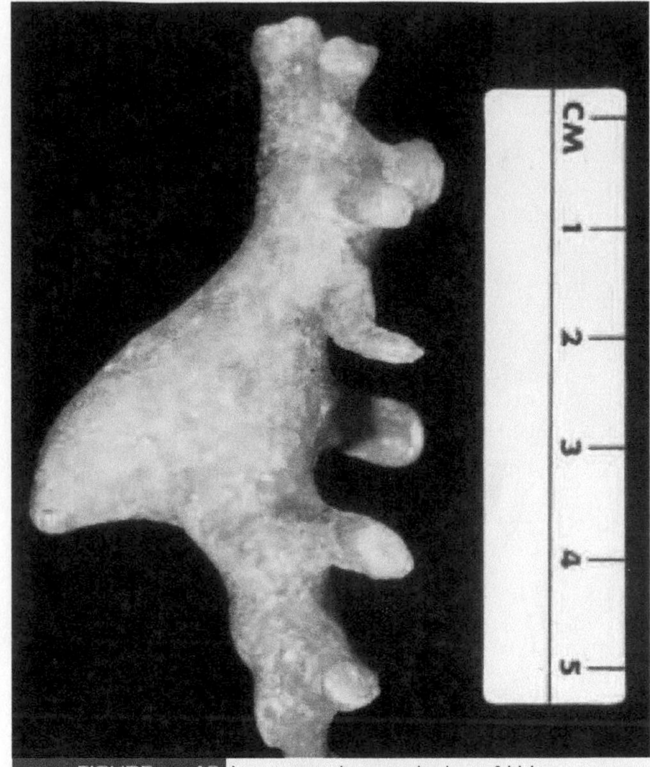

FIGURE 13 Large staghorn calculus of kidney.

Sometimes, stones form in the bladder. Usually, this stone formation is secondary to the combined effect of infection and stasis of urine, which decrease the solubility of dissolved salts in the urine. Sometimes bladder calculi can be removed through the bladder by means of a cystoscope. The stones are first broken up by an instrument passed through the cystoscope into the bladder and are then flushed out.

Shock wave lithotripsy (lith-o-trip′sē) *A method for removing stones from the urinary tract by breaking them into small bits that can be excreted in the urine.*

Foreign Bodies

It is not uncommon for people to insert various foreign bodies into the urethra and bladder either accidentally or as a means of sexual stimulation. Such objects must be removed because they may induce infection and may perforate the bladder wall. Frequently, the objects can be removed by means of a cystoscope passed into the bladder through the urethra. Sometimes, however, it is necessary to perform an operation in which the bladder is opened and the object is removed. The following two cases illustrate some of the clinical problems presented by intravesical (*intra* = within + *vesica* = bladder) foreign bodies (FIGURE 14).

CASE 3

An elderly woman was admitted to the hospital emergency room complaining of lower abdominal pain and burning on urination. An x-ray of the abdomen revealed a rectal thermometer lying horizontally within her bladder. A cystoscope was inserted into the bladder, and the thermometer was manipulated into a vertical position and then extracted through the urethra.

CASE 4

A 15-year-old boy inserted a long piece of stiff electrical wire into his bladder through his penis. The wire coiled within the bladder and could not be extracted. It was necessary to open the bladder and remove the wire through the bladder. Fortunately, neither the urethra nor the bladder were damaged by the wire, and the patient made an uneventful recovery.

Hydroureter
*A dilatation of the ureter secondary to obstruction of the urinary drainage system, often associated with coexisting dilatation of the renal pelvis and calyces (*hydronephrosis*).*

Hydronephrosis
(hydro-nef-rō′sis)
A dilatation of the urinary drainage tract proximal to the site of an obstruction.

Obstruction

In order for urine to be excreted normally, the urinary drainage system that transports the urine must permit free flow of urine. Obstruction or marked narrowing of the system at any point (stricture) causes the system proximal to the blockage to dilate progressively because of the pressure of the retained urine. Dilatation of the ureter is called **hydroureter**. Dilatation of the renal pelvis and calyces is called **hydronephrosis** (*hydro* = water + *nephros* = kidney + *osis* = condition) (FIGURE 15). The distention of the calyces and pelvis in turn causes progressive

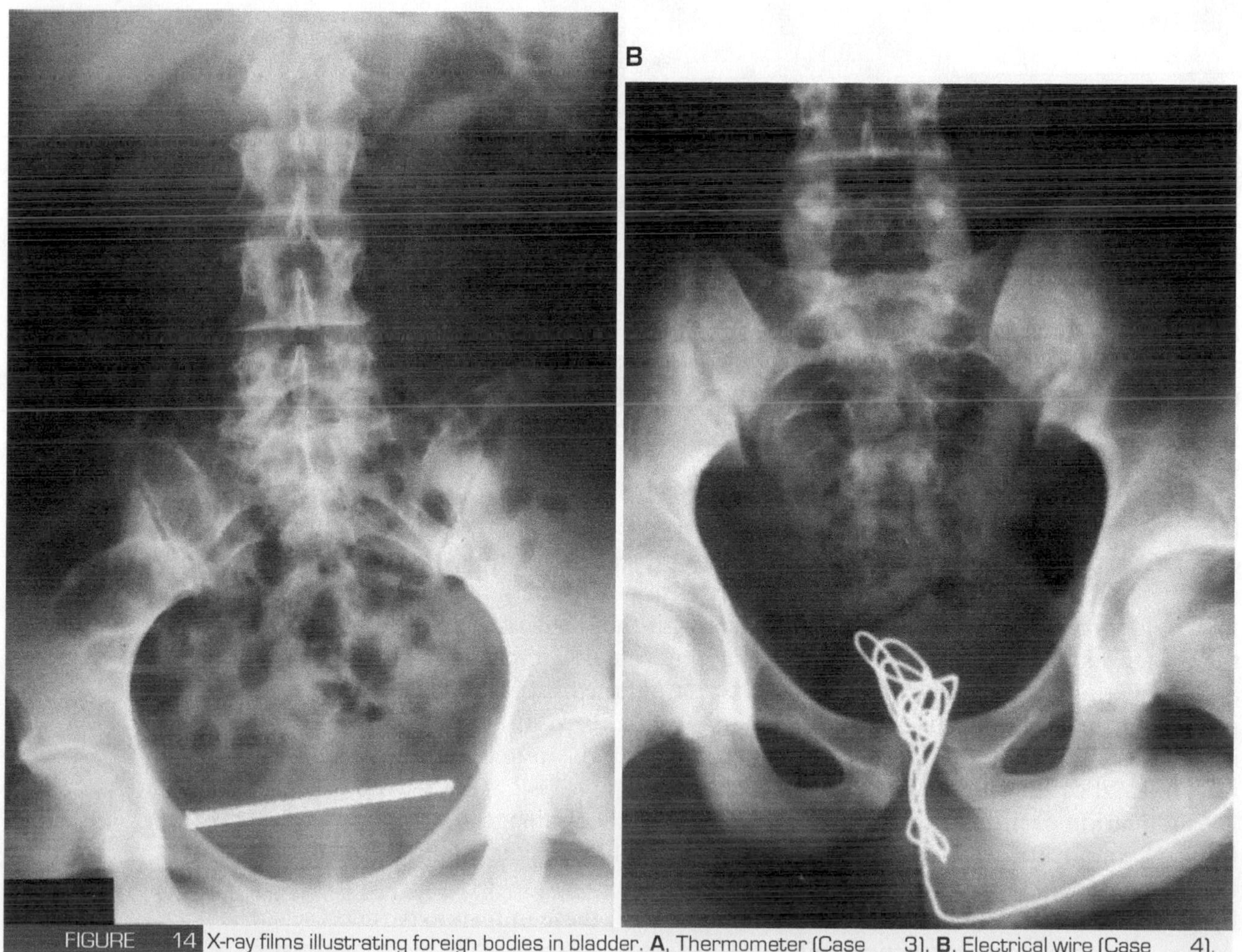

FIGURE 14 X-ray films illustrating foreign bodies in bladder. **A**, Thermometer (Case 3). **B**, Electrical wire (Case 4).

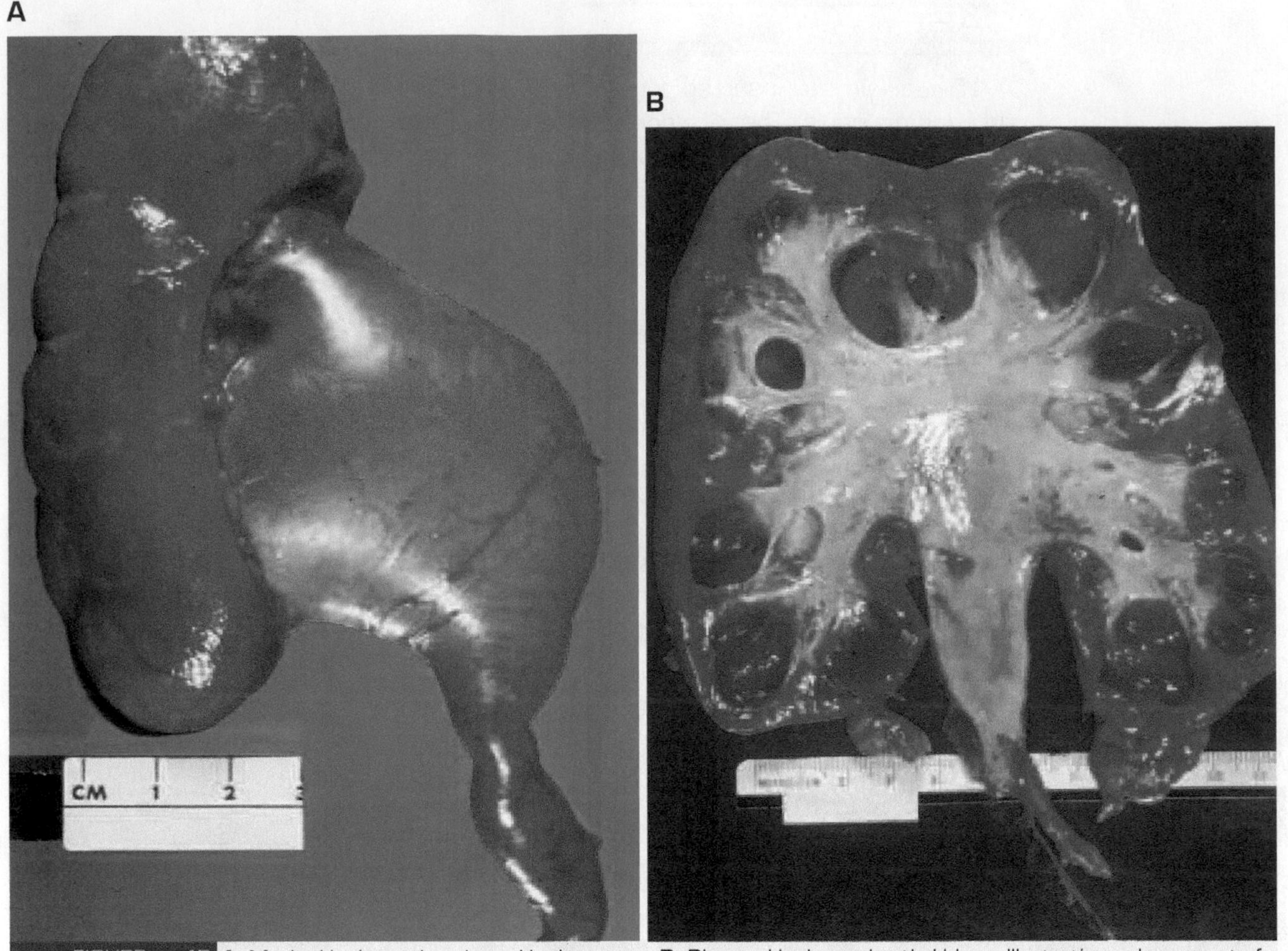

FIGURE 15 **A**, Marked hydronephrosis and hydroureter. **B**, Bisected hydronephrotic kidney, illustrating enlargement of calyces with atrophy of the renal parenchyma caused by the increased pressure exerted by the urine within the distended renal pelvis and calyces.

atrophy of the kidney on the affected side because of the high pressure of the urine within the obstructed drainage system. Eventually, if the obstruction is not relieved, the affected kidney is reduced to a thin shell of atrophic parenchyma covering the overdistended pelvis and calyces.

Which part of the drainage system is affected by the obstruction depends on the location of the block. Obstruction to the outflow of urine from the bladder, as by an enlarged prostate gland or stricture in the urethra, leads to bilateral hydronephrosis and hydroureter, as well as causing overdistention of the bladder (FIGURE 16A). Hydronephrosis and hydroureter are unilateral if the obstruction is located low in the ureter, as might be caused by an obstructing calculus impacted in the ureter or an obstructing tumor of the ureter (FIGURE 16B). If the obstruction is located at the junction of the renal pelvis and ureter, as might be caused by scarring of the ureter in this area, a unilateral hydronephrosis develops, but the ureter on the affected side is of normal caliber (FIGURE 16C).

Stagnation of urine secondary to obstruction of the drainage system may lead to further complications. Stagnation predisposes to infection and to stone formation caused by precipitation of urinary salts. A cycle may become established in which hydronephrosis leads to infection and urinary calculi; these in turn may increase the degree of urinary tract obstruction and cause further progression of the hydronephrosis.

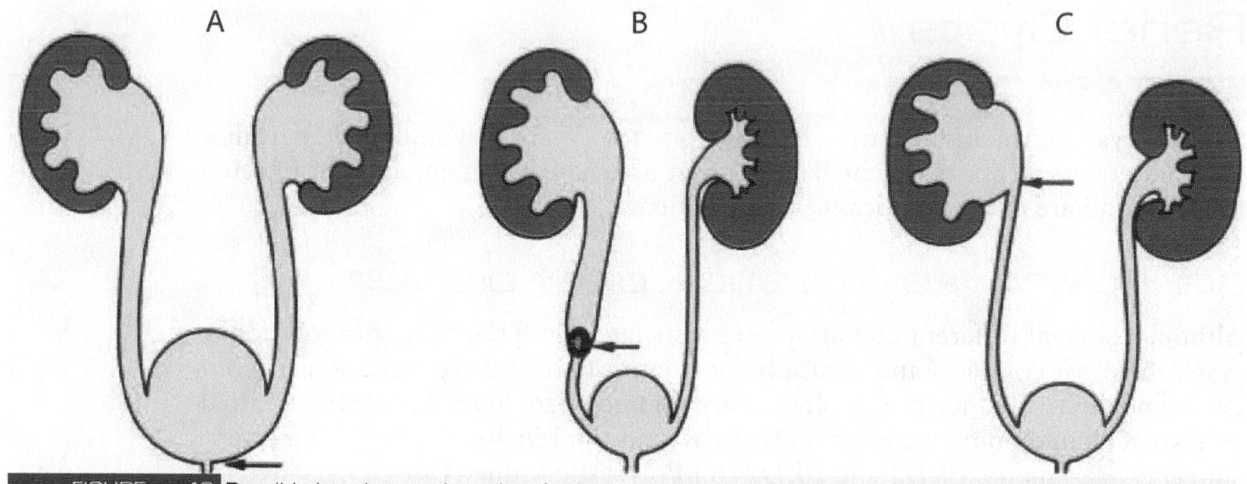

FIGURE 16 Possible locations and results of urinary tract obstruction. The *arrows* indicate sites of obstruction. **A**, Bilateral hydronephrosis and hydroureter with distention of the bladder caused by urethral obstruction. **B**, Unilateral hydroureter and hydronephrosis caused by obstruction of the distal ureter. **C**, Unilateral hydronephrosis caused by obstruction at the ureteropelvic junction.

Diagnosis of urinary tract obstruction is usually made by means of a pyelogram or by CT scan (procedures described in the discussion on general concepts of disease: principles of diagnosis). These procedures demonstrate the dilatation of the urinary tract. Treatment is directed toward relieving the obstruction by appropriate means before the kidneys are irreparably damaged.

Renal Tubular Injury

The blood supply to the renal tubules is derived from the efferent glomerular artery, and minor degrees of tubular injury are seen in many diseases affecting the renal glomeruli. Renal tubular injury in the absence of glomerular disease may be encountered in two situations: tubular necrosis as a result of impaired renal blood flow and tubular necrosis caused by toxic drugs and chemicals. Any condition associated with shock and marked drop in the blood pressure leads to impaired blood flow to the kidneys, which often causes degeneration and necrosis of renal tubules. Many drugs and chemicals that are ingested or absorbed by the body are excreted by the kidneys. Thus, they may cause direct toxic injury to the tubular epithelium.

Acute tubular necrosis causes severe impairment of renal function characterized by a marked decrease in urine output (oliguria) or complete suppression of urine formation (anuria). This condition is called acute renal failure. The reason why urine output is reduced is not well understood. Apparently, marked constriction of renal arterioles reduces blood flow to the kidneys and decreases glomerular filtration. Other factors also may contribute to the reduction of urine output. Many of the tubules are blocked by casts and necrotic debris. The damaged tubular epithelium also has lost its capacity for selective tubular reabsorption, and the glomerular filtrate diffuses back through the damaged tubular epithelium into the adjacent peritubular blood vessels. After a period of several weeks, tubular function is slowly restored by regeneration of the damaged epithelium, but several months may be required before renal function returns completely to normal. During the period of acute renal failure, waste products must be removed from the blood by means of dialysis (described in a later section) until tubular function has been restored.

Renal Cysts

SOLITARY CYSTS

Solitary cysts of the kidney are relatively common. They vary in diameter from a few millimeters to about 15 cm. They are not associated with impairment of renal function and are of no significance to the patient.

CONGENITAL POLYCYSTIC KIDNEY DISEASE

Although several different conditions are associated with the formation of kidney cysts, the most common and clinically most important of these conditions is congenital polycystic kidney disease. It is a very common hereditary disease transmitted as a Mendelian dominant trait that affects as many as 1 in 400 persons. Two different genes, designated *PKD1* and *PKD2* (for **P**olycystic **K**idney **D**isease), located on separate chromosomes are involved. About 85% of cases result from mutation of *PKD1*. In most of the others, the mutation involves *PKD2*, which is associated with later onset and slower progression of the disease. A few unfortunate persons have mutations of both *PKD1* and *PKD2*, which causes severe and rapidly progressive disease. The disease is characterized by disturbed proliferation of tubular epithelial cells, leading to the formation of cysts that become detached from the tubules. The epithelium lining the cysts secretes fluid that accumulates within the cysts and causes them to enlarge. As the cysts gradually increase in size, they cause progressive enlargement of both kidneys, where they compress and destroy adjacent renal tissue. Eventually, almost no normal kidney tissue remains, and renal failure supervenes (FIGURE 17). Sometimes small numbers of cysts also form in the liver, but usually they do not disturb liver function. Some affected persons also have small cystlike outpouchings extending from the cerebral arteries at the base of the brain, which are called congenital cerebral aneurysms. Because congenital cerebral aneurysms may rupture and cause a brain hemorrhage, some physicians have advocated routine magnetic resonance screening of all patients with autosomal dominant polycystic kidney disease, but the Mayo Clinic experience favors more limited screening only in a select group of polycystic kidney patients (see the reference by Torres and others in the list of Supplementary Readings). Congenital aneurysms and their complications are described in the discussion on the nervous system.

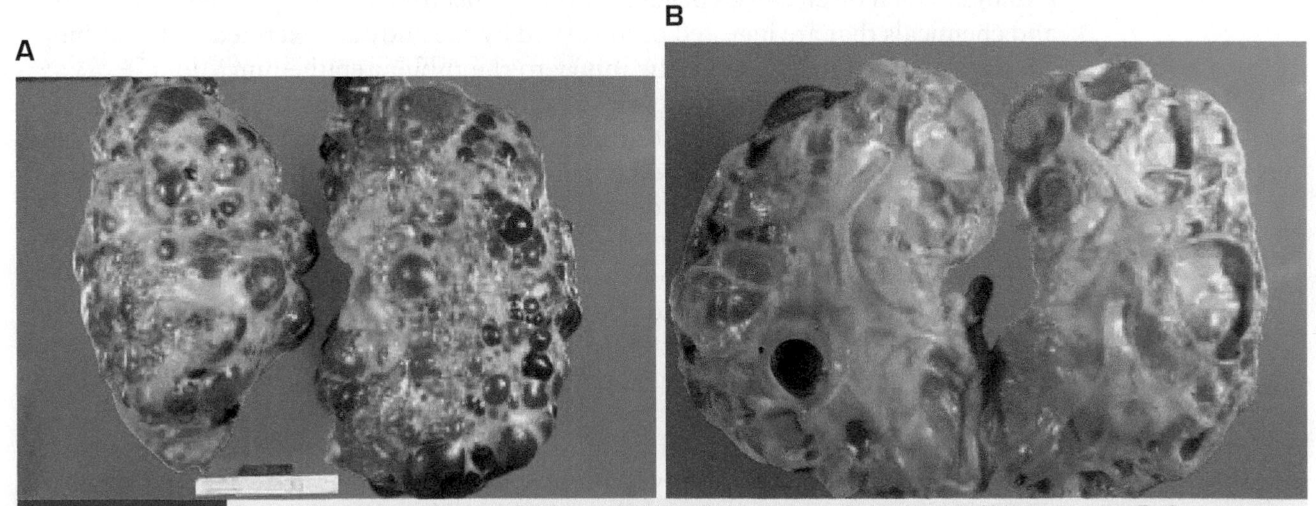

FIGURE 17 **A**, Greatly enlarged abnormal kidneys characteristic of congenital polycystic kidney disease. **B**, Cut surfaces of diseased kidneys, illustrating multiple large cysts. No normal renal tissue remains.

Because renal tissue is destroyed slowly, renal insufficiency does not usually occur until the patient reaches middle age, and some patients do not experience problems until they are in their 60s. Many persons with congenital polycystic kidney disease are free of symptoms until onset of renal failure, but some experience periodic urinary tract infections or episodes of bloody urine (hematuria) caused by bleeding into one of the enlarging cysts. Some patients also develop hypertension, which often accompanies renal failure.

Polycystic kidney disease can often be suspected by physical examination, which reveals the greatly enlarged kidneys. The diagnosis can be confirmed in several ways. Ultrasound examination or CT scan of the abdomen reveals the large cystic kidneys. An intravenous pyelogram (IVP) reveals the distortion of the pelves and calyces caused by the cysts. There is no specific treatment. When the kidneys fail, dialysis treatments or a kidney transplant may be required.

The following case illustrates some of the characteristic features of congenital polycystic kidney disease.

CASE 5

A 67-year-old man was admitted to the hospital after having sustained a severe heart attack. Marked enlargement of both kidneys was detected on physical examination, and there was also clinical and laboratory evidence of severe renal insufficiency. The patient had seven brothers and sisters, four of whom had died between the ages of 40 and 60 of renal failure as a result of congenital polycystic kidneys. The patient eventually died in the hospital of heart failure in conjunction with chronic renal failure. The autopsy revealed greatly enlarged polycystic kidneys. There were also a few cysts within the liver.

Tumors of the Urinary Tract

Tumors may arise from the epithelium of the renal tubules in the cortex of the kidney, from the transitional epithelium lining the urinary tract, or rarely from remnants of embryonic tissue within the kidney.

RENAL CORTICAL TUMORS

Benign tumors called renal cortical adenomas sometimes arise within the kidney. Usually, a benign adenoma is small, well circumscribed, located within the renal cortex, and can be removed by a limited resection. Some well-differentiated kidney carcinomas are also slowly growing, well-circumscribed tumors confined to the renal cortex, which can be removed along with adjacent normal kidney tissue without removing the entire kidney (partial nephrectomy). Unfortunately, less well-differentiated carcinomas are larger, grow more rapidly, extend into the renal medulla, and exhibit aggressive behavior (FIGURE 18). Often, the first manifestation of an aggressive carcinoma is blood in the urine (hematuria) as a result of ulceration of the epithelium of the pelvis or calyces caused by the growing tumor. Often, the tumor eventually invades the renal vein and gives rise to distant metastases. The tumor can be diagnosed by means of a pyelogram (discussion on general concepts of disease: principles of diagnosis), which reveals the distortion of the pelvis and calyces caused by the tumor, or by means of the CT scan, which demonstrates a mass within the kidney. Treatment is by resection of the kidney (nephrectomy).

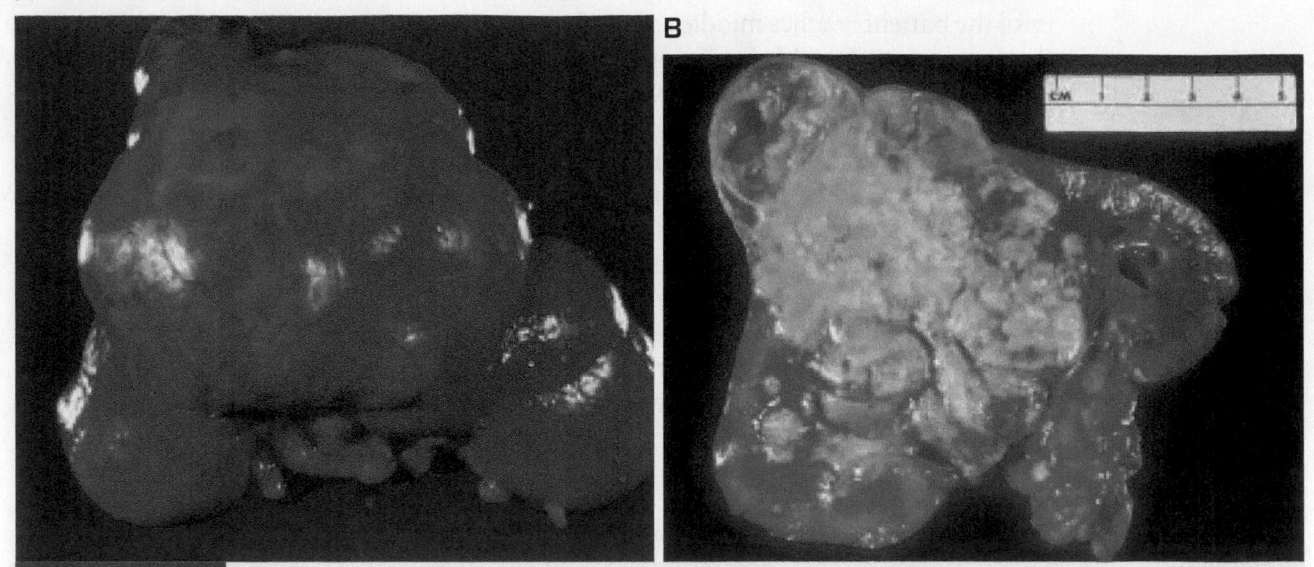

FIGURE 18 Large renal cortical carcinoma. **A**, External surface. **B**, Longitudinal section of kidney and tumor.

TRANSITIONAL CELL TUMORS

Almost all tumors arising from the transitional epithelium of the urinary tract are malignant and are called transitional cell carcinomas. Most arise from bladder epithelium, are of low-grade malignancy, and carry a good prognosis. The tumors are often quite vascular, and they tend to bleed; so hematuria may be the first manifestation of the neoplasm. Bladder tumors can be visualized by means of a cystoscope inserted into the bladder through the urethra and often can be resected by means of a similar type of instrument inserted through the urethra. Sometimes it is necessary to resect part of the bladder in order to remove the tumor completely.

NEPHROBLASTOMA (WILMS TUMOR)

An unusual highly malignant tumor composed of primitive cells sometimes arises in the kidney of infants and young children. Histologically, the tumor bears some resemblance to the structure of an embryonic kidney and is called a nephroblastoma or Wilms tumor. The neoplasm often metastasizes widely. Treatment is by nephrectomy followed by radiotherapy and anticancer chemotherapy.

Diagnostic Evaluation of Kidney and Urinary Tract Disease

A variety of methods are used to detect disease of the kidneys and urinary tract, to evaluate the degree to which renal function is disturbed, and to define the type of disease present.

URINALYSIS

The most widely used diagnostic test is an examination of the urine, which is called a **urinalysis**. The examination is useful for detecting whether urinary tract disease is present and for detecting other systemic diseases that alter renal function. The examination includes determinations of urine pH (acidity) and specific gravity (a measure

Urinalysis
(ur-in-al′i-sis)
A commonly performed chemical and microscopic analysis of the urine.

of urine concentration) and simple tests for glucose and protein. The urinalysis may also include tests for bile pigment, acetone, and other constituents that may appear in the urine in association with various diseases. A sample of the urine is also centrifuged, and the sediment is examined microscopically. If the urinalysis is normal, renal disease is unlikely. Alternatively, the presence of red cells and protein in the urine may indicate that damage to the glomerular filter has permitted these substances to leak into the glomerular filtrate or that bleeding is occurring somewhere in the urinary tract. Renal casts, which are collections of protein and cells molded into the shape of the kidney tubules, are an indication of glomerular disease. Leukocytes and bacteria in the urinary sediment indicate urinary tract infection.

Additional tests may be performed on the urine as indicated by the patient's clinical condition. If a urinary tract infection is suspected, for example, the urine is cultured for pathogenic bacteria and sensitivity tests are performed if bacteria are present.

CLEARANCE TESTS

Clearance test
(klēr′ans)
A test of renal function that measures the ability of kidneys to remove (clear) a substance from the blood and excrete it in the urine.

Impairment of renal function can be recognized by measuring the concentration in the blood of various substances, such as urea and creatinine, which are waste products excreted by the kidneys. Elevated levels indicate impaired renal function, and the degree of elevation is a measure of the degree of impairment. Even before elevated levels of waste products are present in the blood, impaired renal function can be detected by means of renal function tests called **clearance tests**. Clearance tests provide a rough estimate of the degree of kidney damage, and periodic clearance tests can be used to follow the progress of renal disease. A gradual fall in the renal clearance of a substance means that renal function is declining.

Clearance tests measure the ability of the kidneys to remove various substances from the blood and excrete them in the urine. To determine the clearance of a substance, one calculates how much blood plasma must flow through the kidney each minute and be completely cleared of the substance in order to provide the quantity of the substance that appears in the urine within the same period of time. For example, if the concentration of a substance in the plasma is 1 mg per milliliter (mg/ml) and 50 mg of the substance is excreted in the urine in 1 minute, then 50 ml of blood must flow through the kidneys each minute and be cleared of the substance to obtain a urinary excretion of 50 mg per minute (mg/min).

Clearance is expressed in milliliters of plasma cleared of the constituent per minute and is expressed by the following formula:

$$\text{Clearance} = \frac{UV}{P}$$

where U is the concentration of the substance excreted in milligrams per milliliter of urine; V is the volume of urine excreted, expressed in milliliters per minute; and P is the concentration of the substance in the plasma expressed in milligrams per milliliter.

Creatinine
(krē-at′in-ēn)
A waste product derived from the breakdown of a compound present in muscle (phosphocreatine) that is excreted in the urine.

The most frequently used clearance test measures the clearance of the waste product **creatinine**, which is derived from the breakdown of a compound present in muscle, called phosphocreatine. In the original method used to determine creatinine clearance, the urine output is measured for a specific period of time and the average output per minute is calculated. The concentrations of creatinine in the urine and in the blood also are determined, and clearance is calculated by means of the standard formula. For example, if the urine output is 2 ml/min, the concentration of creatinine in the urine is 0.15 mg/ml, and the concentration of creatinine in the blood is 0.003 mg/ml, the creatinine clearance is

$$\frac{UV}{P} = \frac{0.15 \times 2}{0.003} = \frac{0.3}{0.003} = 100 \text{ ml/min}$$

The test result, expressed as milliliters of plasma cleared of creatinine per minute, represents the glomerular filtration rate. Although simple in principle, the test is rather cumbersome in practice and also had some other disadvantages. Now the clearance is usually determined from a formula using the serum creatinine, along with the person's age, gender, and lean body weight, as illustrated in the formula:

$$\text{Creatinine clearance} = \frac{(140 - \text{age in years}) \times (\text{lean body weight in kilograms})}{72 \times \text{serum creatinine in mg/dl}}$$

For women, in whom the clearance is lower than in men, the result is multiplied by 0.85 to take into account the slightly lower clearance rate in women. The normal creatinine clearance is 85–105 ml per minute. It is not necessary to remember the formula or perform the calculations as long one understands what the test is measuring and its significance.

ADDITIONAL TECHNIQUES

Many other specialized procedures can be used to study the kidneys and urinary tract, including various x-ray examinations, ultrasound examinations, and cystoscopy. These examinations are described in the discussion on general concepts of disease: principles of diagnosis. Their specific diagnostic applications have also been considered in conjunction with the various renal and urinary tract diseases in which they provide useful information. X-ray examination of the abdomen, for example, can identify the size and location of the kidneys and can detect radiopaque calculi in the kidneys or urinary tract. CT scans and pyelograms can detect anatomic abnormalities within the kidneys, such as cysts and tumors, and many abnormalities of the urinary drainage system, such as hydronephrosis. Other specialized procedures using radioisotopes can measure renal blood flow and renal excretory function. Renal arteriograms, with the use of techniques similar to those used to study the coronary arteries, can determine the caliber of the renal arteries, can detect segmental areas of narrowing in the renal arteries, and can identify areas of increased vascularity within the kidney, which often occur when a tumor is present.

Sometimes the clinician cannot make an exact diagnosis concerning the type of renal disease without resorting to biopsy of the kidney. This can be accomplished without undue difficulty or serious risk to the patient by introducing a small biopsy needle through the skin of the flank directly into the substance of the kidney. A small bit of kidney tissue is removed for histologic study. Examination of the biopsy material by the pathologist often permits an exact diagnosis as to the nature and extent of the renal disease, which serves as a guide to proper treatment.

Renal Failure (Uremia)

Renal failure is an inability of the kidneys to adequately perform their normal regulatory and excretory functions. Function may decline rapidly, which is called acute renal failure, or slowly but progressively, which is called chronic renal failure.

ACUTE RENAL FAILURE

This condition results from necrosis of renal tubules caused by impairment of blood flow to the kidney or by the effects of toxic drugs that damage the kidney tubules, as described previously in the section dealing with renal tubular injury.

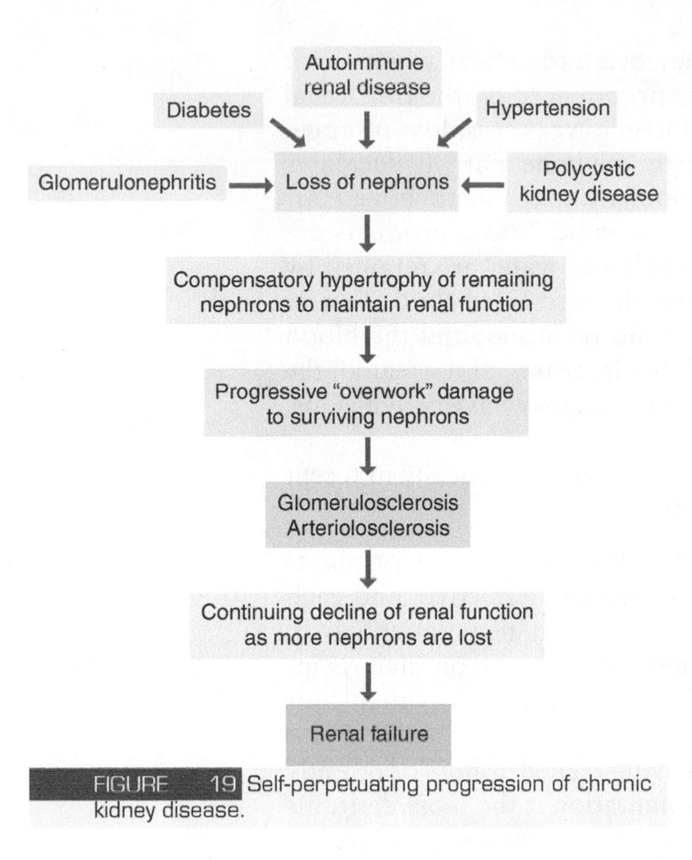

FIGURE 19 Self-perpetuating progression of chronic kidney disease.

CHRONIC RENAL FAILURE

In contrast to acute renal failure, this condition is a gradual deterioration of renal function resulting from chronic renal disease. Approximately 50–75% of all cases of chronic renal failure result from diabetes and hypertension. Chronic pyelonephritis, congenital polycystic renal disease, chronic glomerulonephritis, and autoimmune diseases involving the kidney account for most of the remainder.

A normal kidney contains about one million nephrons. In chronic renal failure, renal function declines as the population of nephrons decreases, although relatively normal renal function can be maintained until the number of functioning nephrons falls below 20–30% of normal. Unfortunately, all types of chronic renal disease tend to progress because of the way the surviving nephrons respond to the declining renal function (FIGURE 19). The surviving nephrons are forced to "work harder" in order to accomplish the functions previously performed by a full complement of nephrons. Each of the remaining nephrons receives a larger volume of blood to process at a higher than normal pressure. The high blood volumes and pressures damage the arterioles and glomerular capillaries, which leads to thickening of the walls of glomerular arterioles with narrowing of their lumens (arteriolosclerosis) along with glomerular capillary injury followed by scarring (glomerulosclerosis). The tubules are also damaged because the blood vessels that supply the glomeruli also supply the tubules. Consequently, a vicious cycle is created in which the reduced number of functioning nephrons indirectly damages the overworked surviving nephrons, many of which become scarred and cease to function. As more nephrons are lost, an additional burden is placed on those that still survive, which eventually causes many of them to fail. As this process continues, progressively more nephrons are lost at an increasing rate, until eventually renal function deteriorates to the point where the kidneys are no longer able to perform their regulatory and excretory functions. The patient experiences severe derangements of fluid, electrolyte, and acid–base balance. Various acids that would normally be excreted by the kidneys are retained, which disturbs the normal pH of body fluids, leading to a condition called metabolic acidosis described in the discussion on water, electrolyte, and acid–base balance. The failing kidneys cannot produce erythropoietin to stimulate bone marrow function, and the patient becomes anemic. Renal failure is sometimes called **uremia**. This term refers to the characteristic retention of urea in the blood when the kidneys fail. **Urea** is a normal by-product of protein metabolism and is excreted in the urine. It is not a toxic compound and is only one of many substances that accumulates in the blood when the kidneys fail. The amount of urea in the blood, however, correlates with the degree of retention of other waste products and with the clinical manifestations of deteriorating renal function. Therefore, measurement of the concentration of urea in the blood (blood urea nitrogen test or BUN) provides a rough estimate of the severity of the kidney failure. Another commonly used measure of renal functional impairment is the level of creatinine in the blood.

Uremia
(ur-ē′mi-yuh)
An excess of urea and other waste products in the blood, resulting from renal failure.

Urea
(ū-re′yuh)
The nitrogen waste product derived from protein metabolism and excreted in the urine.

Symptoms of renal failure are nonspecific. They begin to appear when about 80% of renal function has been lost and are quite pronounced by the time renal function has fallen to 5% of normal. Symptoms include weakness, loss of appetite, nausea, and vomiting. Production of red cells by the bone marrow decreases because the failing kidneys cannot produce erythropoietin to stimulate bone marrow function, and the patient becomes moderately anemic. Waste products are not eliminated and increase to toxic levels. Excess salt and water are retained by the failing kidneys, resulting in weight gain as a result of retained fluid ("water weight"). The blood volume increases because of fluid retention, and the blood pressure also tends to rise as the intravascular volume increases. If untreated, the patient in chronic renal failure eventually lapses into coma, may have convulsions, and eventually dies.

The outlook for patients with renal failure has improved dramatically in recent years because of two effective methods of treatment:

1. Hemodialysis and peritoneal dialysis, which remove waste products from the patient's blood. Both methods are equally effective, and each has advantages and disadvantages. Every year, many new patients with advanced renal disease begin dialysis. Some will continue on dialysis indefinitely. Others will rely on dialysis until a kidney becomes available for transplantation.
2. Renal transplantation, using kidneys from living related donors or recently deceased persons (cadaver donors). Transplantation is the most desirable option; however, kidneys for transplantation are in very short supply.

HEMODIALYSIS

Hemodialysis substitutes for the functions of the kidneys. Waste products from the patient's blood diffuse across a semipermeable membrane into a solution (the dialysate) on the other side of the membrane. The rate of diffusion is determined by several factors: the concentration of the substances on the two sides of the membrane, the rate of blood flow and flow of the dialysate through the dialyzer, and the characteristics of the dialyzer membrane. Waste products, which are present in high concentrations in the patient's blood, diffuse from the blood into the dialysate because of differences in the concentration on the two sides of the membrane. Usually, the patient's blood is dialyzed by an "artificial kidney" machine. This type of hemodialysis is called extracorporeal hemodialysis (*extra* = outside + *corpus* = body) because the blood is transported outside the patient's body for dialysis in the artificial kidney and then returned by means of a system of tubes connected to the patient's circulatory system.

Hemodialysis (hēm-ō-dī-al′i-sis) *A dialysis procedure by which waste products are removed from the blood of patients in chronic renal failure, usually by means of an artificial kidney machine.*

Hemodialysis is usually performed in an outpatient dialysis center 3 times per week for 3 or 4 hours during each dialysis session, but it can be performed at home with the assistance of a family member who has been given special training along with the patient. The patient's blood flows along one side of a synthetic semipermeable membrane that restricts the passage of blood cells and protein but permits the passage of water and small molecules. The dialysate flows on the other side of the membrane in a direction opposite to the flow of blood. This type of flow pattern, which is called countercurrent dialysis (*counter* = against + *current* = blood flow), promotes more efficient removal of waste products than when dialysate and blood flow in the same direction.

During dialysis, plastic tubes connect the patient's circulation to the dialyzer in the artificial kidney machine. One tube transmits blood to the dialyzer unit where the blood is cleansed and excess fluid is removed, and the other tube conveys the blood from the dialyzer back to the patient's circulation. Before dialysis begins, the clotting time of the patient's blood is prolonged by administration of heparin to prevent the blood from clotting as it flows through the dialyzer.

In order to perform hemodialysis on a regular basis, one of the patient's arteries and a large vein must be easily accessible so that the tubes that transport blood to and from the dialyzer unit can easily be connected to the patient's blood vessels. Although several methods have been devised to gain access to the patient's circulation, the preferred method consists of surgically interconnecting the radial artery in the wrist and an adjacent vein, forming an artificial communication called an arteriovenous fistula (FIGURE 20A). After the fistula has been created, arterial blood is short-circuited directly into the vein instead of flowing through the peripheral capillaries. The vein, which now receives blood directly under high pressure, becomes much larger and develops a thick wall.

After it has been determined that long-term dialysis will be needed, the arteriovenous fistula is created several months before the first dialysis treatment so that the vein has time to enlarge and thicken. When the vein has become suitable for use, dialysis treatments are begun. Two needles are inserted through the skin directly

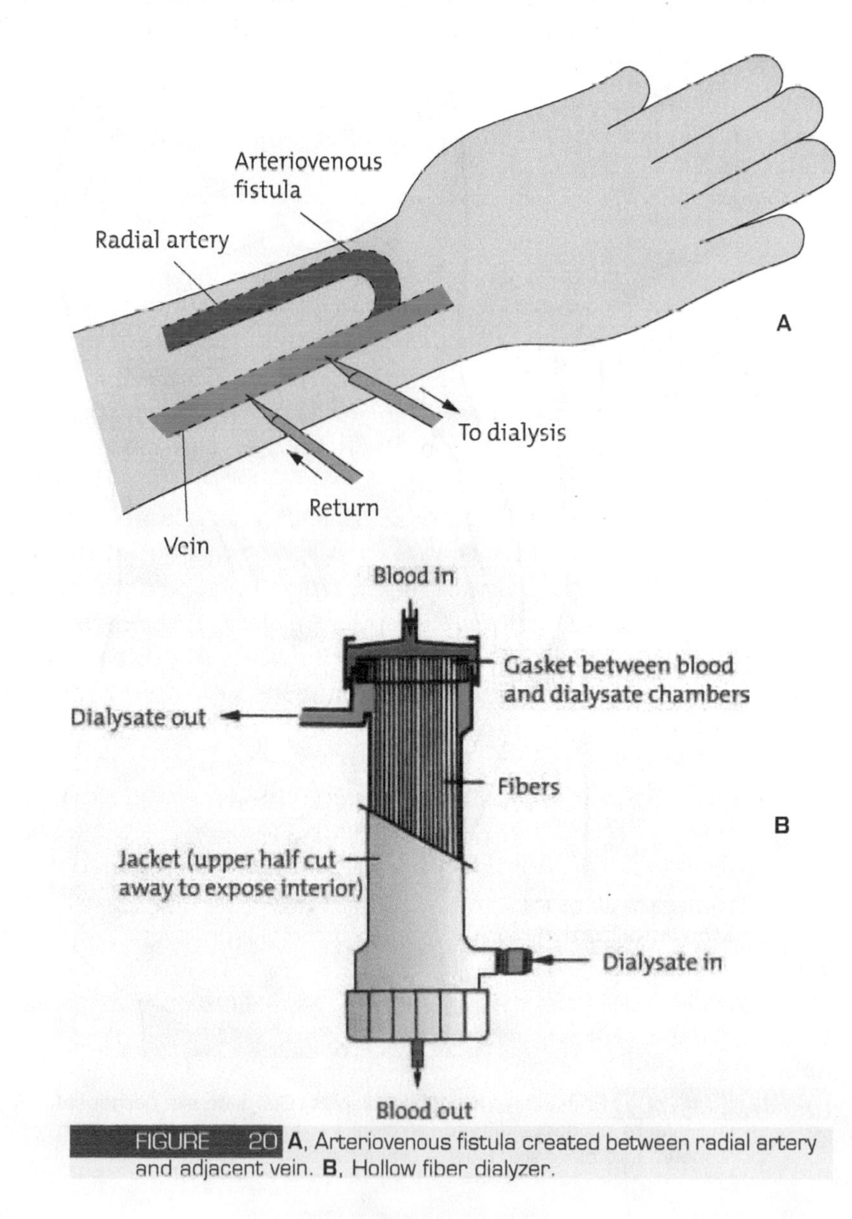

FIGURE 20 **A**, Arteriovenous fistula created between radial artery and adjacent vein. **B**, Hollow fiber dialyzer.

into the vein. One needle is attached to the tube that delivers blood to the dialyzer, and the second needle is attached to the tube that returns the blood to the patient (FIGURE 20A). Less commonly, other procedures are used to gain access to the patient's circulation for dialysis.

There are many types of artificial kidney machines. Many are quite compact, and portable units are available. Improvements in the design and operation of the machines are being made continually. The essential component of the artificial kidney machine is the dialyzer. Attached to it are the tubes that carry blood to and from the patient and the tubes that carry dialysate to and from the unit. A hollow fiber dialyzer, which is quite compact and efficient and is the most commonly used type, consists of a bundle of hollow synthetic fibers through which the blood passes. The dialysate circulates around the outside of the fibers in the opposite direction (FIGURE 20B).

PERITONEAL DIALYSIS

Peritoneal dialysis uses the patient's own peritoneum as the dialyzing membrane (FIGURE 21). In order to perform peritoneal dialysis, a large plastic tube must first be inserted into the patient's abdominal (peritoneal) cavity and fixed in position by

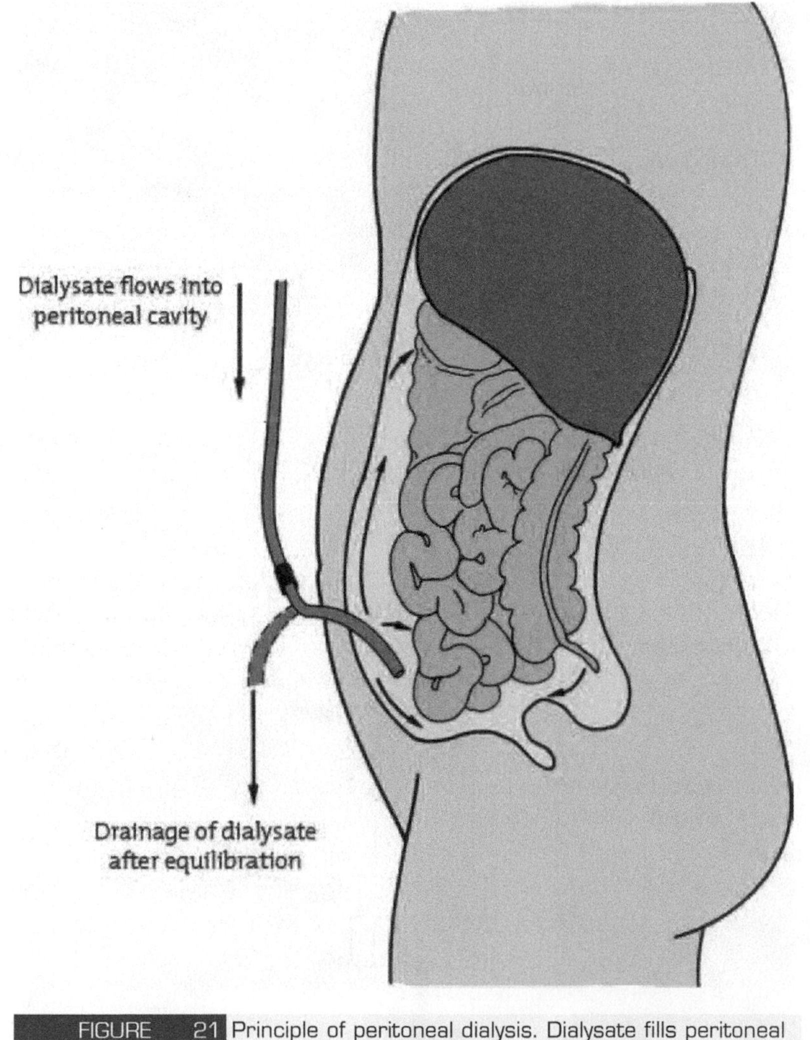

FIGURE 21 Principle of peritoneal dialysis. Dialysate fills peritoneal cavity. Waste products diffuse (*arrows*) from blood vessels beneath peritoneum into dialysate. Fluid is drained after equilibration.

suturing it to the skin. The dialysis procedure consists of instilling several liters of dialysis fluid through the tube into the peritoneal cavity and allowing the fluid to remain within the peritoneal cavity for a variable time. During this time, waste products diffuse across the peritoneum from the underlying blood vessels into the dialysis fluid that fills the peritoneal cavity. Dialysis fluid is then withdrawn and fresh fluid is instilled. Peritoneal dialysis can be performed by means of an automated system in which the machine automatically fills and drains the peritoneal cavity at night while the patient is asleep. Another similar method is called continuous ambulatory peritoneal dialysis. In this procedure, 2 liters of fluid remain within the peritoneal cavity all the time. The patient replaces the fluid with fresh dialysis fluid four or five times a day. Patients carry out their usual activities when they are not draining and refilling their peritoneal cavities.

Peritoneal dialysis is used less frequently than extracorporeal hemodialysis. Not all patients requiring dialysis are suitable candidates for peritoneal dialysis, but the procedure offers an advantage to patients who wish to continue working full time or part time, as they do not have to spend several daytime hours 3 days each week at a dialysis center, and many patients who choose peritoneal dialysis are quite satisfied with their choice. However, peritoneal dialysis has disadvantages. It is less efficient at removing waste products and carries some risk of peritonitis, which can result if bacteria gain access to the peritoneal cavity around the tube that extends from the skin surface directly into the peritoneal cavity.

RENAL TRANSPLANTATION

When the kidneys fail, a normal compatible kidney sometimes can be transplanted from a close relative, an unrelated volunteer donor, or a recently deceased person (cadaver donor). The best results are obtained from a living kidney donor.

In any kidney transplantation, the transplanted kidney must be matched as closely as possible with the donor in order to give the transplant the best chance of survival in the recipient. The ABO blood group antigens of the proposed donor must be compatible with the blood group antibodies in the blood of the proposed recipient because the ABO blood group antigens are present in body tissues (including the kidney) as well as red cells. For example, one could not give a kidney from a group A donor to a group O recipient because the recipient's blood contains anti-A and anti-B antibodies that would attack and destroy the donor kidney. The principles are the same as when selecting blood for a blood transfusion.

The next group of important antigens are the HLA antigens. Unless the transplanted kidney comes from an identical twin whose tissues contain identical HLA antigens, the transplant will invariably contain foreign HLA antigens that the patient lacks. (The HLA system is considered in chromosomes, genes, and cell devision discussion.) Consequently, the patient's immunologic defenses will respond to the foreign antigens and attempt to destroy (reject) the foreign kidney unless the patient's immune system is suppressed by drugs or other agents (discussion on immunity, hypersensitivity, allergy, and autoimmune diseases).

The likelihood that a transplanted ABO blood group compatible kidney will survive depends on how closely the HLA antigens match those of the patient. The more closely they resemble one another, the better the chances of survival. More than 90% of transplanted kidneys survive for 5 years when the transplanted kidney is obtained from a close relative whose HLA antigens very closely resemble those of the patient. The survival rate of cadaver transplants has improved greatly in recent years and now is almost as good as transplants from living related donors.

In the transplant operation, the transplanted kidney is usually placed in the iliac area outside the peritoneal cavity. The renal artery of the transplanted kidney is connected to the internal iliac (hypogastric) artery. The renal vein is connected to the iliac vein, and the ureter is connected to the bladder (FIGURE 22). In the great majority of patients, the transplant is successful and "takes over" for the patient's own nonfunctional kidneys. Some patients, however, reject the transplant despite intensive immunosuppressive therapy. Most rejections occur within the first few months after transplantation. Should this occur, the patient resumes dialysis treatments until another kidney suitable for transplantation becomes available.

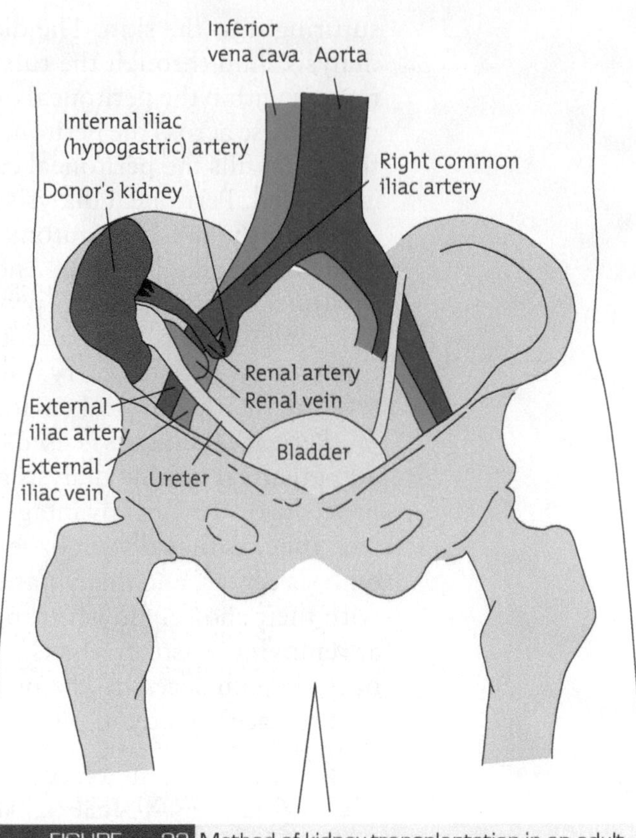

FIGURE 22 Method of kidney transplantation in an adult. A transplanted kidney is placed in the iliac region. Artery and vein of transplant are connected to patient's iliac artery and vein, and the ureter of the transplant is connected to the bladder.

Although a well-functioning transplanted kidney permits the patient to lead a relatively normal life, the patient with a renal transplant may have other problems. Immunosuppressive drugs may need to be continued indefinitely to prevent rejection of the foreign kidney, and adverse side effects sometimes result from these drugs. The immunosuppressed patient is also more susceptible to infection because the body's immune defenses have been weakened so that the transplant can survive. Occasionally, the disease that destroyed the patient's own kidneys, such as glomerulonephritis, also destroys the function of the transplanted kidney.

Based on new studies on a selected group of transplant patients, in the future, it may not always be necessary to continuously suppress the immune system in order to prevent rejection of the transplant. These studies indicate that the immune system can be "taught" to recognize the foreign HLA antigens as part of the patient's own antigens. The key to success involves suppressing the patient's own immune system first before the kidney is transplanted, and then administering bone marrow from the proposed kidney donor into the circulation of the patient. The kidney donor blood cells become established in the patient's bone marrow because the weakened immune system is unable to reject the foreign blood cells. Eventually, the patient ends up with two different blood cell populations, the patient's own blood cells and the transplanted donor blood cells. As a result, the patient's immune system "learns" that the HLA antigens in both the donor blood cells and the patient's own blood cells must be the patient's own self-antigens. Consequently, continuous suppression of the immune system may no longer be required when the kidney from the donor whose blood cell HLA antigens have already been accepted by the patient's immune system. In some other dialysis patients, transplanted kidney cells can be manipulated so that they may no longer be recognized as foreign by the patient's immune system. In these initial studies, several patients have been followed for up to 5 years without requiring drugs to suppress the immune system, which is a remarkable accomplishment. Hopefully, continued progress at inducing the transplant cells and those of the recipient to live together in harmony will do much to simplify the life of the transplant recipient.

QUESTIONS FOR REVIEW

1. What is the difference between glomerulonephritis and pyelonephritis? What is the relationship between glomerulonephritis and beta-streptococcal infection? What factors predispose to urinary tract infection?
2. What is the difference between nephrotic syndrome and nephrosclerosis? Why does edema develop in a patient with nephrosis?
3. What are the common causes of urinary tract obstruction? What are its effects on the kidneys and lower urinary tract?
4. What conditions lead to renal tubular necrosis? What are its clinical manifestations?
5. What is uremia? What are its manifestations? How is it treated? What is the role of urea in producing the clinical manifestations of uremia?
6. What methods does the clinician use to establish a diagnosis of renal disease?
7. What is congenital polycystic kidney disease? What are its clinical manifestations? What is its pattern of inheritance? How is it treated?
8. What is the difference between acute and chronic renal failure?
9. What is the difference between hemodialysis and peritoneal dialysis? How is the patient's circulation connected to the artificial kidney for hemodialysis?
10. Why does a kidney transplant from a donor who is a close relative usually have a greater likelihood of survival than does a cadaver transplant?
11. How does diabetes affect the kidneys? What are the clinical manifestations? How does gout affect the kidneys?

SUPPLEMENTARY READINGS

Chertow, G. M. 2004. A 43-year-old woman with chronic renal insufficiency. *Journal of the American Medical Association* 291:1252–9.

▶ A case discussion dealing with the problems and treatment of a patient with chronic renal disease, based on the pathophysiology of renal failure.

Grantham, J. J. 2009. Clinical practice. Autosomal dominant polycystic kidney disease. *New England Journal of Medicine* 359:1477–85.

▶ An excellent article on the important concepts regarding this disease, including pathogenesis, genetics, associated conditions, complications, clinical manifestations, monitoring disease progression, and treatment.

Himmelfarb, J., and Ikizler, T. A. 2010. Hemodialysis. *New England Journal of Medicine* 363:1833–45.

▶ Patients with end-stage kidney disease often have significant cardiovascular complications such as hypertension, atherosclerosis, cardiac hypertrophy, and congestive cardiac failure related in part to loss of normal kidney function. Death rate among U.S. patients is approximately 20% per year after maintenance dialysis is begun. Arteriovenous shunts are preferred for obtaining vascular access, and hollow fiber dialyzers are recommended. The usual treatment time is about 4 hours and usual frequency is 3 times per week. More frequent dialysis and longer dialysis time reduce cardiovascular complications and improve survival.

Ibrahim, H. N., Foley, R., Tan, L., et al. 2009. Long-term consequences of kidney donation. *New England Journal of Medicine* 360:459–69.

▶ Survival and risk of end-stage renal disease (ESRD) in carefully screened kidney donors appears to be similar to those in the general population. However, the study has certain limitations. Only the donors who are still alive and could be contacted were able to participate in the study, which is less than 15% of the total donor population.

- Removal of a kidney is followed by a reduction in the glomerular filtration rate (GFR) of the remaining kidney to about 70% of the prenephrectomy value. There has been a concern that kidney donors who have a 50% loss of kidney tissue may experience "overwork" (hyperfiltration) damage to the remaining kidney in addition to the normal progressive loss of kidney function that occurs with age. ESRD occurred in 11 of 3698 kidney donors contacted who donated kidneys in the period from 1963 to 2007.

Meyer, T. W., and Hostetter, T. H. 2007. Uremia. *New England Journal of Medicine* 357:1316–25.

- Current concepts and discussion of the pathophysiology of chronic renal failure.

Mulley, A. G., Jr. 1986. Shock-wave lithotripsy: Assessing a slam-bang technology. *New England Journal of Medicine* 314:845–7.

- Lithotripsy is a well-engineered, highly selective application of brute force. Applications in fracturing gallstones are also described.

Rubin, H. R., Fink, N. E., Plantinga, L. C., et al. 2004. Patient ratings of dialysis care with peritoneal dialysis vs hemodialysis. *Journal of the American Medical Association* 291:697–703.

- New patients beginning dialysis must choose between hemodialysis and peritoneal dialysis. Although not all patients requiring dialysis are suitable candidates for peritoneal dialysis, those who chose peritoneal dialysis were more likely to be working full time or part time and were more satisfied with their care than were hemodialysis patients.

Starzl, T. E. 2008. Immunosuppressive therapy and tolerance of organ allografts. *New England Journal of Medicine* 358:407–11.

- The author reviews three landmark articles in the same issue of the January 24, 2008, *Journal* in which combined kidney and bone marrow stem cells induced formation of two cell populations that "tricked" the immune system into recognizing the antigens of both cell populations as normal antigens for the patients, so the immune system did not respond, and immunosuppression was not required to maintain the transplants. Details of the other cases reported are also provided.

Stevens, L. A., Coresh, J., Greene, T., et al. 2006. Assessing kidney function—measured and estimated glomerular filtration rate. *New England Journal of Medicine* 354:2743–83.

- Clearance calculated from serum and urine creatinine values overestimate the glomerular filtration rate because of tubular secretion of creatinine. The Cockcroft-Gault formula provides a reasonably good estimate. A reduction of GFR to less than 60 ml per minute (related to body surface area) defines chronic kidney disease.

Torres, V., Pirson, Y., and Wiebers, D. O. 2006. Cerebral aneurysms. *New England Journal of Medicine* 355:2703–4.

- In Mayo Clinic studies on patients with polycystic kidney disease, prospective screening detected intracranial aneurysms in 16% of 77 patients with a family history of intracranial aneurysms, and in 6% of patients without such a family history. All of the aneurysms were small (mean diameter 3.5 mm with range from 1–7 mm diameter). According to the International Study of Unruptured Intracranial Aneurysms, the expected rupture rate of such aneurysms is very low. Current Mayo Clinic indications for screening are limited to those who have a family history of an intracranial aneurysm, a previous rupture of an aneurysm, contemplated major elective surgery, a high-risk occupation where an aneurysm rupture would be a major catastrophe, or extreme patient anxiety about the possibility of rupture.

OUTLINE SUMMARY

Structure and Function of Urinary Tract

KIDNEYS

Bean-shaped organs below diaphragm adjacent to vertebral column.

Divided into outer cortex and inner medulla.

Latter contains pyramids and renal columns.

EXCRETORY DUCT SYSTEM

Ureter conveys urine to bladder by peristalsis.

Pelvis: expanded upper end of ureter.

Major calyces: subdivisions of pelvis.

Minor calyces: subdivisions of major calyces into which renal papillae (apices of pyramids) discharge.

BLADDER

Stores urine.

Discharges urine into urethra during voiding.

Anatomic configuration of bladder and ureters normally prevents reflux of urine into ureters during voiding.

FUNCTION OF THE KIDNEYS

Excretory organ.

Regulates mineral and water balance.

Produces erythropoietin and renin.

THE NEPHRON

Composed of glomerulus and renal tubule.

Material filtered by three-layered glomerular filter.

Inner: fenestrated capillary endothelium.

Middle: basement membrane.

Outer: capillary epithelial cells (with foot processes and filtration slits).

Mesangial cells: contractile phagocytic cells that hold the capillary tuft together and regulate the caliber of the capillaries, which influences the filtration rate.

RENAL REGULATION OF BLOOD PRESSURE AND BLOOD VOLUME

Renin released in response to reduced blood volume, low blood pressure, or low sodium concentration.

Angiotensin II formed.

Functions as vasopressor.

Stimulates aldosterone secretion.

REQUIREMENTS FOR NORMAL RENAL FUNCTION

Free flow of blood through glomeruli.

Normal glomerular filter.

Normal tubular function.

Normal outflow of urine.

Developmental Disturbances

NORMAL DEVELOPMENT

Kidneys develop from mesoderm along back body wall of embryo.

Bladder derived from lower end of intestinal tract.

Excretory ducts (ureters, calyces, pelves) develop from ureteric buds that extend from bladder into developing kidneys.

Kidneys develop in pelvis and ascend to final position.

DEVELOPMENTAL ABNORMALITIES

Renal agenesis.

Bilateral: rare and associated with other congenital abnormalities. Usually incompatible with postnatal life.

Unilateral: relatively common and usually asymptomatic.

Duplications of the urinary tract.

As a result of abnormal development of ureteric buds.

Complete duplication: extra ureter and renal pelvis.

Incomplete duplication: only upper part of excretory system duplicated.

Malpositions.

Caused by failure of kidneys to ascend to normal position.

Kidneys may be fused.

Horseshoe kidney: fusion of lower poles.

Fusion of upper pole of one kidney to lower pole of other kidney.

Glomerulonephritis

IMMUNE-COMPLEX GLOMERULONEPHRITIS

Usually follows beta-streptococcal infection.

Circulating antigen–antibody complexes are filtered by glomeruli and incite inflammation.

Most patients recover completely.

ANTI-GBM GLOMERULONEPHRITIS

An autoimmune disease.

Autoantibodies directed against glomerular basement membranes.

Nephrotic Syndrome

CLINICAL FEATURES

Loss of protein in urine exceeds body's capacity to replenish plasma proteins.

Low plasma protein leads to edema and ascites.

PROGNOSIS

In children: minimal glomerular change, with complete recovery.

In adults: manifestation of more severe progressive renal disease.

Arteriolar Nephrosclerosis

PATHOGENESIS

Develops in hypertensive patients.

Renal arterioles undergo thickening.

Glomeruli and tubules undergo secondary degenerative changes.

Diabetic Nephropathy

PATHOGENESIS AND STRUCTURAL CHANGES

A complication of long-standing diabetes.

Nodular and diffuse thickening of glomerular basement membranes (glomerulosclerosis).

Usually coexisting nephrosclerosis.

MANIFESTATIONS

Impaired renal function.

Nephrotic syndrome may result from protein loss in urine.

May lead to renal failure.

Gout Nephropathy

PATHOGENESIS

Elevated blood uric acid leads to increased uric acid in tubular filtrate.

Urate may precipitate in Henle's loops and collecting tubules.

Tubular obstruction causes kidney damage.

MANIFESTATIONS

Impaired renal function

Common problem in poorly controlled gout.

May lead to renal failure.

Urinary Tract Infections

PATHOGENESIS

Usually caused by gram-negative bacteria ascending the urethra.

Free urine flow, large urine volume, complete emptying of bladder, and acid urine protect against infection.

Impaired drainage of urine, injury to mucosa of urinary tract, and introduction of catheters or instruments into bladder predispose to infection.

MANIFESTATIONS

Cystitis: bladder infection.

Causes pain and burning on urination; bacteria and leukocytes in urine.

Common in young, sexually active women and older men who are unable to empty their bladders completely owing to enlarged prostate.

Usually responds promptly to antibiotics.

Pyelonephritis: infection of upper urinary tract.

Usually ascending infection. May be hematogenous.

Stagnation of urine or obstruction or both predispose.

Usually responds to antibiotics.

Some cases become chronic and may lead to kidney failure.

Role of Vesicoureteral Reflux in Urinary Tract Infections

Urine normally prevented from flowing retrograde into ureters during voiding.

Failure of mechanism allows bladder urine to reflux into ureter during voiding.

Urine forced into ureter flows back into the bladder after voiding, preventing complete emptying of bladder.

Reflux predisposes to urinary tract infection because of residual urine.

Urinary Tract Calculi

PREDISPOSING FACTORS

Increased concentration of salts in urine.

Uric acid in gout.

Calcium salts in hyperparathyroidism.

Infections: alter solubility of salts.

Urinary tract obstruction: promotes stasis and infection.

CLINICAL MANIFESTATIONS

Renal colic associated with passage of stone.

Obstruction of urinary tract causes hydronephrosis-hydroureter proximal to obstruction.

Predisposes to infection.

Foreign Bodies in the Urinary Tract

INCIDENCE AND MANIFESTATIONS

Usually inserted by patient.

May injure bladder.

Predispose to infection.

TREATMENT

Usually removed by cystoscopy.

Occasionally necessary to open bladder by surgical operation.

Obstruction of Urinary Tract

PATHOGENESIS

Blockage of urine outflow leads to progressive dilatation of urinary tract proximal to obstruction.

Eventually causes compression atrophy of kidneys.

MANIFESTATIONS

Hydroureter: dilatation of ureter.

Hydronephrosis: dilatation of pelvis and calyces.

COMMON CAUSES

Bilateral: obstruction of bladder neck by enlarged prostate or urethral stricture.

Unilateral: ureteral stricture, calculus, or tumor.

COMPLICATIONS

Stone formation.

Infection.

DIAGNOSIS AND TREATMENT

Pyelograms or CT scans or both demonstrate dilatation of drainage system.

Treat cause of obstruction.

Renal Tubular Injury

PATHOGENESIS

Caused by toxic chemicals.

As a result of reduced renal blood flow.

CLINICAL MANIFESTATIONS

Oliguria or anuria.

Tubular function gradually recovers.

Treated by dialysis until function returns.

Renal Cysts

SOLITARY CYSTS

Relatively common.
Usually asymptomatic.

CONGENITAL POLYCYSTIC KIDNEY DISEASE

Incidence one per thousand.
Mendelian dominant transmission.
Cysts enlarge and destroy renal function.
Onset of renal insufficiency in middle age or later.
May be complicated by infections or bleeding into cysts.
Relatively common cause of renal failure.

Tumors of the Urinary Tract

RENAL CORTICAL TUMORS

Arise from epithelium of renal tubules.
Adenomas small and asymptomatic.
Carcinomas more common.

May cause hematuria as first manifestation.
Tumor may invade renal vein and metastasize through bloodstream.
Treated by nephrectomy.

TRANSITIONAL CELL TUMORS

Arise from transitional epithelium lining urinary tract.
Most are of low-grade malignancy and have good prognosis.
Hematuria may be first manifestation.
Diagnosis by cystoscopy.
Treated by resecting tumor.

WILMS TUMOR

Uncommon, highly malignant renal tumor of infants and children.
Treated by nephrectomy, radiotherapy, and chemotherapy.

Diagnostic Evaluation of Kidney and Urinary Tract Disease

URINALYSIS

Detects abnormalities in urine.
Widely used screening test.

URINE CULTURE AND SENSITIVITY TESTS

Where appropriate.

BLOOD CHEMISTRY TESTS

Measure retention of waste products normally excreted by kidneys.
Urea and creatinine commonly measured.
Degree of elevation correlates with degree of renal insufficiency and clinical condition.

CLEARANCE TESTS

Measure ability of kidneys to remove constituent from blood and excrete it in the urine.
Calculated by formula.
Creatinine clearance commonly used to monitor renal function.

X-RAY STUDIES

X-ray of abdomen: determines size and location of kidneys, radiopaque calculi.
Pyelograms: evaluate drainage system and distortion of calyces caused by renal cysts or tumors.
CT scan: detects renal cysts, tumors, hydronephrosis.
Arteriogram: detects abnormalities of renal blood flow, narrowing of renal arteries, increased renal vascularity associated with tumors.

ULTRASOUND EXAMINATION

Identifies cysts and tumors.

CYSTOSCOPY

Visualizes interior of bladder.

RENAL BIOPSY

Small biopsy of kidney obtained by needle inserted into kidney through flank.
Invasive procedure performed when nature of renal disease uncertain.
Histologic diagnosis serves as guide for proper treatment.

Renal Failure (Uremia)

CLASSIFICATION

Acute:

Caused by tubular necrosis from impaired renal blood flow or toxic drugs.
Renal function returns when tubules regenerate.

Chronic:

As a result of progressive chronic kidney disease.
No recovery of renal function.

MANIFESTATIONS

Nonspecific symptoms.
Anemia: as a result of reduced red cell production.
Toxic manifestations: caused by retained waste products.
Retention of salt and water.
Hypertension.

TREATMENT

Hemodialysis.

Patient's circulation connected to artificial kidney machine (dialyzer).
Access to patient's circulation facilitated by creation of arteriovenous fistula between radial artery and adjacent vein.
Blood cleansed and excess fluid removed.
Several types of dialyzers used.
Treatments last from 4 to 5 hours three times per week.

Peritoneal Dialysis.

Patient's own peritoneum used as dialyzing membrane.

Indwelling tube placed in peritoneal cavity and fixed to skin.

Dialysis fluid fills peritoneal cavity, is allowed to equilibrate, and is then drained. Cycles repeated.

Less efficient than hemodialysis and carries risk of peritonitis.

Kidney transplantation.

Kidney obtained from close relative, volunteer donor or recently deceased person (cadaver donor).

Survival of ABO-compatible transplant depends on similarity of HLA antigens between donor and recipient.

http://health.jbpub.com/humandisease/9e

Human Disease Online is a great source for supplementary human disease information for both students and instructors. Visit this website to find a variety of useful tools for learning, thinking, and teaching.

Index

A
Abscess, 49
Acetoacetic acid , 326
acetylcholine, 422-424
Achondroplasia, 408
Acid_base balance
  diagnosis of, 402
Acquired hydrocephalus, 386
actin, 420-421
Actinic keratoses, 64
Acute hemorrhagic pancreatitis, 319
Adhesions, 46, 386, 410
AIDS (acquired immune deficiency syndrome)
  complications of, 243, 419
  distribution of, 399
  prevalence of, 244
  tumors, 234, 398-403, 415-416
alkaline phosphatase, 406
Allergy, 229
alpha fetoprotein (AFP), 385
Amenorrhea
  exercise-induced, 417
Amnionic fluid, 141, 385
Amyloid protein, 396
anaerobic bacteria, 351
anaphylactic shock, 146
anemia
  aplastic, 231
Anemia
  bone marrow replacement, 231
  etiologic classification of, 230-231
  hemolytic, 231
anemia
  hypochromic, 227
Anemia
  hypochromic microcytic, 230-231
  iron metabolism, 231
anemia
  iron-deficiency, 245
Anemia
  morphologic classification of, 230
  of chronic disease, 231
  pernicious, 239
  sickle cell, 236-237
Aneurysms
  arteriosclerotic, 390-391
  cerebral, 379-380
Angiogram
  coronary, 389-390
Angioma , 57
Angiotensin-converting enzyme , 433
Anicteric hepatitis , 287
annulus fibrosus, 418
Antibiotics for bacterial infections
  adverse effects of, 243-244
Anticancer drugs , 75
Antihistamine drugs , 104
Aorta
  dissecting aneurysm of the, 419
Arbovirus infections, 394
Arteriolar nephrosclerosis, 439
Arthritis
  osteoarthritis, 410
astrocytes, 395-396
Atheroma, 178
Autoimmune diseases
  lupus erythematosus, 238

B
B lymphocytes, 241, 410
Bacilli, 415
Bacteria
  classification of, 243
  gram-negative, 415
barium enema, 370
biopsy, 242
Blood
  composition and function of, 227
  platelets, 227-229
  pressure, 236-237, 383, 418
  tests, 233, 403
  vessels, 237, 380, 418
Blood coagulation disturbances
  laboratory tests to evaluate, 233
Body fluids
  regulation of, 230
Body Mass Index, 373-374
Bone
  formation, 236-237, 407
  fractures, 409
  growth, 231-232, 407
  osteomyelitis, 415
  osteoporosis, 405
Bone marrow replacement anemia, 231
Bone marrow suppression, 234
Bowel
  Crohn disease, 234
Brain
  cerebral aneurysm, 391-392
  cerebral hemorrhage, 387-388
  cerebral injury, 382
  cerebral thrombi and emboli, 388
brain
  development of, 381
Brain
  encephalitis, 393-394
  parts of, 381
Brain hemorrhage , 195
Breast carcinoma
  clinical manifestations, 241, 399-400, 415
  treatment of, 233, 400
Bronchogram, 11

C
Caged-ball valve , 174
Calcium
  metabolism, 423
Candida albicans, 342
cardiac output, 418
Cardiac system
  blood supply, 383
  blood vessels, 237, 380, 418
  chambers, 239
Cardiovascular abnormalities, congenital
  Marfan syndrome, 418-419
Cardiovascular disease
  congenital, 239, 379, 405
  rheumatic, 412
Carotid endarterectomy, 390-391
Cells
  alpha, 229, 385
  beta, 229
  chromosomes, 238
  delta, 229
  division, 399
  injury, 238, 382, 415
  mast, 229
  organization of, 402
  out of, 236, 380, 415
  swelling, 411
Centers of ossification, 406
Cerebral aneurysm, 391-392
Cerebral injury, 382
Cerebral thrombi and emboli, 388
Cerebrospinal fluid (CSF)
  hydrocephalus, 379
Chest wall abnormalities, 418
Chloride, 34
chondrosarcoma, 416
Chromosomal abnormalities
  sex, 417
Chromosomes
  analysis, 237
Chronic infection, 415
Clostridium difficile, 350
Clubfoot, 408-409
Collagen fibers, 418
Condylomas , 65
Congenital and hereditary diseases
  multifactorial inheritance, 383
Congenital heart disease
  cause of, 234-235, 387, 426
  pathogenesis and manifestations of, 379
  prevention of, 412
Congenital hydrocephalus, 385
Conjugated bilirubin, 284
Coronary angiogram, 181
Coronary angioplasty, 195
coronary arteries, 389
Coronary heart disease
  manifestations, 236, 379, 405
  risk factors, 403, 424
Countercurrent dialysis , 454
Creutzfeldt-Jakob disease, 395
Cryptococcus neoformans, 400
Cysts
  renal, 415
Cytokines, 410
cytoplasm, 84, 178, 229-230, 293, 396, 420-421
Cytoskeleton, 235

D
Degenerative diseases, 398
Dermatomyositis, 421
Diabetic glomerulosclerosis , 440
Diagnosis, principles of
  physical examination, 240
  treatment, 227, 379, 423-425
Diagnostic tests and procedures
  amniocentesis, 237
  magnetic resonance imaging, 390
  radioisotope, 417
  ultrasound, 385, 419
  x-rays, 419
Disease(s)
  characteristics of, 423
  classifications of, 230
  functional, 234, 390, 421
Dissecting aneurysm of the aorta, 419
Disseminated intravascular coagulation syndrome , 140
DNA (deoxyribonucleic acid)
  structure of, 424
  viruses, 244, 401
DNA repair genes , 65
Drugs
  anticancer, 235, 399
duchenne muscular dystrophy, 422
Dura, 380
Dwarfism, 408
dysplasia, 36
Dystrophin, 422-423

E
Ecchymoses, 240
Ectoderm , 30
Elastic fibers, 418-419
Endochondral bone formation, 406
Endocrine glands
  parathyroid glands, 407
Endovascular aneurysm repair , 212
Entoderm , 30
epithelium, 56, 300, 346
Epstein-Barr virus, 241
Erythroblasts, 229
erythropoietin, 230
Esophagus, diseases of
  obstruction, 401
etiology, 231, 421
Extracorporeal hemodialysis , 454

exudate, 47, 393

F
Factor V Leiden , 140
Fetal hemoglobin, 229-230
Fetus, 9
Fibrillin, 418
Fibrous tissue , 322
Folic acid deficiency, 231, 383
Fractures, 408-409
Fungal infections
  treatment for, 394

G
gastric bypass, 234, 359
Gastrointestinal tract
  obesity, 234
Genes
  dominant, 237
  inheritance and, 236
  recessive, 236
Genetic diseases
  achondroplasia, 408
  hemochromatosis, 239-240
  multiple neurofibromatosis, 398
  screening for, 425
  sickle cell anemia, 236-237
  sickle cell trait, 237
  transmitted, 237-239, 394-395, 408
Germ layers , 29
Glioma, 399
gluconeogenesis, 330
Gonadotropic hormones, 417
Gout
  secondary, 412-415
Gouty arthritis, 410
Gram-negative, 415
Granulocytic leukemia , 68
Granulomas, 263
Granulomatous inflammation , 260
Growth hormone
  overproduction of, 414

H
Heart
  abnormalities, 239, 418
  attack, 238, 401-402
  failure, 401-402
Hematogenous osteomyelitis, 415
Hematopoietic system
  iron metabolism and, 231
Hemiplegia, 391
Hemochromatosis, 296
Hemoglobin
  A1C, 322
  abnormal, 230-231
Hemophilus, 393
hepatic encephalopathy, 300
Hepatitis D (delta hepatitis) , 292
Hereditary
  hemolytic anemia, 231
  spherocytosis, 235-236
Herpesvirus, 65
Histocompatibility complex
  system , 30
HIV (human immunodeficiency virus)
  infections, 241, 393-394
  manifestations of, 227, 393-395
hormones
  adrenal, 417
Hormones
  gonadotropic, 417
  pituitary, 417
Huntington disease, 398

I
Idiopathic scoliosis, 418
Immune complexes, 410
Infants and newborns
  fetal hemoglobin, 229-230
  neural tube defects, 383
Infection(s)
  maternal, 385-386
  nervous system, 393-394
  opportunistic, 400
Infectious mononucleosis, 227
Inflammation
  of the intestine, 241
  reaction, 395, 411
Intervertebral disks, 405
Intramembranous bone formation, 406
Iron metabolism, 231
Isotonic solution , 34

J
Juxtaglomerular apparatus, 430

K
keratin, 26
keratinocytes, 62

L
L-Dopa, 397
Lentigo maligna, 64
lesions, 421
Leukemia
  lymphocytic, 242
Leukoplakia, 64
lupus erythematosus, 238
Lymph nodes
  inflammation of, 241
  neoplasms affecting, 242
Lymphadenitis, 241
Lymphatic system
  infectious mononucleosis, 227
  neoplasms affecting lymph nodes, 242
Lysosomes, 47

M
mad cow disease, 395
Matrix, 27, 406-407
Megakaryocytes, 229
Megaloblasts, 234
Meningomyelocele, 384-385
Mesangial cells, 430
Mesoderm , 30
metastasis, 57
Mitochondria, 230
mononucleosis, 227
Multifactorial inheritance, 383
Multiple neurofibromatosis, 71, 398
multiple sclerosis, 379
Muscle
  paralysis, 382, 422
  skeletal, 380-381, 420-421
  tissue, 380, 411
Musculoskeletal system
  arthritis, 405
  bone formation, 406
  bone growth, 407
  chest wall abnormalities, 418
  clubfoot, congenital, 408
  gout, 414
  myasthenia gravis, 405
  myositis, 423-424
mutation, 395, 418-419
myosin, 420-421

N
Neoplasia, 40
Nephroblastoma , 450
nerve tissue, 380
Nervous system
  HIV, 400
  mad cow disease, 395
  multiple sclerosis, 379
  muscle paralysis, 382
  Parkinson disease, 379
  stroke, 379
  structure and function, 380, 405
  transient ischemic attack, 401-404
Neural tube defects
  anencephaly, 383-384
  prenatal detection of, 385
  spina bifida, 383-385
Neuroglia, 380
Neuron, 28
Nonalcoholic steatohepatitis , 294

O
Oligodendroglia, 380
Oncogene , 67
Oral cavity
  inflammation, 393, 406
Organelles, 230
organs, 29
osteoclasts, 406
osteocytes, 406
osteogenesis imperfecta, 409
Osteoid, 406-407
osteomalacia, 408
osteosarcoma, 416

P
Papilloma, 57
Parathyroid glands, 407
patent ductus arteriosus, 166
Pathogen, 400
Pathogenesis, 379, 405
Pathogenic, 243, 394, 415
Pectus excavatum, 418-419
Periapical abscess , 341
Peripheral nerves
  disorders, 399, 421
Peripheral neuritis, 399-400
Physical examination, 238
Pia, 380
Pituitary gland
  hormones, 417
  hypothalamus, 417
pleural cavity, 141, 252, 418
Podocytes, 429
Poliomyelitis
  postpolio syndrome, 394-395
Polyneuritis, 399-400
Prenatal development
  detection of neural tube defects, 385
  of heart , 190
  stages of, 240
Prion, 395
Prognosis, 379
prostaglandins, 47
Pulmonary embolism
  small, 228, 386-388, 419
Pulmonary emphysema, 239
pulmonary fibrosis, 239
Pulse deficit , 157
Pyloric obstruction, 376
Pyorrhea , 341

R
Red cells
  enzyme deficiencies, 235
  polycythemia, 227
Renin, 429
Respiratory distress syndrome
  adult, 399, 417
  infant, 394
Respiratory system
  pleural cavity, 418
  pulmonary fibrosis, 239
  tuberculosis, 401, 425
  ventilation, 418
Reticulocyte
  count, 237
Rheumatoid factor, 410
rickets, 407

S
Sarcoma
  breast , 64
scoliosis, 405
Sex hormones
  production of, 74, 271, 330
Shock
  lung, 418-419
Skin tumors, 398
Small cell carcinoma , 275
Spinal cord
  poliomyelitis, 382
Spine
  scoliosis, 405
Splenectomy, 227
Staphylococci, 415
Stroke
  rehabilitation, 391
stroma, 29
Suppression of immune response
  methods of, 235, 403
synapse, 380

T
Talipes, 408-409

Thalassemia, 230-238
Thrombolytic therapy, 402
Tissues
    muscle, 381-382, 412
    nerve, 384
Toxoplasma gondii, 400
Transient ischemic attack, 391
Transmural infarct , 188
Treatment, 227, 379, 405
tumors
    benign, 398-399, 416
Tumors
    bone, 234-235, 414-417
    bowel, 234
    brain, 12, 379-380, 422
    breast, 242, 399, 415
    colon, 233, 399, 423
    kidney , 14, 449
    leukemia, 235, 415
    liver, 234, 424
    lymphomas, 242, 399-400
tumors
    malignant, 234, 398-403, 416
Tumors
    malignant
        noninfiltrating , 64
        types of, 3-4, 24-26, 53, 106-107, 273, 463
    multiple myeloma, 416
    peripheral nerves, 398-399
    prostate, 415
    skin, 61, 241, 398, 415
    spinal cord, 380, 417
    stomach, 234
Tyrosine kinase , 89

U
Urate nephropathy, 414, 440
Urinary tract infections
    diagnostic tests, 233
urine, 449

V
varicocele, 217
Vasculitis, 111
vasodilator, 46
Viral infection, 240, 394
Vitamin B, 400
Vitamin B12
    deficiency, 231-234, 407-408

X
X, 389-390, 409
X-rays
    chest, 418-419